Essential Paediatrics
and Child Health

T0176966

This book is dedicated to the coming generations of students and their patients

Essential Paediatrics and Child Health

Fourth Edition

Mary Rudolf
Professor of Population Health
Azrieli Faculty of Medicine
Bar Ilan University, Safed, Israel
Former Professor of Child Health
University of Leeds, Leeds, UK

Anthony Luder
Director of Paediatrics, Ziv Medical Centre, Safed, Israel
Professor of Paediatrics, Azrieli Faculty of Medicine
Bar Ilan University, Safed, Israel

Kerry Jeavons
Consultant in Paediatric Medicine
Leeds Teaching Hospitals NHS Trust
Yorkshire, UK

WILEY Blackwell

This edition first published 2020 © 2020 by John Wiley & Sons Ltd

First published by Blackwell Publishing Ltd 1999.
Reprinted 2000
Second edition 2006
Third edition 2011

Registered Offices
John Wiley & Sons, Inc., 111 River Street, Hoboken, NJ 07030, USA
John Wiley & Sons Ltd, The Atrium, Southern Gate, Chichester, West Sussex, PO19 8SQ, UK

Editorial Office
9600 Garsington Road, Oxford, OX4 2DQ, UK

For details of our global editorial offices, customer services, and more information about Wiley products visit us at www.wiley.com. Wiley also publishes its books in a variety of electronic formats and by print-on-demand. Some content that appears in standard print versions of this book may not be available in other formats.

Library of Congress Cataloging-in-Publication Data
Names: Rudolf, Mary, author. | Luder, Anthony, author. | Jeavons, Kerry, author.
Title: Essential paediatrics and child health / Mary Rudolf, Anthony Luder, Kerry Jeavons.
Other titles: Paediatrics and child health
Description: Fourth edition. | Chichester, West Sussex, UK ; Hoboken :
    Wiley-Blackwell, 2020. | Preceded by: Paediatrics and child health /
    Mary Rudolf. Third edition. 2011. | Includes bibliographical references and index.
Identifiers: LCCN 2019033004 (print) | LCCN 2019033005 (ebook) | ISBN
    9781119420224 (paperback) | ISBN 9781119420248 (adobe pdf) | ISBN
    9781119420231 (epub)
Subjects: MESH: Pediatrics | Child Welfare
Classification: LCC RJ45 (print) | LCC RJ45 (ebook) | NLM WS 200 | DDC 618.92–dc23
LC record available at https://lccn.loc.gov/2019033004
LC ebook record available at https://lccn.loc.gov/2019033005

Cover Design: Wiley
Cover Images: Courtesy of Micha de Vries

Printed in Great Britain by Bell & Bain Ltd, Glasgow

Set in 10/12pt Adobe Garamond by SPi Global, Pondicherry, India

Contents

Companion website
This book is accompanied by a companion website:

www.wiley.com/go/rudolf/paediatrics

- multiple-choice questions
- interactive patient scenarios
- illustrations from the book for download
- examination instruction videos

Foreword

Paediatrics and medical education have changed radically over the last 40 years. When I was a medical student in the early 1970s the student was expected to have a wide knowledge of every specialty including rare and abstruse conditions. Times have changed and now we expect students to know the basics of the subject and to be able to know how to obtain more information if required. Now the newly qualified doctor is a mere beginner in the process of assessing, diagnosing, and treating patients and receives progressive training in his or her own area of interest over years before they are experienced enough to be appointed to a specialist post. Medical education has changed to match the recalibration of what the student is required to know and paediatrics has led the way in this respect. The latest edition of *Paediatrics and Child Health* reflects the core knowledge that is required by a British medical student at the end of their paediatric rotation.

When I was a student we mostly used the textbook written by Hugh Jolly *Diseases of Children*. This was first published in 1964 and it rapidly became a core text for medical students studying paediatrics. When I undertook my paediatric rotation at medical school in 1972, the book was in its second edition and when I did my first house position post in paediatrics at Charing Cross hospital, London where Hugh was a consultant it was in its third edition. Paediatrics was changing considerably, particularly in respect to advances in neonatal medicine and the introduction of more modern investigation techniques. Hugh asked me to assist him in updating the fourth edition and kindly added me as a co-author on the fifth edition published in 1985 when I was a newly appointed consultant paediatrician.

Hugh sadly died in 1986 and knowing that he was dying had asked me to continue his book, and in 1990 I published as editor the sixth edition of the renamed *Jolly's Diseases of Children* with the assistance of a number of colleagues. At that time undergraduate education in paediatrics was changing enormously; students were spending less time on children's wards and many children were being seen by doctors based in the community, an area previously relatively neglected in textbooks.

I had the great pleasure of working in Leeds at that time with Mary Rudolf who had been appointed as a community paediatrician and we decided to produce a totally new undergraduate textbook on the basics of paediatrics including the way that children presented to doctors both in primary care and at hospital. In particular, a section on the adolescent was added. This book was entitled *Paediatrics and Child Health* and was published in 1999. It grew from Hugh Jolly's vision of holistic child health and understanding how children reacted to their environment, but took a modern approach to the way that paediatrics has evolved in the modern medical undergraduate curriculum. The second edition was published in 2006 and Dr Tim Lee joined us in collaboration with the third edition in 2011. Although I am no longer involved in writing, this fourth edition continues Hugh's legacy of showing how health and disease in children are closely related and is an up-to-date book for undergraduates to learn from.

Malcolm Levene
Emeritus Professor of Paediatrics
July 2018

Preface to the fourth edition

He who studies medicine without books sails an uncharted sea, but he who studies medicine without patients does not go to sea at all.

William Osler

In the preface to the third edition of this book, Benjamin Disraeli was cited as saying that one 'cannot learn men from books'. William Osler, one of the fathers of modern Medicine, endorses this view but balances it with the notion that books provide the charts needed for the navigation of the stormy seas of suffering and disease. Even though more than a century has passed since these words were written, the truth behind them was never so compulsively true as now. Witness the increasing flow of quality publications in every sphere of Medicine, not least in Paediatrics.

Since the last edition of this book was published, advances in the understanding of human biology and medical practice have accelerated at a dizzying pace along with society and people's expectations. Today's patients are increasingly informed by instant on-line communication and information, and technology is transforming the practice of Medicine and its management. These developments and more, constitute huge challenges for the traditional doctor–patient relationship and the bioethical environment in which it exists, and from which it derives its acceptance in society and its professional legitimacy. These challenges have to be met by equally fundamental, and responsible, changes in the way that Medicine is taught and learnt. In this new and revised edition, we have tried to reflect these seismic shifts in a manner that presents to the student a clear, comprehensive and up-to-date reflection of contemporary Paediatrics.

Chapters have been revised and extensively re-written to ensure that the latest information about diagnosis, investigation and management is discussed. New chapters have been added on communication and prescribing, together with a new introduction. New additions include reference to national guidelines and flow charts and diagrams. The recent emphasis on outcome-based education has been reflected through clear highlighting of the key competences expected of students. Scientific aspects that strengthen the book include new imaging techniques, genetics and epigenetics, environmental medicine, aspects of emergency paediatrics, paediatric pharmacology, toxicology and lifestyle paediatrics. The sections on student experience, learning and self-assessment have been recast, through chapters on doing well in paediatrics and practice multiple-choice questions.

The on-line edition of the book is now an independent, although closely linked, entity. It continues to include the printed version as well as physical examination instruction videos, but now also provides new experiences: two 'mock' examinations are provided, which students can use to test their skills in taking a time-limited challenge in the same way as their final examinations are given; and a complete set of interactive patient scenarios are presented, which provide readers with an on-line simulation opportunity to work through real-life clinical problems, with extensive feedback discussion provided at every point and for every choice. These both test clinical knowledge and judgement and also provide opportunities for curious and enquiring students to broaden their knowledge and deepen their reading into more detailed and specialised channels. We hope that students of every ability will find a fascination with paediatrics stimulated and their interest awakened. If we achieve this, then our purposes will have been fulfilled and this new edition of our book will take its place as a landmark in the education of students in paediatrics.

Acknowledgements

We acknowledge the considerable energy and time that Professor Malcolm Levene and Dr Tim Lee invested in writing the first three editions of this textbook. We are grateful to the following who have contributed significantly to chapters in the book: Dr Michael Harari, Professor Eric Shinwell, Dr Mervyn Jaswon and Kim Roberts, and Dr Micha De Vries for photographs for the cover. We are grateful too to the following who have contributed illustrations: Dr Elizabeth Morris, Dr Rosemary Arthur, Mr P.D. Bull, Dr Tony Burns, Professor Martin Curzon, Dr Mark Goodfield, Dr Phillip Holland, Mr Tim Milward, Dr P.R. Patel, Dr John Puntis, Mr Mark Stringer, Dr David Swirsky, Ms Clare Widdows, Dr Susan Wyatt, Dr Jane Wynne and Matteo Gray and his mother Tina Meharry.

We would like to thank the Royal College of Paediatrics and Child Health and Harlow Printing for permission to reproduce their growth charts. We would like to thank the following: The extract of 'Henry King who chewed string and was cut off in dreadful Agonies' from *Cautionary Verses* by Hilaire Belloc (Copyright © The Estate of Hilaire Belloc 1930) is reproduced by permission of PFD (www.pfd.co.uk) on behalf of the Estate of Hilaire Belloc. Extract of 'Rebecca who slammed doors for fun, and perished miserably' from *Cautionary Verses* by Hilaire Belloc (Copyright © The Estate of Hilaire Belloc) is reproduced by permission of PFD (www.pfd.co.uk) on behalf of the Estate of Hilaire Belloc. Extract from 'Now We Are Six' © A.A. Milne. Published by Egmont UK Limited, London and used with permission. Published by Dutton's Children's Books, a division of Penguin Young Readers Group, a member of Penguin Group (USA) Inc, 345 Hudson Street, New York, NY 10014, and used with permission. All rights reserved. Extract from *When We Were Very Young* © A.A. Milne. Published by Egmont UK Limited, London and used with permission. Published by Dutton's Children's Books, a division of Penguin Young Readers Group, a member of Penguin Group (USA) Inc, 345 Hudson Street, New York, NY 10014, and used with permission. Quote from Janusz Korczak Permission from Sandra Joseph https://www.korczak.org.uk/contact.html. All rights reserved.

How to get the best out of your textbook

Welcome to the new edition of *Essential Paediatrics and Child Health*. Over the next two pages you will be shown how to make the most of the learning features included in the textbook

An interactive textbook ▶

Your textbook comes with free access to a **Wiley E-Text: Powered by VitalSource** version – a digital, interactive version of this textbook. Your **Wiley E-Text** allows you to:

Search: Save time by finding terms and topics instantly in your book, your notes, even your whole library (once you've downloaded more textbooks)

Note and Highlight: Colour code, highlight and make digital notes right in the text so you can find them quickly and easily

Organise: Keep books, notes and class materials organized in folders inside the application

Share: Exchange notes and highlights with friends, classmates and study groups

Upgrade: Your textbook can be transferred when you need to change or upgrade your computer or device

Link: Link directly from the page of your interactive textbook to all the material contained on the companion website.

To access your Wiley E-Text:

- Find the redemption code on the inside front cover of this book and carefully scratch away the top coating of the label.
- Go to https://online.vitalsource.co.uk and log in or create an account. Go to Redeem and enter your redemption code to add this book to your library.
- Or to download the Bookshelf application to your computer, tablet or mobile device go to www.vitalsource.com/software/bookshelf/downloads
- Open the Bookshelf application on your computer and register for an account.
- Follow the registration process and enter your redemption code to download your digital book.
- If you have purchased this title as an e-book, access to your **Wiley E-Text** is available with proof of purchase within 90 days. Visit http://support.wiley.com to request a redemption code via the 'Live Chat' or 'Ask A Question' tabs.

Videos showing you how to ▶ examine children

A unique feature of the textbook is a detailed video taking you step by step through the examination of the child. Salient features are captured, and the correct technique demonstrated for each organ system – essential for eliciting signs, coming to a diagnosis and showing your competence in OSCE examinations.

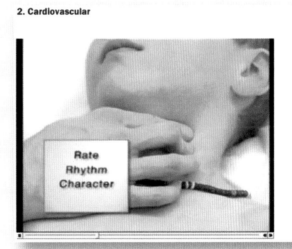

2. Cardiovascular

Rate
Rhythm
Character

Look out for the examination instruction videos icon

FREE companion website

Your textbook is also accompanied by a FREE companion website that contains:

- Multiple-choice questions

- Illustrations from the book for download

- Examination instruction videos

- For the first time a complete set of interactive clinical scenarios, which will take you through the clinical thinking required for the evaluation and management of some common problems. These questions also open up the possibility of deeper reading and learning for those who wish.

Online Interactive Questions [Online Interactive Qs]

These icons notify you when there is a related interactive patient scenario on the companion website.

Log on to **www.wiley.com/go/rudolf/paediatrics** to find out more.

Features contained within your textbook ▶

Chapters are organized by organ system. Each opens with the competences you need to acquire as well as the key topics covered. The first part of each chapter goes through the most important symptoms and guides you through the differential diagnosis and the features of the history, examination and investigations that will help you come to a competent diagnosis. Full details of common and important conditions and disorders follow.

Throughout your textbook you will find a series of icons highlighting the learning features in the book: ▶

Online Interactive Questions: These icons notify you when there is a related interactive patient scenario on the companion website.

Red flags: Worrying symptoms and signs indicative of serious conditions that you must not miss are highlighted with red flags.

Clues to the diagnosis boxes: The conditions you need to consider when encountering a sick child are shown with clues for key symptoms and signs that will help you come to the correct diagnosis.

At a Glance boxes: These boxes concisely summarize the aetiology, clinical features, investigations and management of common and important conditions for quick re-cap.

Key points boxes: Key points boxes highlight the 'take-home' messages you need to remember.

Examination instruction videos: These icons notify you when there is a related step-by-step patient examination instruction video.

NICE guidelines: These icons indicate links to evidence-based guidelines for key paediatric conditions

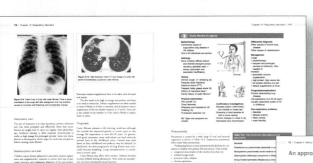

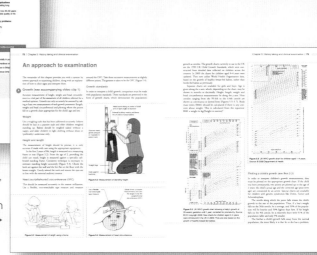

▲ Your textbook is full of useful photographs, illustrations, and tables. The Wiley E-Text version of your textbook will allow you to copy and paste any photograph or illustration into assignments, presentations and your own notes. ▶

We hope you enjoy using your new textbook. Good luck with your studies!

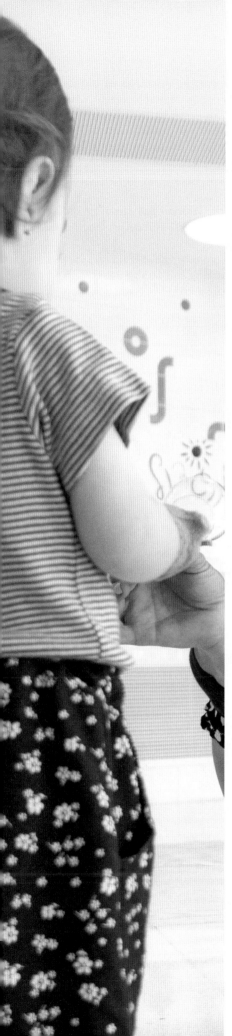

INTRODUCTION: Doing well in paediatrics

How this book can help you learn paediatrics and acquire paediatric skills:

- It guides you step by step on how to work up common symptoms and signs
- Important and common conditions are described in detail
- It helps you prepare for OSCE examinations through
  - Videos on how to examine each organ system
  - Downloadable examination checklists for use by the bedside
- You can test your knowledge through a bank of examination questions and two, timed practice examinations
- Links are provided to key evidence-based guidelines
- There are interactive questions if you wish to go into paediatric problems in further depth

Essential Paediatrics and Child Health, Fourth Edition. Mary Rudolf, Anthony Luder and Kerry Jeavons.
© 2020 John Wiley & Sons Ltd. Published 2020 by John Wiley & Sons Ltd.
Companion website: www.wiley.com/go/rudolf/paediatrics

Background

Paediatrics is a relatively young specialty in Medicine. Although the medical problems of infancy and childhood were discussed in ancient times, the first hospitals for children in the Western world were opened only in the nineteenth century, and the professional specialty developed into its modern form during the twentieth. Thus, paediatrics is still very much a work in progress; and what progress there has been! Beginning as a branch of internal medicine, paediatrics has like a child, gone through its growth stages and is today a mature and critical part of any health system.

We have seen the emphasis shift from hospital-based treatment, through social concerns and preventative initiatives, to today's complex picture of hospital-based intensive and surgical care working side-by-side with fully developed ambulatory and community health services including rehabilitation, palliative and health maintenance programmes. There have been revolutionary changes of approach where it is recognised today that most common paediatric problems can and should be managed outside the hospital, with admission being often a last resort and then only for as short a time as possible. In this respect paediatrics is a leader in Medicine.

There has also been an increasing awareness that health and disease in childhood has important implications for adults, family and society. Thus we now know that many of the 'big killers' in adult life like hypertension, handicap, immune disorders, addiction, diabetes, heart and vascular disease, obesity and even cancer, have their origins and beginnings in the paediatric age group, and that the paediatrician's responsibility is far wider than simply treating individual children, important as that is. The scientific underpinning of this holistic understanding has expanded rapidly in recent decades with the explosion of knowledge in genetics, epigenetics, bioenergetics, therapeutics and, most recently, microbiomics.

The aim of this book is to present you with the essential principles and practice of paediatrics in a clear and consistent way that will aid learning, develop skills, arouse interest and hopefully inspire love for this fascinating profession.

How to get the most out of your paediatric rotation

The aim of the paediatric rotation is to provide you with a broad understanding of the common and important illnesses and disorders of childhood, child health and its maintenance, and child growth and development. The underlying purpose is to make sure that all medical graduates, whatever specialty they ultimately choose, know when children need investigation or intervention and the principles of correct management. The focus is on how children present, and management, rather than specialist areas in detail. The ability to take a good paediatric history and conduct an effective paediatric physical examination are fundamental skills that you need to acquire.

As with any clinical placement, you will get the most out of your time in paediatrics by:

1. Becoming familiar with the location and layout of the wards, departments and clinics you will be working in, including academic and other areas.
2. Getting to know nursing and other allied healthcare staff as well as the principal teaching and administrative staff, with necessary contact details and on-line communication resources.
3. Attending registration formalities and obtaining required means of identity.
4. Learning the structure of the rotation including the time and place of activities.
5. Making sure you have all the necessary materials to hand, including syllabi, curricula, skills list, any learning aids and logbooks, and personal equipment.
6. Making sure that you understand how to access library and other academic resources you will need.
7. Most importantly – making your own learning schedule and keeping to it. Remember that after intensive activity like preparing a seminar, doing a test or even being on-call in the evening you need time for rest and recreation.

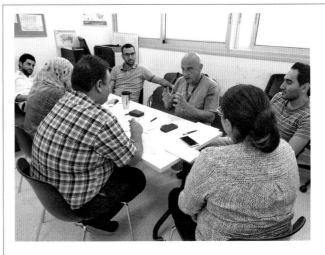

Figure 1 Senior clinical teacher and medical students discussing patients at a ward meeting.

Relating to children of all ages and understanding their developmental status are important skills which are most easily acquired on the wards where young patients and their parents are 'captive', often with time to spare. Take every opportunity to relate to them informally or simply observe them. Playing with them, talking to them and helping with their care by feeding and offering to assist in changing nappies will help you appreciate child development in a way that you can never learn from books. Try 'guessing' children's ages from what you observe. Observing behaviour, activity, colour and respiration from a distance will also help you develop your clinical skills in identifying sick children who may not participate in a formal examination.

Combining reading with clinical experience is the most effective way to learn. This book has been laid out so that each clinical chapter is in two parts: the first part provides you with the work up of common and important symptoms and presentations, guiding you through the history, physical examination and investigations, and leading you to make a coherent differential diagnosis. The second half covers key conditions in detail required at the undergraduate level. Any duplication of coverage is deliberate, as we recognise that learners do not generally read whole chapters but rather sections that they need at a particular time.

The chapter on physical examination shows you how to examine each organ system and is accompanied by purpose made video clips demonstrating the correct technique you require to elicit signs competently. Downloadable reminders or checklists for each system allow you to easily check in real time whether there were features you have omitted.

For those of you who wish to learn more in depth there are a series of on-line interactive questions you can access, which offer you the opportunity to work through, in a realistic manner, actual clinical cases that mimic what you are likely to see in the emergency department, clinics and wards. The purpose is to introduce you to some core topics and the associated clinical thinking at a more advanced level than required for examination purposes alone but based on your studies and teaching during your rotations. The cases are designed to lead you through logical steps in the evaluation of clinical problems in which correct and incorrect possible choices are both explained. They are based mainly on history, physical examination and investigations, but some diseases or pathophysiologic details that are not necessarily included in the main book are discussed, since they are necessary for the management of real-life situations. Finally, there is a denouement in which some details of management and follow-up are described.

Ways you may be assessed

There are a variety of ways you may be assessed to judge your progress. Departments should provide you at the start of the rotation with the types of assessment that will be used. These may include:

- *Student logbooks.* Logbooks record your various educational experiences; for example, procedures, activities and conditions that you have witnessed and clinics you have attended. They may need to be countersigned by supervising clinicians or other staff and submitted at the end of the course to demonstrate that you have achieved appropriate clinical experience.
- *Workplace-based assessments (WPBA).* Students are often required to conduct a number of clinical examinations – for example, a respiratory examination, developmental examination, etc. – under direct observation of a supervising clinician, who then fills out a formal WPBA feedback form. You are required to submit these forms at the end of the course to demonstrate that you have acquired good clinical examination skills.
- *Multi-source feedback (MSF).* Occasionally you will be asked to arrange a multi-source feedback, where members of a multidisciplinary team provide feedback that focuses on your clinical skills, communication skills and professional attitude.
- *Written case reports.* Case reports require a detailed history and examination, followed by a list of key problems and concerns, an investigation plan, the differential diagnosis and initial management plan. They are generally written in a similar way to entries made in children's medical records. Case reports allow for assessment of many of the key skills that you are expected to acquire during the attachment.
- *Written feedback from supervising clinicians/course teachers.* These reports are often helpful in identifying the quality of your skills and attitudes, as well as when you are struggling with the course.
- *Written examination.* Most courses have some form of written examination, usually extended matching questions (EMQ), or multiple-choice questions (MCQ). Some of the questions may be based on images, or on written stems. Stem questions usually focus on testing diagnostic reasoning, and you are required to choose the most likely diagnosis or next intervention, based on a short clinical description or 'stem'. The electronic version of this book now includes examples of interactive clinical questions for extended learning and practice.
- *Objective Structured Clinical Examination (OSCE).* OSCEs consist of a circuit of short 5- to 15-minute stations, mostly with an examiner at the station and a real or simulated parent and/or child. They focus on key clinical skills such as history taking, counselling or clinical examination. Some may include video clips, photographs or investigations that you need to interpret. Students rotate through all of the stations in turn.

Preparing for examinations

In order to make sure that you perform well in written examinations, you need to work at acquiring a broad knowledge of the whole syllabus (Box 1). The best way to prepare is to attend

Box 1 Tips for performing well in paediatric assessments and examinations

- Read the course material carefully at the start of the attachment
- Check through all the ways you will be assessed and how these assessments contribute to your final mark
- Take every opportunity to meet children and parents, and take a history and perform an examination as often as you can
- Use the bedside checklist to make sure you do not omit key aspects of the examination
- Attend all of the available course seminars and workshops, as these will often cover much of the course syllabus
- When you have seen a child with a particular condition, read the appropriate section of this textbook and consider the differential diagnoses
- Watch the video on the companion website showing how to examine children section by section and practise the technique on children on the ward
- Try and complete your in-course assessments as soon as you can, rather than doing them all in a rush at the end of the attachment
- Practise written exam questions (MCQ, EMQ) and read through the topics for questions you get wrong
- Practise OSCE scenarios with colleagues and give feedback to each other

the whole course and its seminars and workshops. It is especially worthwhile to spend a good amount of time seeing children in any setting – community and hospital, acutely via the accident and emergency department, and in outpatient clinics. Remember, what you see you tend to remember, so do maximize every possible opportunity to extend your clinical exposure.

Many multiple-choice questions (MCQs) and extended matching questions (EMQs) test your ability to link symptoms and signs to particular diagnoses. Reading through the chapters in this book will be good preparation. The 'symptoms and signs' section of each chapter, guides you systematically to link particular presentations to relevant diagnoses. A box lists the most significant symptoms and signs providing you with clues as to how to come to a differential diagnosis.

An important skill to master is the exam technique itself. Read the stem carefully and do not skim; often single words or nuances can alter the significance of the question and this can cause misunderstanding and lead to an incorrect answer. Remember that your first considered response is likely to be the correct one; changing answers later is usually counterproductive. Timing is critical. Look at the whole paper and do not dwell over long on hard questions, there may be a few simpler ones you can get credit for in the same time. Lastly, do not try to second guess the results; self-evaluation is notoriously unreliable. After the exam, relax!

An important aspect of preparation is to practise answering exam questions, such as those provided in this book. Many courses will also provide mock questions or past papers. This enables you to familiarize yourself with the question structure and technique, as well as checking your knowledge. In order to learn from questions that you get wrong, you should try to understand why you chose the wrong answer. Reading through the section of this book appropriate to the question stem will help. Chapter 26 – 'Practice MCQ and examination questions' – provides you with a bank of sample questions to try. If you get any wrong, you are guided to the section of the book that will provide you with the correct answer. You also have two exam papers provided which you can use to time yourselves as well as

providing you with a mark. Try to do these within the recommended time only, as this will provide the best simulation of an actual examination experience.

Preparing for Objective Structured Clinical Examinations

OSCEs assess basic clinical skills. At each of the stations you are asked to interact with a patient or a simulated patient. Your performance is scored by an examiner with a checklist or rating scale. Often an actor or simulated patient may also give a score. Scores may be awarded for content and style separately.

Many students get exceptionally nervous prior to OSCEs. The rigid time limits for each station, and the need to move on rapidly to a completely new station tend to fill students with apprehension, especially if there has been a mishap on a previous station.

The key to OSCEs is to ensure that during the paediatric course you practise all the skills you may have to perform in the OSCE in real life, with real children and parents. It helps if you

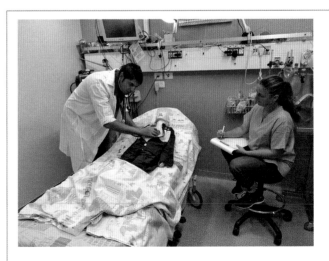

Figure 2 A simulation exercise during an OSCE examination.

aim to perform at least one detailed history and examination every day during your paediatric attachment, so that the skill becomes second nature by the time of the examination. The website associated with this book provides videos to demonstrate the correct technique for examining children, and you will find it most helpful if you watch it section by section rather than in one go. In addition, the specific aspects of the history and physical examination relevant to each presenting symptom and sign are provided for you at each chapter's opening and as a downloadable checklist. Remember, too, it is always helpful to spend time observing how experienced clinicians counsel parents and children.

Try to practise the scenarios with student colleagues prior to the exam. Common counselling scenarios should be listed in your course documentation; they often include immunisation, enuresis, soiling, febrile convulsion, asthma and constipation. Remember that marks are given not only for appropriate content, but also for good counselling skills such as active listening, eye contact and emotional empathy. Practise by counselling a student colleague and then asking them to give you feedback.

On the day of the OSCE, try to channel your nerves into performing well. Often there is a 'change-over' minute between each station, so make the most of this by trying to forget your performance on the previous station, and focusing on the next station. There may be some written information outside the station for you to read. If so, use this to plan how you will approach the next station. For example, if the written information suggests the station concerns the examination of the lower limbs in a child with an abnormal gait, then think what the differential diagnosis might be. Plan to ask if the child is able to walk for you to demonstrate the gait, as well as planning to observe the child's legs and assess tone, power and reflexes. Remember, as you enter the station, to take time to introduce yourself well to both parents and children, as a good friendly start really helps the rest of the station go well and will help you make the most of the time available. And always wash your hands!

Endnote

Learning paediatrics should be an enjoyable, inspiring and interesting experience for every student, not least because children are naturally fun to work with, even if ill. They often have a more innocent or optimistic attitude than their parents. In this chapter we have given you practical tips on how to get the most out of your rotation. There may seem a lot to learn but once you are in the thick of things it should fall into place. If you are diligent, the evaluation tests and examinations should not pose any special problem; especially if you do not leave everything to 'cramming' at the end. We hope this book is useful in guiding your learning through your paediatrics rotation and, perhaps for some, may lead to a lifelong attachment to this very special specialty.

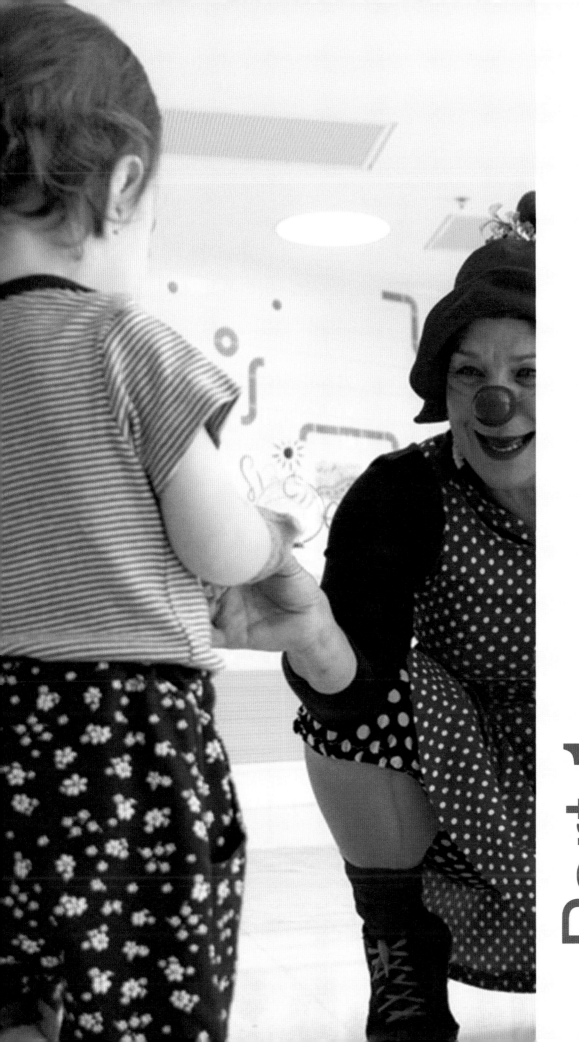

Part 1
About children

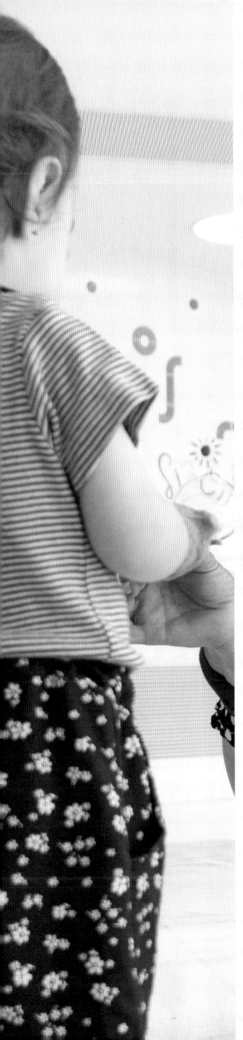

CHAPTER 1
Nature and nurture

And one man in his time plays many parts,
His acts being seven ages. At first the infant,
Mewling and puking in the nurse's arms.
And then the whining schoolboy, with his satchel,
And shining morning face, creeping like a snail
Unwillingly to school.

William Shakespeare

KEY COMPETENCES

YOU MUST...

Know and understand

- How babies develop and socially interact over time
- Factors that influence physical growth through the life course
- The advantages of, and how to encourage, breast-feeding
- How to promote optimal bottle feeding
- The components of healthy nutrition and healthy eating behaviours through childhood
- The importance and recommendations for physical activity
- The development of sleep patterns at different ages

Be able to

- Make up a formula feed
- Support a mother wishing to breast-feed
- Hold and undress a baby

Appreciate

- The importance of the early years for long term health and wellbeing
- The challenges of parenting and the influence that its quality has on a child's development
- The critical role that the internal, psychosocial and external physical environment has on child health
- The impact that social determinants have on health
- The importance of encouraging breast-feeding

Essential Paediatrics and Child Health, Fourth Edition. Mary Rudolf, Anthony Luder and Kerry Jeavons.
© 2020 John Wiley & Sons Ltd. Published 2020 by John Wiley & Sons Ltd.
Companion website: www.wiley.com/go/rudolf/paediatrics

This chapter describes children's neurological, psychological, emotional and physical development. It discusses the importance of the early years and parenting, children's nutritional, physical activity and sleep needs, and the impact that social determinants have on children's health.

The importance of the early years

The early years are a period of enormous growth and development. Much of the infant brain develops after birth, shaped by events in the first years of life. Babies have relatively few synapses at birth. Over the next few years synapses develop and are refined by stimulation and experience: nature interacting with nurture.

The formation of synapses follows a 'bottom-up' sequence, with lower level brain 'circuits' wired first. The skills and abilities that emerge in young babies reflect this sequence. From a focus on bodily functions such as hunger and the need for sleep, babies rapidly start to explore the world around them, develop emotional bonds and then manifest higher brain functions such as reasoning, language, self-control and language.

Neuronal circuits strengthen the more that experiences (positive or negative) are repeated. Over time they stabilize, making alteration harder at a later date. By the age of six years 'pruning' starts where infrequently used synapses are eliminated and well-used ones are retained (see Figure 1.1). Pruning ensures that the most important networks of synapses grow and become more complex.

The developmental process is not uniform and there are periods, or windows, of opportunity when specific parts of the brain are particularly developmentally sensitive. Vison and hearing develop first, peaking in the first few months, followed by language circuits later in the first year and higher cognitive function peaking during the second year of life (see Figure 1.2).

Influences on early development

Responsive caregiving and positive stimulation are essential for development:

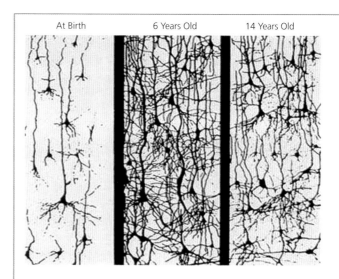

| At Birth | 6 Years Old | 14 Years Old |

Figure 1.1 Synaptic density in children at birth, 6 years and 14 years old. *Source:* Reproduced with permission from Families and Work Institute (1997) New York.

Relationships

Attachments through one-to-one interaction with adults begin developing at birth. Babies who form secure attachments develop a secure sense of self and a lifelong ability to form healthy relationships, while those whose earliest attachments are negative or insecure may have continuing difficulty in developing positive relationships.

Nutrition

A balance of nutrients is needed for healthy brain growth and development. Undernourished children grow more slowly and have less energy for learning and exploring. When there is severe undernutrition, brain growth may be slowed and affect physical and emotional development.

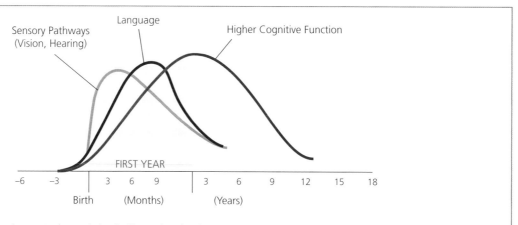

Figure 1.2 Sequence of development of neural circuits illustrating developmentally sensitive periods.

Stress

Stress can have a profound effect. Three different levels of stress are described:

- *Positive stress* – everyday events such as minor injuries, meeting new people or experiencing frustration are inevitable and contribute to building emotional resilience.
- *Tolerable stress* – time-limited events such as moving home, parental separation, changing child care or a sibling's birth can profoundly affect a child but are usually tolerable if there is a nurturing adult supporting the child emotionally.
- *Toxic stress* – when a child experiences physical and emotional abuse, neglect or severe parental mental health problems, long-term damage can occur resulting in learning, behaviour and emotional problems.

Figure 1.3 shows structural changes in the brain that were found in a child suffering from severe neglect.

Poverty

Children growing up in extreme poverty are particularly susceptible to stress, poorer nutrition and less nurturing stimulation. MRI scans show that in these circumstances the brain's grey matter is reduced, with lags in the development of areas of the brain responsible for language, cognition and spatial perception.

If babies and young children's life circumstances are not ideal for optimal development, it does not inevitably mean that brain development is affected. The brain has a good degree of plasticity, so some effects of early deprivation can be subsequently mitigated. It is, however, more difficult for the child to develop skills once specific periods of sensitivity have passed and, in some areas, such as vision, emotional stability and language, early damage can never be completely repaired.

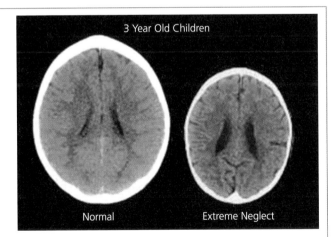

Figure 1.3 Abnormal brain development following neglect in early childhood: The CT scan of a healthy 3 year old (left) and a 3 year old suffering from severe sensory-deprivation neglect, showing microcephaly, enlarged ventricles and cortical atrophy. *Source:* Permission obtained from Springer Nature.

The parent–child relationship

The relationship between baby and parent has a particular impact on the emerging capacity for rational thought, empathy and self-control, which develop almost entirely in response to social experiences. How parents talk and listen to their baby, play with them, comfort them and cuddle them influences their development. When babies and young children experience consistent emotionally responsive parenting, it helps to develop neurological pathways that, over time, help them to manage their feelings and calm themselves as they grow older.

Babies need stressful experiences managed for them. Being held and cuddled regulates babies' arousal system, triggering a hormonal response to reduce the stress they are experiencing. If they do not get the soothing they need in early life, children can grow up with an over-sensitive stress response – prone to experiencing the world as a hostile and threatening place and making them more vulnerable to depression, anxiety and stress-related physical illnesses in later life.

Attachment

Attachment has been defined as the propensity to make strong emotional bonds and is a basic component of human nature. A human baby is extremely immature and dependent at birth and has to rely on motivating adults to protect, feed, care for and comfort them. From the moment they arrive in the world, they are focused on the adults around them – showing a preference for faces and face-like patterns, and quickly learning to show a preference for their mother's voice, smell and face. They quickly develop an understanding of facial expressions, distinguishing surprise, fear, sadness, anger and delight, and express this by making corresponding expressions of their own.

The fact that babies are able to make connections between what they do and the response they get primes them to learn from early interactions. Children whose early interactions communicate that they matter and are loveable are more likely to grow up with self-respect and confidence in their own worth and trust others. Babies and young children with secure attachment feel able to rely on their parents as a source of comfort and safety in times of upset and stress. This is related to greater self-confidence, improved social skills and higher school achievement.

Parenting styles and their influence

How parents respond to their children has an enduring impact on children's sense of self, relationships and wellbeing. Studies of parent–child interactions describe four core parenting styles that are based on the extent to which the parent is more or less responsive to their child, and is in charge as an adult (see Figure 1.4).

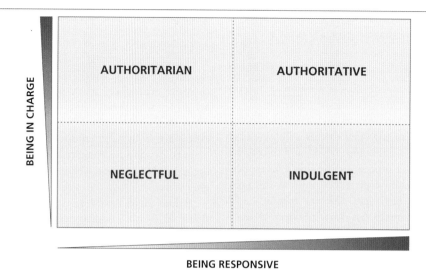

Figure 1.4 Styles of parenting: the four styles relate to how responsive parents are to the child and how much they are in charge within the family.

Authoritative style The optimal style is authoritative where the parent is sensitive and responsive to their child's needs and emotions, yet maintains appropriate boundaries for behaviour. Authoritative parenting is linked to a number of positive outcomes such as social development, self-esteem, mental health, higher academic achievement, lower levels of problem behaviour, less depression and less risk taking.

Authoritarian style Parents with a largely authoritarian style exercise a high degree of control and tend to be very restricting without taking children's needs, feelings and preferences into account. Children raised in this way are likely to become anxious and withdrawn, or rebellious and defiant.

Indulgent style The indulgent style is a kind but weak approach to parenting, in which the parent is responsive to the child's wishes and demands but is unable or unwilling to set limits and maintain boundaries. Children as a result may tend to become demanding and lack security.

Neglectful style A neglectful parenting style differs in that the parent is disengaged, neither in charge nor responsive to the child. Parents may be unaware of the child's needs and set few boundaries. Children as a result may be confused or resort to extreme behaviour as a way of attracting attention.

Parenting is influenced by many factors. How comfortably parents relate to a baby depends on their mental health, ability to provide for the baby, confidence and self-esteem, levels of support, emotional maturity and their cultural background. Health professionals have a key role in supporting parents, particularly as parents are so often bombarded with conflicting advice from family and friends. Common parenting difficulties and how they can be addressed are discussed in Chapter 21.

Psychomotor development and social interaction

Babies are born into a social world and through interacting initially with their parents, then other close carers and eventually other children and adults achieve full social development.

Early social development is divided into discrete periods corresponding to developmental landmarks; each period being an important milestone. More detail about developmental milestones and how to assess them are covered in Chapter 6. Here you are provided with an outline of a child's development through the stages of childhood. Development cannot be accelerated from outside, but external factors, particularly environment and to a lesser extent illness, can retard it.

Babyhood and the preschool years

0-2 months

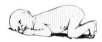 Mothers of new babies 'bond' with their baby during the first hours and days after birth. This is not an automatic process and is facilitated by close physical contact. Mothers who are separated from their babies after birth (e.g. because they are sick or premature and require admission to a neonatal unit) find bonding more difficult. For this reason, parents should be encouraged to handle their babies even when their baby is receiving intensive care.

Infants are born with a variety of needs that must be met by their parents. In the first 2 months babies start to adapt their behaviour into states of arousal. Sleep and wake cycles begin to emerge and are influenced by routine in the house. The longest period of sleep usually occurs in the night.

Infants show a great degree of alertness and are particularly attracted to human faces and the spoken word. Contact is achieved with the mother particularly during feeding. Mothers and babies coordinate their behaviour and take turns to initiate contact by means of alternating sucking with pauses for eye contact. It appears that infants are programmed to respond to their carers in particular ways, and in turn carers are profoundly influenced through their own programming to stimulate the infant and to respond to the baby's contact. A major milestone in the development of babies as social beings in these early weeks is the start of the first smile (at around 6 weeks).

2-5 months

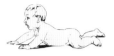

A major developmental change that occurs in the first weeks is the infant's visual development. At 2 months a baby can sustain eye contact, and this is a vital stimulus for parent–child interaction. Over time infants show progressively more gaze interaction, and parents respond with facial expression, speech and intonation.

Another important milestone is the beginning of vocalization. When babies start to babble, carers respond as if engaging in 'conversation'. They respond to their baby's sounds by questioning or talking to the infant, with pauses for a response. Although infants do not understand the meaning of their carer's speech, the pattern and interaction are essential for the child's own language and social development.

5-8 months

At this age babies begin to pay more detailed attention to objects. They begin to reach for toys and so start to explore the inanimate world. Through interaction with their carers, simple play starts to emerge. At 6 weeks of age babies spend about 70% of contact time regarding their carers, but by 6 months two-thirds of the time is taken up with regarding the rest of the world. First contact with objects is by gaze and later by pointing.

At this stage too, infants transform from being egocentric to realizing that they live in a world which is shared with people and objects.

8-18 months

During this period mobility rapidly develops and children start to leave the safety of their carer to interact further with the environment. They begin to initiate contact rather than simply reacting to it, and the concept of reciprocation begins to emerge. They can play 'peek-a-boo' and control the game by adapting their response to the adult's. They begin to 'learn the rules' of games and of social interaction in general. They begin to use carers to obtain a desired object, and can also manipulate objects to attract adults' attention.

At this stage, babies also learn to associate their cry with response and, for example, know that if they are uncomfortable

due to a dirty nappy, relief will be provided. Babies who are institutionalized become apathetic if their cries are unanswered, because communication has been extinguished.

In the first half of the second-year babies begin to take more interest in other children. Initially children play side by side, occasionally sharing a toy. By 18 months they may play together, but there is less vocal contact than when they are engaged with an adult. Carers, particularly parents, are the principal influence on social development at this stage.

18 months and beyond

By 18 months children begin to communicate verbally using speech to describe an event or effect a wish. Make-believe play develops by 2 years, when children use familiar objects to reconstruct events. Examples include using a brush to brush their hair or 'cooking' with pots and pans. They also develop the ability to recognise shapes, including letters (which is the first stage of reading), and then to copy shapes with a pencil.

School-age children

Motor, language and social skills continue to develop rapidly during the school years. Horizons are broadened by starting school, and often for the first time, children need to learn to function outside the security and safety of their own home. Expectations for appropriate behaviour in a variety of situations increase. During school years children also begin to develop a conscience and an understanding of right and wrong.

Socialization is particularly important at this age, and children need to learn to relate to a variety of other children and adults. Play is an extremely important part of this process and brings benefits far beyond its impact on physical development and motor skills. It is necessary for children's happiness and well being, impacts on the quality of friendships, cultural understanding, and social, emotional and cognitive functioning, and allows the development of imagination, creativity and exploration. Through play children practise adult roles, learn a variety of competences, enhance their academic performance, and work out how to handle challenges, work in groups, make decisions and develop leadership skills.

Adolescence

Adolescence bridges childhood and maturity and is a period of biological, psychological and sociological maturation. This is discussed in detail in Chapter 25.

Physical growth

Growth and development are intimately related but are not necessarily dependent on one another. *Growth* is a combination of increase in the number of cells (hyperplasia) and in the size of cells (hypertrophy). *Development* is an increase in complexity of the organism due to the maturation of the nervous system. A child may develop normally but be retarded in growth, and vice versa. Brain injury does not necessarily cause impaired growth, although many children who have severe intellectual disabilities are small due to malnourishment.

Factors that affect growth

Growth is influenced by a number of semi-independent factors (see Box 1.1):
- *Genetics*. Growth patterns and final height are largely genetically determined. A normal child's final height can be predicted to fall close to the centile midway between the parents' centiles.
- *Hormones*. The principal hormones influencing early growth are growth hormone and thyroid hormone. The sex hormones play an important part in the pubertal growth spurt. Disturbance of any of these affects a child's growth.
- *Nutrition*. World wide, malnutrition is an important factor that influences growth, and is the major factor accounting for differences in height observed between developing and more developed countries. Overnutrition, a leading cause of obesity, is on the increase.
- *Illness*. Illness causes a child's growth to slow down. If the illness is short-lived, rapid catch-up occurs. Chronic illness can affect growth profoundly and irreversibly.
- *Psychosocial factors*. Sociodemographically, children and adults from higher socioeconomic classes are taller than their peers from lower classes. An adverse psychosocial environment, particularly if there is emotional neglect, can have a profound effect on a child's growth.

Growth through the life course

Growth in infancy

The rate of growth in the first year of life is more rapid than at any other age. Between birth and 1 year of age, children on average increase their length by 50%, and triple their birthweight. Head circumference increases by one-third. During the second year of life the rate of growth slows down and babies change so their shape takes on the leaner and more muscular appearance of childhood.

> ### Box 1.1 Factors necessary for normal growth
>
> - Genetic potential (mid-parental height)
> - Optimal intrauterine nutrition
> - Appropriate postnatal nutrition
> - Good health
> - Normal psychosocial factors (nurture)
> - Normal hormonal milieu

Growth in the preschool and school years

In the preschool years a child continues to gain weight and height steadily. Beyond the age of 2 or 3 years until puberty, the growth rate is steady at about 3–3.5 kg and 6 cm per year.

Growth in adolescence

Adolescence is characterised by a growth spurt which occurs under the influence of emerging sex hormone levels. During the 3 or 4 years of puberty, boys grow about 25 cm and girls 20 cm. Growth in the pubertal years is discussed in Chapter 25.

Catch-up growth

During a period of illness or starvation the rate of growth is slowed. After the incident children usually grow more rapidly, catching up towards, or actually to, their original growth ('catch-up growth'). The degree to which catch-up is successful depends on the timing of onset of slow growth and its duration. This is particularly important in infants who have suffered intrauterine growth retardation (see pp. 434–6), and who may have reduced growth potential.

In nutritionally compromised children, weight falls before height is impaired, and head growth is the last to be affected. If growth has been slowed for too long or into puberty, complete catch-up is not achieved. Early detection of children with abnormal growth velocity patterns has important therapeutic implications. Early treatment is more likely to ensure that acceptable adult height is achieved.

Organ growth

Not all body systems grow at the same rate, and in some respects the growth rates of some organs are independent of others. Full maturation is not complete until the end of the second decade.

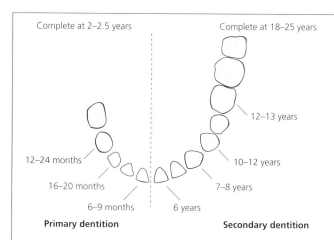

Figure 1.5 Dental development, showing the age at which teeth generally erupt.

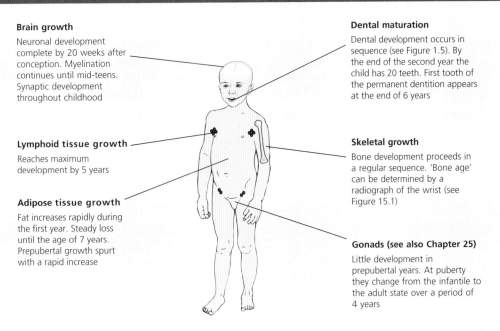

Differential organ growth at a glance

Brain growth

Neuronal development complete by 20 weeks after conception. Myelination continues until mid-teens. Synaptic development throughout childhood

Dental maturation

Dental development occurs in sequence (see Figure 1.5). By the end of the second year the child has 20 teeth. First tooth of the permanent dentition appears at the end of 6 years

Lymphoid tissue growth

Reaches maximum development by 5 years

Skeletal growth

Bone development proceeds in a regular sequence. 'Bone age' can be determined by a radiograph of the wrist (see Figure 15.1)

Adipose tissue growth

Fat increases rapidly during the first year. Steady loss until the age of 7 years. Prepubertal growth spurt with a rapid increase

Gonads (see also Chapter 25)

Little development in prepubertal years. At puberty they change from the infantile to the adult state over a period of 4 years

Nutrition

Milk is the food of babies and is capable of meeting the infant's entire nutritional needs for the first 6 months of life. Breast milk is the ideal food for human babies, but may be unavailable for some infants, in which case alternative formulae are available.

Nutrition – breast-feeding

Breast-feeding (see Figure 1.6)

Breast milk contains all the fluid, energy and nutrients a baby needs in the first 6 months of life. It protects both the mother's and baby's health, and supports emotional bonding. Although infant formula can adequately meet nutritional needs, it is not able to replicate the unique, dynamic composition of breast milk, and does not contain antibodies that provide protection against infection. Long-term protection has also been demonstrated against a number of medical conditions including sudden unexplained death in infancy and childhood (SUDIC), leukaemia, diabetes and coeliac disease. There is also evidence that breast-feeding provides some protection against obesity. Breast-fed babies have more diverse gut bacteria, and it is thought this may play a role in obesity prevention.

The World Health Organization (WHO) recommends exclusive breast-feeding for the first 6 months, followed by a mix of breast milk and solid foods. Mothers are encouraged to continue breast-feeding for longer, and at least to 12 months. In the UK, 74% of women are breast-feeding at birth, but only 45% are still breast-feeding at 6–8 weeks and less than 1% are exclusively breast-feeding at 6 months.

In order to support breast-feeding more widely, the World Health Organization and UNICEF established the Baby Friendly Initiative as a worldwide programme to encourage maternity hospitals and community services to promote successful breast-feeding and to practise in accordance with the International Code of Marketing of Breastmilk Substitutes.

In developed countries, the benefits of breast-feeding are psychological as much as physical. In developing countries, the argument for breast-feeding is very strong: formula feeds may easily be contaminated by polluted water used in making up the feed, with the risk of fatal gastroenteritis. Everywhere, breast-feeding has the advantages of being free of cost, and convenient.

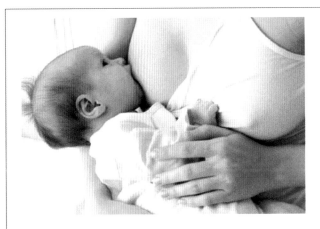

Figure 1.6 Mother breast-feeding her 6-week-old baby.

Physiology of lactation

During pregnancy there is a marked increase in the number of ducts and alveoli within the breast, in response to changes in maternal and placental hormones. The size of the nipple also increases. In the third trimester prolactin sensitizes the glandular tissue, causing small amounts of colostrum to be secreted.

At birth, oestrogen levels fall rapidly while prolactin rises. This is stimulated further by the infant's sucking at the breast. The prolactin secretion from the anterior pituitary maintains milk production from the breast alveoli. The volume of milk produced relates to the frequency, duration and intensity of sucking.

The flow of milk from the breast is under the control of the let-down reflex. The baby's rooting at the nipple causes afferent impulses to pass to the posterior pituitary, which secretes oxytocin. This acts on the smooth muscle fibres surrounding the alveoli so that milk is forced into the large ducts. As the baby takes less milk, the stimulus for prolactin production reduces and lactation is inhibited. The hormonal maintenance of lactation is summarized in Figure 1.7.

The let-down reflex is stimulated by contact with the baby, including hearing the baby cry and handling the child. Anxiety and embarrassment suppress the reflex by action of the sympathetic nervous system. Every step possible should therefore be taken to put the mother at her ease and avoid unnecessary anxiety.

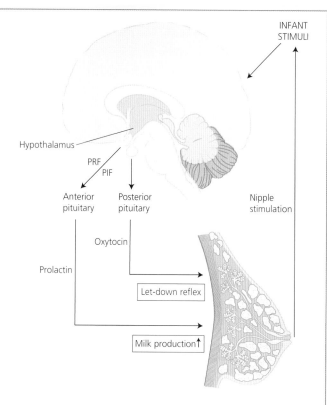

Figure 1.7 Physiology of lactation. PIF, prolactin-inhibiting factor; PRF, prolactin-releasing factor.

Colostrum   The milk produced in the first few days after birth is called colostrum and is a thick, yellowish fluid. It is particularly valuable for the establishment of lactobacilli in the bowel and contains less fat and energy but more immunoglobulins than later milk.

The constituents of milk do not reach their mature proportions until 10–14 days after birth. The secretion from the breast between colostrum and mature milk is referred to as transitional milk.

Technique of breast-feeding

Most of the milk taken by a baby from the breast is consumed in the first 5 minutes of the feed. Much of the rest of the time at the breast is spent in non-nutritive sucking. Mothers should be aware of the feeling of her breast being 'emptied' by her baby shortly after commencement of suckling, but the time spent at the breast following this is also very important.

Mothers should be encouraged to put the baby to the breast directly after birth. A normal baby immediately attempts to suck. Little milk is produced, but the stimulation is important in the establishment of lactation. Mothers should then be encouraged to put the baby to the breast on demand and should also feed the baby during the night. The time the baby spends on the breast should be gradually increased so that the nipples become accustomed to the baby sucking.

Trauma to the nipple in the first few days after birth has to be minimized. The baby exerts strong suction on the nipple and a baby should never be pulled off the breast. The mother should be shown how to release the baby by using her finger to depress the breast away from the corner of the baby's mouth. Babies are often given complementary formula feeds in the early days of life by well-meaning staff in order to let the mother rest, but this is counterproductive and should be avoided.

It is common for mothers to encounter difficulties in establishing breast-feeding in the first weeks, and to feel that their milk is inadequate. The difficulties often relate to positioning of the baby, and expert support from breast-feeding counsellors can often help resolve the problems.

It is now common for women to pump breast milk and give it by bottle, especially when they are proposing to return to work. Some choose to do this exclusively. This choice sometimes follows time spent in neonatal intensive care, where feeding may be harder to establish, and anxiety may follow about not 'seeing' the quantity of milk the baby consumes. A variety of breast pumps are available on the market

Advantages of breast-feeding

The advantages of breast-feeding are summarized in Table 1.1, and ways to encourage successful breast-feeding are shown in Box 1.2.

Breast-fed infants have a significantly lower risk of respiratory and gastrointestinal infections in the early months of life

Table 1.1 Advantages of breast-feeding
Perfect balance of milk constituents
Little risk of bacterial contamination
Ideal food for brain growth and optimal development
Establishes a healthy microbiome
Anti-infective properties
Convenience
No expense to purchase milk
Psychological satisfaction
Possibly reduces risk of atopic disorders
Exposes baby to a variety of flavours
Some protection from obesity
Possible IQ enhancement

Table 1.2 Role of anti-infective agents in breast milk	
Cells	Milk is teeming with white cells, mainly macrophages, polymorphs and both T- and B-lymphocytes
Immunoglobulins	Secretory IgA is the predominant immunoglobulin. Particularly high concentration in colostrum
Lysozyme	Lyses bacterial cell walls
Lactoferrin	Binds iron necessary for the replication of some bacteria and reduces bacterial growth
Interferon	Present in low concentrations in breast milk and has antiviral properties
Bifidus factor	The carbohydrate bifidus factor encourages lactobacilli to flourish in the bowel, inhibiting overgrowth of *Escherichia coli*

Box 1.2 Ways to encourage successful breast-feeding

- Introduce the concept to both parents antenatally
- Place the baby on the breast immediately after delivery
- Allow the baby to feed on demand, in the early days especially
- Avoid offering any formula feeds
- Ensure the mother receives good nutrition and plenty of rest

compared with formula-fed infants. Breast milk has a number of important anti-infective properties which are summarized in Table 1.2.

Contraindications to breast-feeding

For healthy infants there are no disadvantages to breast-feeding. Infants born with anomalies such as severe cleft lip and palate and obstructive bowel problems may not be able to feed, although every effort should be made to provide them with expressed breast milk rather than formula feeds.

There are very few contraindications to breast-feeding. The most important reason is if the mother is HIV-positive: the risk of transmitting the HIV virus to her baby is doubled by breast-feeding. A mother who is excreting *Mycobacterium tuberculosis* should also not breast-feed. Mastitis (inflammation of the breast) is a common problem but, far from being contraindicated, it is alleviated by continued and frequent breast-feeding.

Drugs in breast milk

Most drugs given to the mother are excreted to some degree in her milk, but the exposure to the infant is usually so little that the risk is minimal. Examples of drugs that are clearly contraindicated are tetracyclines (which stain developing teeth), antimetabolites (impair cell growth) and opiates (drug addiction). If in doubt, the Drugs in Breastmilk Information Service provides valuable information.

Nutrition – formula feeds

Parents who feed their babies using infant formula must know how to use infant formula safely and need non-judgemental support. It is important that they understand about responsive bottle feeding so they neither under- or overfeed their baby.

Formula milks are based on cow's milk, but are highly adjusted to meet the basic nutritional requirements of growing immature infants. A variety of components are utilized. Skimmed milk is produced by removing the fat content, and the curd can be separated, leaving whey and lactose together with minerals. These are the building blocks of infant formula.

Virtually all formula feeds have added carbohydrate, usually lactose or maltodextrins. Most milk manufacturers replace the fat with polyunsaturated vegetable oil or butterfat blend. This alters the fatty acid profile to resemble breast milk more closely. The protein base of formula milk is usually demineralized whey to which the appropriate mixture of minerals, vitamins and trace elements are added.

Although there are similarities between breast and formula milks, the constituents are chemically quite different. The protein in formula milk is based on cow's milk protein and the fat content is quite different to breast milk fat content.

Preparation of feeds

The preparation of formula feeds is summarized in Figure 1.8. Parents need to understand and be instructed to use a level measure of powder and not a heaped one, as this would produce too concentrated a feed, especially in its electrolyte content,

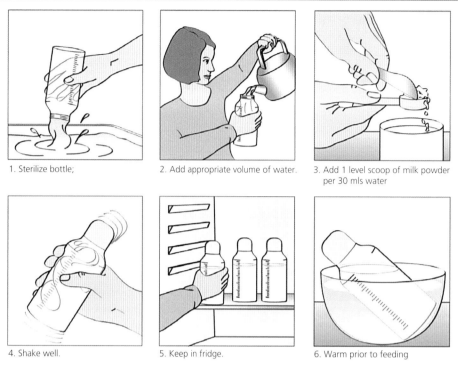

1. Sterilize bottle;

2. Add appropriate volume of water.

3. Add 1 level scoop of milk powder per 30 mls water

4. Shake well.

5. Keep in fridge.

6. Warm prior to feeding

Figure 1.8 Preparation of formula feed.

and could lead to hypernatraemic dehydration (see p. 113). To obtain a level measure, the excess powder is removed with the blade of a knife.

Scrupulous attention should be paid to sterility: bottles and teats should be sterilized either in a microwave, by boiling or by a cold-water sterilizing solution (such as Milton®). It is essential that the bottles are filled with the solution and the teats are totally immersed. The solution should be made up each day according to the manufacturers' instructions.

Most parents like to give the milk warm. To ensure that it is not too hot it should be tested by shaking out a little onto the back of the hand. The teat should not be touched, or it will

become contaminated. The hole in the teat should be large enough so that when the bottle is inverted, milk comes out rapidly in drops, but not in a stream. Too large a hole causes the baby to choke on the feed, and too small a hole leads to excessive air swallowing as a result of the baby's vigorously sucking to obtain the milk.

Promoting optimal bottle feeding

If families are using infant formula it is important that they feed the baby 'responsively' and mimic the body closeness that is natural when breast-feeding. Table 1.3 shows ways to promote optimal bottle feeding.

Table 1.3 Ways to promote optimal bottle feeding	
Bonding	• Baby fed predominantly by parent(s) in early days/weeks • Treat feeding as 'special time' of closeness • Encourage skin-to-skin contact
Avoiding overfeeding and excess weight gain	• Follow baby's signs of fullness and stop feeding even if there is still milk in the bottle • If the baby seems hungry, but has recently fed, try comforting before feeding again • Don't sweeten or add cereal/rusks to milk • Avoid hungry infant formula or follow-on milk, which are not recommended in the UK
Avoiding tooth decay	• Feed baby in a semi-upright position rather than lying down • Do not 'prop' bottle • Do not sweeten infant formula
Reducing risk of gastro intestinal infections	• Sterilize bottles and teats before and after use • Make up bottles freshly for each feed and discard any leftover milk • Use made-up formula within 2 hours at room temperature, or within 4 hours in a cool bag with an ice pack

Nutrition – weaning

See Boxes 1.3 and 1.4. Breast or formula milk provide all infants' nutritional requirements in the early months. WHO recommendations are that solid foods should not be started until 6 months when their gastrointestinal and renal systems are mature enough and the swallowing reflex is adequately developed. Early introduction has been linked to obesity and may increase risks of infection.

By 6 months most babies can manage a range of textures and a wide array of foods. Developmentally they should be able to sit with support. By 7 months most are adequately coordinated to pick up food, and put it in their mouths themselves, move it to the back of their mouths and swallow it. As most of the nutritional needs in the first year of life are provided by milk, the main goal in weaning is to help babies to accept and enjoy a wide range of textures and flavours. On starting new foods, babies commonly screw up their faces, look worried and spit out new foods. This should not be interpreted as dislike. If babies are only given bland, sweet and familiar foods, they are more likely to eat a limited repertoire as they grow older.

Box 1.3 The weaning process

0–6 months	Breast or formula milk only
6 months	Introduce solid foods – pureed and finger feeds. Start with less sweet tastes and accustom babies to: • Vegetables such as broccoli, avocado, carrots, parsnip, green beans • Starch foods such as potato, rice, oats mixed with milk • Full fat dairy foods such as plain yoghurt • Once readily eating these, move on to soft fruits
7–9 months	Give more soft feeds before milk feeds Encourage finger feeding Give water in a cup Gradually move to three meals per day
9–12 months	Mash food with a fork or chop it Three meals a day, at least one with the family
1 year and beyond	Undiluted cow's milk in a cup (no need for formula milk) Baby should be eating family meals (provided they are healthy) Add two healthy snacks between meals Continue breast-feeding as long as mother wants

Box 1.4 Principles of infant nutrition

- Breast milk is the optimal and exclusive feed for the first 6 months
- Continue breast or formula milk for the first year
- Introduce solid foods from 6 months
- Once a baby is able to chew, mashed and then cut up food can be given
- Babies can usually feed themselves biscuits or rusks at 7 months and use a spoon by 15 months
- Cup feeds should replace breast-feeds, and bottles be discouraged beyond the age of 1 year
- Vitamin supplements (Vitamins A, C and D) should be given to all breast-fed babies from 6 months to 5 years, with Vitamin D supplementation from birth. Formula-fed infants will also need daily vitamin supplements once they change to normal cow's milk, rather than supplemented infant formula. Iron supplementation is also recommended (WHO) between 6 and 23 months of age in countries with a high incidence of iron deficiency

Although there are commercial foods, simple home prepared fresh foods, such as mashed, unsalted vegetables are cheaper and often more nutritious. They should be introduced gradually, starting with vegetables and introducing fruit after the baby has accepted a range of savoury foods. Food may be started blended but can rapidly move onto being mashed by fork and then given as finger foods. It is important to encourage independence in eating and give babies control of eating as soon as they are ready to pick up food themselves. In recent years there has been a move towards 'baby-led' weaning where food is put into the mouth by the baby alone. This prevents undue pressure to eat and overfeeding. Some professionals are concerned by baby-led weaning as nutritional needs may not be met when the only foods consumed are those that can be held by a baby.

Certain foods should be avoided in babies and toddlers as shown in Table 1.4.

The principle of responsive feeding (Figure 1.9) is especially important when it comes to weaning as the risk of overfeeding is higher when babies start solid foods. Carers should be encouraged to recognise signs of fullness and hunger which differ at different ages. Ensuring babies learn to respect their satiety cues teaches them to avoid eating beyond when they are full.

Table 1.4 Food and drinks to avoid in babies and toddlers	
Food and drinks	**Reason to avoid**
Salt	Renal system too immature to cope. Primes taste for salty foods
Sugar	Encourages preference for sweet foods Tooth decay
Honey	May be contaminated with botulinum toxin
Nuts and chunks of food	Choking hazard
Low fat foods	Fat is needed for growth and development
High fibre foods, e.g. bran	Inhibits absorption of other nutrients
Additives	Certain E numbers in sensitive individuals. Implicated in hyperactivity
Fruit juices, cordials	Unnecessary sugars
Rice milk	Contains arsenic at levels that may be harmful for babies
Coffee, tea, cola etc.	Stimulants

Box 1.5 Principles of good nutrition in children

- Allow no more than 350 mls milk each day.
- Give three meals and two nutritious snacks each day.
- Try to ensure that children eat with others in a social setting.
- Avoid grazing outside of meals and snack times.
- Encourage a diet with food from each of the basic four food groups.
- The majority of foods should be fruit, vegetables and starchy carbohydrates with the rest made up of foods high in protein and dairy foods.
- Drink 6-8 cups of water or milk and limit juices to < 1 cup per day.
- Choose unprocessed foods if possible, and choose those lower in saturated fat and free sugars.
- Avoid added salt.
- Avoid sugar in the form of sweet drinks and sweets.
- Limit snacking on crisps, sweets, biscuits and cake.
- Avoid an excess of fat.
- Avoid foods which are likely to be aspirated, e.g. nuts, boiled sweets.

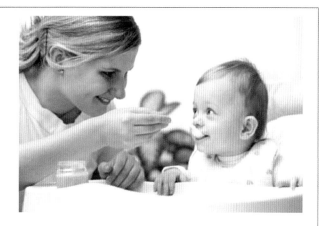

Figure 1.9 Mother feeding her 6-month-old baby. She is seated so she can interact with him and pick up on his hunger and fullness cues, ensuring that she does not under- or over-feed him.

Nutrition – the preschool and school years

Nutrition in the preschool years

See Box 1.5. As toddlers become increasingly dextrous and coordinated, they should be encouraged to eat independently using a spoon and drinking from a cup. Alongside this independence comes a change in eating habits where toddlers tend to eat unpredictably, consuming large amounts on some occasions and almost negligible at others. It is also usual for a wariness of new foods to develop and 'pickiness' is very common.

Although milk is no longer the main source of nutrition, children should still drink 350 mL of milk per day. It is important to ensure that the child becomes used to eating a well-balanced diet, including foods from the four basic food groups:
- meat, fish, poultry and eggs;
- dairy products (milk and cheese products);
- fruits and vegetables;
- cereals, grains, potatoes and rice.

Children of this age have different requirements from adults. A diet low in fat and high in fibre is unlikely to provide the calorie content that is essential for active, rapidly growing children. For this reason, whole-fat milk rather than semi-skimmed milk should be given until the age of 2 years. It is also important to discourage a taste for sweet and salty foods.

The development of independence and inconsistent eating habits often causes problems within the family (see pp. 385–6). Parents may become very anxious and resort to a variety of tactics to make their child eat. This can be extremely stressful for all concerned and may be associated with weight faltering (see pp. 283–5).

The other common problem of this period is iron deficiency anaemia (see p. 374) resulting from a low intake of iron-rich foods. Excessive milk intake may contribute by leading to a reduction in appetite for other nutrients, and may also be responsible for poor weight gain.

Nutrition in the school years

The Food Standards Agency has produced the 'Eatwell Guide' (see Figure 1.10) to guide families on how to balance their diet.

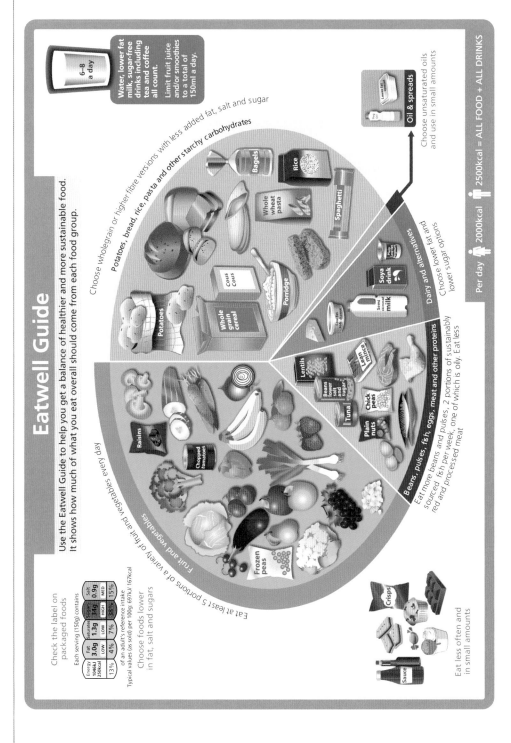

Figure 1.10 The Eatwell Guide, showing how a balanced diet is made up of foods from each of the five food groups. *Source*: Public Health England in association with the Welsh Government, Food Standards Scotland and the Food Standards Agency in Northern Ireland © Crown copyright 2016.

Table 1.5 How different food groups support young children's health and growth

Food group	Needs	No. of portions: < 5 years	> 5 years
Fruit and vegetables	At least five types of fruit and vegetables needed to accustom children to a wide range of tastes	5	5+
Potatoes, bread, rice, pasta and other starchy carbohydrates	A mix of whole grain and refined starchy foods. Excessive fibre can reduce intake of energy and other nutrients	4	5
Beans, pulses, fish, eggs, meat and other proteins	Important for growth Omega 3 and other essential fatty acids needed for brain development	2-3	2-3
Dairy and alternatives	Calcium, vitamins A and D, riboflavin, zinc and iodine needed in growing children	3	2
Oils and spreads (fats)	Energy needs for growth and activity but excess leads to obesity. Saturated fats (in meat, butter cakes) should be limited. Fats for absorption of Vitamin A and D	Minimal	Minimal

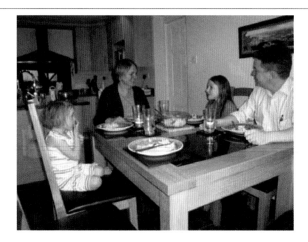

Figure 1.11 A family mealtime. Eating regularly together as a family is associated with a broad range of benefits in such areas as social behaviour, language development and academic achievement.

It visually emphasises how prominent fruit and vegetables should be in the diet, and how little fat and sugar are required relative to the other foods. Maintaining healthy eating is often a challenge, particularly compounded when children are introduced to snacking on sugary and salty foods by their peers. Schools are well placed to educate about nutrition and provide well-balanced meals, and regulations are in place to make sure that food eaten on the premises is nutritious.

Table 1.5 shows the key food groups, the needs they meet and the number of portions recommended daily.

As important as *what* children eat is *how* they eat. Family mealtimes (Figure 1.11) are associated with many benefits including enhanced language development, psychosocial well-being, fewer high-risk behaviours, reduced obesity levels and lower academic dropout rates.

The adolescent years bring increased requirements for energy, calcium, nitrogen and iron. Unfortunately, in this criti-cal period, when good nutrition is so important, young people often develop lifestyles which lead to a very poor nutritional intake. Particular problems include an increase in snacking and skipping meals, inappropriate consumption of fast foods, dieting, and restrictive cult diets. The problems of obesity (see pp. 292–4) and eating disorders (see pp. 462–4) often have their onset at this time, while teenage pregnancy has nutritional consequences for both the baby and the mother.

Active play and physical activity

In the past children were engaged in active play, often outdoors, for much of the day. Nowadays many spend much of the day being sedentary. Building physical activity into daily routines is important as it increases fitness, improves emotional health, and reduces the risks of heart disease and diabetes. Benefits also include musculoskeletal strengthening, mental alertness, reduced risk of illness and effects of stress, and maintenance of healthy weight. Active play also improves behaviour, and encourages children to take safe risks. Table 1.6 shows recommended levels of activity at different ages.

TV and other screen time

Television and other screen time are often used by busy parents to occupy and entertain their children. Unfortunately, it easily becomes habitual. Too much TV and screen time is harmful as it:

- affects brain and language development
- reduces time playing and being active
- is habit-forming
- is often accompanied by snacking
- contributes to excessive weight gain

The National Institute for Health and Care Excellence recommends no more than 2 hours/day spent watching TV or engaged in other screen time, with some TV-free days. The American Academy of Paediatrics goes further and recommends that children under 2 years should have no screen time.

Table 1.6 Recommended levels of activity at different ages

Infants who are not yet walking	Under 5s	Children aged 5-18 years	Adults
• encourage physical activity from birth through 'tummy time' • minimise time spent being restrained for extended periods	• physically active for at least 3 hours a day, spread throughout the day	• at least 1 hour of physical activity every day • strength-based exercises 3 times a week – hopping, skipping, jumping	• at least 150 minutes of physical activity a week (moderate intensity); or 75 minutes of vigorous exercise • activity to improve muscle strength on at least 2 days a week – weights or heavy loads

Sleep

Sleep is restorative, and crucial for the maintenance of physical, emotional and cognitive functioning. Sleep disruption affects children's ability to concentrate and learn; children who do not get enough sleep cope less well with daily life and stress, and are more likely to have behavioural difficulties. Lack of sleep is also associated with excess weight gain and obesity, partly because the more hours a child is awake, the more food and drink they are likely to consume.

Parents whose children wake frequently in the night are also likely to suffer from sleep deprivation, making it much harder to cope well. Children's lack of sleep can dominate family life, resulting in exhaustion, stress, relationship conflict, affecting physical and mental health, as well as ability to work.

Sleep patterns at different ages

Sleep rhythms are irregular in the first few months of life, but become more regular as a child grows older (see Table 1.7).

Struggles around bedtime are one of the most common challenges of family life. Establishing consistent and effective bedtime routines can help both parents and children:
- Starting the bedtime routine at the same time each day.
- A sequence of 'wind-down' activities that signal it is bedtime and help children to relax: having a bath; a milk feed; brushing teeth; a bedtime story or song.

- Having objects that a child associates with bedtime, such as a blanket or cuddly toy.

How parents approach daytime naps and bedtimes has a big influence on a baby's sleep patterns. It is very tempting to feed, hold, rock or take the baby into the parental bed – even if this does not help establish good sleeping habits in the long-term. 'Sleep training' can be helpful but should not be started before the age of 4-6 months. The methods include:
- 'Controlled crying' which involves putting the baby down to sleep at regular times and leaving them to go to sleep. Parents leave the room and return periodically to settle the baby, or stay without removing the baby from the cot.
- The 'no tears' approach which is more gradual, with the parent offering comfort right away when their child cries, but slowly changing how this is provided so that the child becomes used to getting to sleep on their own.

Child care and education

Not so long ago, children were cared for by their mothers until they started school. Now, most parents work outside the home and arrange alternative care for their young children. Options may include a nanny or minder in the home, or child care outside the home. Child minders who take other children into their own home have to be legally approved and registered with the Department of Social Services.

Table 1.7 Sleep patterns at different ages and stages

Age	Optimum sleep	Sleep patterns
0–3 months	16–17 hours	Newborns sleep a lot in the early weeks – broken by the need for frequent feeds.
3–6 months	15 hours	Sleep patterns start to settle at about 4 months into shorter daytime naps and longer periods of night-time sleep.
6–12 months	13–15 hours	Most babies start to follow a daytime schedule with morning and afternoon naps. By 10 months most babies sleep through the night or wake for one feed.
1–2 years	12–15 hours	By 18 months many toddlers nap just once a day for 1–3 hours.
3–4 years	11–13 hours	Most children drop their daytime nap by the age of 5.
School age	9–11 hours	Children may get less sleep than they need and/or have difficulty getting to sleep.
Teens	9 hours	Many teenagers stay up late but need as much sleep.

Alternative care is available in **day nurseries** staffed by nursery nurses. These may be run by Social Care, privately or by voluntary organisations. Unfortunately, they are in limited supply and are often expensive. In disadvantaged areas family centres may be provided, which not only provide child care, but are also attended by parents with the aim of improving parenting skills.

The majority of children grow up away from an extended family network, and many parents appreciate the opportunities for their children to mix with other children from a young age. **Mother and toddler groups** and **playgroups** are available in most areas. The former are attended by children accompanied by a carer. Playgroups are run by trained and registered leaders, where children attend for a few sessions per week and have the opportunity to meet, play and socialize with others.

School education

In Britain compulsory education begins at the age of 5 years, although there is limited availability of **nursery school** places from the age of 3 years. From 5 to 11 years children attend **primary school,** then move to **secondary school** until the school-leaving age of 16 years. At 16 years teenagers have the option to continue their education in a **secondary school sixth form, sixth form college,** or **college of further education, or to start an apprenticeship or traineeship**.

Educational provision for children with special needs is discussed on pages 50–1.

Determinants of health in children

Children's health is affected by a wide range of factors that operate at many different levels, from within the child (such as genetics) to broader conditions in the home and in society. Socioeconomic and environmental factors play a very large part and account for much of the variation in children's lives and their health. When considering a child's health, it is important to bear these in mind. A helpful framework for identifying and understanding the interaction of various determinants affecting children's health is the Dahlgren and Whitehead model (Figure 1.12) which places the child at the centre, surrounded by the other influences on their lives.

Inequality and social disadvantage

A large and increasing number of children, in both developed and developing countries, grow up socially disadvantaged. Disadvantage may arise as a consequence of poverty, poor housing, homelessness, inadequate parenting and problems resulting from immigration. It is important to appreciate that these all have a significant impact on children's health and extend to affect their health and wellbeing throughout their lives.

Alleviation of these problems is mainly a political issue for society, but doctors need to understand the impact of the problems and, where necessary and possible, to act as the child's advocate in improving their circumstances. Table 1.8 shows some of the factors that impact on children that are associated with long-term adverse outcomes.

Poverty

It is hard to bring up a family on a low income. Not only is it hard to feed and clothe children and provide them with the care and conditions required for them to develop and thrive, but poverty also often diminishes the capacity of parents to be supportive, consistent and involved with their children.

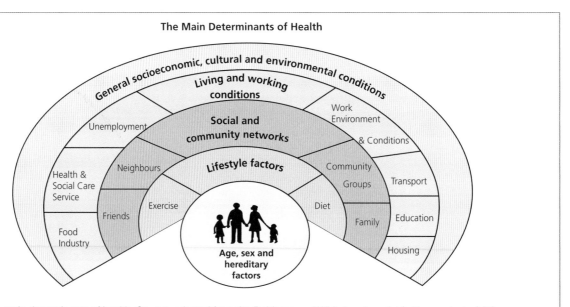

Figure 1.12 The main determinants of health. *Source:* adapted from the Dahlgren and Whitehead model (with permission) [3].

Table 1.8 Adverse factors in childhood and their long-term outcomes

Factor	Long-term outcomes
Poverty	Unemployment, low income, low working hours
Abuse and neglect	Depression, anxiety, drug abuse, suicidal behaviour, STIs, health issues, trust problems
Early mental health problems	Emotional problems, leaving school early, criminal justice system contact, poor physical health
Conduct problems	Anti-social and criminal behaviour
Poor health and nutrition	More health problems; poor academic achievement, not graduating on time

Box 1.6 Morbidity associated with poverty

- Low birthweight
- Poor growth
- Obesity
- Respiratory infections
- Iron deficiency anaemia
- Lead poisoning
- Sudden unexplained death in infants and children (SUDIC)
- Hearing disorders
- Psychological problems
- More and longer hospitalizations
- Lower survival in some malignancies (e.g. leukaemia)
- Lower educational attainment and learning disabilities

Poverty also has a strong effect on the physical health of children, and children from poor families have higher than average rates of death and illness from almost all causes (Box 1.6). Many factors are responsible for the increased morbidity, including overcrowding, poor hygiene and health care, poor diet, environmental pollution, poor education and stress.

Housing

Housing conditions have a profound effect on children's health and development. Dampness and mould are associated with an increase in a wide variety of symptoms and illnesses. Overcrowding and poor sanitary conditions are related to the spread of gastroenteritis and respiratory infections. Inadequate housing may lead to parental depression, affecting a child's psychosocial development and behaviour. Poor housing is also linked to a higher rate of accidents, including road traffic accidents as a result of a lack of safe supervised areas for play outside.

Homelessness

Homelessness exacerbates the problems of poverty. Homeless families have very restricted facilities, often living in bed and breakfast or hostel accommodation, with little space or privacy and little possibility of cooking. Moves are frequent, with disruption in the provision of health and social services and schooling for the children. Homeless children suffer from increased frequency of illness (infections, anaemia), neurological conditions and learning disorders, fits, mental illness, dental problems, trauma and substance abuse, and are more likely to be victims of abuse and neglect.

Family structure

There have been major changes in the structure of society in recent years. Fewer children in developed countries now live with both natural parents, and there are increasing numbers of parents bringing up children single-handedly. Although this does not necessarily imply that the children are disadvantaged, single parenting is difficult, particularly if it is associated, as it often is, with a reduced income, lack of support with resultant stress and depression, and family tensions and arguments. These all may have an effect on the child.

Ethnic minorities and immigrants

The other major change that has occurred in developed countries is absorption of a variety of different ethnic and cultural groups. While immigrant families are often well supported within their cultural framework, children may be disadvantaged in a variety of ways of which health professionals need to be aware.

Language and cultural barriers often lead to high degrees of social stress and isolation, and families may find it difficult to access services including health care. Specific health problems affecting some groups include nutritional deficiencies, higher perinatal and infant mortality rates, and inherited diseases if consanguinity is common practice.

To test your knowledge on this part of the book, please see Chapter 26.

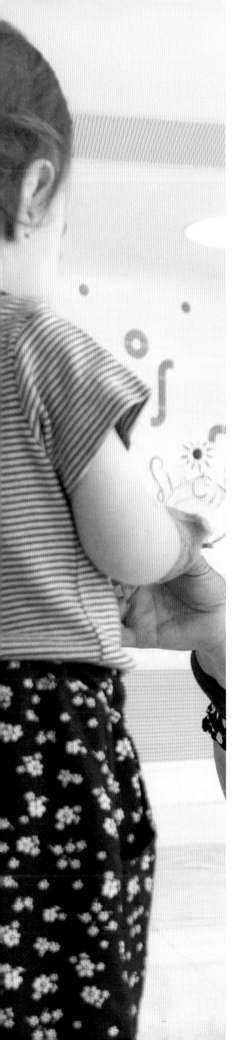

CHAPTER 2
Health care and health promotion

> The fundamental objective of paediatrics is to guide children safely and happily through childhood so that they will become healthy, well adjusted, normal young adults—to enable them to achieve their maximum potential physically, intellectually, psychologically and socially.
>
> *James G. Hughes, MD*

KEY COMPETENCES
YOU MUST …

Know and understand

- What is meant by new paediatric morbidities
- The composition and components of paediatric services and the UK Healthy Child Programme
- The screening tests offered routinely for children
- Which immunisations are recommended for children and any contraindications
- The role that child health care providers have in safeguarding children

Be able to

- Undertake health promotion discussions with parents
- Physically examine babies for newborn anomalies, developmental dysplasia of the hips and testicular descent

Appreciate

- The principles underlying the UK Healthy Child Programme
- That vulnerable groups of children have particular health needs
- The special ethical issues and dilemmas involved in child health care
- That professional liaison is central to providing good health care
- That health professionals have an obligation to report suspected child abuse

Essential Paediatrics and Child Health, Fourth Edition. Mary Rudolf, Anthony Luder and Kerry Jeavons.
© 2020 John Wiley & Sons Ltd. Published 2020 by John Wiley & Sons Ltd.
Companion website: www.wiley.com/go/rudolf/paediatrics

Box 2.1 New morbidities in child health

- Emotional and behavioural problems
- Childhood obesity
- Accidents and injuries
- Child abuse and neglect
- Sexually transmitted disease and teenage pregnancy
- Increase in disabilities and chronic illness
- Substance misuse
- Suicide and self-harm
- Social and health inequalities
- Poor vaccine uptake

A century ago infection was the major cause of morbidity and mortality in childhood. Improvements in the environment and housing began the trend for advancement in population health, and this was accelerated by the introduction of immunisations and antibiotics. Educational standards, social support, health care and knowledge about child development have all improved and child abuse is less well tolerated. The face of health care has changed, and children are presenting with a range of new morbidities (see Box 2.1)

Paediatric and child health services

With the changing face of childhood disease, health professionals need to be competent at managing a broad variety of conditions. They include the following broad categories:

- Acute illnesses such as bronchiolitis, respiratory infections and anaphylaxis
- Chronic illnesses such as asthma, epilepsy, diabetes and cancer
- Disabilities – both physical and intellectual
- Injury, accidental and nonaccidental
- Disorders of eating and nutrition including weight faltering, obesity and anorexia
- Mental health disorders such as attention deficit disorder, challenging behaviour, depression and anxiety

More children are now admitted to hospital, but the experience of hospitalization has changed. Once visiting hours for parents were limited to 30 minutes per day, and now the norm and expectation is that parents stay with their child. Where possible, every effort is made to keep children out of hospital and many aspects of specialised complex care have become available in the community. Even for acutely ill children, day case observation now allows serious causes of illness to be excluded with discharge to recover at home. A significant proportion of admissions are more for social than medical reasons, if there are concerns that the family is unable to cope or lives too far away to send the child home.

Health services for children can be seen as a pyramid of care (see Figure 2.1)

A variety of professionals and agencies are involved in health care (see Box 2.2)

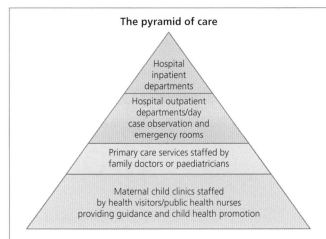

The pyramid of care

Figure 2.1 The paediatric pyramid of care.

Box 2.2 Individuals involved in services for children

A variety of agencies are involved:
- Parents have the central role
- Child care providers and minders
- Teachers

Nurses
- Health visitors/public health nurses
- School nurses
- Practice nurses
- Specialist nurses

Doctors
- General practitioners
- Paediatricians

The Healthy Child Programme

The Healthy Child Programme is the national child health promotion programme in the UK, which provides health practitioners with guidance covering pre-conception, pregnancy and care of children aged 0-19 years. It aims to promote children's health and development, prevent illness and work in partnership with parents to achieve physical, social and emotional well being for all children. The Programme is underpinned by the principle of progressive universalism, whereby all children receive a basic package of care which is increased progressively according to the needs of the child and family. Recognizing the significance of health inequalities, the rights of every child are described, along with the package of progressive input that should be provided for children in greater need because of biological, family or societal influences.

The Healthy Child Programme (see Table 2.1) has many facets which include:
- guidance on important child health topics, such as parenting, development, behavioural problems, nutrition and the use of services for children;

Table 2.1 The Healthy Child Programme

Age	Health guidance	Observation and examination	Screening procedure
Newborn	Feeding and nutrition Parenting Injury prevention Baby care Crying and sleep problems Passive smoking Car seats Reducing risk of SUDIC	Full physical examination Weight Head circumference	Hip examination Testicular descent Red reflex Cardiovascular examination Phenylketonuria Thyroid Haemoglobinopathies Cystic fibrosis Other rare inherited metabolic diseases Oto-acoustic emissions test
6 weeks–6 months	Parenting Maternal mental health Nutrition and weaning Development Play Immunisation Recognition of illness in babies Accidents: fires, falls and scalds, baths	Weight, length at 6–8 weeks (and 3–4 months if concern) Head circumference Eyes Development Cardiac examination	Hip examination at 6–8 weeks Testicular descent at 6–8 weeks
6 months–1 year	Children's physical, emotional and social needs Parenting Accident prevention Nutrition Passive smoking Developmental needs, language and play Behaviour problems Dental health	Monitor growth Evaluate development	
1–3 years	Children's physical, emotional and social needs Parenting Behaviour Language development Nutrition, play and sleep Dental care Accident prevention Toilet training	At 2-year review: • monitor growth • evaluate development	
3–5 years	Parental and teacher concerns Nutrition, play and sleep Accident prevention Dental health Medical or developmental problems that may interfere with education Review immunisation status		
Primary school	Health education in school	Height and weight for the National Child Measurement Programme at school entry and at age 11 years	At school entry: • vision (Snellen chart) • hearing (sweep test)
Secondary school	Health education in school Self-referrals to school doctor or nurse Careers advice		Visual acuity in disadvantaged areas *Chlamydia*

- a focus on vulnerable children, with identification of children in need, whether socially disadvantaged or with disabilities;
- monitoring of developmental progress;
- prevention of disease by immunisation;
- detection of abnormalities through physical examination and screening tests, and facilitating early recognition by parents;
- measurement and recording of physical growth;
- health promotion and education.

Professionals involved in child health promotion in the UK

Health visitors

Health visitors are nurses who are specially trained in child care and development. They generally work within the framework of a health centre, often with GPs or children's centres, and carry out the bulk of the child health promotion programme for preschool children. This includes running child health clinics, visiting at home and providing support, particularly for those children and families identified as being in need or at risk.

School nurses

School nurses are specially trained nurses who work in the framework of schools. They are responsible for identifying children with medical needs, facilitating their care at school, providing liaison between professionals and supplying medical information to school staff. As school doctors are no longer required to see every child at school entry, the school nurse is now responsible for reviewing all children and selecting those who need to be seen by the community paediatrician.

Community paediatricians

Community paediatricians are doctors who specialize in working in the community. They are responsible for evaluating children identified through the child health promotion programme or school as having problems. Some have specialised roles such as audiology, child protection or developmental paediatrics.

General practitioners

In recent years GPs have taken over responsibility for the routine aspects of most of the preschool child health promotion programme.

Parents

Parents have a central role in enhancing the health of their children and they should be seen as partners in child health promotion.

Child health records

Parent-held child health records

Every child is issued a child health record at birth which is kept by the parents. The advantages of this are that the child's record is available wherever and whenever the child is seen, confidentiality rests with the parents and, most importantly, it involves parents centrally in child health promotion. The parent-held record consists of a record of child health checks, the child's growth chart, parental observations, a record of primary care and dental and hospital visits, and health education and advice. Parents have welcomed this development and have been shown to be effective in ensuring that the record is kept up to date. (see Chapter 4, Figure 4.2).

Other records

In addition to the parent-held record, each professional keeps their own record of contact with the child. Computer-based systems are increasingly being used and are particularly effective in child health promotion.

Special registers

Many districts keep registers of children with special needs or chronic illness. They are useful in providing parents with information about services, keeping track of referral and review, anticipating needs and auditing the service.

Detection of medical and developmental problems

An important part of child health promotion involves identification of subtle or latent defects and disorders that may seriously affect the child later in life. These defects and disorders are usually identified in one of the following ways:

- Child health checks.
- Follow-up of infants and children who have suffered various forms of trauma or illness.
- Detection by parents or relatives, who are often the first to recognise that their child has a problem. When such suspicions are reported to a health professional they should be taken seriously, as parents are often right.
- Detection by other professionals such as nursery nurses, playgroup leaders and teachers. Playgroup leaders and nursery nurses play an important part in child care, particularly in deprived areas, and become expert at recognizing the child whose health or development requires further evaluation.

Health education and promotion

Increasingly, young families are growing up isolated and without the support of an extended family. Parenting skills and confidence are often lacking, and the Healthy Child Programme is therefore particularly valuable in providing information and advice to inexperienced parents. In disadvantaged areas this may take place through Children Centres (p. 24), although these are now under threat due to lack of funding.

The following issues are addressed by the programme:

Baby care

Young parents are likely to need advice about simple issues such as clothing, bathing, handling and positioning their baby. They need to know about common medical problems, and to learn the appropriate responses when the baby is unwell. As time goes by, they need to know about normal development, what to expect from their child, how to promote learning and how to recognise developmental difficulties.

Nutrition (see Chapter 1)

If a good nutritional environment is provided in the early years, the ground is laid for healthy eating later in childhood and beyond. Addressing nutritional issues is a major focus of a health visitor's work. It includes promoting breast-feeding, advising about weaning, dealing with toddlers' eating difficulties and education about healthy diets for the entire family.

Behavioural problems

Behavioural concerns are universal. Advice and support in the early stages can avoid development into major problems. Crying, sleep problems and temper tantrums are particularly common issues of concern.

Dental care

Information should be provided about dental hygiene and regular dental check-ups.

Passive smoking

Children exposed to passive smoking are at greatly increased risk of respiratory disorders. Avoidance of passive smoking is an important health promotion issue.

Unintentional injury

Accidents are the commonest cause of mortality in the childhood years and an important cause of morbidity. The term 'accident' is actually inappropriate as it implies the injury occurred by chance. In fact, most accidents are predictable and could be avoided with appropriate strategies. As most accidents occur in the home, education of parents has an important impact on the prevention of accidents. Areas which should be addressed in the course of health education are shown in Table 2.2.

Table 2.2 Strategies for the reduction of injuries in childhood

Injury	Prevention strategy
Road traffic injuries	Use of car seats and belts
	Road safety instruction from age 2 years
	Cycle helmets
Falls	Gate on stairs
	Guards on windows
	Safe playground surfaces
Burns	Exercise caution in the kitchen
	Reduce home hot water temperature
	Install smoke detectors
	Install fire guards
	Have flameproof clothing
	Cover electric sockets
	Avoid trailing flexes on kettles and irons
Drowning	Never leave young children alone in bath
	Fence pools
	Swim only with lifeguard present
Poisoning	Keep medicines/poisons out of reach
	Have locks on cupboards
	Have safety caps on bottles
Choking	Keep small toys away from toddlers
	Do not give nuts before age 5 years
	Secure window-blind and curtain cords
	Teach Heimlich manoeuvre (p. 407)

Health promotion in school

School provides an invaluable opportunity to educate the young about healthy living. The school years are a time when adjustments in lifestyle can be made more easily than later on in life. Issues of particular importance which are addressed are:
- nutrition;
- physical activity;
- drugs and alcohol abuse;
- contraception and safe sex;
- sexually transmitted diseases;
- smoking;
- healthy relationships;
- parenting skills.

Screening (see Figure 2.2)

Screening is the identification of unrecognised disease or defects by the application of tests, examinations and other procedures. Screening tests sort out apparently well children who may have a problem from those who do not. A screening test is not intended to be diagnostic.

Various criteria have been established to determine whether there is a value in screening for a particular condition. These criteria include a recognizable latent or early symptomatic stage of the condition, and the availability of some form of treatment or intervention that can influence the course and prognosis. Cost inevitably must be considered and needs to be balanced against the cost of medical care as a whole and the cost of treatment if the patient does not present until later.

The following screening tests have been incorporated into the child health promotion programme in the UK.

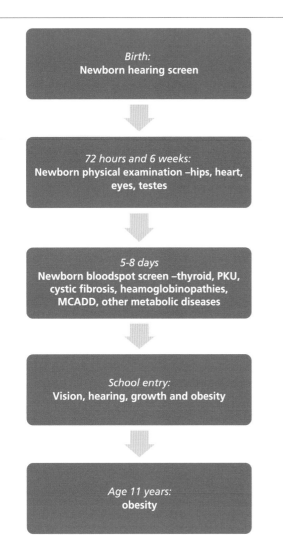

Figure 2.2 The screening timeline.

Congenital hypothyroidism

- *Age at which the test is performed.* Neonates (5–8 days of age).
- *The test.* A few drops of blood are obtained by heel prick, dripped onto a filter paper and sent to a central laboratory for analysis of thyroid-stimulating hormone (TSH) (Figure 2.3).
- *Significance of the test.* Approximately one in 4000 infants is born with congenital hypothyroidism. If untreated, congenital hypothyroidism results in severe learning disability. (see p. 294). If treated early with thyroid hormone, the child grows and develops normally.
- *Action if the test is abnormal.* The baby must be referred urgently to a paediatric endocrinologist.

Phenylketonuria

- *Age at which the test is performed.* Neonates (5–8 days of age).
- *The test.* The test is carried out on the same sample as that taken for thyroid testing. The baby must be on full milk feeds for 3 days prior to testing.
- *Significance of the test.* One in 10000 babies is born with phenylketonuria (PKU). This causes severe learning disability (mental retardation). Introduction of a low-phenylalanine diet prevents the build-up of phenylalanine metabolites which cause brain damage.
- *Action if the test is abnormal.* Referral to a metabolic clinic for dietary advice and long-term follow-up.

Other newborn screening tests

Cystic fibrosis. Immunoreactive trypsin levels in blood are used as a screening test for cystic fibrosis.

Haemoglobinopathies (sickle cell disease and thalassaemia). These are common in some ethnic communities. Screening is carried out in some parts of the country.

Medium-chain acyl-coA dehydrogenase deficiency (MCADD). A metabolic disorder where there is a deficiency of a mitochondrial enzyme, making it difficult for the body to break down fatty acids and produce energy. It can cause hypoglycaemia and sudden death in infants. Treatment involves ensuring that children do not go for long periods without food.

Other inherited metabolic diseases. These include Maple Syrup Urine Disease (MSUD), isovaleric acidaemia (IVA), glutamic aciduria (GAI) and homocystinuria (HCU).

Eliciting the red reflex using an ophthalmoscope (see also p. 97)

- *Age at which the test is performed.* Neonates, 6–8 weeks.
- *The test.* The examiner looks through an ophthalmoscope, held approximately 50 cm from the baby, and directs the light into the baby's eyes. A red reflection is normally seen

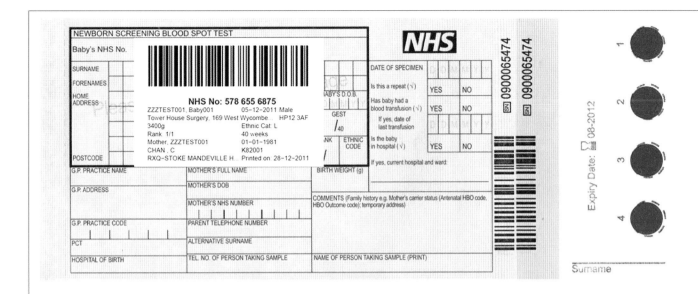

Figure 2.3 Newborn heel prick test (in the UK).

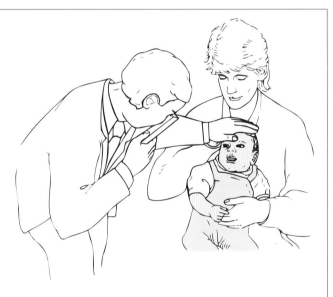

Figure 2.4 Eliciting the red reflex using an ophthalmoscope.

as the light is reflected back from the vascular retina (Figure 2.4).

- *Significance of the test.* If white light is reflected instead of red, it is a serious sign and suggests the presence of a cataract or other intraocular pathology, preventing the reflex from being elicited.
- *Action if the test is abnormal.* Immediate referral to an ophthalmologist is required, as in those conditions that are treatable, amblyopia (p. 250) can only be avoided if treatment is given early.

Examination for developmental dislocation of the hips

- *Age at which the test is performed.* Neonates, 6–8 weeks.
- *The test.* The Ortolani and Barlow procedures (see Figures 24.10, 24.11) for babies up to the age of three months are described on p. 453. Limited hip abduction, shortening of the leg and limp (once walking) are found beyond 3 months. Ultrasound is recommended if the birth was breech, premature or the pregnancy was multiple, or if there is a family history of childhood hip abnormalities.
- *Significance of the test.* Approximately three babies per 1000 are born with dislocated, subluxed or dysplastic hips. Orthopaedic treatment given early is likely to be more effective in preventing limp in childhood and painful disability later in life.
- *Action if the test is abnormal.* Ultrasound is recommended if the clinical exam is not normal and orthopaedic referral is required. Treatment involves the use of a harness or splint to maintain the hip in flexion and abduction. If this conservative treatment fails, surgery is required.

Palpation for testicular descent

- *Age at which the test is performed.* Neonates, 6–8 weeks.
- *The test.* The testes are palpated when the baby is relaxed (Figure 2.5).
- *Significance of the test.* Non-palpable testes suggest maldescent (see p. 342). If corrected early, the risks of the sequelae of infertility and malignancy are minimized.
- *Action if the test is abnormal.* If on repeat examination the testes are impalpable, referral to a paediatric surgeon is required. Surgery should be performed before the age of 2 years.

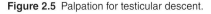

Figure 2.5 Palpation for testicular descent.

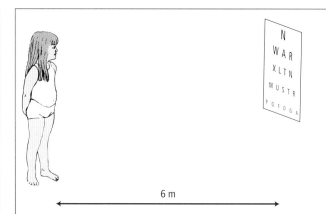

Figure 2.6 Testing visual acuity using a Snellen chart.

Hearing test (oto-acoustic emissions)

Oto-acoustic emission testing to identify hearing impairment is carried out on all babies throughout the UK.

- *Age at which the test is performed.* Neonates.
- *The test.* An ear probe is attached to a portable computer. A 'cochlear echo' is detected if the cochlea is functioning normally.
- *Significance of the test.* Significant sensorineural hearing loss occurs in one to two babies per 1000. If it is not identified early before language is acquired, permanent impairment of language development can result.
- *Action if the test is abnormal.* A diagnostic brainstem evoked response test is carried out by the audiology service. If neurosensory deafness is confirmed, hearing aids and speech and language therapy are provided (see pp. 272–4). Cochlear implants may be required if hearing aids give inadequate amplification

Later hearing screening

- *Age at which test is performed.* School entry.
- *The test.* Sweep audiometry tests the child's ability to hear sounds at a set level across the main speech frequencies.
- *Significance of the test.* As most cases of sensorineural deafness have already been detected through neonatal screening or distraction testing, this test principally identifies children with hearing impairment caused by secretory otitis media (see p. 146) that may have educational implications.

- *Action if the test is abnormal.* The ears should be examined for otitis media. Referral to an ear, nose and throat (ENT) surgeon and more sophisticated audiological evaluation is required.

Visual acuity using a Snellen chart

- *Age at which the test is performed.* School entry, and repeated through the school years in some parts of the country.
- *The test.* The child's visual acuity is tested 6 m from the Snellen chart, with each eye occluded in turn (Figure 2.6). In young children a letter-matching card can be used instead of asking them to name the letters.
- *Significance of the test.* Myopia is very common in childhood. If the child can only read letter size 6/12 or less, he or she is likely to be myopic.
- *Action if the test is abnormal.* Referral to an optician for prescription of spectacles is required.

Growth and development

Growth during childhood is discussed in some detail in Chapter 15, and monitoring of children's growth is a part of child health promotion. Normal growth reflects a child's well-being, and any deviation may be indicative of adverse physical or psychosocial factors.

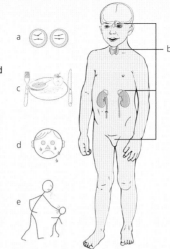

Growth at a glance

General

Growth reflects a child's wellbeing and deviation suggests abnormal physical or psychosocial factors

Between the age of 2 years and puberty, growth is usually steady along a centile

Factors that affect growth
- Genetics (**a**)
- Hormones (**b**)
- Nutrition (**c**)
- Illness (**d**)
- Psychosocial factors (**e**)

Growth standards

Charts for boys and girls give centile lines ranging from the 99.6th to the 0.4th centile

National Child Measurement Programme (NCMP)

The NCMP was introduced in 2006 to monitor the rising problem of obesity

Children are measured at school entry and at the age of 11 years

Parents are provided with information if their child is overweight or obese

Plotting a child's growth

Correction for gestational age must be made up to the age of 24 months

Growth monitoring

Benefits include:
- identification of endocrine conditions
- identification of other treatable conditions
- identification of eating disorders
- monitoring chronic diseases
- focus for discussion of health issues with parents
- access to children at risk
- public health issues

Guidelines for concern beyond the age of 2 years

Height or weight > 99.6th or < 0.4th centile

Crossing of centiles

Discrepancy between height and weight

Discrepancy with parental heights

Parental or professional concern

BMI > 98th centile (obesity)

BMI between 91st and 98th centile (overweight)

Normal growth

A baby's weight and length at birth are influenced by intrauterine and to a lesser extent by genetic factors and so do not correlate well with parental heights. Over the next year or two the baby's growth adjusts, so that by the age of 2 years most children have attained their genetically destined centile. From the age of 2 years until the onset of puberty it is usual for a child to grow steadily along their centile with little deviation. During puberty it is normal for centiles to be crossed again until final height is achieved.

Growth monitoring

In the past, growth monitoring through childhood has been an important part of routine child care. It is still maintained elsewhere, but in Britain it has been pruned down so that it is principally carried out only in the younger years, and as a means for identifying those at risk of obesity. Current recommendations for monitoring of growth are shown in Table 2.1. Growth monitoring has a number of benefits:

- *Identification of endocrine conditions.* Conditions leading to hormone excess or deficiencies profoundly affect growth, and may be missed if growth is not monitored.
- *Identification of other treatable conditions.* Although chronic illness usually presents with obvious signs and symptoms, some may only be detected by a fall-off in growth.

- *Identification of obesity and excessive weight gain.* A principal purpose of the National Child Measurement Programme is to monitor the prevalence of obesity and identify children at most risk (see pp. 286–8).
- *Identification of eating disorders.* Growth monitoring can identify the child with an eating disorder, whether anorexia (see p. 463) or excessive eating (see pp. 286–6).
- *Monitoring chronic diseases.* Chronic disease affects growth as a result of a number of factors. In some diseases, monitoring growth is an important part of management, e.g. in diabetes it reflects the adequacy of diabetic control.
- *Focus for discussion of health issues with parents.* Most parents are interested in their children's growth, particularly in the early years, and this can provide a good opportunity to discuss a variety of health issues with them.
- *Access to children at risk.* Children at risk may be identified through monitoring growth, which also serves to provide acceptable access to a family that might not otherwise welcome contact.
- *Public health issues.* The growth of a population reflects the population's health, and growth records can be an important source for epidemiological studies.

Guidance as to when one should become concerned about a child's growth is given in Chapter 15. In general, height or weight beyond the dotted lines on a growth chart

Table 2.3 Problems seen in growth monitoring
Common problems
Short stature (see p. 279)
Failure to thrive (see p. 283)
Obesity (see p. 286)
Less common problems
Tall stature
Fall-off in height
Weight loss

(>99.6th or < 0.4th centiles, see Figure 15.1) are outside the normal range and an evaluation needs to be considered, particularly if they are outside the range expected for parental height. Crossing of centile lines are of particular concern and a cause should be sought. In addition, a good clinical evaluation should be carried out in any child where the parents or other professionals are concerned about growth. Where a child is obese or overweight (BMI > 98th centile or between the 91st and 98th centile, respectively), guidance needs to be given about risk and the special importance of a healthy lifestyle.

Common growth problems

Common problems identified through growth monitoring are shown in Table 2.3.

Developmental evaluation

Evaluation of a child's development involves a developmental history, observation of the child's behaviour and the assessment of developmental skills (pp. 99–105). The purpose is to ensure that the child's development is progressing at a normal rate, and to recognise deviations from the normal pattern; it is usually performed by the health visitor. Beyond early infancy developmental screening is no longer routine, but is targeted at needy or at-risk families, or where there is parental concern. If the child is delayed or is demonstrating abnormal development, referral is made to the appropriate therapist or, if difficulties seem to be complex, to a child development team (see p. 49–50).

Immunisation

Immunisations have changed the entire picture of paediatrics. In the past, family life and medical care were dominated by epidemics of infectious diseases that caused serious morbidity and mortality for the childhood population. These diseases are now rare, but if immunisation rates fall, they re-emerge. A high level of uptake of immunisations is important to ensure both protection for the individual and also, for some diseases, herd immunity.

An important example where a disease has made a recurrence is measles. Some years ago unfounded concerns were raised that the measles component of the MMR (measles, mumps, rubella) vaccine was responsible for increasing numbers of children suffering from autism and inflammatory bowel disease. As a result many parents declined immunisation, and as a result, immunisation rates fell to worryingly low levels. Major efforts were required to inform the public of the situation, yet again measles cases have dramatically risen with several recent outbreaks in the UK.

General immunisation guidelines

- Immunisations should not be given at a younger age than indicated in the schedule.
- Vaccines which require repeat immunisation should not be given at shorter intervals than indicated.
- If for any reason a child misses an immunisation or immunisations, it should be given at a later stage. There is no need to restart the course.
- Immunisations should not be given if a child is acutely unwell with fever.
- Immunisations should not be given if there has been a serious reaction following a previous dose of the same vaccine.
- Live attenuated vaccines (e.g. measles, mumps, rubella, BCG) should not be given to immunodeficient children such as those on cytotoxic therapy or high-dose steroids because of the risk of severe generalised infection.

Routine immunisations (see Figure 2.7)

Diphtheria

Diphtheria is now very rare in developed countries. It is caused by the organism *Corynebacterium diphtheriae*. Infection occurs in the throat, forming a pharyngeal exudate, which leads to membrane formation and obstruction of the upper airways. An exotoxin released by the bacterium may cause myocarditis and neuritis with paralysis.

The vaccine. The vaccine is an inactivated toxin (toxoid), given as an intramuscular injection combined with tetanus, pertussis, polio, HiB and hepatitis B (6-in-1) vaccines at 2, 3 and 4 months, with boosters at school entry and in secondary school. A more dilute form is given to individuals over the age of 10 years.

Tetanus

Tetanus is caused by an anaerobic organism, *Clostridium tetani*, found universally in the soil, which enters the body through open wounds. Progressive painful muscle spasms are caused by a neurotoxin produced by the organism. Involvement of the respiratory muscles results in asphyxia and death.

The immunisation schedule

6-in-1 infant vaccine DTaP/IPV/Hib
- Primary immunisation given intramuscularly three times in infancy, with boosters preschool and in high school
- Protects against the six following diseases:
  - Diphtheria (D)
  - Tetanus (T)
  - Pertussis (aP)
  - Polio (IPV)
  - *Haemophilus influenzae* type B (Hib)
  - Hepatitis B
- Pertussis should not be given to a child with a progressive neurological condition
- Possible side effects within 12–24 hours include the following:
  - Swelling and redness at site
  - Fever
  - Diarrhoea and/or vomiting
  - Papule at injection site lasting a few weeks
  - Irritability for 48 hours
  - Rarely high fever, febrile convulsions, and anaphylaxis

4-in-1 preschool booster DTaP/IPV
- Protects against diphtheria, tetanus, whooping cough, polio

3-in-1 teenage booster Td/IPV
- Protects against tetanus, diphtheria and polio

Men B and Men C
Given IM. Protects against infection by meningococcal groups B and C bacteria respectively—meningitis and septicaemia. It does not protect against any other form of meningitis

Pneumoccoccal
Given IM. Protects against pneumococcal infection—pneumonia, septicaemia and meningitis

Tetanus
- Given IM in infancy as part of the 5-in-1 infant vaccine, with boosters preschool and in high school
- *Dirty wounds:* Give tetanus immunoglobulin, with booster if last vaccination was >10 years previously (or give full course if not immunised)

NATIONAL IMMUNISATION SCHEDULE IN THE UK*

Infant

Birth	Hepatitis B and BCG for infants at risk
2 months	6-in-1; pneumococcal; meningitis B; rotavirus
3 months	6-in-1; pneumococcal; rotavirus; meningitis C
4 months	6-in-1; pneumococcal; meningitis B
12–13 (months)	Hib/ Men C; MMR; pneumococcal; meningitis B

Preschool

3 years 4 months	4-in-1 preschool booster; MMR
2–8 years	Children's flu (annual)

Secondary school

12–13 years	HPV
14 years	3-in-1 teenage booster; Men ACWY

*schedules are similar in USA, Australia.

Rotavirus
- Given orally at 2 and 3 months
- Protects against rotavirus gastroenteritis
- Side effects: irritability and mild diarrhoea

Men ACWY
Given IM. Recommended for adolescents and students. Protects against infection by four strains of Meningococcus — meningitis and septicaemia.

MMR
- Live attenuated vaccine against:
  - Measles
  - Mumps
  - Rubella
- The vaccine is a live attenuated virus given at 12–13 months and at school entry. Children who are severely immunosuppressed should not receive the vaccine, or pregnant girls. Advice is needed if the child is severely allergic to eggs (the vaccine is grown on chick embryo tissue)
- There is no evidence that it is related to autism and bowel disease
- Side effects:
  - Common to have rash and fever 5–10 days later
  - Mild mumps 2 weeks later

BCG (Bacille Calmette–Guérin)
Protects against tuberculosis. Given to babies living in areas with a high rate of TB or to children recently arrived from countries with high levels of TB or who have come into close contact with somebody infected with respiratory TB
  - A live attenuated bacterium strain of *Mycobacterium bovis*
  - Given intradermally
  - Papule forms and often ulcerates
  - Heals over 6–8 weeks with a scar

HPV (human papillomavirus virus)
Given to girls aged 12–13 years
Two injections 6–24 months apart
Protects against common causes of cervical cancer, and offers some protection for genital warts too

Figure 2.7 The immunisation schedule.

The vaccine. The vaccine is an inactivated toxin (toxoid) given combined with diphtheria, pertussis, polio, Hib and hepatitis B vaccines (6-in-1) at 2, 3 and 4 months by intramuscular injection. After a primary course of three injections in infancy and a booster at school entry, a further two boosters 10 years apart are required. If a dirty wound is incurred more than 10 years after the last injection, a further booster is required. If an unimmunised individual sustains a dirty wound, tetanus immunoglobulin is given and a full course of the inactivated toxoid initiated.

Pertussis (whooping cough)

Whooping cough is caused by the bacterium *Bordetella pertussis*. It is an upper respiratory illness which lasts for 6–8 weeks, consisting of three stages: catarrhal, paroxysmal and convalescent. The child experiences paroxysms of coughing, followed by a whoop (a sudden massive inspiratory effort against a narrowed glottis), with vomiting, dyspnoea and sometimes seizures. Manifestations are most severe in children under the age of 2 years, where there is a high morbidity and mortality. Complications include bronchopneumonia, convulsions, apnoea and bronchiectasis. The diagnosis must be suspected clinically, and confirmed by special culture of nasopharyngeal swabs. Erythromycin given early in the catarrhal stage shortens the illness, but is ineffective if given when the whoop is heard.

The vaccine. The vaccine is made from highly purified components of the organism, given in three doses with diphtheria, tetanus, polio, HiB and hepatitis B (6-in-1) vaccines at 2, 3 and 4 months, and at school entry. Mild reactions consisting of local pain and swelling, irritability and pyrexia are common. The risks of naturally acquired pertussis far exceed any risks of the vaccination and it is recommended for all babies, other than when a severe reaction has followed a previous immunisation or if a progressive neurological disease is present. The vaccine is also offered to women in pregnancy between 16 and 32 weeks gestation, to protect infants prior to their first vaccinations.

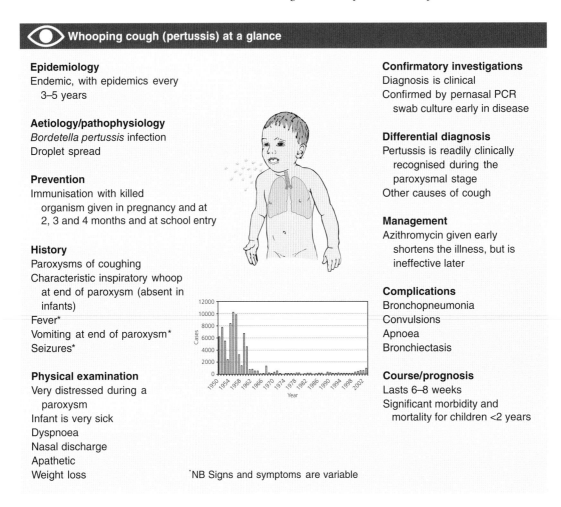

Whooping cough (pertussis) at a glance

Epidemiology
Endemic, with epidemics every 3–5 years

Aetiology/pathophysiology
Bordetella pertussis infection
Droplet spread

Prevention
Immunisation with killed organism given in pregnancy and at 2, 3 and 4 months and at school entry

History
Paroxysms of coughing
Characteristic inspiratory whoop at end of paroxysm (absent in infants)
Fever*
Vomiting at end of paroxysm*
Seizures*

Physical examination
Very distressed during a paroxysm
Infant is very sick
Dyspnoea
Nasal discharge
Apathetic
Weight loss

*NB Signs and symptoms are variable

Confirmatory investigations
Diagnosis is clinical
Confirmed by pernasal PCR swab culture early in disease

Differential diagnosis
Pertussis is readily clinically recognised during the paroxysmal stage
Other causes of cough

Management
Azithromycin given early shortens the illness, but is ineffective later

Complications
Bronchopneumonia
Convulsions
Apnoea
Bronchiectasis

Course/prognosis
Lasts 6–8 weeks
Significant morbidity and mortality for children <2 years

Polio

Polio is caused by the poliomyelitis virus, which produces a mild febrile illness, progressing to meningitis in some children. Paralysis in association with pain and tenderness develops as a result of anterior horn cell damage, and may lead to respiratory failure and bulbar paralysis. Residual paralysis is common in those who survive.

The vaccine. The IPV (inactivated polio vaccine) has now replaced the oral live vaccine and is given in three doses with diphtheria, tetanus, pertussis, HiB and hepatitis B (6-in-1) vaccines at 2, 3 and 4 months, followed by boosters preschool and as a teenager. The vaccine can cause irritability and fever within 12–24 hours.

Haemophilus influenzae B

Haemophilus influenzae type B was the main cause of meningitis (p. 235) in young children, leading to severe neurological sequelae such as profound deafness, cerebral palsy and epilepsy in 10–15% of cases and death in 3%.

The vaccine. The HiB vaccine consists of the polysaccharide capsule of the killed organism conjugated with a protein, and is given with diphtheria, tetanus, pertussis, polio and hepatitis B (6-in-1) vaccines at 2, 3 and 4 months and again at 1 year with MenC. It is only effective against type B infection. The vaccine is highly effective with a low incidence of side effects.

Hepatitis B

Hepatitis B is transmitted when blood, semen or another body fluid from a person infected with the Hepatitis B virus enters the body through sexual contact, sharing needles or other drug-injection equipment or from mother to baby at birth. For some, hepatitis B is an acute, or short-term illness but it can become a long-term, chronic infection leading to cirrhosis or liver cancer. Approximately 90% of infected infants become chronically infected.

The vaccine. The hepatitis B vaccine contains the HepB surface antigen and is given with diphtheria, tetanus, pertussis, polio and Hib B (6-in-1) vaccines at 2, 3 and 4 months. Side effects are minimal.

Meningococci

Meningococci (*Neisseria meningitidis*) cause a purulent meningitis in young children with a purpuric rash and septicaemic shock. Mortality is as high as 10% and morbidity includes hearing loss, seizures, brain damage, organ failure and tissue necrosis.

The vaccine. The vaccines are conjugated polysaccharide antigens which are combined with tetanus toxoid as a carrier protein. MenB is given at 2, 4 and 12 months; MenC in combination with Hib at 12 months and Men ACWY at the age of 14 years. The vaccine may cause some local swelling, fever, vomiting and irritability.

Pneumococcal infection

Invasive pneumococcal infection is a cause of pneumonia, septicaemia and meningitis, which carry a high mortality and morbidity, particularly in babies.

The vaccine. The vaccine is a polyvalent vaccine containing purified capsular polysaccharide from each of the 23 types of pneumococcus. It is given at 2, 4 and 12 months. These 23 types are responsible for the vast majority of serious pneumococcal infections seen in this country. The vaccine may cause a sore arm and fever.

Measles

Measles is characterised by a maculopapular rash, fever, coryza, cough and conjunctivitis (see p. 149). Complications include encephalitis leading to neurological damage and a high mortality rate.

The vaccine. The vaccine is a live attenuated virus given at around 13 months and again at 3 years 4 months with mumps and rubella (MMR), and before school entry. It is common for children to develop a rash and fever 5–10 days after the immunisation. Children who are immunodeficient and those severely allergic to eggs (the vaccine is grown on chick embryo tissue) should not receive the vaccine.

Mumps

Mumps causes a febrile illness with enlargement of the parotid glands (see p. 148). Complications include aseptic meningitis, sensorineural deafness and orchitis in adults.

The vaccine. The vaccine is a live attenuated virus grown on chick embryo tissue and is given with measles and rubella (MMR) at around 13 months and again at 3 years 4 months. It should not be given to immunodeficient children or those severely allergic to eggs.

Rubella (German measles)

Rubella is a mild illness causing rash and fever (see p. 150). Its importance lies in the devastating effects it has on the fetus if infection occurs in the early stages of pregnancy. These include multiple congenital defects such as cataracts, deafness and congenital heart disease.

The vaccine. The vaccine is a live attenuated virus given with measles and mumps vaccines (MMR) at around 13 months and again at 3 years 4 months. A mild form of rubella sometimes occurs following vaccination. The vaccine, like all live virus vaccines, is contraindicated in pregnancy.

Tuberculosis

Tuberculosis (TB) remains a major problem in many developing countries and still occurs in developed countries, particularly in immigrant communities from endemic areas such as Asia and Africa. Most children are identified because they are contacts of infected adults. Tuberculosis affects many organs including the lungs, meninges, bones and joints. The diagnosis is not always easy, and often relies on demonstration of tuberculin sensitivity, which develops within 4–8 weeks after infection. This is demonstrated by Mantoux testing where purified protein derivative (PPD) is injected into the skin. The result is read 3–10 days later. Tuberculin sensitivity causes severe induration at the site and if this is found the child requires a chest X-ray and follow-up. Active TB requires treatment which must be continued over many months.

BCG vaccination. BCG (bacille Calmette–Guérin) is a live attenuated virus strain of *Mycobacterium tuberculosis*, which is given intradermally. It causes formation of a papule that enlarges over a few weeks and may ulcerate. It heals over 6–8 weeks, leaving a residual scar. It is given at birth to babies who are likely to come into close or prolonged contact with family members who have TB, and to children who have arrived from a country where TB is prevalent or who have had close contact with an individual with TB.

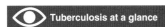

Tuberculosis at a glance

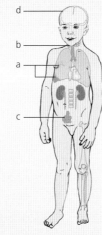

Epidemiology
TB still occurs in the UK, especially in the Asian community

Aetiology/pathophysiology
Infection with *Mycobacterium tuberculosis*
Primary infection may occur in the lung, skin or gut
Miliary TB (bloodstream spread) is the most serious complication in childhood

Prevention
Bacille Calmette–Guérin (live attenuated virus) given intradermally at birth to babies from high-risk families

History
Prolonged fever
Malaise
Anorexia
Cough
Weight loss
Contact with infected adult*

NB *Signs and symptoms are variable

Physical examination
Signs depend on focus of infection:
• primary in lung – signs of bronchial obstruction, pleural effusion, etc. (**a**)
• primary in tonsils – cervical adenitis (**b**)
• primary in small bowel – malabsorption, peritonitis (**c**)
• miliary TB – meningitis, chest signs, hepatosplenomegaly (**d**)

Confirmatory investigations
Demonstration of tuberculin sensitivity by Mantoux testing
Chest X-ray evidence of pulmonary TB
Culture of gastric washings

Management
Even if asymptomatic, tuberculin-positive children require treatment
Active TB requires treatment over many months

Prognosis/complications
Postprimary TB may present as local or disseminated (miliary) disease affecting:
• bones
• joints – arthritis
• kidneys – haematuria, renal failure
• pericardium – constrictive pericarditis
• CNS – mental retardation, hydrocephalus
• Morbidity and mortality is significant if TB is detected late

Cervical cancer

Infection with human papillomavirus (HPV) is common, with over 50% of sexually active women infected over the course of their lifetime. Two strains of HPV (16 and 18) are the cause of cervical cancer in over 70% of cases.

The vaccine. The HPV vaccine protects against HPV 16 and 18 and is given to 12–13-year-old girls in two injections 6-12 months apart. It does not protect against any other sexually transmitted infections or against pregnancy. Side effects include swelling, redness and pain at the injection site and other very mild side effects, such as fever and dizziness. Very rarely anaphylaxis can occur.

Safeguarding children

In any aspect of paediatrics and child health care, concerns often arise regarding the possibility that a child is the victim of neglect, non-accidental injury, or emotional or sexual abuse. In this circumstance, it is the duty of the professional (and indeed any individual) to report these concerns to the authorities so that appropriate investigations can be made. Child health promotion goes beyond detecting abuse and also includes its management and prevention.

In a preventive role guidance and support are provided for families, reducing the likelihood of children becoming victims of abuse and neglect. The health visitor is ideally positioned to follow children who are at risk. She is usually seen as being a non-threatening and supportive professional, who is a visitor to all homes. Social Care also provides essential support for families in need, but may be viewed less positively.

When a child is found to be in need of child protection the health visitor, school nurse and community paediatrician have an important role in determining how the interests of the child are best met (p. 395). This involves close liaison with the family and other professionals. If the child is placed in care or has a Child Protection Plan, the child health service provides continuous surveillance and support to ensure that the needs of the child are met.

The clinical presentation and care of children presenting actual or suspected child abuse or neglect is covered in detail in Chapter 22 ('Social paediatrics').

The role of the child health service in safeguarding children

- Reporting suspected victims of abuse and neglect.
- Following children at risk of abuse and neglect.
  Health visitors are particularly well placed for this.

- Providing guidance to reduce the risk of abuse.
- Liaison with social services.
- Following children in care and on the child protection register.

Ethical issues in paediatrics

Ethics is the science of morals, and morals are the personal framework that dictates right and wrong. The law defines what an individual in a society may and may not do, and a moral approach to a situation depends on an individual's conscience, religious views and previous experience.

Paediatrics is a speciality where there are many ethical issues to be considered, such as withdrawal of intensive care, consent and parental rights. You need to be aware of some of these issues, and it is the responsibility of every practising doctor to have established his or her own *modus vivendi* for working in these difficult areas (see Box 2.3).

Three important concepts underlie an understanding of ethical issues. These are the sanctity of life, the concept of omission vs. commission, and the quality of life. Each is briefly discussed here.

Sanctity of life

Life is sacred, and any act intended to end a life is illegal. Those with some particular religious points of view think that every effort must be made to preserve life, under all circumstances, but this is not accepted by others. Most people would agree that to offer an anencephalic baby intensive care would be wrong because the prognosis for life is so poor: intensive care simply delays the time when the heart will stop beating. Others believe that it is acceptable not to feed a patient in a persistent vegetative

---

Box 2.3 Principles of medical ethics

- The clinician can only act within the legal code
- Ethical decisions usually do not need to be made rapidly, only after full discussion and consideration
- It is usually inappropriate to make decisions which conflict with the views of the patient's relatives
- All members of staff must be involved in discussions before a decision is made
- Discuss all options with the parents so that they know that all the possible courses of treatment have been considered
- Where the child is mature enough, he or she should be involved in ethical decisions
- Adolescents may receive treatment without parental knowledge, provided they are deemed mature enough to appreciate its consequences
- Where dispute remains between clinical staff and parents, the courts should be asked to make a final decision

---

state, so that the patient dies of dehydration, albeit appropriately sedated. The concept of the sanctity of life alone is thus too broad to be the ultimate benchmark, and there is much scope within the law for making decisions that affect life and death.

Omission vs. commission

This concept considers the method of a patient's death. It is illegal to undertake an act that kills a patient: this is an *act of commission*. An example would be giving a patient a lethal injection: this is both illegal and immoral.

There is a moral difference between causing someone to die by a positive action and allowing death to occur by failing to act. An example of the latter is leaving septicaemia untreated in a patient on a ventilator who has a very poor prognosis, knowing that death will occur as a result of non-treatment with antibiotics. This is legal and, most would argue, ethical. An *act of omission* may be illegal if failure to treat causes a patient to die who might otherwise have fully recovered.

Both acts of commission and omission may therefore be acceptable in one framework and unacceptable (and illegal) in another.

Quality of life

Most people would agree that ventilating a baby who has no chance of independent survival without a ventilator is wrong. The quality of life the child would have if he or she were to survive is a factor to be considered. This is usually what causes the most controversy within an ethical context.

'Quality of life' is a nebulous concept. It has been suggested that the quality of life is encapsulated within the idea of individual 'humanhood'. The qualities of humanhood are those that make us individual. These include:

- awareness of oneself;
- concept of time, both future and past;
- ability to communicate;
- care and concern for others;
- curiosity.

Withdrawal of intensive care

Uncritical application of intensive care is one of the most frequent areas of ethical uncertainty in medicine and is particularly relevant to paediatrics. The physician must consider the following issues within the ethical context of offering or continuing intensive care:

- *What is the prognosis?* Intensive care that only acts to put off the time of death is unlikely to be in the best interest of the patient, but this may help relatives come to terms with the impending death. Long-term intensive care of a patient with a hopeless prognosis is often thought to be wrong. Withdrawal of intensive care should be considered, refocusing the emphasis of care from the child to the family, to help the parents with the process of mourning.

- *Quality of life*. If the patient survives, will the quality of life be acceptable? The answer to this question often depends on the family. Some parents may say that life of any quality is acceptable, even if their child is very severely damaged with blindness, severe spasticity and very low intelligence. Other parents may find a child with only moderate disability unacceptable.
- *Pain and suffering*. One may question whether treatment which is very painful or where the child has to suffer severely to overcome a life-threatening disorder is justified. The management of cancer is an example of a protracted course of unpleasant and distressing treatment. If the ultimate prognosis is good then this may be easy to justify, but if the prognosis is uncertain or poor then it may be unfair to put the child through the distress of treatment.
- *Use of scarce resources*. In most developed health care services there is an unequal balance between demand on facilities and their availability. There may only be one intensive care ventilator with two patients needing it. This often causes major dilemmas in neonatal intensive care, where a less acceptable form of therapy must be given because the resources are limited. A judgement may have to be made as to which patient is most likely to benefit from the treatment.

Guidelines from the Royal College of Paediatrics and Child Health

Recommendations have been produced by the Royal College of Paediatrics and Child Health to help doctors decide when medical treatment should be withdrawn from children (although not intended for the newborn). The situations when withdrawal should be considered include:
- when the child is brain dead;
- when the child is in a permanent vegetative state;
- when care delays death without easing suffering;
- when the child survives so physically or mentally impaired that it is unreasonable to expect him or her to suffer further;
- when the illness is so progressive and irreversible that further treatment is intolerable.

Consent and parental rights

Another area of ethical concern is the issue of consent. For adults, it is accepted that a competent patient has the right to accept or refuse health care. Many paediatric patients are not competent to make their own decisions and therefore parents traditionally have made such decisions on their behalf. This is acceptable in most situations and the majority of parents act in the best interests of their child, but the issue arises regarding the age at which an individual becomes competent to make his or her own decisions.

Whereas many people feel that a child's views should be taken into account, it is not possible to define a precise age at which a child will have the maturity to decide whether he or she wishes to be investigated or treated for an illness, particularly if this is at variance with the parents' views. An important concept regarding children's ability to give their own consent is that of 'Fraser' competence' – where the law recognises that if a doctor considers that a child under 16 years is mature enough to understand the implications of a procedure or treatment, he or she does not have to inform the parent.

The issue causing particular controversy in this regard relates to the prescription of contraceptives to adolescents. Strict requirements for parental consent may deter adolescents from seeking health care, with consequences in terms of teenage pregnancies and sexually transmitted disease. However, in Britain legal precedent allows a physician to prescribe contraceptives without parental consent, provided the adolescent is deemed mature enough to understand the risks and benefits.

Another difficult issue concerns situations where parents fail to act in the best interests of their child. Not many years ago it was accepted that parents had absolute rights over their child and that these rights should not and could not be interfered with by external agencies. In fact, the first court case prosecuting a parent for abusing a child had to be brought on the grounds of cruelty to an animal as there was no procedure for prosecuting a parent who was abusing a child. Society has changed its views and laws now exist whereby children can be protected and parental rights and authority curtailed (p. 395). However, debate continues as to the extent to which society and the law can intervene in parental practices, particularly where cultural issues are involved.

Ethical conflicts

The nature of ethical dilemmas means that there can be no right or wrong answers. Each case is different and its circumstances must be carefully reviewed. The parents' wishes must be very carefully considered and it is, in general, unwise to act against their wishes. Sometimes, however, it is necessary to do so if the parents' wishes are clearly unreasonable or unrealistic. In these circumstances it is usually appropriate to take the legal precaution of making the child a ward of court so that the decision is taken out of the clinician's direct control.

A second major source of ethical conflict arises when one clinical view conflicts with another. An example may be in withdrawing care, when the doctor thinks it a reasonable option but a senior nurse disagrees. These differences must be reconciled; it is a failure of clinical management if major disagreement continues to exist. It is important that the opinion of every member of the clinical team is heard and that no-one feels left out of the process. Ultimately a decision must be made by the senior clinician, but it is his or her role to ensure as far as possible that no-one feels that the decision is wrong. Local ethics committees and legal advisors can be of assistance if there is conflict.

The essence of decision making in medical ethics is effective communication. Communication should involve the child (when appropriate), parents, other relatives and staff, and, if necessary, lawyers and possibly clergy. Decisions cannot be made by committee but neither can they be made by diktat. Sometimes prolonging intensive care with no prospect of the patient surviving is the appropriate course of management in order to buy time for relatives to accept the appropriateness of the decision. Nevertheless, this carries the price of using valuable resources to no medical purpose and possibly denying resources to a more deserving patient.

To test your knowledge on this part of the book, please see Chapter 26

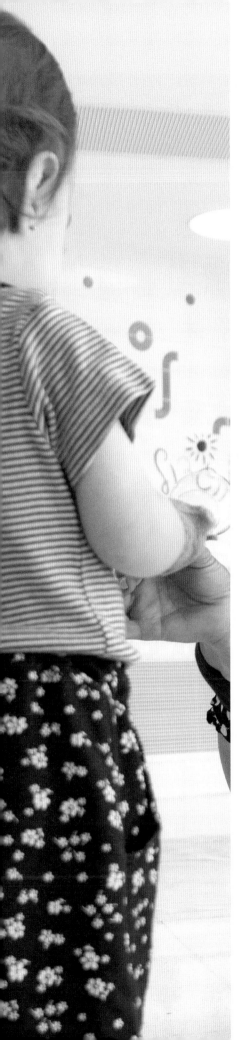

CHAPTER 3
Children with long-term medical conditions

Physicians of the utmost fame
Were called at once; but when
they came
They answered, as they took their fees,
There is no cure for this disease.
'Henry King', Cautionary Tales,
Hilaire Belloc

KEY COMPETENCES

YOU MUST...

Know and understand

■ What is meant by 'chronic illness'
■ The principles involved in the paediatric care of children with chronic illness or disabilities
■ How 'bad news' is best broken
■ How the major disabilities in childhood present
■ The role of health professionals in the care of children with disabilities
■ The pros and cons of mainstream vs. special education for children with disabilities
■ The impact that cancer has on the child and the family, and the long-term issues for the child
■ The principles involved in paediatric palliative care

Be able to

■ Take a full and sensitive history from a child with a long-term medical condition, including psychosocial circumstances
■ Make a clinical and functional evaluation of a child with a chronic condition
■ Draw up a medical and social management plan for discussion with family and health professionals

Appreciate

■ The impact that disability or a chronic illness has on the child and the family
■ The principles involved in managing long-term medical conditions
■ That some chronic conditions still attract stigma
■ The difficulties and stress involved in bringing up a disabled child
■ The doctor's role in supporting the family
■ The importance of multidisciplinary team work and the physician's particular role

Essential Paediatrics and Child Health, Fourth Edition. Mary Rudolf, Anthony Luder and Kerry Jeavons.
© 2020 John Wiley & Sons Ltd. Published 2020 by John Wiley & Sons Ltd.
Companion website: www.wiley.com/go/rudolf/paediatrics

The child with a chronic illness

There is no universally accepted definition of childhood chronic conditions; however, the following definition is useful:

a chronic illness is a physical condition that lasts longer than 3 months and is of sufficient severity to interfere with a child's ordinary activities to some degree.

According to the UK General Household Survey, one in four children experience a long-standing medical condition at some point in childhood, with 5–10% having a moderately to severe long-term illness or disability (Table 3.1).

Children with chronic disease have many needs in common with each other, irrespective of what disease they may have. It is important to understand the impact that chronic illness has on a child and the family, and the physical, emotional and social stresses which may result. These psychosocial factors not only affect how the child functions in the family, with peers and at school, but can also affect the very course of the medical condition.

Effects of chronic illness on children

The impact that a chronic illness has on a child varies depending on the age of the child and the age at which the condition developed. Factors other than the severity and prognosis of the condition can affect the child's adjustment. In fact, there appears to be little relationship between the severity of the condition and the degree of psychosocial difficulties encountered. Children with mild disabilities may suffer as much or more than those in whom the condition is severe. Factors which may influence a child's adjustment are shown in Table 3.2.

Given the impact that chronic illness has on a child, it is perhaps not surprising that chronically ill children are two to three times more likely to experience emotional, behavioural and educational difficulties than their healthy peers. Low self-esteem,

Table 3.1 Chronic conditions in childhood

Condition	Epidemiology
Asthma	Commonest long-term condition in childhood with 1 in 10 children diagnosed as having asthma
Epilepsy	1 in 220 children have a diagnosis of epilepsy
Diabetes mellitus	28 children per 100 000 are diagnosed with new onset diabetes per year
Cancer	The most frequent medical cause of death in childhood with 1700 diagnosed each year
Disability and additional learning needs	14–23% of children and young people are identified as having special or additional educational needs; 2.8% have complex needs with a 'statement' of their needs

Table 3.2 Factors affecting children's adjustment to chronic illness

The child

The age of the child

The age at which the illness developed. School entry and adolescence are particularly vulnerable periods

Low intelligence or physical disfigurement increase the probability of maladjustment

The illness

Conditions with unpredictable flare-ups or recurrences are more stressful than stable conditions

'Invisible' conditions (e.g. diabetes) may be concealed by the family and lead to lack of acceptance

The family

The family's attitude and ability to function is the most critical factor in determining the child's adjustment

impaired self-image, behavioural problems, depression, anxiety and school dysfunction are all common. These problems may occur as a result of the child's own reaction to his or her chronic illness or the reaction of parents, peers, professionals and society as a whole.

Chronic illness and school

School is a central part of any child's life. Acquiring academic and vocational skills, and the development of work-related habits are only one component. An equally important part is the development of social interactions with peers and adults outside the family.

When ability to perform at school is affected by illness, children are placed at risk of becoming underachievers and failures in their own eyes and the eyes of their peers. This can be compounded by the amount of school missed through acute exacerbations, outpatient appointments and hospitalizations. If the child has adapted poorly, further days may be missed.

Chronic illness affects social aspects of school life too. Frequent illness episodes and restrictions can exclude children from activities. Physical appearance, acute medical problems, taking medications at school and special diets all make the child different. As a result, children can be made fun of, and come to feel inferior to and isolated from their classmates.

In addition to contending with the special problems of the condition and the reaction of others, children are also likely to experience the concerns and difficulties in aggravated form that beset all children at school, such as peer acceptance, competition, anxiety about academic achievement and athletic prowess and concerns about physical appearance and sexual development.

Effects of chronic illness on the family

The development of a long-term medical condition in a child can affect a family on a number of levels: practical, social and psychological. Altered daily routines, outpatient visits and hospitalizations, unexpected exacerbations and the administration of medications require organization, time and energy. Socially, the family may experience isolation from neighbours and friends, difficulty in finding babysitters, and may have to forgo activities and holidays and even change career plans.

The parents

Parents usually have a common response on learning that their child has a chronic illness, which is comparable to bereavement. The initial reaction is one of shock or disbelief, which is followed by denial, anger and resentment. These feelings often induce a sense of guilt and then sadness. Acceptance eventually follows, although this may not occur if the parent gets stuck at an earlier stage.

It is not surprising that clinical anxiety, depression, guilt and grief are commonly experienced by parents, and that marital problems are also common.

Siblings

Although siblings often develop kind and considerate relationships, they may also suffer. Parents are likely to be less available, and they may neglect, overindulge or develop unrealistic expectations for their healthy children. Anxiety, embarrassment, resentment and guilt are common, as are fears about their own well being and the cause and nature of their sibling's health problems.

In discussing chronic illness in childhood, the focus is often on psychopathology and psychosocial problems; however, it must be emphasised that the impact is not always negative. Some families seem to grow closer to each other, and in working with families the question often arises: 'How do some families of chronically ill children survive so well?'.

Paediatric care of children with chronic illness

When seeing children with chronic illnesses it is essential to develop rapport with the parents and the child and to acquire the skills needed to assess psychosocial consequences of the condition. It is important to allow adequate time for this, particularly at the onset of the condition, and when important transitions occur, such as at school entry and in adolescence. If there are problems, parents must be given the opportunity to express themselves without the child being present, and adolescents should be offered the possibility to be seen alone as well as with their parents. This is important, not only to allow the adolescent to talk about problems, but also as it transmits the message that they should begin to be responsible for their own health care.

When evaluating children at an initial or follow-up visit a full picture of the child's physical, emotional and behavioural condition must is needed. Key points in the assessment are shown in Box 3.1.

Principles of management

Too often the management of chronic illness by medical professionals focuses on the relatively simple clinical management alone.

> ## Box 3.1 Key points to address when seeing children with chronic conditions
>
> - What is the extent of the disease and its complications?
> - What understanding does the child have of the condition and the difference treatment makes?
> - What are the physical effects (e.g. poor growth, delayed puberty) of the illness on the child?
> - How has the illness affected the child's performance at home, at school and with peers?
> - How has the child adjusted to the illness?
> - What impact does the child's illness have on the family and its members?
> - How has the family adjusted to the special impact or burden of the illness?

> ## Box 3.2 Principles in managing chronic illness
>
> - Try to confine the consequences of the condition to the minimum manifestation
> - Encourage normal growth and development
> - Assist the child in maximizing his or her potential in all possible areas
> - Prevent or diminish the behavioural and social consequences of a chronic condition

---

It cannot be emphasised enough that the child must be seen as a whole. If this is ignored, the child's and family's needs are not met, thus increasing their difficulties, which in itself is likely to impact adversely the course of the illness.

Counselling

In an age of technological medical advances there is still no substitute for the old-fashioned quality of caring for the child and the family. It is always remarkable how a thorough assessment is in itself a therapeutic intervention, and concern and empathy go a long way in assisting the family to make the best of the circumstances they face. It is important to note that it is rarely helpful to try to conceal chronic conditions (where this is possible), as it encourages the child to believe that the illness is a secret and something of which to be ashamed.

Education

A vital aspect of management is education of the family about the condition. Gone are the days when doctors paternalistically 'protected' their patients from knowing about the condition and its prognosis. Including the parents and young person increases their trust and also provides them with the skills to self-manage many aspects of the condition. This is particularly critical in conditions such as asthma, cystic fibrosis and diabetes.

Coordination and liaison

Very often in chronic illness the child is looked after by a variety of health professionals: consultants, therapists and dietitians, not to mention teachers and social workers. Liaison and coordination is very important as differing opinions and advice can be very confusing for the family. The development of specialist clinics for the more common medical conditions has improved this problem, especially as clinics usually include specialist nurses whose role is one of support, education and liaison.

Genetic issues

Most parents have questions regarding genetic implications for subsequent children and the affected child's own chances of fertility. It is important that these are addressed and, where necessary, the family is referred to a geneticist.

Support

An assessment of support available to the family must be made. Chronic illness can be an isolating experience and many families do not have the support of an extended family and friends. Referrals to a social worker may be needed in order to advise on benefits and services offered by social services (see p. 40). If the child has emotional and behavioural difficulties, referral for counselling may be required. Self-help and voluntary organisations such as Diabetes UK or the Epilepsy Society can be helpful and often run support groups and activities allowing families with similar problems to meet.

Increasingly families find support through social media but may need guidance for reliable sources.

School

Involvement of the child's school is essential for a number of reasons.
- *Medical.* The school staff need to understand the child's condition well in order for them to cope competently with problems arising. The greatest concern is usually the handling of acute exacerbations, but other requirements such as dispensing medication and dietary restrictions must be discussed. Asking teachers to report untoward events such as symptoms or drug side effects can be helpful.
- *Educational.* Children with long-standing medical conditions are at risk of underachieving, for the reasons explained above. This risk can be minimized with appropriate support, such as help in making up with school work lost through illness or hospital visits, or providing preferential seating in class. Children may need extra encouragement, but care must be taken that this does not result in preferential treatment, which may have social repercussions. Some children may have special educational requirements that need to be met (see p. 46).
- *Social.* Teachers can be instrumental in helping children cope and integrate socially into school life. Emotional and behavioural difficulties are likely to be expressed at school, and the teachers need to be sensitive to this. For children whose family is failing to cope effectively, the school has a particularly important role.

 The child with a chronic medical condition at a glance

Epidemiology
1 in 4 children have a chronic medical problem at some time in childhood, 5–10% have a severe or moderate condition

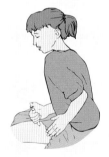

Effect on the child
Chronic illness:
- Impacts on the child psychologically
- Increases the risk of emotional, behavioural and educational difficulties
- Is associated with dysfunction at school

Effect on the family
The initial parental response is akin to bereavement. Parents must cope with:
- demands of appointments
- drug administration
- unexpected exacerbations
- social difficulties
   Siblings may suffer from altered attention and expectations, and experience more emotional and behavioural problems

Effect on the child at school
Academic performance, achievements and social life may be affected
Concerns and difficulties experienced by any child are likely to be aggravated

Approach to the child
Time, rapport and skill required
A holistic approach is essential

Management
Management must extend beyond the medical to:
- counselling and support
- education
- coordination and liaison between professionals
- genetic issues
- medical, educational and social issues at school

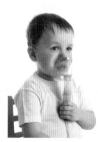

The child with a disability

One in 20 children in the UK have a long-term condition of which nearly half are long-term neurodevelopmental problems. In this section the child with long-lasting and complex needs is considered. The commoner causes of disability are shown in Table 3.3.

How disability presents

Children with disabilities are identified as a result of parental suspicion, concern by health professionals or child health surveillance. This occurs at different times, depending on the problem. A syndrome or central nervous system abnormality may be identified in the antenatal period or at birth. Deafness, motor handicaps and severe disabilities often become apparent during the first year. Moderate or even severe developmental impairments, language disorders and autism may not be recognised until the child is 2 or 3, when the family or health visitor question the child's developmental progress. Finally, children may present after life-threatening events such as head injury or encephalopathy.

Assessment of disability

Identifying the underlying medical problem is only one aspect of the child's diagnosis. A detailed assessment of the child's development and how the difficulties are likely to impinge on his or her life is also needed. When the difficulties are complex, the paediatrician alone is unlikely to be able to make a sufficiently detailed assessment, or advise on appropriate management. In this circumstance the child should be referred to a child development team.

The child development team

The child development team is a multidisciplinary team of professionals who are involved in assessing and managing children with complex difficulties (Figure 3.1). The members of the team (see Table 3.4) and the manner in which they work vary from centre to centre, and their roles often overlap considerably in practice.

Table 3.3 Commoner causes of disability among school children
Physical and multiple disabilities
Cerebral palsy
Spina bifida
Muscular dystrophy
Severe learning disabilities
Chromosomal abnormalities
Central nervous system abnormality
Idiopathic
Special senses
Severe visual handicap
Severe hearing loss

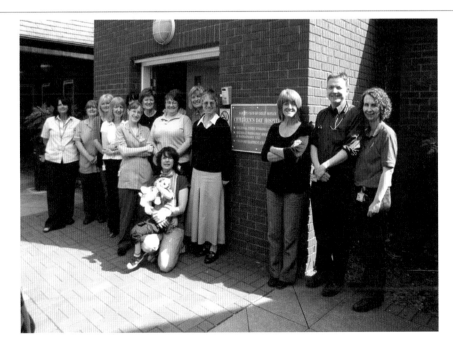

Figure 3.1 Example of multidisciplinary team, consisting of specialist nurses, dietitian, physiotherapist, psychologist and clerical staff as well as medical staff.

Table 3.4 The child development team

Professional	Role
Developmental paediatrician	Diagnosis of medical problems
	Advice on medical issues
Physiotherapist	Assessment and management of gross motor difficulties, abnormal tone and prevention of deformities in cerebral palsy
	Provision of special equipment
Occupational therapist	Assessment and management of fine motor difficulties
	Advice on toys, play and appliances to aid daily living
Speech and language therapist	Advice on feeding
	Assessment and management of speech, language and all aspects of communication
Psychologist	Support and counselling of family and team
Special needs teacher	Advice on special educational needs
Social worker	Support for the family
	Advice on social service benefits, respite care, etc.
Health visitor	Support for the family
	Liaison with local health visitor

Principles of management

Management of children with disabilities goes beyond making a diagnosis, explaining the problem and providing therapeutic input. It involves supporting the family while they come to terms with the child's difficulties and learn how to cope. It also involves a great deal of liaison work with other professionals both medical and non-medical.

The major benefit of the team approach lies in the coordination of care, so ensuring that the various professionals communicate with each other well and that the family does not receive a mixture of contradictory advice.

Breaking the news

The diagnosis of a disability is usually devastating, and the way that the news is initially broken is of long-lasting importance to the family. The session should be conducted in private by a senior doctor in the presence of both parents. There should be plenty of opportunity for questions, and a follow-up session should be arranged shortly after. If a baby is born with congenital anomalies, the first session should take place directly after birth, when possible with the baby present.

Box 3.3 Managing a child with a disability

- Obtain a detailed assessment of the child's difficulties and abilities
- Explain the nature and possible causes of the child's disability
- Devise a programme to cover the needs of the child and the family
- Help the family cope practically and emotionally
- Advise on educational needs and schooling

Medical management

Once the child's difficulties have been fully assessed, appropriate therapeutic input is required. This may be delivered in the child development centre, at home or at nursery. Once the child is in full-time school, the services are delivered there by community therapists, whose task is not only to work with the child but also to advise school staff.

Genetic counselling

When a child has been diagnosed as having a disability, the family will want to know the genetic implications for themselves and their relatives. Many disabilities have a genetic basis, in which case informed advice must be provided. However, even if there is no specific underlying genetic cause, the family will need to discuss the risk of further children being affected.

Provision of services

Agencies other than health agencies are involved in providing services to the family:

- *Education services.* Education services are responsible for assessing learning difficulties, providing preschool home teaching, nursery schooling and education in both mainstream and special schools.
- *Social Care.* Social Care is responsible for providing preschool child care, relief/respite care, advice about benefits and assessment for services needed on leaving school. Child protection concerns also fall into its remit.
- *Voluntary organisations.* Voluntary organisations provide support and information for families, run play facilities and provide educational opportunities and sitting services. Some are large national agencies with numerous local branches, others are smaller groups concerned with a local issue or a single diagnosis.

Education

Schools are required to provide extra provision for children with special educational needs and disabilities (SEND) and to make reasonable adjustments to provide additional help, whether individual or in small groups. When children fail to make progress with local provision a more detailed assessment is required, including a medical report and reports from any other involved professionals such as therapists and the child's nursery or school. The child's educational needs and the provision which must be made to meet them are clearly outlined in a legally binding document known as the Education and Health Care Plan (EHCP).

Mainstream and special schools Where possible, children with SEND are educated in mainstream schools, with extra help provided in the classroom as needed. This often involves the employment of an assistant for the child, along with physiotherapy, occupational therapy and speech and language therapy support. Mainstream placement has the advantage of integrating children with special needs into a normal peer group in their own locality, and encouraging their adaptation to normal society at an early age. It is also advantageous for other children to learn to live alongside children with disabilities. However, there are some disadvantages as mainstream schools usually suffer from comparatively large classes, may have inadequate support and the buildings may be poorly adapted for the child with physical difficulties.

Special schools, on the other hand, provide expert teaching in small classes, by staff who have an understanding of developmental impairment. Transport and health service support are also often provided. The disadvantage lies in the child's limited exposure to 'normal life'. Often, a good compromise between mainstream and special schooling is to establish special units for children with disabilities in the mainstream setting.

 The child with a disability at a glance

Presentation and how the diagnosis is made
Antenatally or at birth if anomalies are present
In the first year for motor handicaps and severe learning disabilities
In the second or third year for moderate learning disabilities, language disorder and autism
After cranial insults

Assessment of the disability
- Detailed assessment of the child's abilities
- Recognition of the child's underlying medical problem
- Assessment of the likely long-term effects
- When difficulties are complex, a multidisciplinary approach is needed.
  This involves the **child development team**: paediatrician, physiotherapist, occupational therapist, speech and language therapist, psychologist, teacher, social worker, health visitor

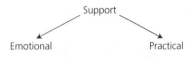
Support
Emotional   Practical

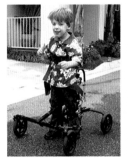
Child with CP walking in Hart walker

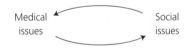
Medical issues   Social issues

Issues for the family
The initial impact is similar to bereavement
The impact of disability is similar to that of chronic illness (see pp. 46–8)

Issues for the school
School needs information and guidance, and may need to make adaptations

Breaking the news
Must be done by an experienced senior professional

Medical management
Usual paediatric care
If therapeutic input is needed, it should be provided initially at home, and then in nursery and school

Genetic counselling
Required for many families, even if no genetic cause is identified

Provision of services
Additional services are provided by education, social services and voluntary agencies

Education
The Education and Health Care Plan describes the provision that must be made for children with disabilities
Where possible, children with disabilities should be integrated into mainstream school

Support
Includes informal support, voluntary organisations, sitting services, respite care, home help and social service allowances

Support

Having a child with a disability places extra pressure and stresses on any family. It is important, therefore, to determine how much support is available. Informal support in terms of family and friends can be variable, and additional support is often appreciated. This may take a number of forms. Voluntary organisations and parent support groups give families the opportunity to meet others in similar circumstances and so can reduce the sense of isolation. Sitting services and respite care give parents a break from the burden of constantly caring for the child, and help in the home can also be provided. As regards financial benefits, families may be eligible for Disability Living Allowance and Carer's Allowance.

Issues for the family

Families differ greatly in their reaction to having a child with a disability. On first receiving the news, however, they all tend to pass through similar emotional stages to those experienced in coping with bereavement. The first reaction is one of shock, when often only a small proportion of what is said is taken in. Negative feelings of fear and loss, anger and guilt then follow. Gradually adaptation follows, and leads to the final stage of acceptance. Some parents have difficulty in reaching this last stage, in which case supportive counselling by a psychologist may be necessary.

The family needs to adapt again at each stage of the child's development. Independence becomes an issue at each step, but particularly so at adolescence. An important part of the child's education is to foster independence, and this is usually addressed well at special schools. Young adult disability teams provide a service to advise about options beyond secondary school.

Issues for the school

When a child with a disability is accepted at a mainstream school, the school needs to be prepared and informed about any anticipated difficulties. If the child needs occupational therapy, physiotherapy or speech and language therapy, the staff will need to work with the therapists in order to implement their recommendations. In some circumstances the school may need to make alterations to accommodate physical disabilities. Special guidance or counselling may be required and help may be needed to integrate the child into the classroom.

The child with cancer

Cancer is a rare occurrence in childhood, and in the majority of cases the prognosis is good. Nonetheless, the diagnosis is inevitably one of the hardest for a family to come to terms with. Given its rarity, the requirements for complex investigation and treatment, and the need for long-term monitoring, paediatric cancer care only takes place in specialist centres. The management of cancer in children presents unique challenges as treatment with chemotherapy, surgery and radiation can adversely affect growth and development.

Prevalence

In the UK, 1700 children are diagnosed with cancer each year. Throughout childhood and adolescence, the commonest malignancies are acute leukaemia, followed by brain tumours, lymphomas and soft tissue sarcoma. Other cancers in childhood include germ cell, neuroblastoma, eye, kidney liver and bone. Overall, there has been a significant decrease in mortality in recent years, although this is very dependent on the type of malignancy. The various types of cancer are shown in Table 3.5.

Aetiology and pathophysiology

In most cases of cancer, environmental and host factors are involved. In children, host factors may be more important than environmental factors, as cancers tend to occur in tissues (e.g. the haemopoietic and the nervous tissue) that are not exposed directly to the environment. The majority of solid tumours are embryonic in appearance, presumably because they are caused by malignant transformation of embryonic tissues.

Initial presentation of the child with cancer

The presenting clinical features differ for each type of cancer (Table 3.5). However, certain less specific signs can be suggestive of malignancy. These include atypical courses of apparently common childhood conditions, unexplained or prolonged fever (>3–4 weeks), and unexplained (and especially growing) masses, particularly when associated with weight loss.

A tentative diagnosis can often be inferred from the presenting symptoms, the location of the tumour and the age of the child, and then confirmed by biopsy. It is usually appropriate to search for metastatic disease first, so allowing the surgeon/oncologist to judge whether diagnostic biopsy or complete resection is the best procedure. The studies carried out depend on the tumour, and may be non-invasive or invasive.

Staging

At the time of diagnosis it is critical that the extent of disease be accurately defined. This delineation is called staging. A system of staging has to be designed for each tumour on the basis of the extent of the disease at diagnosis and the subsequent clinical course. Staging helps to determine prognosis and treatment plans.

Histology

At the core of diagnosis is the histological examination. The surgeon has to search carefully at biopsy, excision or

Table 3.5 Childhood cancers

Type	Site	Peak age	Presentation
Acute lymphoblastic leukaemia (pp. 379–80)	White cell precursors	Throughout childhood. Peak 5 years	Non-specific anorexia, lethargy, pallor, fever, bleeding
Hodgkin disease	Lymph tissue	Late childhood, adolescence	Enlarged lymph nodes, systemic upset
Non-Hodgkin lymphoma	Lymph tissue	Young children	Rapidly enlarging lymph node
Neuroblastoma	Any part of the sympathetic nervous system	First 2 years	Failure to thrive, abdominal mass, bleeding
Brain tumours	Infratentorial, supratentorial, hypothalamic–pituitary axis	School age	Cerebellar/brainstem dysfunction, endocrine/visual impairment, epilepsy/hemiplegia
Wilm tumour	Kidney	Under 5 years	Abdominal mass
Rhabdomyosarcoma	Muscle	<5 years, late adolescence	Painful mass
Osteosarcoma	Femur, humerus	Adolescents	Bone pain, limp
Ewing sarcoma	Bone	<10 years	Bone pain
Retinoblastoma	Retina	<2 years	White pupil, squint
Gonad/germ cell tumours	Ovaries/testis	<3 years, puberty	Scrotal mass, vomiting, nausea, pain in girls

exploration for evidence of regional dissemination to lymph node groups or adjacent organs. If an attempt is made to remove the whole tumour, the pathologist has to examine the margins of the specimen to ensure that no microscopic residue remains.

Goals of management

The goal of medical management is to eradicate the malignancy whenever possible. In so doing, the minimum of damage should be inflicted on normal tissues. As cancer therapy is invariably toxic, the child must be actively sustained through the effects of the treatment, and special attention paid to nutritional status. The diagnosis of malignancy is always devastating, and management must include good support for

the child and family. Once treated, the child must be followed up long term for development of sequelae to the cancer or the treatment.

Treatment

The most appropriate place for management of children with cancer is a specialised paediatric oncology centre. Centralizing care allows for the systematic assessment of new treatments, collaborative trials and the specialised support that families need. The treatment of childhood cancer rests on the initial diagnostic studies, and involves surgical removal, irradiation and/or chemotherapy. In many children all three therapies are necessary.

Surgery

Surgery used to be the first-line treatment for most solid tumours. Chemotherapy is now usually initially used to shrink the tumour and so permit more limited and successful resection. Surgery is also required for insertion of indwelling central venous lines giving access for intensive chemotherapy, fluids and blood sampling.

Radiotherapy

Radiotherapy is effective in the region to which it is applied, and so is principally used to treat areas of known disease. It is also used in total body irradiation in conjunction with bone

---

Box 3.4 Goals in managing cancer

- Eradicate the malignancy whenever possible, inflicting the least damage on normal tissues
- Sustain the child through the toxic effects of treatment
- Ensure that the nutritional status of the child is maintained
- Provide support for the family
- Follow the child for development of late sequelae related to the malignancy or the treatment

marrow rescue techniques. Unfortunately, it damages local tissue, and local effects can not only be disfiguring but also affect function (see Prognosis, below).

Chemotherapy

The drugs used in chemotherapy kill cancer cells by interfering with the replication and division of DNA during cell division. They are most commonly given intravenously, although some individual agents are given orally, topically or intrathecally. Their effectiveness depends on their being more cytotoxic to the malignant cells than they are to normal dividing cells. The use of several agents simultaneously reduces the likelihood of chemoresistance developing. Chemotherapeutic agents are toxic substances. The common side effects are hair loss, and bone marrow and immune suppression.

Bone marrow transplantation

Haemopoietic suppression is the side effect that limits the use of many cytotoxic agents. The technique of bone marrow transplantation overcomes this problem, and so allows high doses of these agents to be used. Bone marrow is either harvested from a histocompatible donor or from the patient prior to treatment and then implanted after chemotherapy has finished. Profound immunosuppression, organ toxicity and graft-vs.-host disease are hazards. Nonetheless, this treatment has been successful, particularly now it is being used earlier for patients in remission rather than with florid disease. Peripheral blood stem cell harvest and re-infusion is a similar procedure being used more frequently.

Management of acute problems and supportive treatment

Management of the effects of cancer and therapy

Metabolic consequences. The breakdown of malignant tissue either before or as a result of therapy can precipitate uric acid crystals in the renal tubules, causing impaired renal function ('tumour lysis'). Uric acid and creatinine levels must therefore be closely monitored and adequate hydration and allopurinol (a xanthine oxidase inhibitor) given to maintain uric acid in the normal range. Phosphates and potassium can also be released into the circulation and symptomatic hypocalcaemia and hyperkalaemia can be a problem.

Bone marrow suppression. Bone marrow suppression with consequent pancytopenia can occur as a result of bone marrow invasion in some cancers, or as a result of therapy. Anaemia is treated by transfusion of packed red cells, and thrombocytopenia by infusion of platelets. Granulocyte infusions, however, are toxic and rarely used. The febrile neutropenic (<500 cells/mm³) patient needs appropriate cultures and intravenous broad-spectrum antibiotic coverage.

Immunosuppression. Immunosuppression is a consequence of some tumours and treatment regimens, and may persist for months after treatment has stopped. Viruses normally of low pathogenicity can then produce serious disease. As a result, patients should not be given vaccines containing live virus, and if exposed to live varicella should receive immunoglobulin. If chicken pox develops they must be hospitalized and treated with aciclovir. Fungal infections are common, particularly candida, and opportunistic organisms such as *Pneumocystis jiroveci* can produce fatal disease.

Nutrition

Patients undergoing cancer therapy commonly lose weight, particularly if undergoing intensive chemotherapy, total body irradiation or radiotherapy to the head and neck. Attention must be paid to their nutritional status. Parenteral nutrition is sometimes required.

Symptom management

Cancer and its investigation and treatment produce distress, discomfort and sometimes pain. The effective use of analgesics, local anaesthetics and chemotherapy/radiotherapy should ensure control of almost all distressing symptoms.

Emotional support

The child and family need support in coming to terms with the diagnosis. This process is helped by being told as soon as possible about the nature of the cancer, its prognosis and treatment. The child should be told all that he or she can understand and would find useful to know. Explanations may have to be repeated several times before distraught families feel that they really understand. Support is particularly essential for the dying child, who should wherever possible receive care at home with the back-up of a palliative care service and ready access to a familiar children's hospice or ward.

Monitoring and the management of relapses

The child needs monitoring both for relapse of the malignancy and the adverse effects of treatment. Acute problems include febrile neutropenia, bone marrow suppression and immunosuppression.

Patients who have been successfully treated for childhood cancer should be examined annually and should be carefully assessed for the late effects of therapy (see 'Prognosis' below). The principles involved in the follow-up of any child with a chronic medical condition (p. 47) are particularly important for the child with cancer.

Prognosis

The patient's prognosis varies with the type of tumour and the extent of disease at the time of diagnosis, as well as with the adequacy of treatment. More than 70% of the

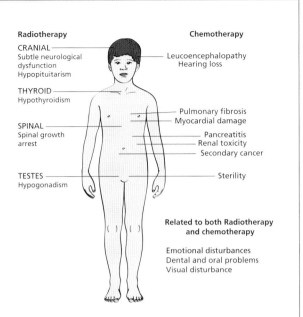

Figure 3.2 Late consequences of cancer treatment.

patients diagnosed today will be cured, and approximately 80% survive more than 5 years following diagnosis.

The late consequences of therapy may result in serious morbidity (Figure 3.2), which may only become evident when the child is fully grown. Radiotherapy may produce irreversible damage to organs, so that irradiation to one extremity can cause marked asymmetry. Spinal irradiation can cause spinal growth arrest and along with growth hormone deficiency contribute to short stature. Cranial radiation can cause subtle neurological dysfunction such as short-term memory defects, difficulties with mental arithmetic and poor attention span. Repeated radiation for relapses of leukaemia, or high-dose radiotherapy for intracranial malignancies, may damage the hypothalamic–pituitary axis, leading to a variety of endocrine disturbances such as growth hormone deficiency or pubertal delay. Irradiation of endocrine organs such as the thyroid gland or testes can destroy their endocrine function. Chemotherapeutic agents can also have long-term effects such as leucoencephalopathy, sterility, myocardial damage, renal toxicity, pulmonary fibrosis, pancreatitis and hearing loss.

Another late problem is the occurrence of second cancers in patients successfully cured of a first. This is probably caused by a combination of factors including an underlying genetic predisposition and the carcinogenic effects of radiotherapy and chemotherapeutic agents.

Issues for the family

There are intense issues for the family of both a practical and emotional nature. The diagnosis and treatment of cancer demand the involvement of the parents at all stages. Although centralizing the care of paediatric oncology results in a superior

service, the distances involved in reaching the centre can be problematic for many families. Residential facilities are often available, but these do not resolve the problems of child care for siblings, and separate families from normal family and friend support systems. Financial difficulties are common, and in many families a parent may have to give up or change jobs. Input from community nurses and social workers is important.

The emotional needs of the family are likely to be greater than the practical. The child and family need expert help to contend with facing life-threatening illness, ongoing fears of relapse and, for some, the process of dying and death. Relationships within a family are bound to be disturbed, and feelings of anxiety, depression, guilt and anger are common in all members.

The child has to cope not only with the effects of the cancer, but also with the debilitating effects of treatment and changes in appearance, such as alopecia, which can make reintegration into normal life all the more difficult.

Issues at school

Whenever possible the child should remain in school and with classmates. Because most treatment regimens are intensive, considerable amounts of schooling are usually missed in the first year or two after diagnosis. Help should be provided so that the child does not fall too far behind.

School staff need preparation to help them understand the child's condition and prognosis, and to enable them to help the child reintegrate socially as well as academically.

Palliative care

Palliative care is the active total care of patients whose disease is no longer curable and whose prognosis is limited. Its aim is to ease the symptoms, discomfort and stress of serious illness for children and their families, and enhance children's quality of life. Palliative treatment may involve radiotherapy, chemotherapy or surgery if these are helpful in symptom control.

Children with cancer comprise the largest paediatric group in need of palliative care. But care is also available for children and teenagers living with other serious illnesses, such as neurologic disorders, genetic disorders, heart and lung conditions, and others. Palliative care is important for children at any age or stage of serious illness.

The approach taken is to acknowledge the sadness that results from life-threatening illness and help parents attend to the needs of the ill child and the rest of the family too. Parental grief for the loss of their expected normal child starts from the time of diagnosis. For some parents, continued hope for cure, no matter how unlikely, may be an important coping mechanism or may conform with deeply held religious or cultural beliefs.

Principles of palliative care

While acknowledging uncertainty, families benefit from a realistic appraisal of prognosis and the time range in which death

👁 The child with cancer at a glance

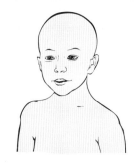

Epidemiology
1700 children are diagnosed with cancer each year in the UK.
  Commonest cancers are acute lymphoblastic leukaemia, lymphoma and brain tumours

Aetiology/pathophysiology
Host factors may be more important than environmental factors in childhood cancers

How the diagnosis is made
The presentation depends on the individual malignancy. Non-specific signs include unexplained or prolonged fever, unexplained (especially growing) masses and weight loss. Diagnosis is confirmed by histology. Staging is needed to determine treatment and prognosis

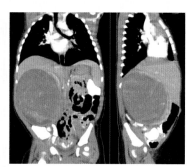

MRI showing Wilm tumour of the right kidney

General management
Treatment must take place in a paediatric oncology centre

  Specific treatment involves a combination of:
- Surgery
- Radiotherapy
- Chemotherapy
- Bone marrow transplantation
- Biological and targeted agents; Immunotherapy

Supportive treatment
required for:
- Effects of cancer and Rx
- Metabolic disturbances
- Immunosuppression
- Bone marrow suppression
Nutrition
Symptom management including pain
Emotional support

Liaison with school
Missed schooling
Reintegration following treatment

Management of acute problems
Fever — cultures and IV antibiotics
Immunosuppression — no live vaccines, treat chicken pox
Bone marrow suppression — packed red cells and platelet transfusion
Relapse

Points for routine follow-up
Close monitoring is required for relapse of cancer and adverse effects of treatment. Once in full remission, annual routine follow-up is required indefinitely

Prognosis
Varies with type and extent of cancer. Some 70% are cured. Overall, 80% survive > 5 years. Late effects of treatment can be debilitating. Second cancers are not uncommon

---

is likely to occur. Parental disappointment, anger, grief and suffering associated with the child's illness need to be acknowledged. This grief is often the first step toward facing the reality of the child's illness and acceptance is likely to help parents focus on the quality of the child's remaining life.

Children's feelings need acknowledgement too and they should be encouraged to talk or express themselves through other means about feelings of anger, sadness, fear, isolation and guilt. Key principles include:
- Honesty and openness: always important but especially when families try to protect the child, as trust can be so easily damaged
- Quality of life and symptom control: shifting away from the focus on cure

- Considering the needs and wishes of the child: according to the child's age and maturity

Organization of care

Palliative care involves a multidisciplinary team who work together to support the family. The approach should be one of partnership between the child, the parents and the health care team. An important role includes listening to preferences and helping the family think through the care options.

Palliative care is different from hospice care. Hospice care focuses on a person's final months of life, whereas palliative care is available at any time during a serious illness. Palliative care can be provided wherever the child is: in the hospital, during clinic visits, or at home. Some children receive palliative care for many years.

The palliative care team commonly involves a variety of professionals:

- Paediatrician supported by the GP
- Specialist nurse
- Social worker
- Psychologist
- Play therapist
- Pharmacist
- Religious and spiritual support e.g. Chaplain

Care also includes practical support for families such as providing respite care for parents to be able to spend time with their other children, assistance in including siblings in conversations, and locating community resources for services such as counseling and support groups. Care is especially needed at times of transition when children move from hospital to outpatient care or care at home.

Symptom control

Palliative care or referral to palliative care specialists should not be delayed until curative options have been exhausted. By contrast with curative treatments which are given to reverse the disease process, palliative treatments focus on relieving symptoms, and common symptoms that are amenable to control are shown in Box 3.5. At times their management may impact on the underlying disease process. Treatment may involve pharmacological and non-pharmacological measures.

Pain relief is a major component of palliative care. In general a stepwise approach is used starting with paracetomol or NSAIDs and leading to opioids of increasing strength.

Box 3.5 Types of symptoms ameliorated by palliative care

- Pain
- Shortness of breath
- Fatigue
- Depression
- Anxiety
- Nausea
- Loss of appetite
- Problems with sleep

A combination of different medications is more effective than an escalating dose of one analgesic. The oral (or transdermal) route is used with subcutaneous infusion reserved for terminal care. Adjuvants may include medications for neuropathic pain, antispasmodics muscle relaxants and steroids

The palliative care plan

In developing a palliative care plan, children should participate to the fullest extent possible, taking into account their illness experience, developmental capabilities and level of consciousness. Regardless of the prognosis, children need a developmentally appropriate description of the condition along with the anticipated burdens and benefits of management options. They need to be listened to and their preferences solicited. Factors that need to be considered when discussing death with a child include the disease experience and developmental level of the child; the child's understanding of and prior experience with death; the family's religious and cultural beliefs about death; the child's usual patterns of coping with pain and sadness; and the expected circumstances of death.

Decisions to forgo life-sustaining medical treatment do not necessarily imply an intent or choice to hasten death. Although a child's life may be shortened by avoiding burdensome treatment or providing sedation for otherwise unrelieved symptoms, the goal is to optimize the quality of the child's experience rather than hasten death. Dying with dignity and without pain or distress is the primary goal. An adolescent nearing death may refuse further life-sustaining medical treatment and the ethical issues are discussed in Chapter 2.

In the UK most children die at home but the family may opt for hospital, an intensive care unit or another institution. The decision depends on a number of factors such as the family's wishes, the ability of staff to be involved, and the availability of bereavement counselors and clinicians with palliative care expertise. Wherever death takes place, the family must have the opportunity to carry out important family, religious or cultural rituals and to hold the child before and after death. Members of the extended family, friends, primary care physicians and religious advisors need to be included, if the family chooses. It is often helpful if the team works with the school or youth organisations to assist other children affected by the death of the child.

To test your knowledge on this part of the book, please see Chapter 26

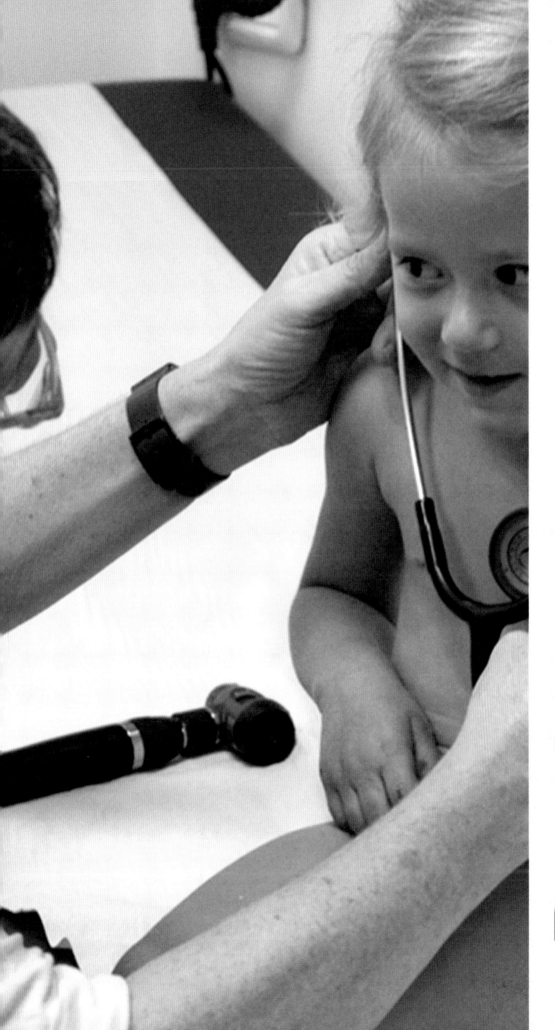

Part 2
A paediatric tool kit

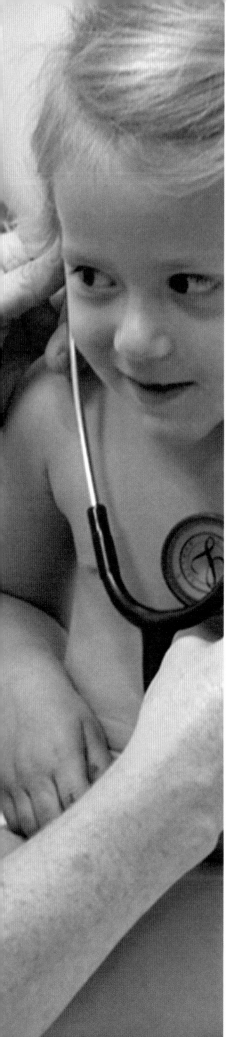

CHAPTER 4

Communicating with children, their families and colleagues

"Children are not the people of tomorrow, but are people of today. They have a right to be taken seriously, and to be treated with tenderness and respect."
Janusz Korczak
1878–1943

KEY COMPETENCES

YOU MUST...

Know and understand

- About parental responsibility regarding children's health care and how this may alter in child protection and adolescent health
- How to involve children of differing maturity in decisions about their health care
- The value of the Personal Child Health Record
- The principles of supporting families over time

Be able to

- Communicate with children, young people of differing ages and abilities, and their parents
- Explain common and important medical conditions
- Explain common procedures and investigations

Appreciate that

- Communication is central to paediatric care and requires practice to improve
- Communicating with parents and children differs from adult care
- Illness often has a profound emotional impact on both parent and child, and that good communication skills can improve the family's experience of illness
- Team working is an important aspect of paediatric care

Essential Paediatrics and Child Health, Fourth Edition. Mary Rudolf, Anthony Luder and Kerry Jeavons.
© 2020 John Wiley & Sons Ltd. Published 2020 by John Wiley & Sons Ltd.
Companion website: www.wiley.com/go/rudolf/paediatrics

Communication skills and their importance

Communication is at the heart of medical care. Good communication not only leads to patient satisfaction, health care is more effective and health outcomes are also improved. Much greater emphasis is now placed on communication skills and their assessment in medical education. Despite this, doctors too often fail to introduce themselves or look at their patients when discussing sensitive issues, talk in jargon, or use technical words and talk about patients as if they were not there. Patients are clear about what they wish from their doctor (see Box 4.1).

Professional qualities and skills

Respect for others is at the core of communication and is key to all interactions with patients and their relatives, as well as colleagues and others involved in patient care. Knowledge of cultural and local customs is vital to establish a therapeutic relationship with a family. Listening and the ability to empathise is valued, and it is essential in order to tailor care while taking the patient's perspective, feelings and circumstances into account. It is important to communicate empathy rather than simple sympathy; the latter often being misinterpreted as non-professional (see later on page 64, Supporting families over time). Poor communication and lack of respect are still consistently prevalent in complaints against doctors.

Communicating with patients requires skill and the ability to discuss sensitive issues, including difficult, embarrassing and stigmatized topics, such as death and bereavement, mental illness, abortion, domestic violence and child abuse. It also demands the ability to understand and respond to the emotional impact of illness, responding to reactions such as distress, fear and anger, as well as discussing mistakes and complaints.

Box 4.1 What patients say they want from communication with their doctor

- Greeting me in a way that makes me feel comfortable
- Treating me with respect and showing interest in my ideas about my health
- Letting me talk without interruptions and understanding my main health concerns
- Paying attention to me (looking at me, listening carefully), talking in terms I can understand, checking to be sure I understood and giving me as much information as I want
- Encouraging me to ask questions
- Involving me in decisions as much as I want and discussing next steps, including any follow-up plans
- Showing care and concern
- Spending the right amount of time with me
- Summarizing to show he/she understood everything I said

One of the most challenging skills involves delivering bad news and discussing with patients and those close to them their diagnosis and prognosis. This is especially hard when the condition is serious, long-term, life-changing or life-limiting, and when there are no effective treatments, a risk of serious adverse effects or when treatment ceases to be effective. Doctors also often need to cope when there is uncertainty about diagnosis, prognosis and the 'correct' treatment option to meet patients' needs. It is vital to be honest and open while maintaining an optimistic tone. One should never leave the patient without hope.

Communicating with children and their parents

Communicating in paediatrics follows the same principles as adult care, but requires additional skills. By its nature, consultations are 'triadic' involving the child, the parent or carer, and the doctor. Two types of paediatrician have been described, those who work well with parents and others who work well with children. In reality doctors need to be skilled in communicating with both parents and children. If the child is made to feel at ease the parents' confidence is gained, and when parents feel comfortable children are more likely to relax and be more cooperative.

Communication is facilitated by the setting and atmosphere. Young children do not have a full understanding of the role of health professionals, and are likely to be anxious and uncertain in an unfamiliar environment. They do not necessarily understand all of the language in the consultation but they quickly detect a sense of personal warmth, friendliness and relaxed mood in adults around them. This is helped by making the room child-friendly with toys available for children of different ages, so that they can play during consultations.

At times it may be better if parents can talk to the doctor on their own. Doctors need to anticipate parents' wishes not to talk in front of the child, particularly as parents may feel too embarrassed to ask, and so may withhold important information. Children should be allowed to leave the room to play rather than hear themselves being discussed. This requires adequate supervision of the waiting room and an accompanying family member is ideal. In order to allay anxiety, it needs to be clear that the child can always return to the consulting room.

The nature of consultations inevitably varies according to the age and understanding of the child. When the patient is a young baby the discussion is entirely with the carers (usually parents) but thereafter the child needs their own explanations pitched at an age-appropriate level. Adolescents require particular sensitivity, and ideally both parent and child should have the opportunity to talk to the doctor alone. Time often does not permit this, but there are circumstances where it is essential that this occurs, and the aspects of the session that are confidential need to be made clear. The consultation needs to conclude with coming back together to plan the next steps.

Procedures

Special attention is required when children need to undergo practical procedures, such as venupuncture and investigations, as well as more invasive procedures such as lumbar punctures and surgery. This is especially important when they are likely to be repeated in the future. When children are clear about what is involved anxiety is reduced, making the procedure easier to carry out for everyone.

Children should never have painful or unpleasant procedures undertaken in their hospital bed and should be taken to the treatment room. They need to feel that their bed is a place of safety. It is no longer acceptable to perform painful procedures without adequate pre- and post-procedure analgesia and often sedation, at all ages, and the child and family need to be reassured about this.

Communicating during procedures should involve:
- explaining the procedure in age-appropriate language
- ensuring the child agrees before proceeding where possible
- responding effectively to questions, concerns and emotions
- providing an appropriate commentary

It generally helps to have the parent in the room, although a nurse may need to substitute if the parent does not feel they can cope. In recent years many hospitals have introduced medical clowns ("dream doctors") into the wards (see Fig 4.1). They can play an important role in easing pain and anxiety, providing and obtaining information and making procedures and indeed the whole admission a more positive experience.

Diversity in communication

There is a duty to provide equitable care to all, and services need to work towards achieving health equality and inclusion, and cater for diversity. Doctors must be able to communicate effectively regardless of patients' circumstances, whether due to age, nationality, physical impairment, ethnic or cultural background, religious beliefs, intellectual ability, socio-economic status, education or family background.

Paediatrics is a setting where these principles are extremely important. Developing communication skills to a variety of populations demands skill and is fostered by openness in exploring one's own cultural beliefs and practices. Language barriers are always challenging and in paediatrics children of recent immigrants may have better local language than their parents. Although tempting to use them as interpreters, this is generally inappropriate and professional interpretation needs to be available.

Patients' notes and the Personal Child Health Record (PCHR)

In recent years parents have been given responsibility for looking after their children's health records. In the UK and many other countries every child has a Personal Child Health Record (see Figure 4.2 and p. 30) held by their parents. The PCHR (or 'red book' as it is popularly called in the UK) is maintained as

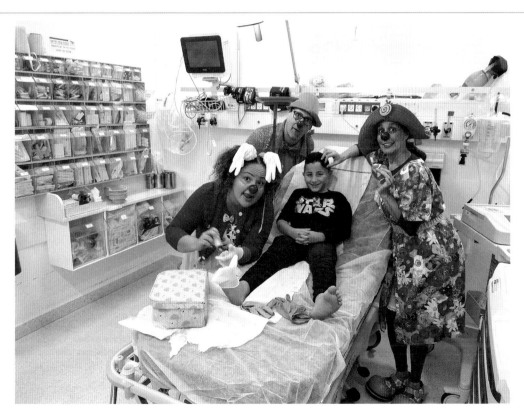

Figure 4.1 Medical clowns on a paediatric ward.

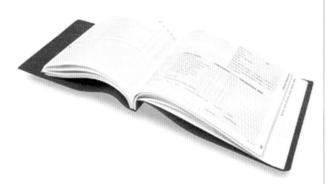

Figure 4.2 The 'Red Book' – the Personal Child Health Record in use in the UK. *Source:* reproduced with permission from Harlow Printing Limited ©.

an individual record of the child's health, growth and development, as well as a record of contacts with doctors and health professionals. The record is particularly useful when a child is newly referred to a doctor. Parents are expected to bring the record to appointments to foster communication between different professionals as well as to ensure details of immunisation, growth and development are readily available.

Technology

The challenge of managing virtually any medical encounter has been increased by the presence of the 'third party' in the room - the computer. In paediatrics the computer is the 'fourth party' and too often overrides the patient narrative and the interaction between doctors and their patients. Apart from the issue of a computer in the consultation, most families now have access to internet and smartphone based medical information and the doctor needs to know how to enable patients to interpret this kind of information, which may be misleading or stress extreme situations.

Consent

Children (defined as below 18 years) in general do not make their own decisions about their health care and parents make decisions on their behalf. However it is important to understand children's concerns, and children as they mature have a right to be included in discussion and involved in decisions. It is practically very difficult to treat an adolescent for example who actively resists medical intervention.

At times, if a child's views are at variance with their parents', a decision has to be made whether they are mature enough to decide whether they are investigated or treated for an illness. Legally, older children who are deemed competent to understand the significance of the issues are permitted to consent to examination and treatment without their parents' knowledge (see Chapter 2). It is undoubtedly best practice to encourage the young person to involve their parents for support. In Britain legal precedent allows a physician to prescribe contraceptives without parental consent, provided the adolescent is deemed mature enough to understand the risks and benefits.

When parents do not act in the child's best interest

A difficult situation arises when parents fail to act in the best interests of their child. Not many years ago it was accepted that parents had absolute rights over their child but society has changed its views. Children by law can be protected and parental authority curtailed (p. 395). In any aspect of paediatrics and child health care, when concerns arise regarding the possibility that a child is the victim of neglect, non-accidental injury or emotional or sexual abuse, it is the professional's duty (and indeed any individual's duty) to report these to the authorities so that appropriate investigations can be made.

Supporting families over time (see Figure 4.3)

Doctors have an important and influential role in supporting families in promoting their children's health, whether this relates to taking medications consistently, their health behaviors or planning the care ahead. The support is most effective when efforts are made to build and maintain a trusting relationship, strengths and concerns are explored,

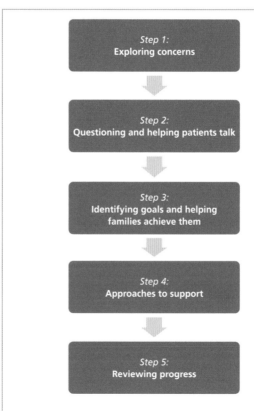

Figure 4.3 Steps in supporting families over time.

goals and how to achieve them are identified and reviews occur on a regular basis.

A relationship based on trust and a desire to understand is the starting point for quality care and is best built by understanding the family's views rather than imposing thoughts about what they need. If parents feel they are being judged, hostility or defensiveness is often the result. Being aware of this allows for response in a way that helps, rather than reacting to the behaviour.

Exploring concerns

Exploring issues involves two key skills: encouraging patients to talk, and listening well to what they say. Active listening requires concentrating fully on the other person, noticing their facial expression and body language, as well as their words. Empathy is key and requires one to focus on the other person's experience and to listen with a desire to truly understand. As well as building trust, empathy is a powerful catalyst for change. When people sense they have been heard and understood, they are more able to think, problem solve and start to tackle the issues they are facing.

Questioning and helping patients talk

How professionals talk, as well as how they listen, has a major impact on how likely patients are to open up, think and talk about their own experiences and ideas. Combining helpful questions and truly listening, without interrupting, commenting or disagreeing, allows patients the opportunity to explore their own issues and develop confidence and motivation.

When taking a history, doctors generally use closed questions which can be answered with yes, no or factual one-word answers. They are an efficient use of time when making an assessment, but are not the best way to support patients in managing their health. By contrast, open questions help patients to think and reflect. Examples of open questions include 'where would you like to start?' 'how do you react when…?' 'how do you feel when that happens?' 'what do you think might be going on…?'

Identifying goals and helping families achieve them

Managing health concerns is facilitated by setting goals and working out how to achieve them. Doctors often feel that their role is to use their expertise to make suggestions, but the process should be parent-led rather than doctor-led. Parents know best what will work for their family, and if well managed the experience helps them learn more about the process of finding solutions and increases the chances of success. Most people are more likely to try out new ideas if they have come up with them themselves and thought through what will help put them into practice.

Approach to support

Traditionally, doctors adopt a 'problem-focused' approach to examining issues and difficulties, with the result that both doctor and patient become ever more expert in the details of a problem but not necessarily further forward in taking effective action. A more effective approach is a 'solution-focused' approach which identifies and highlights families' existing strengths and expertise, focusing on what they are already managing to do. Identifying strengths, resources and successes is a powerful way to build parents' belief in their ability to cope and make change. Part of the skill is to balance responding to what parents say while maintaining a positive focus and helping them to develop a plan of action. Using empathy to acknowledge feelings of discouragement, frustration or sadness can help to avoid being dismissive whilst bringing them back to what is going well and what will help them move forward.

Reviewing progress

Periodic review is integral to the process. In some countries child health care involves regular appointments throughout childhood even for healthy children. In other countries, like the UK, follow-up occurs for children with chronic and long-standing health concerns. When reviewing progress, evaluation, support and encouragement are important components. Doctors' interest, reassurance and concern can make a big difference. Empathising with feelings of frustration and disappointment, finding the positive and helping keep focus all increase parents' and children's abilities to cope.

Communicating beyond the patient

Many aspects of paediatrics involve teamwork and liaising with colleagues within health services and beyond. Individual liaison may be required, but multidisciplinary team working is now prevalent and has changed the face of health care, especially for children with chronic medical conditions and disabilities (see Chapter 3). The child development team is a good example of multidisciplinary working (see pp. 49–50).

Communication with other physicians and diligent note-keeping is crucial for good quality care in health systems, especially within hospitals and between hospitals and the community. Caring for patients in hospitals is done by teams and there are frequent opportunities for communication as well as misunderstandings. It is good practice to give and take information according to a standard format (such as the 'SOAP' method – Symptom (patient's complaints), Observation (patient's status), Assessment (trends, investigations), Plan (treatment, management) see p. 71, Chapter 5). The passage of information to the family physician and patient upon discharge is a critical but neglected area. Discharge letters are too often ignored or unread by GPs, and rarely are families given a written summary in everyday language.

Paediatrics by its nature also often involves communication with other health professionals such as health visitors, school nurses and nursery nurses. Other colleagues include social workers, teachers and at times childminders. When children have disabilities or chronic health issues, then direct contact with school is required to make sure their health needs are met during school hours. Professional liaison is always demanding on time, but without it many children 'fall through the cracks' particularly if their parents have poor health literacy.

To test your knowledge on this part of the book, please see Chapter 26

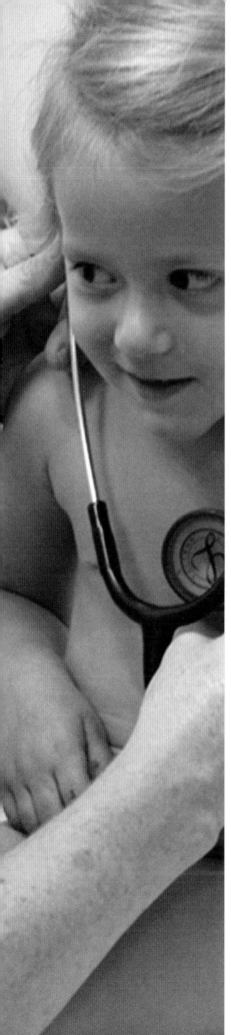

CHAPTER 5
History taking and clinical examination

Observe, record, tabulate, communicate. Use your five senses. Learn to see, learn to hear, learn to feel, learn to smell, and know that only by practice alone you can become expert.

William Osler 1849–1919

KEY COMPETENCES

YOU MUST ...

Know and understand

- How to integrate clinical information and clinical thinking in paediatrics
- How a paediatric history differs from that in adults
- That physical signs in paediatrics are more often appreciated by non-touch observation than in adults

Be able to

- Take a competent and age-appropriate history
- Measure vital signs, weight, height or length, and head circumference
- Carry out an age-appropriate physical examination demonstrating good technique
- Measure vital signs
- Plot measurements accurately on a growth chart
- Write up the history and physical examination in a systematic way
- Evaluate the case, make a problem and differential diagnosis list

Appreciate that

- Over 80% of diagnoses are reached by history
- Children can and want to add important information
- Parents may interpret symptoms rather than report them factually
- Children are likely to be wary of a physical examination and be uncooperative
- You may need to be flexible rather than strictly systematic in your approach
- It is best to leave unpleasant parts of the examination to the end

Essential Paediatrics and Child Health, Fourth Edition. Mary Rudolf, Anthony Luder and Kerry Jeavons.
© 2020 John Wiley & Sons Ltd. Published 2020 by John Wiley & Sons Ltd.
Companion website: www.wiley.com/go/rudolf/paediatrics

In clinical medicine, history taking and physical examination are the keystones of diagnosis and subsequent therapy. The first contact between the child, the family and the doctor sets the scene for the future therapeutic relationship. Very little may be remembered by the child and his or her family about that visit except the first impression, hopefully that the doctor is an approachable and sympathetic person. In paediatrics, the doctor's approach is of special importance and techniques may need to be altered in light of the patient's age (see Chapter 4).

The consultation (see Chapter 4)

Begin gathering information even before the child and the family enter your room. Discreet observation in the waiting room from a distance, of noise, posture, movement, breathing, colour, behaviour, activity and relationships can often be very valuable. Before you start with the formal interview, you need to work at gaining the child's trust and cooperation. Start by introducing yourself to the child and parents, and try to put them at ease. You obviously need to talk to the child in a manner appropriate to their age. While you take the history, observe the child as you can learn a great deal from how he or she looks and plays. It helps to make the room child-friendly and have toys available for children of different ages, so they can play while you talk to the parents.

Parents and children often fail to express their underlying concerns. For example, the development of headache may represent fears about brain tumour, and enlarged glands may arouse anxiety about cancer. It is very important that you are sensitive, anticipate these issues and ask specifically about them. Fears can be elicited by asking questions such as: 'Is there anything in particular you are worried about?' or 'In my experience some parents worry about cancer in a child with tummy pain. Is this something that you have thought of?' 'How do you explain all these problems?' 'What questions have you come here today to ask me?'

At times you may decide it would be better if the child left the room to play rather than hear themselves being discussed, but, in order to allay anxiety, it should be made clear that they can always return to the consulting room. A sensitive doctor should anticipate the parents' wish not to talk in front of the child, as some parents feel too embarrassed to ask, with the result that they may withhold important information.

Adolescents require particular sensitivity. It is ideal practice to offer both parent and child the opportunity to talk to you alone and then come back together to conclude the consultation. Time is usually at a premium, but there are circumstances where it is essential to talk to each alone, making it clear what aspects of the session are confidential.

How to take a history

The history is usually given by the parents, although you should include the child if old enough. It is important to make the family feel they have your full attention and that you are listening to their concerns. It is also important that you develop a structured approach to make sure that you do not miss important points, but do not make this too rigid as it is sometimes necessary to pursue a different line to elicit important information. Use open questions whenever possible rather than those requiring a simple 'yes' or 'no' (see p. 65, Chapter 4). A suggested approach is shown in Box 5.1.

Box 5.1 What to ask about when taking a history

Presenting complaint	Record the main problems in the family's own words as they describe them
History of presenting complaint	Try to get an exact chronology from the time the child was last completely well. Allow the family to describe events themselves, using questions to direct them, and probe for specific information. Try to use open questions: 'Tell me about the cough' rather than 'Is the cough worse in the mornings?'
Past medical history	Ask about all illnesses, hospital attendances, operations including accidents and admissions
Perinatal history	In young children and infants this should start from the pregnancy and include birthweight and details of the delivery and neonatal period, including any feeding or breathing problems
Developmental history	Ask about milestones and school performance. Are there any areas of concern?
Nutritional history	Ask about infant feeding, weaning and eating difficulties. In older children ask if there are food fads or extreme habits. Ask about food allergies
Immunisations	Identify if immunisations are up to date, and if not, why not?
Drugs and allergies	What medications is the child taking and are there any allergies?
Family history	Who is in the family and who lives at home? Ask about consanguinity, as cousin marriages increase the risk of genetic disorders. Ask if there are any illnesses that run in the family. Does anyone have a disability, and have there been any deaths in childhood? Draw up a family tree (see Figure 5.1)
Social history	Which school or nursery does the child attend? Ask about jobs and smoking, and try to get a feel for the financial situation at home. The social context of illness is very important in paediatrics
Review of systems	Ask screening questions for symptoms within systems other than the presenting system (see Box 5.2)

Presenting complaint(s)   The presenting complaints should be listed initially as a list of simple, one or few word headliners without further detail. A separate section then follows containing the full history. Record the chronology of the presenting complaint in a systematic manner with a heading for each date line starting from when the child was last '100%' or 'their normal self':

■ 4 weeks ago: onset of cough;
■ 3 days ago: sore throat;
■ today: seizure.

Do not write the days of the week in the history as they give no indication of the duration of the disease. It is important that you gain a clear idea in your mind of the chronology of the problem, so make sure you have done so by 'playing back' the history to the family. Each symptom should be thoroughly reviewed with severity, onset and duration over time, exacerbating and relieving factors, quality location and radiation (for pain) and response to any treatment all recorded. Any previous investigations should be detailed.

Previous medical history   The GP's referral letter is often helpful in determining previous visits to the doctor's surgery and details of any medications the child has been given in the past. Ask about all admissions to hospital and operations. Enquire about allergies and determine how severe any previous allergic reactions have been. Ask specifically about asthma, eczema and hay fever.

Perinatal history   Ask about birthweight and the duration of pregnancy. Enquire about screening tests done during pregnancy (like ultrasound or genetic tests), medications and immunisations given, any problems during the pregnancy such as hypertension, smoking, drug ingestion, influenza-like illnesses, and details of the birth, type of delivery and condition at birth. If the mother cannot provide medical details, the following questions are helpful:

■ Did the baby need any special treatment at birth, for example, help with breathing?
■ Was the baby taken away from you after birth? If so, for how long?
■ How long was it before you could feed your baby?
■ How old was the baby when he or she went home?
■ Did the baby suffer from any fits in the newborn period?
■ Did the baby have breathing problems requiring oxygen?

Ask about previous pregnancies and their outcome

Development   A full developmental review should be made (see Chapter 6 for more details). In toddlers ask about socialization and preschool activity. For older children enquire about scholastic achievements, school attendance, and physical activity like sport and youth group membership.

Nutritional history   For babies ask whether the baby has been breast-fed, for how long and if exclusively. If not, why not and what formula was given? Later when tastings and then solids were introduced, and in what order? For toddlers, ask about mealtimes and food fads. Determine if there are any intolerances or feeding difficulties. In older children ask if the diet is varied and balanced. Older children and adolescents may develop unusual habits like food obsessions or exclusions like veganism.

Immunisations   Full immunisation is vital for the child's health. Don't rely on memory, ask to see records like the 'red book'. If immunisations have been missed or refused, enquire why. There may have been good reasons like illness or family circumstance; on the other hand, there is an increasing problem of ideological resistance to immunisations based on ignorance and prejudice, and this may endanger the child and his surroundings.

Family history   You should include a family tree (as shown in Figure 5.1) in your notes.

Ask specifically about:

■ Whether there is a member of the family (including second and third degree relatives) with a similar condition to the problem under review or any medical conditions (fear of these may be unrevealed, and reassurance given).
■ Whether there have been any disabled children or deaths in childhood.
■ Consanguinity. This is particularly common in some ethnic groups, and the family's ethnic and religious identity recorded.
■ Establish how the family works. Who is the main carer? What are the parental occupations? If there is a man in the house, is he the father of the patient and/or the other children? What are living conditions like? Is there economic security? Do the parents work, and if so at what? If not, why not?

Social history   Social problems may strongly influence the health of children in a family. An absent father may be a source of unhappiness and you should find out about the relationship the child has with the natural father. School is another potential source of conflict and anxiety. Bullying may be a particular

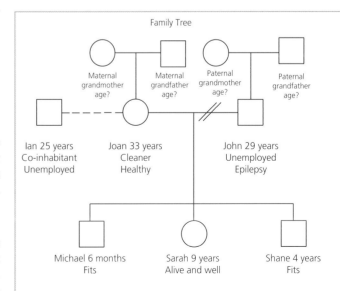

Figure 5.1 Example of a family tree to illustrate family history.

problem which is unknown to the parents. Internet and social media shaming or abuse are now important problems. Find out if the symptoms are related to school days and how much time is missed from school. With adolescents, sexual activity should be sensitively discussed as well as drug and alcohol abuse.

Review of systems   Box 5.2 shows a schema for review of systems. In paediatrics it is not always necessary to run through a full review and the schema can be used judiciously.

Examining the child

When you come to examine the child remember the following principles:

- **Rapport** — Time spent initially gaining the child's confidence is never wasted. With younger children, complimenting them on their shoes or clothes is often a good start

- **Observation** — You should have already gained a good deal of information by informal observation before and while taking the history

- **Undress the child** — The child should usually be undressed down to underwear so that you can maximize your chances of finding physical signs

- **Be systematic** — You need to follow a systematic structure to your examination. Don't dive for your stethoscope but follow the order of:
  - Observation
  - Palpation
  - Percussion
  - Auscultation

  Note that, with the abdomen, auscultation is often done before palpation since spontaneous bowel sounds may be altered by the examination

- **Right side of the bed** — Remember that if you are right-handed you should, where possible, examine the child from the right-hand side of the bed

Older children can be examined like adults, but younger children, particularly if fretful or anxious, must be approached quite differently. Any uncomfortable procedure such as examination of ears and throat should be left until last in order to avoid upsetting the child. It may help if you keep up a 'running commentary' during the examination, asking questions as you go along. However, if the child fails to answer you should immediately move on. Children can become acutely embarrassed by a silence, but may be reassured by continuing chatter.

Box 5.2 Review of systems

General	Activity, tiredness Sleep School absence Weight loss
Cardiovascular	Faints Murmurs Cyanosis
Respiratory	Cough Wheeze
Gastrointestinal	Nutrition Appetite Vomiting Diarrhoea Constipation Abdominal pain
Genitourinary	Enuresis Dysuria Frequency Age at menarche Dysmenorrhoea
ENT	Earache Hearing impairment Recurrent sore throat Enlarged glands
Neurological	Seizures Faints/funny turns Headaches Hearing and vision
Skin	Any lesions or rashes
Musculoskeletal	Joint pain or swelling
Development	Gross motor Fine motor Speech and language Social

To avoid upset, ask the mother to undress the child. Vary your routine to suit the child – it may be necessary to examine the back before the front or the abdomen before the chest. This flexibility in routine means that parts of the examination may get forgotten, but you can avoid this by systematically recording your findings, so that it is immediately obvious if you have overlooked something. Using a standard format helps. Modern computerized systems often require the completion of each item.

Children are sometimes put off by a stethoscope. It is often helpful to put it first on the child's knee, or on a teddy bear, to show that they need not be frightened.

Notes, problem lists and plans of action

When you have taken the history you should write your notes clearly following the systematic approach given above. Take a moment to draw up a provisional problem or issues list.

This allows you to focus on parts of the physical examination that are particularly relevant to the child. Then examine the child and write up your examination in a systematic way, organ system by organ system. Draw up a brief summary paragraph delineating the key points from the history and physical examination.

Now you are in a position to revise your problem list. This should be itemized clearly and should be comprehensive. You should include all the factors taking into account family and school difficulties. For example, a problem list might read:

1. Abdominal pain
2. Constipation
3. Bullying at school
4. Sibling with cerebral palsy
5. Father unemployed

Having developed a problem list, a diagnosis list should be drawn up. This should begin with the most likely diagnosis, followed by important other possibilities (differentials). These will indicate logically what plan of action should follow. Itemize each action so that it is clear to others what you have undertaken to do. Actions should be considered under the following headings:

- Investigations to be carried out
- Treatment initiated
- Plans for follow-up and review

Finally, the parents need a full explanation, which should be recorded in the notes. Ensure that the parents understand what your view of the problem is, agree on what needs to be done and agree if admission is required or when the child should be seen again. It is often helpful to provide information leaflets, and contact for support organisations for families with similar problems where appropriate. If the plan is complicated you should provide the parents with notes, and you should write them a letter outlining what has been decided and what needs to be done.

Hospital notes

Hospital notes serve a number of functions. They are firstly a written record of the consultation and its results. They serve as the principal mode of communication with colleagues and for later review. They are also a legal record. In the past it was important that notes were clearly written and legible, but today computerised notes are almost universal.

The initial intake notes should be laid out as described above. Follow-up notes during admission or in the outpatient clinic should also be structured. It is usually most helpful if these notes follow the format of the problem list. Some doctors use the 'SOAP' method of recording: for each problem they comment on:

- **S**ymptom or Subjective
- **O**bservation or Objective
- **A**ssessment
- **P**lan

An approach to examination

The remainder of this chapter provides you with a system by system approach to examining children, along with an explanation of how to elicit signs and interpret them.

 ## Growth (see accompanying video clip 1)

Accurate measurement of height, weight and head circumference is a vital part of the assessment of all children referred for a medical opinion. Growth can only accurately be assessed by taking at least two measurements of each growth parameter (length, weight and head circumference) and plotting where the points fall on a growth chart appropriate for the child's age and sex.

Weight

Use a weighing scale that has been calibrated accurately. Infants should be laid in a pannier scale and older children weighed standing up. Babies should be weighed naked without a nappy, and older children in light clothing without shoes or (preferably) underwear only.

Height and length

The measurement of height should be precise; it is only accurate if made with care using the appropriate equipment.

In the first 2 years of life, length is measured on a measuring frame or mat (Figure 5.2). From the age of 2, providing the child can stand, height is measured against a specially calibrated standing frame. Consistent technique is necessary to estimate standing height accurately (Figure 5.3). Check the heels are against the wall and the feet flat on the floor with the knees straight. Gently extend the neck and ensure the eyes are in line with the external auditory meatus.

Head (occipitofrontal) circumference (OFC)

This should be measured accurately to the nearest millimetre. Use a flexible, non-stretchable tape measure and measure

around the OFC. Take three successive measurements at slightly different points. The greatest is taken to be the OFC (Figure 5.4).

Growth standards

In order to interpret a child's growth, comparison must be made with population standards. These standards are presented in the form of growth charts, which demonstrate the population's

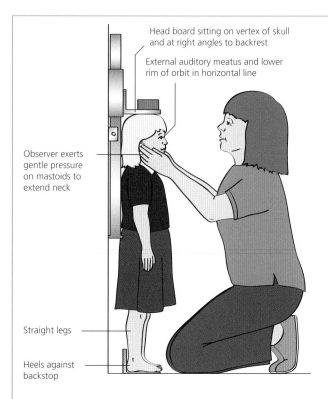

Head board sitting on vertex of skull and at right angles to backrest

External auditory meatus and lower rim of orbit in horizontal line

Observer exerts gentle pressure on mastoids to extend neck

Straight legs

Heels against backstop

Figure 5.3 Measurement of standing height.

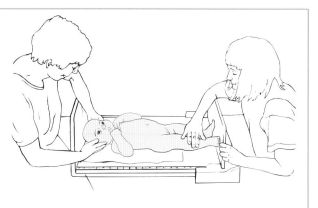

Figure 5.2 Measurement of length using a frame.

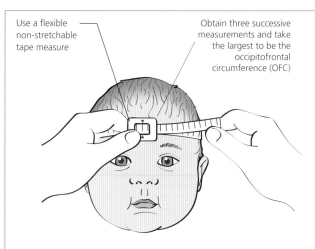

Use a flexible non-stretchable tape measure

Obtain three successive measurements and take the largest to be the occipitofrontal circumference (OFC)

Figure 5.4 Measurement of head circumference.

growth as centiles. The growth charts currently in use in the UK are the 1990 UK Child Growth Standards, which were constructed from detailed data collected on children across the country. In 2009 the charts for children aged 0–4 years were updated. They now utilize World Health Organization data, based on the growth of healthy breast-fed babies, rather than bottle-fed babies as previously.

Separate charts are available for girls and boys. Age is given along the *x* axis, which, depending on the chart, may be shown in months or decimally. Height, length, weight and head circumference measurements lie along the *y* axis. Nine centiles ranging from the 99.6th to the 0.4th centile are shown as continuous or dotted lines (Figures 5.5–5.7). Body mass index (BMI) should be calculated if there is any concern about weight. This is calculated from the equation:

$$BMI = \text{weight in kg}/(\text{height in metres})^2$$

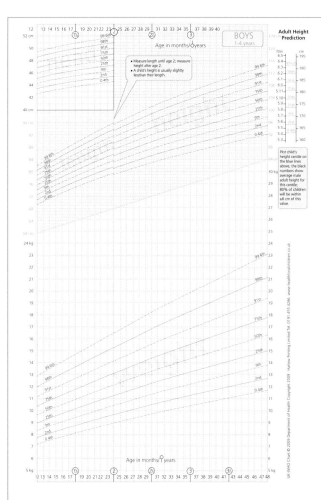

Figure 5.6 UK-WHO growth chart for children aged 1–4 years. *Source*: © 2009 Department of Health.

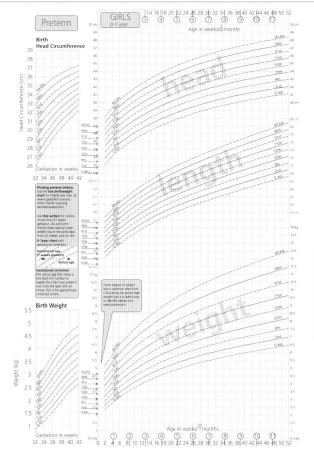

Figure 5.5 UK-WHO growth chart showing a baby's growth at 28 weeks' gestation until 1 year, corrected for prematurity. *Source*: © DH copyright 2009. New charts for children aged 0–4 years were introduced in the UK in 2009. They are now based on the growth of healthy breast-fed babies.

Plotting a child's growth (see Box 5.3)

In order to interpret children's growth measurements, they must be plotted on the appropriate growth chart. If the child was born prematurely, two points are plotted up to the age of 2 years: the child's actual age and the corrected age (post-term age) are connected by an arrow. Special charts are available for children with genetic syndromes like Down, Turner and Achondroplasia.

The centile along which the point falls relates the child's growth to the rest of the population. Thus, if a boy's weight falls on the 50th centile, he is average, and 50% of the population will be heavier and 50% lighter than him. If his height falls on the 9th centile, he is relatively short with 91% of the population taller and only 9% smaller.

The further a child's growth falls away from the normal population, the more likely it is that he or she has a problem.

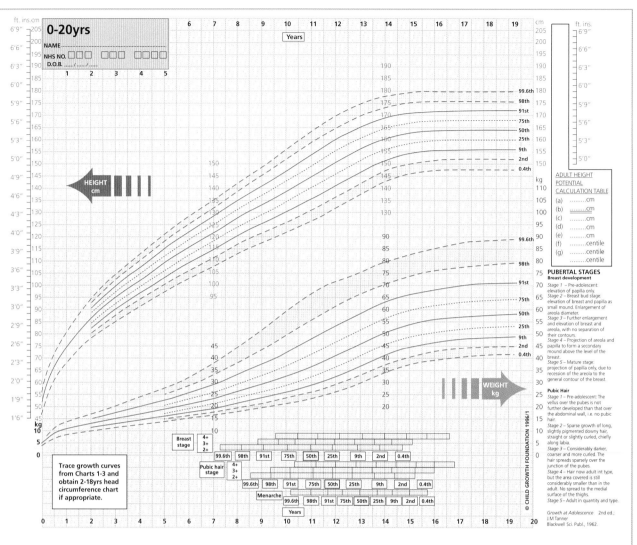

Figure 5.7 UK 1990 growth chart for children aged up to 20 years. *Source*: © 2012/13 Royal College of Paediatrics and Child Health.

Box 5.3 Principles of plotting a child's growth

- Mark the child's measurement with a dot (not a cross or circle)
- If a baby is born prematurely, indicate corrected (post-term) age up to the age of 2 years
- Assess the *rate* of growth by measuring on two occasions at least 4–6 months apart
- Plateauing of growth and weight, or heights below the 0.4th centile, merit evaluation (see p. 280)
- A child's final height is expected to fall midway between the parent's centile lines

Thus, measures falling between the 0.4th and 2nd centiles may be normal, whereas those below the 0.4th centile are more likely to be abnormal. Furthermore, crossing centiles over time is concerning (other than in the first 2 years or at

puberty) and needs evaluation. Interpretation of growth in babyhood and at puberty is important and requires skill. Values for BMI should be plotted in the UK on the UK 1990 BMI charts, which have waist circumference charts on the reverse (see Figure 5.8).

Interpretation of growth charts

After the first 2 years of life, children usually grow steadily along the same centile, but infants in the first few months of life may follow a centile quite different to their subsequent growth centiles. It is important to relate the height to weight and head circumference and so gain an idea of the child's build. In general children reach a final height midway between their parents' centiles. This is sometimes called target height and can either be simply estimated from the parents' positions on the charts or calculated using the formula given on the growth charts. Interpretation of children's patterns of growth is discussed in Chapter 15.

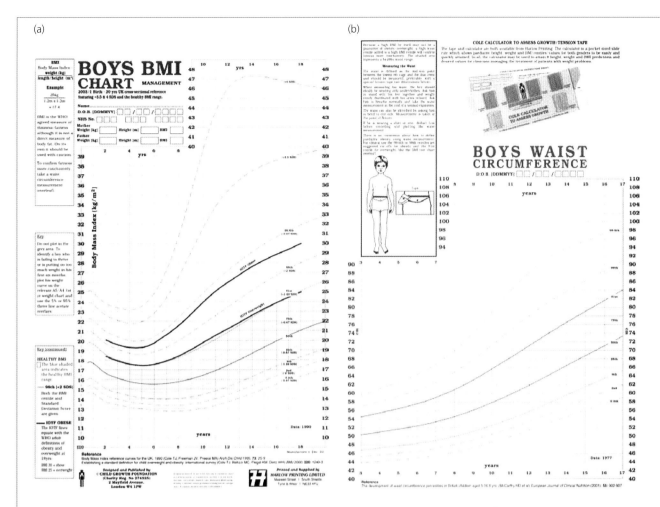

Figure 5.8 UK BMI and waist circumference charts, used for the assessment of obesity. A child whose BMI is above the 98th centile is considered obese, and one with a BMI between the 91st and 98th centile is overweight. *Source*: © 2012/13 Royal College of Paediatrics and Child Health.

 ## General observation (see accompanying video clip 2)

Much can be learnt by watching children while they are being undressed and how they play. Observation starts from before and after the family enters the room, and should not be confined to the physical examination.

Formal observation should include:

- *Well or ill?* The first point to note is whether the child looks ill or well. Is she full of energy or does she prefer to cuddle up against her parent? Does she appear flushed, dehydrated, apathetic or irritable?
- *Dysmorphism* Look for evidence of dysmorphic features or asymmetry. This may be obvious if there are major anomalies, or you may simply have a sense that the features are unusual.
- *Colour* Examine the lips and tongue for central cyanosis and pallor. Evert the lower eyelid to assess the colour of the mucosal membrane for anaemia or the conjunctiva for jaundice.
- *Sounds* Is there noisy breathing, wheezing, stridor, dry or productive cough, hoarseness?

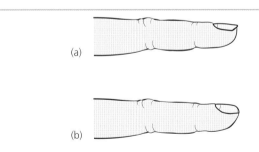

Figure 5.9 Nail bed angle: (a) normal and (b) clubbing.

- *Hands* Examine the hands. Look at the palmar creases, and the nail beds for colour (cyanosis, anaemia). Look for clubbing. The most sensitive way to detect early clubbing is to look at the profile of the nail bed, as the normal nailbed angle is lost very early in the clubbing process (Figure 5.9). You can also appose the index finger nails, nail facing nail. In clubbing you do not see light between the nails. The commoner causes of clubbing are listed in Table 5.1.

Table 5.1 Commoner causes of finger clubbing

Familial	Benign condition
Cardiovascular disease	Cyanotic heart disease, e.g. Fallot tetralogy
Respiratory disease	Chronic suppurative lung disease, e.g. cystic fibrosis
Bowel disease	Chronic inflammatory bowel disease, e.g. ulcerative colitis

Cardiovascular examination (see accompanying video clip 3 and downloadable check sheet)

Observation

When you examine the cardiovascular system (Box 5.4), make sure you take note of growth, as significant heart disease restricts growth and weight gain. Cyanosis is a major sign of cardiovascular disease. It also occurs as the result of respiratory disease, and you should examine both systems sequentially. Central cyanosis is always abnormal and determined by examining the tongue. Lips and fingers may be blue because of non-cardiac causes such as cold, and are not uncommon in babies. Anaemia and clubbing can both be seen by examining the child's hands. Dyspnoea and tachypnoea may be due to cardiac as well as other causes.

Check if the child is pale or sweating as these are further signs of heart failure. Pectus carinatum (see Figure 5.15) is the only abnormal shape associated with heart disease.

Palpation

Pulse

Examine the radial, femoral, brachial and carotid pulses for rate, rhythm, character and volume. It is easier to assess the right brachial pulse in young children than the radial.

- *Rate.* The rate should be timed over 15 seconds and converted to a rate per minute. Normal heart rate depends on the child's age (Table 5.2).
- *Rhythm.* Children often have sinus arrhythmia, where the heart rate varies with the respiratory cycle, and this is normal. Occasional ectopic beats are also normal in children.
- *Pulse character.* This is detected by the pulse volume. A *collapsing pulse* (*waterhammer pulse*) occurs with a wide pulse pressure, most usually in children with patent ductus arteriosus. The increased pulse volume is best felt by elevating the limb. A *slow rising pulse* has a slow upstroke and rapid fall off. It is caused by left ventricular outflow obstruction.
- *Volume.* Is the pulse full, or weak and thready, as in shock?
- *Radiofemoral delay.* It is always important to compare the radial or brachial pulse in the right arm with the femoral pulse. In coarctation of the aorta, either the pulse in the right limb is felt before the femoral (or left radial pulse) or the femoral pulse is absent.

Box 5.4 Bedside checklist for examining the cardiovascular system

Growth Measure the child and plot on to centile charts
Observation Look for
- ☐ Central cyanosis
- ☐ Anaemia
- ☐ Breathlessness
- ☐ Chest shape and scars
- ☐ Clubbing

Palpation
- ☐ Pulse
  - rate
  - rhythm
  - character
  - volume
- ☐ Absent or delayed femoral pulse
- ☐ Praecordium
  - parasternal heave (? right ventricular hypertrophy)
  - thrills
  - apex beat (? left ventricular hypertrophy)
- ☐ Hepatomegaly
- ☐ Oedema
- ☐ Capillary refill

Auscultation
- ☐ Heart sounds
- ☐ Murmurs
  - systolic or diastolic?
  - character
  - grade
  - site of maximum intensity
  - radiation

Blood pressure
- ☐ Right arm
- ☐ 4 limbs if BP raised

Table 5.2 Range of heart rates in normal children

Age	Normal heart rate (beats per minute)
<3 months	100–180
3–24 months	80–150
2–10 years	70–110
>10 years	55–90

Praecordium

- *Parasternal heave.* Right ventricular hypertrophy can be detected by placing the palm of your hand over the lower half of the sternum (Figure 5.10). An abnormal impulse is felt by a heaving sensation under the heel of your hand.

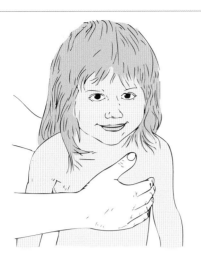

Figure 5.10 Position to place hand to assess for a parasternal heave.

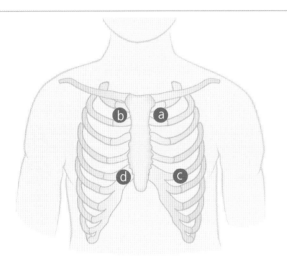

Figure 5.11 Valve areas: (a) pulmonary, (b) aortic, (c) mitral, (d) tricuspid.

- *A thrill.* A thrill is a palpable murmur felt as a vibration and is always abnormal. Place your fingertips over the four valve areas and in the suprasternal notch (Figure 5.11).
- *Apex beat.* Place your hand over the chest with the fingertips in the anterior axillary line (Figure 5.12). The maximal lateral impulse is found with one fingertip. Define its position by counting down the ribs starting at the sternal angle, which corresponds to the second rib. The apex beat is normally in the mid-clavicular line in the fifth intercostal space (fourth interspace in children less than 5 years old). A forceful apex or displacement of the apex to the left suggests left ventricular hypertrophy or lung disease distorting the mediastinal position.

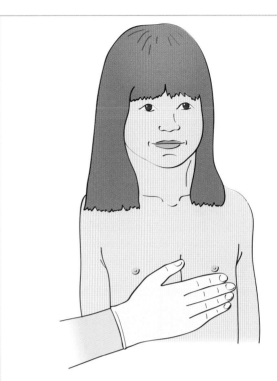

Figure 5.12 Palpation of the apex beat by the index finger.

Liver

Palpate the lower edge of the liver and percuss the upper edge (see p. 82–3). Hepatomegaly suggests heart failure.

Ankle oedema

Look for pitting oedema, although peripheral oedema and raised jugular venous pressure (JVP) are rarely seen in children.

Capillary refill

Poor skin perfusion is a sign of shock. Apply moderate pressure with your finger on a warm periphery for 5 seconds and watch for the colour to return. The normal capillary refill time is up to 2 seconds; a time longer than this is suggestive of poor peripheral circulation or otherwise shock.

Auscultation

Auscultate carefully with both the bell and the diaphragm of the stethoscope. The bell is particularly important in picking up low-pitched murmurs. Listen first for heart sounds and then for murmurs. Listen in the four valve areas (see Figure 5.11) and over the axillae, carotids and back.

Heart sounds

The first heart sound is heard when the mitral and tricuspid valves close and the second when the aortic and pulmonary valves close. When the child breathes in, blood is sucked into the right side of the heart and right pulmonary ejection is prolonged, causing the pulmonary valve to close slightly after the aortic valve. During expiration the two valves close together. Normally, you can hear 'splitting' of the second heart sound in the pulmonary area on inspiration. This is an important sign in paediatric cardiology, and it is worth effort in mastering it. In an atrial septal defect (ASD) there is wide and fixed splitting of the second heart sound (i.e. it does not vary with respiration). Unlike many other congenital lesions, ASD is not usually associated with a a noticeable murmur, yet the consequences of missing it can be very serious. A loud and single second heart sound is heard with a large left-to-right shunt (e.g. a ventricular septal defect) and a soft single sound or paradoxical splitting (widening in expiration rather than inspiration) in significant aortic stenosis. Listen for added sounds such as gallop rhythm in heart failure or ejection click in aortic stenosis.

Murmurs (see also p. 218)

Murmurs are caused by turbulence of blood flow and may be innocent or pathological. If you hear a murmur:

- check for radiation in the axilla, over the carotid arteries and the back
- listen again in inspiration and expiration
- listen with the child lying down and sitting up
- turn the child on the left side, as some murmurs change with position.

Murmurs can be graded according to their loudness and presence of a thrill (see Table 5.3), but the loudness may not correlate with severity. The murmur may occur during systole or diastole. Systolic murmurs may be either ejection (diamond-shaped in intensity) or pansystolic (Figure 5.13). Diastolic murmurs are always pathological, and are caused by increased blood flow through a normal atrioventricular valve, narrowing (stenosis) of an atrioventricular valve or incompetence (leak) of the pulmonary or aortic valves.

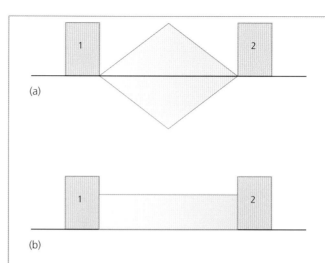

Figure 5.13 Shape of cardiac murmurs: (a) ejection systolic murmur and (b) pansystolic murmur. 1, 2 denote the first and second heart sounds.

Describe the murmur according to the following characteristics:

- Is it systolic or diastolic?
- Character – is it blowing or harsh?
- The grade
- The site of maximum intensity
- The radiation

Most murmurs in children are innocent and you should be able to distinguish them from a pathological murmur (see p. 218).

Blood pressure

Measuring the child's blood pressure (BP) is an essential part of the physical examination, but it is left until last to avoid upsetting younger children. Use an appropriately sized cuff – it should be wide enough to cover two-thirds of the upper arm and the bladder should completely encircle the arm. It is important to have a range of cuff sizes available in every paediatric clinic.

Oscillometric and electronic devices to measure BP non-invasively are now readily available and are easily used even on the smallest child. It is still important to choose the appropriate cuff size. Systolic diastolic and pulse pressures should be recorded.

Table 5.3 Grading of cardiac murmurs. Grades 1 and 2 are usually innocent, grades 5 and 6 are always significant and grades 3 and 4 are suspect

	Murmur	Thrill
Grade 1	Barely audible	None
Grade 2	Soft and variable in nature	None
Grade 3	Easily heard	None
Grade 4	Loud	Present
Grade 5	Very loud	Present
Grade 6	Heard without a stethoscope	Present

🔑 Key points: The cardiovascular system

- Sinus arrhythmia is normal in children
- Radiofemoral delay or absent femoral pulses are always abnormal
- A systolic ejection murmur denotes no cardiac pathology in at least 50% of cases
- A thrill is always abnormal

Table 5.4 Upper limit of normal (above 2 standard deviations from the norm) for systolic blood pressure through childhood

Age of child	Abnormal systolic pressure (mmHg)
Neonate	90
1–12 months	100
1–5 years	110
6–9 years	120
10–12 years	130
13–14 years	140

If a raised BP is consistently obtained in the right arm, the BP should then be measured in all four limbs. Sometimes BP is measured on standing (postural hypotension).

The upper limit of normal for blood pressure in childhood is shown in Table 5.4.

Respiratory system (see accompanying video clip 4)

In children, interpretation of physical signs relating to the respiratory system requires care (Box 5.5). Obvious sounds on auscultation may indicate no significant disease, whereas the child with more subtle signs, such as tachypnoea and intercostal recession, is likely to have a significant respiratory condition even if auscultation is unremarkable.

Observation

Respiratory distress

Observe the child for signs of respiratory distress. Is there an audible wheeze or stridor? Is the voice hoarse? Is there tachypnoea, use of accessory muscles, nasal flaring or recession? Expiratory grunting is a particularly worrying sign associated with severe respiratory distress. Cough if present should be carefully assessed. Is it brassy and dry, as in laryngitis, or wet and productive as in pneumonia? Is it repetitive and short (as in bronchiolitis) or prolonged and spasmodic, perhaps followed by a 'whooping' sound, as in Pertussis? Parents can be encouraged to record cough on a smartphone to aid the physician. The sites of chest recession are shown in Figure 5.14. Restlessness and drowsiness suggest hypoxia/hypercapnoea (increase in pCO_2). Count the respirations when the child is quiet, preferably asleep. A raised respiratory rate may be the single most sensitive sign of significant respiratory pathology in paediatrics. The respiratory rate varies with age and is shown in Table 5.5.

Signs of chronic disease

Examine the hands for clubbing, cyanosis or anaemia. The causes of clubbing are shown in Table 5.1.

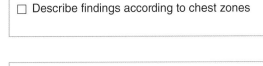

Box 5.5 Bedside checklist for examining the respiratory system

Observation Look for
- ☐ Restlessness or drowsiness
- ☐ Abnormal shape of the chest
- ☐ Count the respiratory rate
- ☐ Audible respiratory sounds
- ☐ Signs of respiratory distress
  - subcostal/intercostal recession
  - use of accessory muscles
  - nasal flaring
  - tachypnoea
- ☐ Cyanosis and anaemia
- ☐ Clubbing

Palpation
- ☐ Mediastinal deviation
  - tracheal position
  - apex beat
- ☐ Chest expansion

Percussion
- ☐ For resonance
- ☐ To define the upper edge of liver dullness

Auscultation
- ☐ Listen for
  - breath sounds
  - any adventitious noises (crepitations, wheezing)
  - tactile vocal fremitus and vocal resonance
- ☐ Describe findings according to chest zones

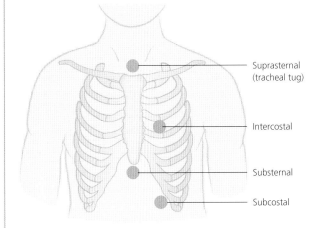

Figure 5.14 Sites of chest recession in a young child with respiratory distress.

Describe the chest shape. The commoner abnormalities are illustrated in Figure 5.15: barrel chest (because of air trapping) has an increased anteroposterior diameter and is best observed

Table 5.5 Normal respiratory rate at different ages

Age	Awake respiratory rate (breaths per minute)
0–12 months	25–40
1–5 years	20–30
6 years and above	15–25

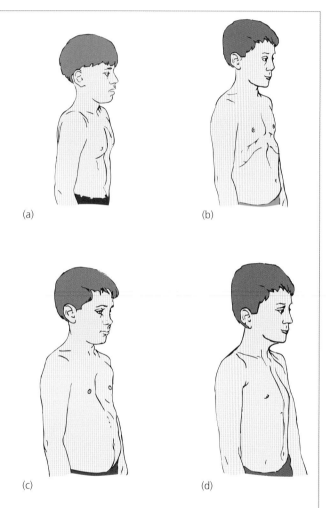

Figure 5.15 Commoner types of chest wall deformity: (a) barrel chest, (b) Harrison's sulcus, (c) pectus excavatum and (d) pectus carinatum.

by looking at the chest from the side. Harrison's sulcus is caused by diaphragmatic overactivity and is shown by grooves parallel to and 2–3 cm above the costal margin. It is seen in chronic asthma. Pectus excavatum (also known as funnel chest) and pectus carinatum (also known as pigeon chest) are relatively common and may cause concern due to their cosmetic appearance, but are usually not associated with underlying respiratory disease.

Chest asymmetry

Look to see if one half of the chest is more prominent. This may be a result of scoliosis and is assessed by examining the spine (pp. 94).

Palpation

Mediastinal deviation

Look for deviation of the trachea and the cardiac apex beat. The tracheal position is palpated by identifying the trachea in the suprasternal notch between two fingers (Figure 5.16). The trachea is in the midline and any deviation may be a sign of serious disease. The apex impulse is detected by the method described on p. 77. Dextrocardia can be associated with chronic chest problems due to primary ciliary dyskinesia.

Chest expansion

Place your hands on the child's chest with your thumbs just touching at the sternum and your fingers lightly resting on the skin over the ribs (Figure 5.17). Ask the child to take a deep breath – the distance your thumbs move apart gives the degree of chest expansion. In a 5-year-old, 1 cm or more is normal.

Percussion

The degree of resonance is assessed by percussion. Place the middle finger of your left hand (if you are right-handed) along the line of the rib and strike the middle phalanx with the first finger of the right hand as if it were a hammer hitting a small nail. Percuss the entire chest back and front in a systematic way, including the clavicles and in the axillae. The percussion note should be resonant across the chest, with normal liver dullness starting just below the nipple.

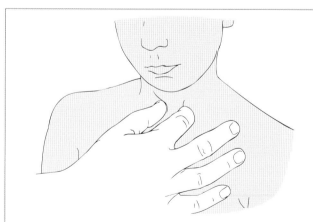

Figure 5.16 Examining the position of the trachea.

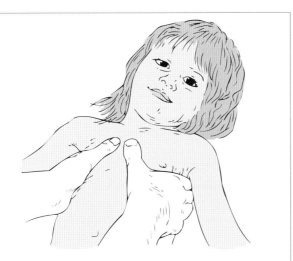

Figure 5.17 Assessing chest expansion.

- *Hyper-resonance* occurs with hyperinflation due to air trapping, particularly seen in chronic asthma or emphysema. Unilateral hyper-resonance is found in pneumo-thorax.
- *Dullness* to percussion is found in consolidation or lung collapse.
- *Stony dullness* occurs with pleural effusion.
  Percussion is not very useful in children below 1 year of age.

Auscultation

Ask the child to breathe in and out through the mouth, or wait until the child is quiet in younger patients. Upper airway sounds are often transmitted over the whole chest in children, but asking the child to cough may clear them. Listen for breath sounds using the diaphragm of the stethoscope. Start at the top of the chest, comparing one side with the other, and then listen over the back and axillae in a similar way. In young children, sounds transmitted from the upper airway may be confused with lower respiratory sounds, particularly wheezes. It may help to listen first to the noise of breathing without the stethoscope. Sometimes, when the upper airway sounds are soft, applying the stethoscope close to the child's mouth, nose or larynx may help to clarify whether the sounds are coming from the upper airway or the chest itself.

Breath sounds

Normal breath sounds are called *vesicular* and there is no distinct interval between inspiration and expiration. *Bronchial breathing* has a distinct break and has a harsher sound; it is heard normally over the trachea, but also occurs pathologically with pneumonia. Reduced breath sounds are a common, sometimes the only, finding in childhood pneumonia and obstruction, for example by an inhaled foreign body.

Added sounds

Crepitations (crackles) sound like the soft rustling of leaves. These are heard with acute consolidation and chronic bronchiectasis, but may clear after coughing. *Rhonchi* (wheezes) indicate bronchial narrowing as heard in asthma and bronchiolitis. They are usually expiratory. Inspiratory stridor is transmitted from the trachea or larynx.

Absent breath sounds

An absence of breath sounds in one area suggests pleural effusion, pneumothorax or dense consolidation.

Tactile vocal fremitus and vocal resonance

If you find signs of consolidation, examine for vocal fremitus and resonance by palpating and listening when the child says 'ninety-nine'. The sounds and vibration are increased over an area of consolidation and decreased or absent over effusion or collapse.

Location in the chest

If you detect any physical signs you should describe them according to their location in the chest (see Figure 5.18).

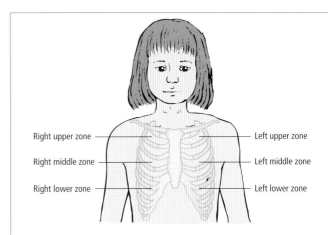

Right upper zone — Left upper zone
Right middle zone — Left middle zone
Right lower zone — Left lower zone

Figure 5.18 How to describe the location of physical signs in the chest.

Key points: The respiratory system

- In children, the observation of respiratory distress is more important than auscultatory findings
- The respiratory rate in infants is normally faster than in older children
- Percussion and auscultation may be unreliable in delineating consolidation in young children
- In children, transmitted sounds from the upper airways may be easily confused with adventitious sounds

The abdomen (see accompanying video clip 5)

This section describes how to examine the abdomen if there is no acute problem (Box 5.6). The child with an 'acute abdomen' requires a different approach, which is described on pp. 196–7.

A particularly important part of examining the gastrointestinal system is to plot the child's height and weight on a centile chart, as this is a critically important measure of gastrointestinal function.

Box 5.6 Bedside checklist for examining the abdomen

Growth Measure the child and plot on to centile charts

Observation Look for
- ☐ General appearance
- ☐ Clubbing
- ☐ Jaundice and anaemia
- ☐ Oedema
- ☐ Mouth
- ☐ Spider naevi
- ☐ Wasted buttocks
- ☐ Abdominal distension

Palpation
- ☐ Ask if the abdomen is tender
- ☐ Palpate lightly for obvious masses, deeply for other masses
  - • liver
  - • spleen
  - • kidneys
  - • groin (for hernia)

Percussion
- ☐ For resonance
- ☐ To define the upper edge of liver dullness ascites
  - • shifting dullness
  - • fluid thrill

Auscultation
- ☐ Note absent or tinkling bowel sounds

Rectal and Genital examination
- ☐ Not routinely performed
- ☐ Inspect visually genito-perineal area
- ☐ In males check penis for rash, discharge, phimosis and hypospadias
- ☐ In males check scrotum for undescended testes, swelling, tenderness and crimasteric reflex (absent in torsion of testis)
- ☐ In young females check vulva for trauma, worms, rash or foreign body

Stool and urine specimens
- ☐ Describe findings according to site in the abdomen

Record findings

In order to examine the abdomen, you must make sure the child is relaxed, otherwise the abdominal muscles contract and palpation becomes difficult. If necessary, small children can be examined on their parent's lap. Older children should lie on a couch. You should be at eye level with the abdomen, which may mean kneeling beside the couch. It may be necessary to examine some children standing up, if the alternative is to have them crying when lying down.

Observation

Look for the following signs:
- *Jaundice and anaemia*. Look at the sclerae and conjunctiva. The colour of the urine should also be observed (p. 114).
- *Oedema*. This has many causes but in relation to the abdomen it may be a feature of renal, bowel or liver disease. In children it is first noticed in the face, and the mother may remark on puffy features. Unlike oedema in adults, it is not usually seen in the feet or over the sacrum.
- *Mouth*. Check the state of the teeth and mucous membranes, and any abnormal smell
- *Skin lesions.* Pruritus is a common feature of cholestatic jaundice, and scratch marks may be very obvious. Look for palmar erythema and spider naevi, seen in children with chronic liver disease. These are small surface blood vessels that radiate out from a central point and sometimes resemble a small red spider. They blanch on pressure on the central point (unlike petechial haemorrhages) and then rapidly refill once the pressure is removed.
- *Wasted buttocks*. Look for loose skin folds over the buttocks, which suggest recent significant weight loss.
- *Abdominal distension*. Any distension (either generalised or localized) and visible peristalsis should be noted in particular. Remember that toddlers normally have a protuberant abdomen because of an exaggerated lordosis and relaxed abdominal musculature. Remember the 5 'F's of abdominal distension: fat, fluid, faeces, flatus, fetus.
- *Hernias*. Umbilical herniae are common particularly in black infants. These usually require no treatment as they rarely obstruct or incarcerate. Examine the groin for the bulge of an inguinal hernia or maldescended testes (see p. 341 and p. 342).
- The lower spine, buttocks and peri-anal area should be inspected for lesions.

Palpation

The aim of palpation is to see if there is tenderness, any masses, or enlargement of the liver, spleen or kidneys. Before touching the child, you should warm your hands and ask if there is any tenderness. Get down to the child's level and watch the child's face for any grimacing or wincing in response to pain. Palpate lightly first and then more deeply, using two or four fingers depending on the child's size. All four quadrants should be palpated in turn and then the peri-umbilical area.

Liver

In children under 2 years old, one can normally palpate the liver 1–2 cm below the right costal margin. The edge should be

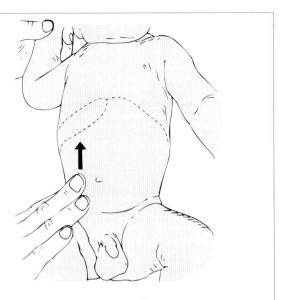

Figure 5.19 Palpation for an enlarged liver.

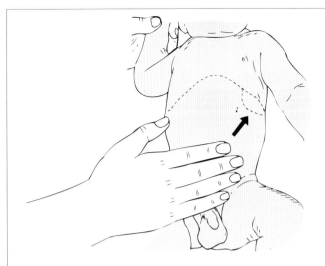

Figure 5.20 Palpation for an enlarged spleen.

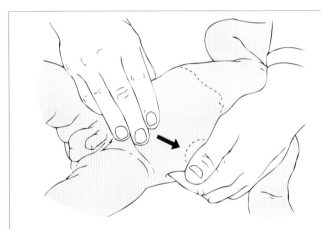

Figure 5.21 Bimanual examination for a moderately enlarged spleen.

smooth and rubbery but not hard or tender. It enlarges down to the right iliac fossa, so start in the right lower quadrant. Use your right hand and palpate with the lateral side of your whole right index finger (see Figure 5.19). Gradually move your hand up towards the right costal margin until you feel the liver edge. If the child is fretful, it may help to place his or her hand under your own and palpate through it. You can confirm liver size by percussing the upper and lower borders. The liver may appear to be large if there is lung over-inflation or if there is a normal variant 'Riedel' right lobe.

Spleen

A normal spleen tip often may be palpated in young infants. Usually the spleen is only modestly enlarged and palpable just under the left costal margin. As it enlarges it extends towards the right iliac fossa. There are two useful techniques to increase the chance of detecting a modestly enlarged spleen.

Start palpating in the right iliac fossa and move your hand up towards the left costal margin (see Figure 5.20), asking the child to take deep breaths. On inspiration you can feel a large spleen being pushed down towards your hand. You can also turn the child on to his or her right side towards you, causing the spleen to drop towards your right hand (see Figure 5.21).

Kidneys

Examine the kidneys by bimanual palpation. Place one hand on the loin and press upwards. Place the other on the abdomen and palpate firmly ('ballottement'). You should be able to feel an enlarged kidney. The lower pole of the right kidney may also be felt in thin, healthy individuals.

Other masses

Carefully palpate for other masses and check for constipation, which you can feel as an indentable mass in the left iliac fossa.

Hernias

Check if there is a hernia present (see p. 341).

Percussion

Percuss the entire abdomen. The note is normally resonant, but hyper-resonant if the bowel is distended with gas. It is dull over the liver and spleen, and their size can be checked this way. It is also dull over a full bladder.

Ascites

Ascites is suspected if you find dullness on percussion in the flanks and a resonant note in the midline. Confirm this by looking for:
- *Shifting dullness*. Roll the child over onto his or her side and percuss in the midline again. If the note is now dull, this indicates that ascitic fluid has shifted with the child's position to give a dull note.
- *A fluid thrill*. Place your hands on either side of the abdomen. Flick your finger on one side. You can feel the movement of

the fluid against your other hand when ascites is present. The thrill can be blocked by asking the parent or child to place their hand firmly in the midline.

Auscultation

Auscultation is useful in children with an acute abdomen (p. 196). The bowel sounds are absent if there is ileus, and increased or tinkling if there is bowel obstruction.

Rectal examination

This is not routinely performed in children, and if needed must be left until last. Look at the anus for fissures or signs of trauma. Lubricate the tip of your index finger and press it flat against the edge of the anus before insertion – this causes less discomfort than inserting direct into the centre of the orifice. Use your little finger for infants. Rectal examination is done to detect impacted stool, worms, blood or mucus, masses or tenderness.

You may need to examine the stool or urine specimens.

Location in the abdomen

Describe any symptoms or signs according to their location in the abdomen (see Figure 5.22).

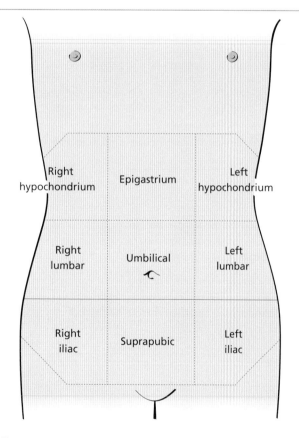

Figure 5.22 How to describe the location of physical signs in the abdomen.

 Key points: The abdomen

- A protuberant abdomen is normal in toddlers
- Light palpation precedes deep palpation to assess areas that are acutely painful
- The liver edge is normally palpable in children below 2 years
- An underdeveloped scrotum suggests undescended testes

Reticuloendothelial system

The reticuloendothelial system consists of the lymph glands, the liver and the spleen. Lymph node enlargement is very common and is usually due to local infection. In preschool children, small, 'shotty' (usually no larger than the size of a pea), firm, mobile and discrete glands are common. If one gland is enlarged, you should check for lymphadenopathy elsewhere and hepatosplenomegaly. Describe a large node in terms of:

- **Size**
- **Position**
- **Texture** – is it hard or rubbery?
- **Mobility** – is it mobile or fixed to other tissues?

General

Look for anaemia and jaundice (Box 5.7).

Neck (see also swellings in the neck, pp. 139–40)

The sternomastoid muscle divides the neck into the anterior and posterior triangles. Examine the lymph nodes in these two

---

Box 5.7 Bedside checklist for examining the reticuloendothelial system

General
- ☐ Anaemia
- ☐ Jaundice

Lymph nodes
- ☐ Neck
- ☐ Axillae
- ☐ Groin
  - size
  - position
  - texture
  - mobility

Focus of infection
- ☐ Throat
- ☐ Limbs

Liver

Spleen

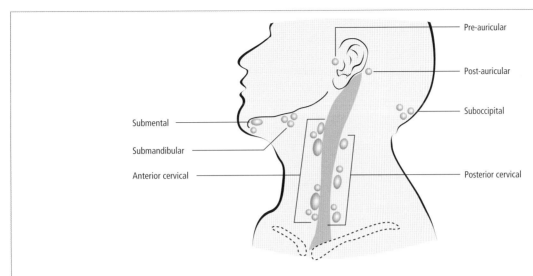

Figure 5.23 The cervical lymph nodes.

Pre-auricular

Post-auricular

Suboccipital

Posterior cervical

Submental

Submandibular

Anterior cervical

triangles (see Figure 5.23). Stand in front of the child to feel the pre- and post-auricular nodes, occipital nodes and those along the anterior cervical chain. Place your hands at the angle of the jaw and work them forward and down. Stand behind the child to feel the submental, submandibular and posterior cervical nodes.

Remember to examine the throat if you find cervical lymphadenopathy. Small cervical nodes may be felt in healthy children between 1 and 5 years and are usually of no significance. Supra-clavicular nodes are always abnormal. Enlarged cervical glands are most commonly caused by tonsil or, less commonly, middle ear infection, and both should be carefully examined. Occipital nodes enlarge as a result of scalp infection (eczema is a common cause), and rubella, now a very rare disease, classically causes posterior auricular and occipital node enlargement.

Axillae

Examine the axillae with the child sitting facing you. Support the child's flexed arm at the elbow, with your left hand holding the right arm. Place your right hand in the right axilla and feel for the presence of enlarged nodes against the chest wall. Reverse the process for the other side.

If there is lymphadenopathy check the hands or arms for a focus of infection.

Groin

Lie the child down and gently palpate the groin for enlarged nodes. They are usually small, discreet and mobile.

If they are enlarged, look for infection in the feet or legs.

Hepatosplenomegaly

Look for liver and spleen enlargement as described in the section on the abdomen.

 Key points: Lymph node enlargement

- *'Shotty' mobile nodes:* are common and of no concern
- *If one gland is found to be enlarged:* carefully examine for lymphadenopathy elsewhere
- *If lymphadenopathy is generalised:* examine for hepatosplenomegaly; blood tests are essential

Genitalia (see accompanying video clip 7)

This is a sensitive area but must not be neglected. In school age and older children the genitalia should be examined only with consent and then usually only visually inspected, unless a particular issue arises. Younger children usually require a formal examination.

Observation

The perineum, groin and external genitalia in both sexes should be assessed for rashes, signs of trauma, swelling or malformations. In males the penis should be assessed specifically for hypospadias and phimosis, and the scrotum for its symmetry and development. An underdeveloped scrotum is found in undescended testis. An absent crimasteric reflex indicates torsion of the testis. In young females, the vulva should be examined for worms, discharge, residue or foreign bodies such as retained tissue paper.

Palpation

Palpate the testes with warm hands. If you cannot feel them, they may have retracted, or they may be undescended. Retracted testes can usually be milked down from the inguinal area into the scrotum. If you are unsuccessful, it may help to examine the child squatting or sitting cross-legged (see Figure 2.5, p. 31) or in a warm bath.

Swelling in the groin is usually caused by enlarged lymph nodes, hernia or a gonad (see also p. 341). You should be able to distinguish them clinically. An *inguinal hernia* extends into the groin and the testis is palpable separate from the swelling. In a *hydrocoele* the testis cannot be palpated through the fluid. Lymph nodes have clear borders.

Transillumination

This is useful to distinguish a hydrocoele from a hernia. When you hold a light to the scrotum, a hydrocoele transilluminates, whereas a hernia does not.

Neurological examination of children (see Box 5.8 and accompanying video clip 8)

Neurological assessment in infants is discussed on p. 90. The interpretation of neurological signs is shown in Box 5.9.

Cranial nerves

I	Smell
II	Fundi and vision
III, IV, VI	Eye movements
V	Clench teeth
	Facial sensation
	(corneal reflex)
VII	Shut eyes
	Show teeth
VIII	Hearing
IX, X, XII	Stick out tongue. Uvular
	deviation (gag reflex)
XI	Turn head against resistance
	Shrug shoulders

Box 5.8 Bedside checklist for examining the nervous system in an older child

Cranial Nerves (see text)
Observation
- ☐ Dysmorphic signs
- ☐ Abnormal movements
- ☐ Gait
- ☐ Gower's sign
- ☐ Posture

Motor examination
- ☐ Muscle bulk
- ☐ Tone
- ☐ Power
- ☐ Coordination

Reflexes
- ☐ Deep tendon jerks
- ☐ Plantar reflex
- ☐ Clonus

Sensation
- ☐ Light touch
- ☐ Pain
- ☐ Temperature
- ☐ Proprioception

Cerebellar signs and coordination
- ☐ Tremor
- ☐ Nystagmus
- ☐ Finger–nose test
- ☐ Heel–shin test
- ☐ Dysdiadochokinesis
- ☐ Ataxia – heel–toe walking
- ☐ Romberg's test
- ☐ Dysarthria

Box 5.9 Interpretation of neurological signs

Cerebellar signs
- ☐ Nystagmus
- ☐ Intention tremor
- ☐ Incoordination
- ☐ Ataxia
- ☐ Dysarthria

Upper motor neurone lesion, e.g. cerebral palsy
- ☐ Hypertonia/spasticity
- ☐ Increased deep tendon reflexes
- ☐ Positive Babinski sign
- ☐ Clonus

Peripheral disease, e.g. muscular dystrophy
- ☐ Hypotonia
- ☐ Weakness
- ☐ Reduced/absent deep tendon jerks
- ☐ Gower's sign
- ☐ Increased calf muscle volume-pseudohypertrophy

Peripheral neuropathy e.g. Guillain Barre syndrome
- ☐ Weakness
- ☐ Hypotonia
- ☐ Absent deep tendon jerks
- ☐ Reduced sensation (mixed and sensory neuropathies)

Observation

Dysmorphic signs

Look for unusual facial or other features that may suggest a genetic disorder or syndrome.

Abnormal movements

These may occur in children with neurological disorders. The commonest is choreoathetosis (writhing movements of the limbs), usually associated with facial grimacing. Sudden jerking movements may be due to myoclonic epilepsy or, in infants, infantile spasms (pp. 237–8). Repetitive complex movements in an alert child may indicate a tic. Tremor is uncommon in children.

Gait

In ambulant children, observing the way they walk (gait) is very important. An abnormal gait can be accentuated by asking the child to walk on tiptoes or run. Abnormal gait patterns include:

- *Stiffness.* This is the commonest major abnormality and suggests an upper motor neurone lesion, usually cerebral palsy (Figure 5.24). In mild cases you may only see it by asking the child to run. The patterns of movement in different types of cerebral palsy are discussed in Chapter 14.
- *Waddling.* The child with spastic diplegia has a more knock-kneed gait (Figure 5.25). The predominant feature is adduction of both thighs, so that the knees are flexed and knock together with the ankles apart. The child tends to take weight on the toes or anterior part of the foot. Waddling is also seen in Duchenne muscular dystrophy or congenital dislocation of the hips.
- *Ataxia.* The child walks unsteadily with a broad-based gait.

Gower sign

Weakness is suspected if the child finds it difficult to get up from a sitting position on the floor. In Gower's sign, the child 'climbs up' his or her legs to a standing position (Figure 14.4).

Muscle bulk

Look for muscle wasting and compare one side with the other. Wasting of muscle groups occurs in both upper motor neurone disorders (cerebral palsy) and in lower motor neurone lesions (spina bifida, nerve palsies). Pseudohypertrophy of calf muscles is seen in Duchenne dystrophy.

Posture

Observe the child's posture and look for evidence of contractures.

Motor examination

Tone

Muscle tone is defined as resistance to passive stretch. Lie the child down and move the major joints through their passive range of movement, feeling for resistance. *Hypertonia* (increased tone) suggests an upper motor neurone lesion and *hypotonia* (reduced tone, floppiness) a lower motor neurone lesion or muscle disease. *Dystonia* is found in basal ganglia disease. *Spasticity* is the term used to describe spasm in a muscle group with increased tone. In cerebral palsy, the thigh adductors in the legs are most affected. To test for this, grasp the ankles (see Figure 5.26), abduct the legs and assess resistance. Then passively dorsiflex and plantarflex the foot. Resistance occurs particularly in dorsiflexion.

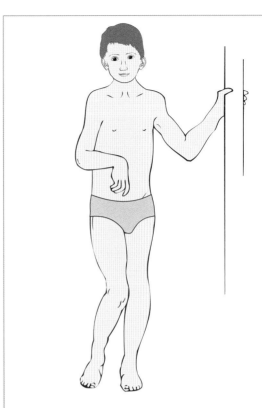

Figure 5.24 A child with hemiplegia. The gait can be exaggerated by asking the child to run.

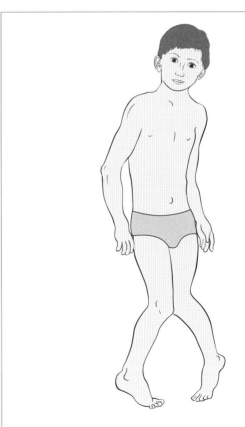

Figure 5.25 A child with spastic diplegia. The gait is waddling.

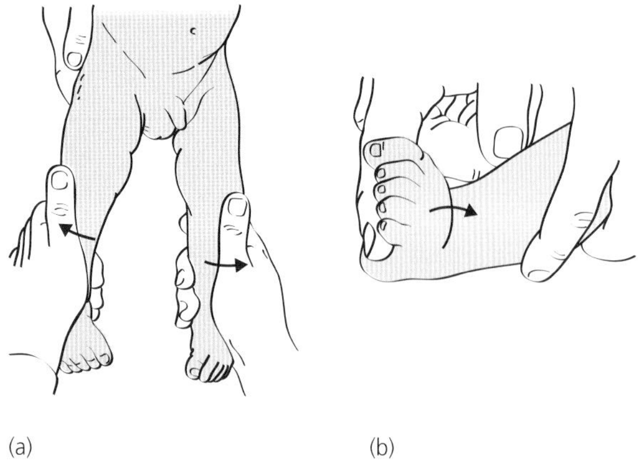

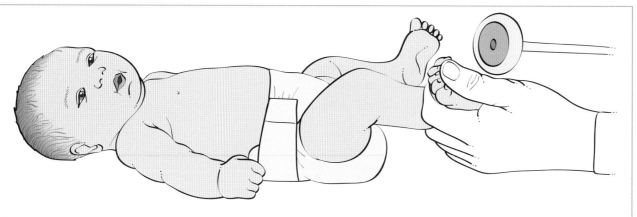

(a)   (b)

Figure 5.26 Assessment of tone in the lower limbs:
(a) assessment of adductor tone and (b) tone assessed at ankle
by dorsiflexion/plantarflexion.

Power

If the child can cooperate, test opposing muscle groups in both
the arms and the legs. The muscle power around each joint
should be assessed Ask the child to do the following manoeuvres against resistance:

Upper limbs
    Arms out to the side
    Bend your elbows
    Push out straight
    Squeeze fingers
    Hold the fingers out straight
    Spread fingers apart

Lower limbs
    Lift up your leg
    Bend your knee
    Straighten your leg
    Bend your foot down
    Cock up your foot

Coordination

Coordination is part of the motor examination and is discussed
below with other cerebellar signs.

Reflexes

The reflexes may be normal, exaggerated (upper motor neurone
lesion), reduced (lower motor neurone lesion) or absent. Before
you conclude that a reflex is absent try *distraction* (reinforcement):
ask the child to clench their teeth hard or to grasp their hands
together and pull them apart, then try to elicit the reflex again.

Check the following deep tendon reflexes:

- Biceps
- Triceps
- Supinator
- Knee
- Ankle

In young children, the ankle jerk is most easily elicited by
gently holding the foot in a slightly dorsiflexed position with
your thumb over the ball of the foot. You tap the hammer on
your thumb and observe the elicited plantarflexion of the foot
(Figure 5.27).

Plantar reflex   Use your thumb nail to stroke the lateral
border of the sole of the foot firmly from the heel to the little
toe. The response may be upgoing in infants until the age of
12 months, but thereafter downgoing is normal. A positive
Babinski sign is an asymmetrical response or an upgoing
response beyond the age of 12 months, and suggests an upper
motor neurone lesion; clonus may also be present.

Abdominal reflexes   should also be elicited. They are absent
in upper motor neurone disease. **The Cremasteric reflex** is
tested if there is suspected testicular disease such as torsion.

Clonus   Grasp the foot and sharply dorsiflex it. Clonus is
present if repetitive jerking movements occur.

Figure 5.27 Eliciting the ankle jerk in young children. The hammer percusses the examiner's thumb.

Sensation

In older, cooperative children, sensation is tested in the same way as it is for adults, but sensory loss is not a common finding in children with upper motor neurone lesions. Compare one side with the other and make sure you ask the child to close his or her eyes so that there are no visual clues. Check for:

- *Light touch* using cotton wool
- *Pain* with a blunt needle
- *Temperature*
- *Proprioception* (position sense). Grasp the sides of the distal phalanx of the toe or thumb between your thumb and index finger. Move it up and down and ask the child which position it is in when you stop.

Cerebellar signs and coordination

Tremor

Ask the child to hold his or her arms outstretched and observe if there is a tremor.

Nystagmus

Ask the child to look at your finger and move it from one side to the other, and up and down. Nystagmus is an involuntary rapid horizontal movement of the eye and is a sign of cerebellar, vestibular or brainstem dysfunction.

Nose–finger test

Ask the child to touch the tip of their nose and then the tip of your finger. Once they have the idea, ask them to do this as quickly as possible while you move your finger. In ataxia the child will find it difficult to touch their nose or your finger accurately. Test both hands separately. *Intention tremor* is characteristic of damage to the posterior lobe of the cerebellum: the child's hand is steady at rest but develops a tremor of increasing amplitude as it approaches the target.

Heel–shin test

With the child lying on their back, ask them to run the heel of one foot down the front of the shin, and see how accurately this is done (see Figure 5.28).

Dysdiadochokinesis

Ask the child to pronate and supinate their forearms quickly and repeatedly slap one hand with the front and back of the other hand. Impairment of rapid alternating movements is called dysdiadochokinesia.

Gait

Observe the gait with heel-toe walking along a line. In ataxia, movements will be clumsy and jerky.

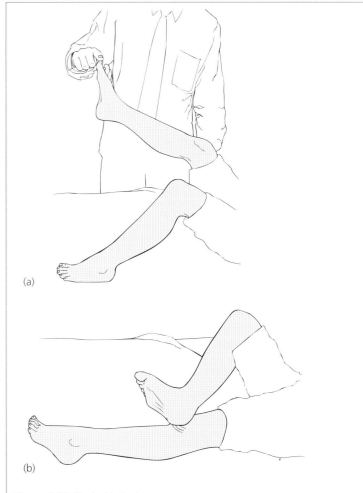

(a)

(b)

Figure 5.28 Heel–shin test.

Romberg's sign

Ask the child to stand with feet together and eyes open and then closed. Romberg's sign is loss of postural sensation with unsteadiness when the eyes are closed (Figure 5.29). Note that in cerebellar disease, the child may be unsteady with eyes open and shut. This is not Romberg's sign.

Speech

Note the quality of the child's speech. A child with a cerebellar lesion may have a halting, jerking dysarthria.

Cranial nerves

In older children the cranial nerves are tested in exactly the same way as they are in adults. Some information about cranial nerve function in young children can be obtained by observation (see below), but it is not always possible to formally examine the cranial nerves in uncooperative children.

EXAMINATION OF THE CRANIAL NERVES

I Olfactory nerve	Ask the child if he/she has a sense of smell, and test with a familiar non-irritant substance
II Optic nerve	Fundi and vision (see pp. 96–7)
III, IV, VI Occulomotor trochlear and abducens nerves	Eye movements (see pp. 96–7)
V Trigeminal nerve	The motor component of the Vth nerve supplies the jaw muscles. Ask the child to open his/her mouth and bite hard. Palpate the masseter muscle. The Vth nerve also provides sensation to much of the face and is divided into the ophthalmic, maxillary and mandibular divisions. Test sensation to light touch in each of these areas. The corneal reflex is not routinely examined in children
VII Facial nerve	Ask the child to screw up his/her eyes as tightly as possible and to show his/her teeth. Inability to bury the eyelashes on one side or close the eye, and drooping of the corner of the mouth, may indicate facial nerve palsy
VIII Auditory nerve	Ask about hearing. If there is any doubt, or speech delay, you should obtain a hearing test
IX, X, XII Glosso-pharyngeal, vagus and hypoglossal nerves	Ask the child to stick out his/her tongue, and look for tongue and uvula deviation. The gag reflex is not routinely examined in children
XI Accessory nerve	Ask the child to turn his/her head to the sides against the resistance of your hand, and to shrug his/her shoulders

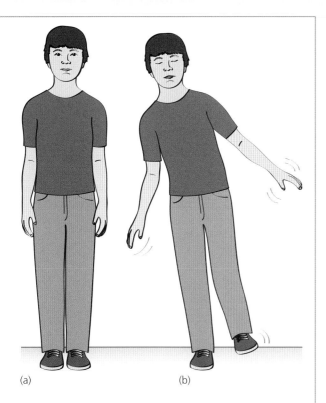

(a)   (b)

Figure 5.29 Romberg's test: (a) child standing with feet together and eyes open; (b) same child unbalanced with eyes closed (positive for Romberg's sign).

Neurological examination in babies (see accompanying video clip 9)

The neurological examination of babies (Box 5.10) is rather different from that of older children. Much is gained by observation and handling the baby, and a good developmental assessment is always required (see Chapter 6).

Observation

Particular points to look for include:
- *Irritability.* Can the baby be consoled by cuddling?
- *Spontaneous movement.* Reduced movement suggests muscle weakness.
- *Position at rest.* See below.
- *Base of the spine.* Examine the base of the spine. A sacral dimple or tuft of hair can be an indication of a spinal abnormality.

Palpation

The anterior fontanelle usually closes by 18 months. A bulging fontanelle suggests raised intracranial pressure and is a late sign in meningitis (p. 235). A pulsatile bulging fontanelle is common in febrile babies.

Tone

You assess tone by picking up and handling the baby. With experience you can identify hypo- and hypertonia. A floppy

Box 5.10 Bedside checklist for examining the nervous system in a baby

Observation
- ☐ Irritability/alertness
- ☐ Position at rest
  - • frog position in hypotonia
  - • opisthotonos, scissoring in extreme hypertonia
- ☐ Reduced spontaneous movement
- ☐ Base of the spine

Palpation
- ☐ Fontanelle
- ☐ Head circumference

Tone
- ☐ Prone

- ☐ Supine
- ☐ Pull to sit
- ☐ Axillary suspension and weight bearing
- ☐ Ventral suspension
- ☐ Passive movements – assess popliteal angle

Reflexes
- ☐ Deep tendon jerks
- ☐ Primitive reflexes

Vision

Hearing

Developmental assessment

baby tends to slip through your hands, whereas a hypertonic baby feels stiffer. You can best assess tone by looking at the baby in a number of positions:

- ▪ *Supine position.* A hypotonic baby lies in a frog's leg position (see Figure 5.30). A hypertonic baby may have a retracted neck (opisthotonos) with scissoring of the legs.
- ▪ *Prone position.* Are the head and shoulders raised (depending on the baby's age)?
- ▪ *Pull to sit.* Pull the baby lying on its back into the sitting position. Head control is gradually achieved by 4 months of age. Head lag persists in a hypotonic baby. Look at the back to see how straight it is held.
- ▪ *Ventral suspension.* This is useful in a baby less than 3 months old. Put your hand under the baby's abdomen and lift him off the couch. A hypotonic baby will droop over your hand.
- ▪ *Axillary suspension.* Pick up the baby under the arms and test weight bearing. A floppy baby tends to slip through your hands like a rag doll. The hypertonic baby may demonstrate scissoring (see Figure 5.31). Babies generally start weight bearing when they are 5 months old.
- ▪ *Passive movements.* If tone is low, there is little resistance to passive movements. You can assess this by assessing the popliteal angle. If tone is high, the leg resists extension (Figure 5.32).

Reflexes

Deep tendon reflexes

Check for these as described for older children. The ankle jerk may be more easily elicited by tapping your thumb over the ball of the foot (see Figure 5.27).

Primitive reflexes

Primitive reflexes (Figure 5.33) appear and disappear at different times, as shown in Table 5.6. If they are absent or persist

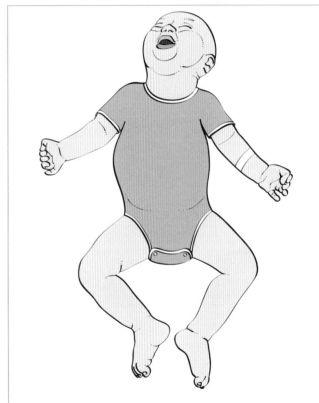

Figure 5.30 A hypotonic child lying in the frog's leg position.

beyond a given period, this suggests neurological dysfunction. The forward parachute reflex appears at 6–9 months of age and is elicited by pitching the baby forward. It comprises extension of both arms with extension of the hands (Figure 5.34). Asymmetry of this reflex may be an early sign of a unilateral upper motor neurone lesion (spastic hemiplegia).

Vision

Check that the baby can fix and follow a silent moving object.

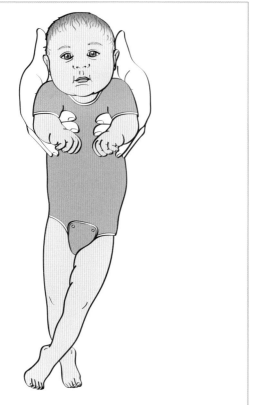

Figure 5.31 Scissoring of the lower limbs.

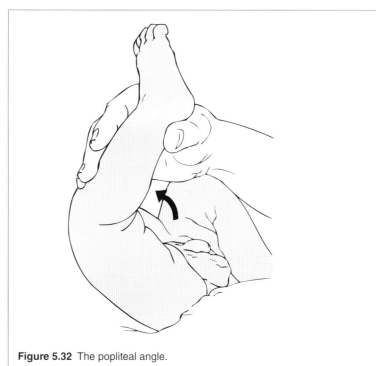

Figure 5.32 The popliteal angle.

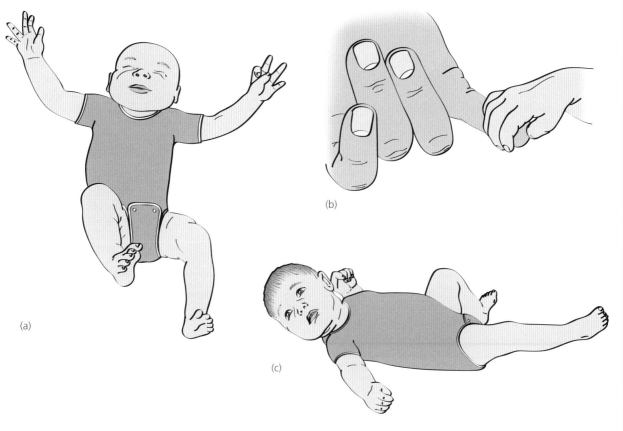

(a)

(b)

(c)

Figure 5.33 Elicitation of primitive reflexes: (a) Moro reflex, (b) palmar grasp reflex and (c) asymmetrical tonic neck reflex.

Table 5.6 Age at which primitive reflexes appear and the latest age by which they should have disappeared. Persistence after this time is definitely abnormal

Reflex	Description	Appearance	Disappearance
Stepping	The baby will step up when the dorsum of the foot touches the surface	Birth	1 month
Moro	Symmetrical abduction and then adduction with extension of the arms when the baby's head is dropped back quickly into your hand (Figure 5.33a)	Birth	3 months
Palmar grasp	Touching the palm with an object causes the baby to grip it (Figure 5.33b)	Birth	3 months
Plantar reflex	Pressing on the ball of the foot causes the toes to curl	Birth	8 months
Asymmetric tonic neck reflex (ATNR)	Turn the baby's head. The arm extends on the side the baby is facing and flexes on the opposite side (Figure 5.33c)	Birth	6 months
Parachute reflex	Develops from 6-9 months and persists; elicit by pitching the baby forward suddenly (Figure 5.34)	9 months	Persists

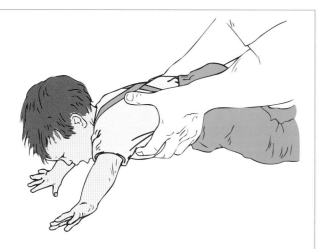

Figure 5.34 The parachute reflex.

Hearing

Screening for hearing is carried out neonatally on all babies (p. 33).

The musculoskeletal system (see accompanying video clip 10)

Examination of the musculoskeletal system is very specialised. As an undergraduate you are only expected to examine a major joint such as the hip and knee, to conduct a pGALS assessment and to assess clinically for the presence of scoliosis.

Examination of a large joint

Observation

- Observe the joint for swelling or redness. An effusion causes loss of definition of the joint. In the knee, the outline of the patella is lost, and if the effusion is mild, the normal concavity is lost first along its medial side.
- Observe the muscle bulk above and below the joint for wasting. Measuring the knee circumference is useful if swelling is suspected.

Palpation

- Palpate the joint for an effusion. This is most likely to be apparent in the knee. First look for the 'bulge sign' by milking fluid in the medial aspect of the knee into the lateral recess. Then firmly stroke the lateral side of the knee downwards to push the fluid back into the medial compartment. You will see a 'bulge' of fluid.
- If the effusion is large, use the 'patella tap' sign. Press firmly on the suprapatellar pouch with one hand to empty any fluid from there, then with the other hand push firmly downwards on the patella. If fluid is present in the knee, the patella will 'bounce'.

Range of movements

Move the joint through its normal range of movements to assess any limitation or contractures.

The paediatric Gait, Arms, Legs and Spine (pGALS) assessment

The examination pGALS is a validated screening examination carried out as an initial assessment for possible rheumatological or musculoskeletal disorders in school-age children. It is similar to GALS in adults, but has some additional manoeuvres.

Screening questions:

- Do you have any pain or stiffness in your joints, muscles or back?

- Do you have any difficulty dressing yourself?
- Do you have any difficulty going up or down stairs?

Inspection (with minimal clothing required for dignity) from the front, back and sides for posture or deformity. The *gait* is assessed by asking the child to walk normally and turn around; then by walking on tiptoes and heels. Note the foot posture as well as the foot and ankle movements.

The *arms* are assessed by asking the child to:
- Put their arms out in front of them to assess the shoulders, elbows, wrists and small joints of the fingers
- Turn their hands up and then make a fist to assess wrist and elbow supination and finger flexion
- Pinch their thumb and index fingers together to review dexterity and grasp
- Touch each tip of their finger to the thumb for dexterity and coordination
- Tell you if there is any pain as you gently squeeze the four fingers at the line of the metacarpophalangeal joints
- Put their hands palm together and then hands back to back for wrist flexion, finger extension and elbow flexion
- Reach up to touch the sky, then look at the ceiling for arm joint extension and neck extension
- Put their hands behind their neck for shoulder abduction and external rotation and elbow flexion

The *legs* are examined through initial inspection (as above) and then lying on a bed or couch. Feel for any effusion at the patellar joint then ask the child to flex and extend the knee while you hold the knee and feel for joint crepitus. With the knee flexed assess the degree of internal hip rotation. Examine both legs separately.

The *spine* is again examined standing up by inspecting from behind and then asking the child to:
- Open their mouth wide and put three of their fingers in their mouth to assess the temporomandibular joint
- Try and touch their shoulder with their ear on each side for cervical spine lateral flexion
- Bend and touch their toes whilst you observe from the side and behind to assess thoraco-lumbar flexion and for scoliosis.

Scoliosis

Scoliosis is common in teenage girls, is usually idiopathic, and if severe can produce life-threatening cardiorespiratory compromise. It may be obvious by inspection of the back while the child is standing upright. The shoulders should be level, and note symmetrical prominence of a scapula.

The best way to examine a subtle scoliosis is to stand behind the child and ask him or her to bend forward at the waist and straighten up slowly. A fixed scoliosis causes prominence of the posterior ribs on the convex side of the bend (Figure 5.35).

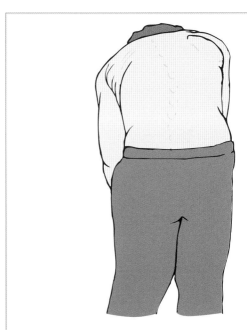

Figure 5.35 Detection of scoliosis by asking the child to bend forward.

The ear, nose and throat (see accompanying video clip 11)

Examination of the ear

Every doctor involved in the care of children should be able to examine ears competently. This is usually left to the end along with examination of the throat, as it is most likely to upset the young child. Ask the mother to hold the child on her lap with the child's head against her chest. To prevent a struggle, the mother's other hand should restrain the arms, and the legs be gripped gently between the mother's legs (Figure 5.36).

Hold the otoscope with your hand resting against the child's temple so that the instrument can move with the child. With your other hand, pull the pinna up to straighten the ear canal, or, in a baby, pull the earlobe down. Choose the largest possible speculum that will comfortably enter the meatus and do not advance it more than 0.5 cm in infants and 1 cm in older children. If wax is present, try to remove it gently.

Look at the tympanic membrane. The normal appearance is shown in Figure 5.37a. The membrane should be pale grey, shiny and translucent, with a light reflex at its anterior lower pole. Some middle ear structures can be seen through the membrane, including the handle of the malleus and the umbo. The normal drum lies in a neutral position. If there is increased pressure in the middle ear, as in otitis media, the drum bulges forward and is inflamed (Figure 5.37b).

In glue ear (secretory otitis media), the drum may be retracted and dull and both the malleus and the umbo are very obvious (Figure 5.37c). The light reflex is also lost. In some cases, a fluid level can be seen through the membrane and air bubbles may also be present. Assessment of drum mobility using a pneumatic bulb is a specialised examination technique. It is easily learned and very useful, but not carried out routinely.

Examination of the nose

For a young child, sit the child as for examining the throat (see below). Examine the nostrils for inflammation, obstruction and polyps.

Examination of the throat

Young children do not like to have their throats examined and this is best done with the child sitting on the mother's lap as shown in Figure 5.38. If the child is uncooperative and will not open his or her mouth, part the lips and teeth gently with the wooden spatula and depress the tongue. If the child cries, this facilitates the examination.

Examine the tonsils for size, redness and exudate. Normal tonsillar size varies enormously. The tonsils are lymphoid tissue and are very small at birth and grow to maximal size by 4–5 years, getting smaller in the early teens. Normal tonsils can appear very large in preschool children. If they meet in the

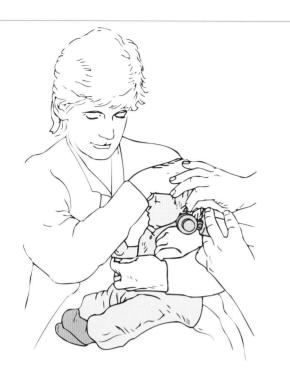

Figure 5.36 Position to hold a baby for otoscopic examination.

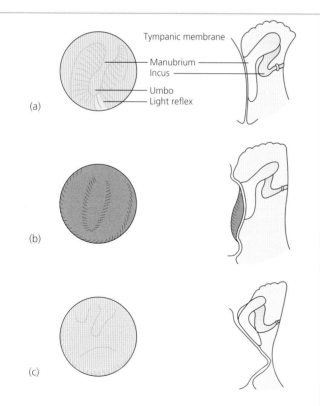

Figure 5.37 Tympanic membrane appearances: (a) normal, (b) otitis media with a bulging drum and (c) glue ear with a retracted drum.

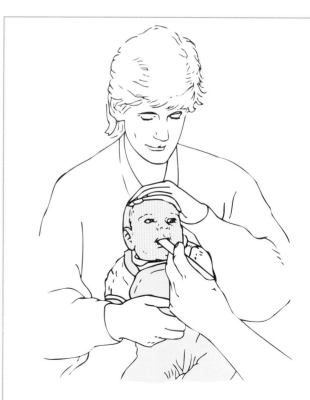

Figure 5.38 Position for holding a child to examine the throat.

midline, they are probably abnormally large. The signs of tonsillitis are discussed on p. 144.

In addition, examine the oropharynx, mucosa, teeth, tongue and palate. Feel for cervical lymphadenopathy.

The visual system (see accompanying video clip 12)

Look for any gross abnormality of the eyes. Note the size, shape and orientation, and examine the corneas, sclera, conjunctiva and iris. Look for a squint. Assess each eye separately: a child who has no vision in one eye may appear to have normal visual function if both eyes are assessed together (Box 5.11).

Visual acuity

Gain visual attention in a newborn using a visually interesting object and move it to see if the baby's gaze follows. See if a toddler is able to see small blocks and tiny beads such as hundreds and thousands. Older children can be asked to count fingers, although it is obviously more accurate to use a Snellen chart. There are formal vision testing kits for young children: the Stycar rolling ball test uses small white balls of different sizes rolled across the floor.

Eye movements

Ask the child to follow your finger through the full range of movement (see Figure 5.39). Note if there is limited movement in any direction. Bring your finger close to assess accommodation.

Visual fields

The 'wiggly finger' test is used to assess children over 5 years, and compares the child's visual field with your own

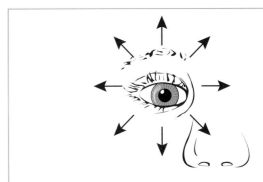

Figure 5.39 The eight positions of gaze.

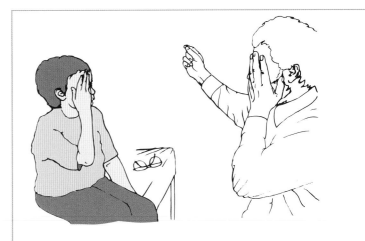

Figure 5.40 'Wiggly finger' test.

as a normal control. Sit 1 meter away from the child. Ask the child to look at your nose and hold his hand over his right eye. Cover your own left eye with your hand. Then gradually bring your finger into the child's range of vision and wiggle it at each of the eight sectors in turn (Figure 5.40). Ask the child to say when he first sees it. He should see the finger at the same point as you do. Repeat with the other eye.

Reflexes

- *Corneal light reflex.* This is a misnomer as it is not really a reflex. The corneal light reflex is the reflection of a light source shone from about half a metre. The reflection should be symmetrically positioned in the centre of both corneas. If it is asymmetric, it indicates a squint.
- *Pupillary reflex.* Shine a bright light into the eye from 10 cm distance. You should see the pupil react and also consensual constriction in the other eye. Pupils also constrict to accommodation which is tested by bringing the examiner's finger toward the nose. Light-accommodation discordance such as the Marcus-Gunn pupil (Relative Afferent Pupillary Defect RAPD), the Adie-Holmes tonically enlarged pupil and the

---

Box 5.11 Bedside checklist for examining the eye

Assess each eye separately

Observation
Visual acuity
Eye movements
Visual fields
Reflexes
☐ Corneal light reflex
☐ Pupillary reflex
☐ Red reflex

Fundoscopy
Cover test

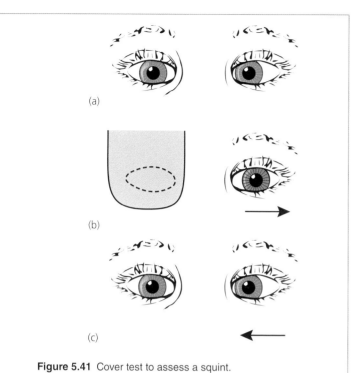

(a)

(b)

(c)

Figure 5.41 Cover test to assess a squint.

Argyll-Robertson contracted pupil, are seen in optic-neurological pathology.

■ *Red reflex.* This is also not a reflex. It is a test usually performed in the newborn period. Look through an ophthalmoscope 45 cm from the child's eye. A red reflection is normally seen. A white reflection suggests a cataract or other pathology.

Includes
- Corneal light reflex
- Ocular movements
- Visual acuity
- Cover test
- Fundoscopy

Fundoscopy

Fundoscopy is difficult in children. Ask the child to focus on a distant point. Approach the eye from the side and adjust the lens setting so that the retina comes into focus.

Cover test

The cover test (Figure 5.41) is used to identify subtle and latent squints. Ask the child to look at an interesting object. Cover the normal eye without touching the face. The squinting eye rapidly flicks to fix on the object. Remove the cover and the squinting eye flicks away again as the covered eye again becomes dominant. In a latent squint the squinting eye moves away when it is covered and flicks back again when the cover is removed.

If you suspect a squint your examination should include the features shown in Box 5.12.

To test your knowledge on this part of the book, please see Chapter 26

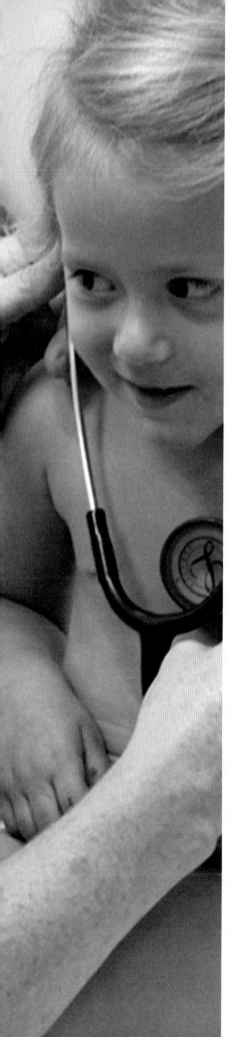

CHAPTER 6
Developmental assessment

When I was One,
I had just begun.
When I was Two,
I was nearly new.
When I was Three,
I was hardly me.
Now We Are Six, AA
Milne

KEY COMPETENCES

YOU MUST ...

Know and understand

- The key developmental milestones and at what age they are usually achieved
- The warning signs indicating delayed development

Be able to

- Engage with young children and establish a rapport
- Carry out a developmental evaluation on babies and children under the age of 5 years by taking a history, examining and observing the child

Appreciate that

- There is variability in the age when developmental milestones are achieved
- 'Quality' of development is as important as 'quantity'
- Repeat evaluations are often needed before concluding that development is concerning
- Developmental abnormality in a single area, in the context of a normal neurological examination is rarely significant

Essential Paediatrics and Child Health, Fourth Edition. Mary Rudolf, Anthony Luder and Kerry Jeavons.
© 2020 John Wiley & Sons Ltd. Published 2020 by John Wiley & Sons Ltd.
Companion website: www.wiley.com/go/rudolf/paediatrics

Developmental assessment (see Figure 6.1) is an integral part of the paediatric examination and carrying out a good assessment requires practice and skill. You need to be systematic in your approach to make sure that you have covered all areas of development and gained a good picture of the child's abilities. As a student you are expected to be able to competently assess preschool children, especially babies and toddlers. Figure 6.2 summarizes the key components.

It is helpful if you divide your developmental assessment into the five major areas:

- gross motor
- fine motor
- speech and language
- social
- special senses (hearing and vision)

and attempt to work through each in turn (child permitting).

It is always hard to remember developmental milestones, but if you make sure that you learn the key landmarks indicated in Table 6.1, you will have a framework for assessing children's skills. When you are with the child, concentrate on the

tasks at hand and record carefully what you see. You can always check later to see the age at which a task is normally achieved.

Look to see whether the child can carry out the task, and also how it is carried out, as this can tell you whether there is a discrepancy between the child's understanding and performance. For example, a child with clumsiness or mild cerebral palsy may not be able to perform a motor task well, but may understand what is wanted, indicating that intellectual capacity is normal.

It is helpful to have a simple kit of tools to test development. A rattle, coloured 1-inch blocks, a ball, a formboard, and crayons and paper are adequate, along with a few dolls or cars and simple pictures of common objects.

Major milestones of development for the first 2 years in each of the four developmental areas are summarized in Figures 6.3–6.6. You may find delay or abnormal development in one or more areas, and it is important that you carry out a thorough neurological examination to sort out whether there are neurological findings in addition.

Delay in two or more areas may indicate significant medical problems and in all four areas usually indicates intellectual disability (p. 258–9), but an isolated delay in any one area is

Figure 6.1 Carrying out a developmental assessment. The most useful tools are small wooden bricks, a ball, a formboard and crayons and paper.

Table 6.1 Milestones that are essential to memorize

Age	Milestone
4–6 weeks	Smiles responsively
6–7 months	Sits unsupported
9 months	Gets to a sitting position
10 months	Start of pincer grasp
12 months	Walks unsupported
	Two or three words
	Tower of two cubes
18 months	Tower of three or four cubes
24 months	Two- to three-word sentences

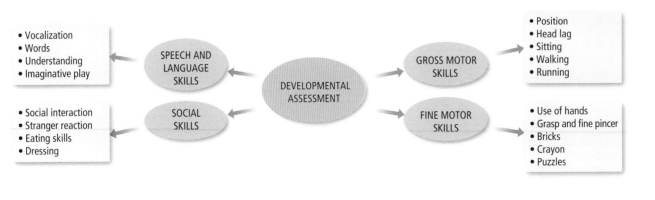

Figure 6.2 Key components of a developmental assessment.

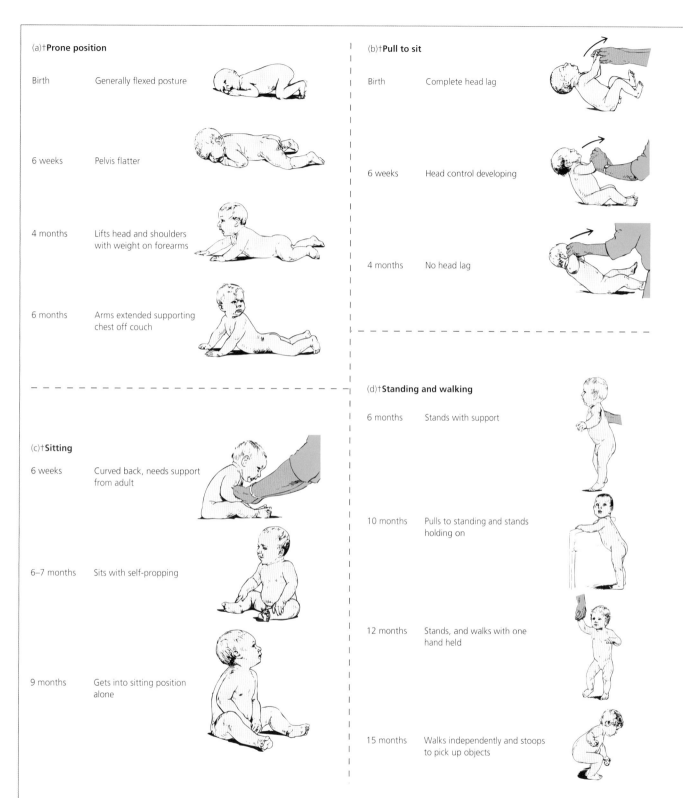

Figure 6.3 Stages in gross motor development.

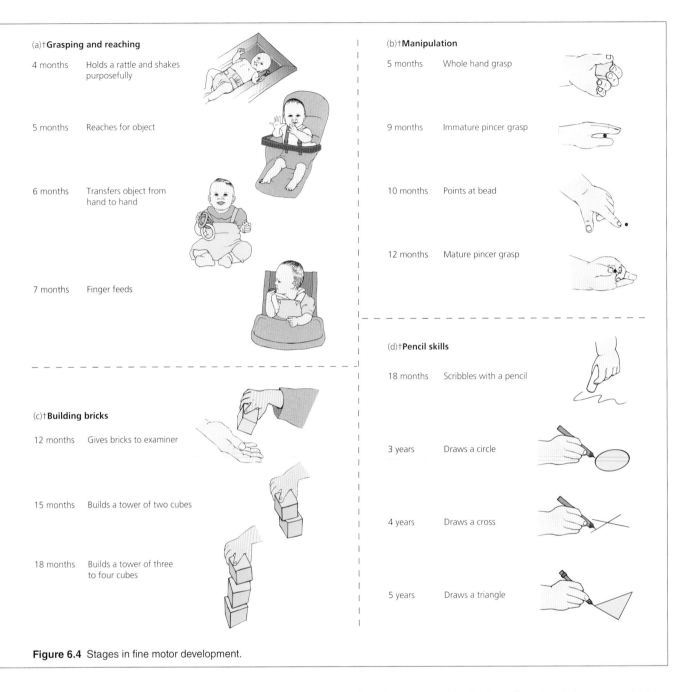

Figure 6.4 Stages in fine motor development.

often not a sign of abnormality in healthy children. Delay in walking alone (p. 231) is common and may have occurred in siblings or parents. Acquisition of speech is another common isolated delay; in all children with speech delay, deafness must be excluded. Remember that the quality of development is as important as the 'quantity'. The interpretation of developmental delay is covered in detail in Chapter 14.

Gross motor development

You should get an idea of gross motor skills (Figure 6.3) from a combination of informal observation and parental report. Start by looking at the baby's position. At birth an infant assumes a flexed posture, with the hips flexed and bottom tucked up when prone. By 6 weeks the pelvis is flatter on the table, and by 4 months the infant can lift the head and shoulders off the couch. At 4 months the baby may begin to roll from prone to supine and at 5 months from supine to prone. By 6 months the arms are held extended, supporting the chest off the couch (Figure 6.3a).

Now, get an idea of head control. Pull the baby to a sitting position and see the extent of head lag (Figure 6.3b). Good head control is achieved by 4 months. Then see how well the baby can sit. Sitting is achieved gradually as neck and trunk tone strengthen. The average age for sitting unsupported is 6–7 months, although at this stage the arms are still used for support.

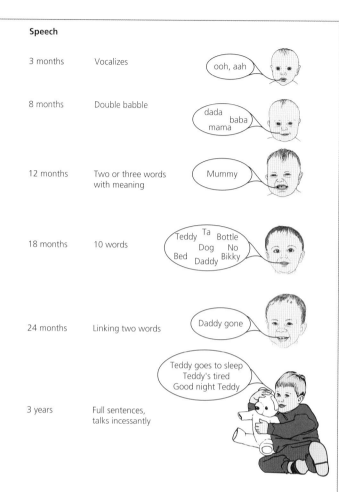

Speech		
3 months	Vocalizes	ooh, aah
8 months	Double babble	dada baba mama
12 months	Two or three words with meaning	Mummy
18 months	10 words	Teddy Ta Bottle Dog No Bed Daddy Bikky
24 months	Linking two words	Daddy gone
3 years	Full sentences, talks incessantly	Teddy goes to sleep Teddy's tired Good night Teddy

Figure 6.5 Stages in speech and language development.

By 9 months the baby can get into the sitting position alone. By 11 months the child can pivot while sitting to reach toys (Figure 6.3c).

The next stage is mobility. A baby can move from sitting to crawling at 7–9 months, but some babies never pass through the crawling phase. Others bottom-shuffle. Pulling up to standing occurs at 10 months, and cruising (walking around while holding onto the furniture) occurs by 11 months (Figure 6.3d). Note that the ability to bear weight on the legs at a very early age may be abnormal and a sign of hypertonia.

At around 12 months the baby walks with one hand held and can stand unsupported. Independent walking is achieved on average at 12–13 months, but this is very variable. At 15 months the baby can stand from crouching and can clamber up stairs.

By 18 months the child can walk upstairs holding the banister and is very steady on the feet. He or she should be able to throw a ball without falling over. Failure to walk independently at 18 months requires investigation (p. 257).

Fine motor development

Fine motor skills (Figure 6.4) require dexterity and cognitive ability. A child who lacks understanding of what he or she is being asked to do will not be able to demonstrate a task; you need to differentiate whether the problem is cognitive or motor.

Start by looking at how the baby uses his or her hands. At 1 month the hands are closed most of the time, but by 2 months they are held open. By 3 months the baby can hold a rattle and shake it. At 5 months he or she can reach out for a toy, and at 6 months can transfer it from one hand to the other. By 7 months the hands are used in play and exploration. The baby can grasp an object and bring it to the mouth. This is the age where finger feeding is a natural development (Figure 6.4a).

By 9 months the finger movements become refined. At first there is a raking grasp using the whole palm, which by 10 months has developed into a scissor grasp using the thumb and first finger and, by 12 months, into finger–thumb apposition, also known as a pincer grasp (Figure 6.4b).

By 1 year, a baby will give a 2-cm square wooden block to you and release it. A child of 15 months can build a tower of two wooden cubes, and one of 18 months a tower of three to four cubes (Figure 6.4c). At this age a child scribbles with a crayon and can turn the pages of a book. Fine motor development advances rapidly after this. By the age of 3 years children can draw a circle, at 4 years a cross and at 5 years a triangle (Figure 6.4d). Note that hand preference (dominance) usually starts between 2 and 4 years and marked dominance before that may indicate a neurological problem.

In the fourth year a child can draw a circle for a face and then progressively add limbs directly from the face, with one or two facial features such as eyes and mouth. It is not until 5 years that the child draws a body to which arms and hands are attached.

Speech and language development

Speech and language development are summarized in Figure 6.5. You can expect young children to be too shy to talk to you directly and you will probably have to rely on a parent's report. In assessing language, you need to try and assess:

- the child's understanding of receptive language
- the child's expressive language (speech)
- the child's play, which reflects their understanding of the world around them

A baby begins to vocalize at about 3 months and starts to enjoy playing with his or her voice. By 6 months he or she can make consonant sounds such as 'da', 'ba', 'ma' and 'ka'. By 8 months these are being combined into 'double babble' (dada, baba, mama).

The first recognizable word is spoken by 12 months, and two or three words are used with meaning. These words may

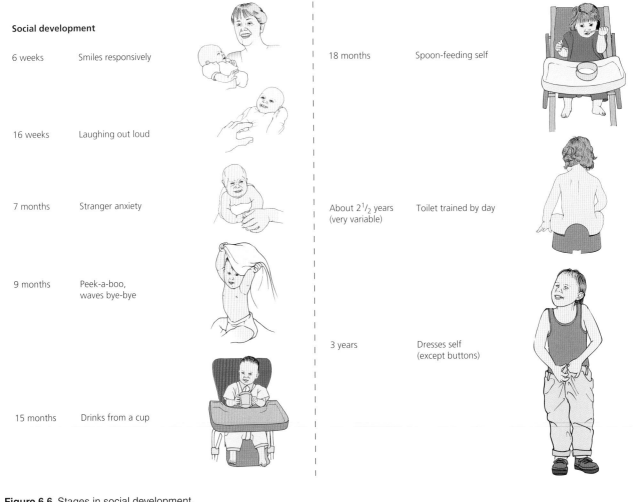

Social development

6 weeks	Smiles responsively
16 weeks	Laughing out loud
7 months	Stranger anxiety
9 months	Peek-a-boo, waves bye-bye
15 months	Drinks from a cup
18 months	Spoon-feeding self
About 2½ years (very variable)	Toilet trained by day
3 years	Dresses self (except buttons)

Figure 6.6 Stages in social development.

be indistinct to anyone other than the mother. Jargon (unintelligible but highly expressive 'language') develops at about 15 months of age. By 18 months the average child has 10–20 recognizable words, and by 24 months these are linked into two-word sentences. From then speech develops rapidly, so that by the age of 3 years the child can form full sentences and talks incessantly.

First get a grasp of how many words the child has. Then try to assess their understanding of language. Do they respond to 'where is daddy'? Can they carry out simple commands such as 'give' and 'take' or 'bring me'? Can they point to their nose or eyes? Lastly, explore their imaginative (or symbolic) play. Are they babying a doll, can they move a toy car forward? If a child hasn't yet started to talk but has rich imaginative play, it is a sign that their intellectual ability is probably unimpaired.

If there is a delay in acquiring language it is essential to test hearing (see below), as if this is not corrected language development can be irreversibly affected. Language delay is covered on p. 255.

Social skills

Social development (summarized in Figure 6.6) refers to how a child interacts with people, and the acquisition of everyday skills such as eating and dressing. You will gain an idea of social skills by observing the child, and also from the parents. Sights and sounds are the most important stimuli that elicit reactions in a baby. By 4 weeks babies quieten to speech, or open their eyes widely in response to the spoken word. At 6 weeks a baby smiles responsively, and this is a major milestone. For this to be considered a social reaction the child must smile in response to your (or a parent's) smile. Failure to smile by 8 weeks is definitely abnormal. Failure to fixate the eyes on the observer's is consistently reported in children who later go on to develop pervasive development disorders. In addition, it is essential to check that the baby can see normally. By 12 weeks a baby squeals with pleasure, and by 16 weeks laughs out loud. By 20 weeks an infant smiles at him- or herself in a mirror.

At 7 months a baby begins to show 'stranger anxiety' and may get upset when you approach him. 'Permanence of objects'

Table 6.2 Some important developmental warning signs

At any age

Maternal concern

Discordance in different developmental areas

Regression in previously acquired skills

At 10 weeks

No smile

Failure to make eye contact

Failure to startle to noise

Weight bearing (indicates hypertonia)

Marked head lag

At 6 months

Persistent primitive reflexes

Not rolling over

Persistent squint

Hand preference

Little interest in people, toys, noises

At 10–12 months

No sitting

No double-syllable babble

No pincer grip

At 18 months

Not walking independently

Fewer than six words

Persistent mouthing and drooling

At 2½ years

No two- to three-word sentences

Abnormal repetitive behaviour

Failure to socialise

At 4 years

Unintelligible speech

develops on average by 9 months – prior to this age, a baby shows no reaction when an object is dropped from view, but at 9 months will search for it. At this time a baby enjoys 'peek-a-boo' and by 10 months can appreciate that when a parent says 'no', he or she is displeased. Other important

social features include waving bye-bye (9 months) and playing pat-a-cake (12 months).

At 15 months a child can drink from a cup, and use a spoon to eat with. At 24 months he or she may indicate toilet needs, with toilet training by day usually achieved by 2½ years (although night wetting is usual for some time beyond this). A baby starts to help with dressing by holding out an arm or leg at 1 year, and by 3 years should be able to dress and undress independently except for buttons and laces.

Special senses

Every baby should have vision checked. At birth the two eyes should be examined for symmetry, pupillary light reflexes and the 'red reflex' (the red colour appearing in the iris when examined with an instrument) (see p. 32). A white colour may indicate serious pathology. Later the baby should fix on faces, smile socially and follow objects and faces. If there is doubt, a specialist ophthalmologist should be consulted. Similarly, the ears should be examined at birth for normal anatomy. The baby will startle at noise (test from behind so vision is not tested inadvertently), although an exaggerated startle response can indicate brain pathology. Later the baby responds to the mother's voice and speech begins (see above). It is now common practice to screen babies' hearing routinely after birth in order to detect hearing disability (see pp. 33–4), and treat it, as soon as possible.

Essential milestones and when to worry

The significance of any abnormal developmental finding is fundamentally related to the child's medical status. Abnormal prenatal, natal or post natal courses can change the interpretation of a developmental concern entirely. Equally, a thorough paediatric and neurological examination, including head circumference, primitive reflexes, and eye and ear examinations, is vital in the assessment of development.

It is impossible to remember all the milestones that children acquire in the course of development, but you do need to know the sequence of the stages for each of the developmental areas. This will help you carry out a developmental assessment thoroughly, and you can check whether the child's development is appropriate for age when you have completed your evaluation. There are some milestones that are essential to know, and these are shown in Table 6.1.

In addition, it is also important that you know when the lack of certain skills becomes abnormal and requires further investigation. These are summarized in Table 6.2.

To test your knowledge on this part of the book, please see Chapter 26

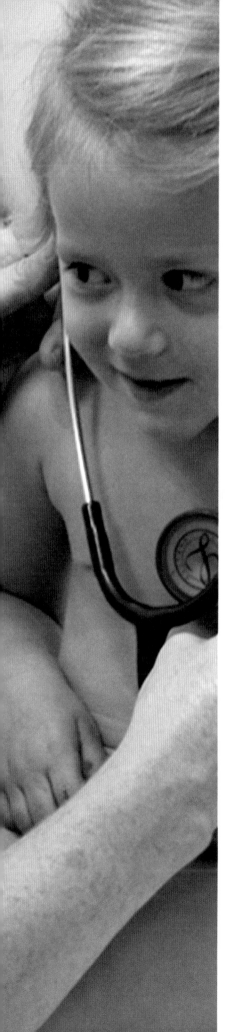

CHAPTER 7

Investigations and their interpretation

> [In the USA] at least $200 billion is wasted annually on excessive testing and treatment…, This overly aggressive care also can harm patients, generating mistakes and injuries that are thought to cause 30 000 deaths each year.
> *Chad Terhune, CNN Money, 2017*

KEY COMPETENCES

YOU MUST …

Know and understand

- When common haematological and biochemical investigations are indicated and how to interpret abnormal results
- The criteria for diagnosing a urinary tract infection
- How to perform and interpret an ECG
- How to interpret the results of a sweat test
- When imaging is helpful, and the advantages and disadvantages of different types of scan

Be able to

- Diagnose children presenting with an anaemic blood film
- Interpret CSF findings
- Measure peak expiratory flow rate
- Recognise biochemical test results indicative of dehydration, DKA and pyloric stenosis
- Interpret blood gases
- Read a chest X-ray
- Dipstick urine

Appreciate that

- Investigations should only be requested to confirm a clinical diagnosis, and 'fishing' for a diagnosis by ordering tests is poor medicine
- The normal range of many tests differs according to age
- Blood tests can be traumatic for children, and local anaesthetic cream and distraction techniques may help reduce the pain of blood taking

Essential Paediatrics and Child Health, Fourth Edition. Mary Rudolf, Anthony Luder and Kerry Jeavons.
© 2020 John Wiley & Sons Ltd. Published 2020 by John Wiley & Sons Ltd.
Companion website: www.wiley.com/go/rudolf/paediatrics

Performing tests in children and infants

Investigations should only be requested to confirm a clinical diagnosis or, if indicated, after taking a careful history and performing a physical examination. 'Fishing for a diagnosis' by ordering a battery of tests is poor medicine, an unacceptable use of resources and not in the best interests of the child.

It is important when performing potential painful procedures on children that consent has been obtained from the parent or carer. Once children are competent to agree (able to understand and weigh up the pros and cons of a test), it is also good practice to gain consent directly from the child (see General Medical Council '0–18 years: guidance for all doctors').

The environment must be thoroughly prepared in order to reduce the stress on the child and to ensure that all equipment is readily available, as children will not remain static whilst vital kit is obtained! The use of distraction techniques, such as picture books, bubbles and play therapists have been shown in research studies to reduce pain and anxiety in children during unpleasant procedures. Children are usually taken into a treatment room for procedures, in order to minimize anxieties associated with their bed space.

Local anaesthetic creams, such as EMLA® and Ametop®, are routinely used to anaesthetize the skin, prior to phlebotomy or cannula insertion. The cream is applied to the area of skin where the vein is visualized and covered with an adhesive dressing. Ametop® takes 30–45 minutes to be effective and should then be removed. The skin will be numbed for 4–6 hours. Local skin irritation and allergy is common with local anaesthetic creams and may preclude their use.

In infants, sucrose drops are frequently used as a form of analgesia prior to painful procedures, and are given as drops directly into the baby's mouth a few minutes before the procedure. Non-nutritive sucking, such as on a dummy or pacifier, is also helpful.

Capillary blood sampling

Blood tests can be carried out in infants and children from capillary samples, avoiding the use of veins. Capillary samples are typically used for blood gases (see below), with arterial sampling usually avoided unless an arterial line is inserted. Blood tests, such as full blood count and urea and electrolytes, can be taken from capillary sampling; however large volume tests, such as clotting tests should be from a venous sample.

In infants the heel is usually chosen for capillary sampling and the sampling area should avoid the base of the heel. Once the foot is cleaned, a lancet is used to make an incision into the skin on the plantar surface of the foot and the blood

drops carefully collected. Sufficient time is required in order to allow the foot to reperfuse, before very gentle pressure is again applied to the sole. Ideally, the thumb is used to 'milk' the blood towards the incision. Occasionally, petroleum jelly is used to help create droplets.

Laboratory tests

It is important to be able to interpret a number of investigations performed on children. In order to do this, you need to know the normal ranges for certain basic investigations. The importance of investigations is not simply to recognise if any value falls outside the normal range, but also to interpret the significance of the abnormality and how it influences diagnosis/management. The normal ranges in childhood for common investigations are listed in the tables below, together with the significance of abnormalities.

Full blood count (FBC)

Normal values for the major haematological indices are shown in Table 7.1.

Haemoglobin

At birth the haemoglobin concentration is high, with a mean of 18 g/dL, but falls rapidly to reach its lowest point at 2 months of age (range 9.5–14.5 g/dL) before increasing to a stable value at about 6 months. A low haemoglobin concentration indicates anaemia (p. 372). Figure 7.1 shows how it should be investigated.

Mean cell volume

Mean cell volume (MCV) is a measurement of size (volume) of the red blood cell. In paediatrics, microcytic anaemia is the

Table 7.1 Approximate normal ranges for the major haematological indices for children of 6 months and older (there may be intra-laboratory variation, and ranges may change depending on gender and age)

	Normal range
Haemoglobin	11–14 g/dL
Haematocrit	30–45%
White cell count	$6.0–15.0 \times 10^9$/L
Reticulocytes	0–2%
Platelets	$150–450 \times 10^9$/L
Mean cell volume	76–88 (fL)
Mean cell haemoglobin	24–30 pg
Erythrocyte sedimentation rate (ESR)	10–20 mm in 1 hour

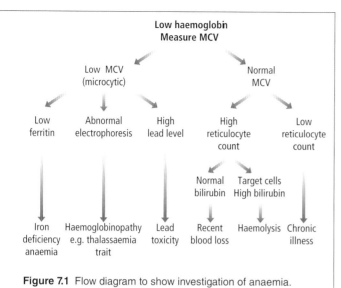

Low haemoglobin
Measure MCV

Low MCV (microcytic) → Low ferritin / Abnormal electrophoresis / High lead level

Normal MCV → High reticulocyte count / Low reticulocyte count

High reticulocyte count → Normal bilirubin / Target cells High bilirubin

Low ferritin → Iron deficiency anaemia

Abnormal electrophoresis → Haemoglobinopathy e.g. thalassaemia trait

High lead level → Lead toxicity

Normal bilirubin → Recent blood loss

Target cells High bilirubin → Haemolysis

Low reticulocyte count → Chronic illness

Figure 7.1 Flow diagram to show investigation of anaemia.

Table 7.2 Distinction between microcytic anaemia and anaemia resulting from haemolysis or blood loss (normal range)

	Microcytic hypochromic anaemia	Anaemia resulting from haemolysis or blood loss
Haemoglobin	Low	Low
Haematocrit	Low	Low
White cell count	Normal	Normal
Reticulocytes	Low	High
Platelets	Normal	Low or normal
Mean cell volume	Low	Normal
Mean cell haemoglobin	Low	Normal

most common abnormality and is a result of iron deficiency anaemia (p. 374), thalassaemia trait (p. 375) or lead toxicity. An abnormally large red cell is rare and is most likely to be a result of folate deficiency, or increased numbers of circulating reticulocytes. The MCV is normally high in the newborn for the first few weeks. A low MCV may precede a fall in haemoglobin level.

Mean cell haemoglobin

Mean cell haemoglobin (MCH) refers to the amount of haemoglobin in the red cell. In iron deficiency anaemia it is usually low (hypochromic) in conjunction with microcytic anaemia.

Examples of pathology

The two most important types of anaemia occurring in paediatrics are discussed below. Table 7.2 shows the important differences in distinguishing the two conditions. Polycythaemia (haematocrit above 65%) is common at birth, particularly if there is IUGR, twin-twin transfusion (recipient twin) or in conditions such as Trisomy 21. Polycythaemia increases the risk of neonatal jaundice, thrombocythaemia and hypoglycaemia, and can also be linked to respiratory distress.

Microcytic hypochromic anaemia

The commonest causes of microcytic, hypochromic anaemia are iron deficiency (see Figure 7.2) and thalassaemia trait, although lead toxicity may also be responsible. To distinguish iron deficiency anaemia from thalassaemia trait, it is necessary to measure serum ferritin (low in iron deficiency anaemia) and perform haemoglobin electrophoresis (abnormal

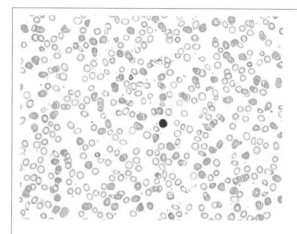

Figure 7.2 A peripheral blood film in severe iron deficiency anaemia. The red blood cells are microcytic and hypochromic with occasional target cells.

in thalassaemia trait). Ferritin is an acute phase reactant, which means that levels are elevated in response to infection and inflammation, therefore testing should wait until the child is well. Iron deficiency is also common, and it is therefore usual to give a therapeutic trial of iron supplementation first, and check ferritin levels when a repeat FBC is obtained. Lead poisoning is rare; although levels should always be checked if there is a history of pica (eating unusual items such as soil, paint).

Anaemia with reticulocytosis

This picture occurs as the result of haemorrhage or haemolysis. The reticulocyte count is increased, indicating an effort by the bone marrow to replenish the destroyed red cells. In haemolysis there may also be evidence of jaundice (p. 201), either clinically or on finding an elevated unconjugated bilirubin (Figure 7.1).

Increased white cell count (leucocytosis)

The white cell count is raised in three circumstances:
- *Viral infection* usually causes only a modest leucocytosis, with a preponderance of lymphocytes. In infectious mononucleosis (glandular fever), characteristic atypical lymphocytes are seen in the peripheral blood film.
- *Systemic bacterial infection* usually causes a higher white cell count (15–30 × 10^9/L). The blood film shows that this is mainly excess polymorphonuclear granulocytes (neutrophils) with a preponderance of immature white cells (a left shift). These changes also can occur as the result of severe stress or administration of corticosteroids.

In *leukaemia* the white cell count is very high, or occasionally very low, and blast cells are usually seen in the peripheral blood film (Figure 7.3). Platelet numbers are often also reduced.

Reduced white cell count (leucopenia)

It is important to consider the constituent cell lines (e.g. neutrophils, lymphocytes, eosinophils, basophils) when a child has leucopenia. Low lymphocytes are often acutely seen with viral infections, and usually spontaneously recover. Chronically low neutrophils, however, are more concerning, and can be caused by viral infection, medication side effects, immunodeficiency syndromes and auto-immune causes. Febrile neutropenia (fever in the context of low neutrophils) is frequently seen in children on chemotherapy or on immunosuppressive treatment, and this requires prompt IV antibiotic administration.

Reduced platelets (thrombocytopenia)

Low platelets (below 150x10^9/L) are a result of either reduced platelet production by the bone marrow or excessive consumption. A platelet level of at least 40x10^9/L is considered essential for lumbar puncture; above 50x10^9/L for any surgical procedure; or above 100x10^9/L for any neurosurgery.
- In conditions affecting marrow production (e.g. CMV, leukemia, myelodysplasia, sodium valproate use) low platelets may be seen. There may also be abnormalities in red or white cell numbers.
- *Disseminated intravascular coagulation* (DIC) is a severe complication of infection, trauma, auto-immune conditions or malignancies, and describes when multiple clots form within the small blood vessels. This leads to intravascular consumption of platelets and clotting factors resulting in low platelets and prolonged clotting; conversely clots have formed within the small vessels, which can lead to end-organ ischaemia. It has a poor prognosis unless aggressively managed. Fibrinogen levels are low, and fibrin degradation products (FDP) are likely to be elevated.
- *Allo-immune thrombocytopenia* – Newborns can experience low platelets if maternally derived platelet auto-antibodies have crossed the placenta.
- *Idiopathic Thrombocytopenia Purpura (ITP)* – this condition usually presents acutely with petechiae, purpura and bleeding (especially epistaxis and gum bleeding). The possibility of physical abuse should always be considered in a child presenting with multiple bruises; however, children with ITP have low platelets as a cause. ITP is an auto-immune disorder, often noted to be triggered by a viral infection, and in most children spontaneously resolves. Advice must be given on avoiding contact sports, minimizing trauma and seeking urgent medical assistance if the child experiences head injury or uncontrolled bleeding. Some children will not spontaneously recover and can go on to develop chronic ITP.
- *Hypersplenism* – conditions which result in excessive splenic sequestration of platelets will cause thrombocytopenia. In children this can be caused by liver disease (e.g. cirrhosis), portal vein thrombosis, sickle cell disease or metabolic storage disorders.

Blood chemistry

Modern analytical blood chemistry investigations can be done rapidly on small volumes of blood by an automated process. One disadvantage of this is that the clinician receives results on all the variables that the machine is programmed to analyse, so the results may contain 12–20 different values. It is not necessary to memorize the normal ranges for all these, but it is important to be familiar with a limited number of them as shown in Table 7.3.

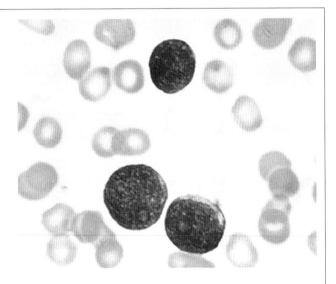

Figure 7.3 Peripheral blood film of a child with acute lymphoblastic leukaemia showing immature blast cells.

Table 7.3 Normal ranges for basic clinical chemistry variables

	Normal range
Sodium	133–145 mmol/L
Potassium	3.5–4.7 mmol/L
Chloride	96–110 mmol/L
Bicarbonate	20–27 mmol/L
Creatinine	20–80 µmol/L
Urea	2.5–6.5 mmol/L
Glucose	3.0–6.0 mmol/L
Alkaline phophatase	Infant, 150–1000 unit/L
	Child, 250–800 unit/L

Blood urea and serum creatinine

Urea and creatinine are an index of renal function and/or vascular hydration.

- *Urea* is a major metabolite of protein breakdown and is both filtered and reabsorbed by the kidneys. Its concentration in the plasma is dependent on protein intake, state of catabolism and renal function. Because its value is dependent on so many variables, it is not a good measure of renal function. The commonest cause of an elevated urea concentration is dehydration.
- *Creatinine* is produced by muscles at a constant rate and is influenced far less by catabolism than urea. It is filtered by the glomerulus, but a proportion is also secreted by the proximal tubules. Nevertheless, creatinine clearance is a reliable measure of glomerular filtration rate, and an isolated serum creatinine measurement is a much better index of renal function than urea. If there are concerns about renal function a formal estimated glomerular filtration rate, based on the child's height, should be calculated.

Sodium

In disease states sodium may be normal, increased (hypernatraemic; $Na^+ > 150$ mmol/L), or low (hyponatraemic; $Na^+ < 130$ mmol/L). These abnormalities are described under dehydration (p. 417). Causes of hypo- and hypernatraemia are shown in Table 7.4.

Potassium

Potassium is the major intracellular cation and is in relatively low concentration in the extracellular spaces. Artefactually high serum potassium levels may be found as the result of red cell haemolysis caused by keeping blood for too long in the container before analysis. If the blood is seen to be haemolysed when it is analysed, the serum potassium level measured will be unreliable.

Hypokalaemia most often occurs as the result of gastroenteritis or pyloric stenosis (see below). Hyperkalaemia results

Table 7.4 Causes of hyper- and hyponatraemia

	Causes
Hypernatraemia ($Na^+ > 150$ mmol/L)	
Dehydration	Diarrhoea
	Fluid deprivation
Excess sodium intake	Inappropriate milk feed preparation
Hyponatraemia ($Na^+ < 130$ mmol/L)	
Sodium loss	Gastroenteritis with hypotonic fluid replacement
	Renal loss (renal failure)
	Cystic fibrosis (p. 175)
Water excess	Excessive IV fluid administration
	Compulsive water drinking
	Abuse of DDAVP for enuresis
	Syndrome of Inappropriate Antidiuretic Hormone secretion (SIADH) as a result of severe infection, pneumonia, head injury etc.

from renal failure and increases as a result of metabolic acidosis. In diabetic ketoacidosis (DKA) the serum potassium is high, but drops rapidly after the DKA is treated.

Alkaline phosphatase (ALP)

Alkaline phosphatase represents a group of isoenzymes arising from bone and liver. It increases as a result of bone growth and is therefore higher in childhood; in neonates the normal range may be up to four times that of the adult.

A very high ALP concentration may represent bone disease (particularly rickets) or, less commonly in children, cholestatic liver disease. A low ALP may be seen in zinc deficiency, such as occurring with coeliac disease.

Blood gases and acid–base balance

Normal acid–base and blood gas values are shown in Table 7.5.

Disturbances in acid–base chemistry occur as the result of either respiratory or metabolic disorders. Table 7.6 lists the causes of acidosis and alkalosis.

Table 7.5 Normal ranges for acid–base and blood gas measurements

Arterial pH	7.35–7.45
Arterial P_{CO_2}	4.0–5.5 kPa
Arterial P_{O_2}	11–14 kPa (lower values in neonates, 8–10 kPa)
Arterial or venous bicarbonate	17–27 mmol/L

Blood pH

The acidity of blood is measured by pH. Normal pH range is 7.35–7.45; measurements above this refer to alkalosis and values below it indicates acidosis. In order to decide if the acidosis or alkalosis is metabolic or respiratory, you need to look at the $P\text{CO}_2$ and bicarbonate levels (see below).

$P\text{O}_2$

The partial pressure of oxygen ($P\text{O}_2$) in arterial blood indicates whether the child is hypoxic (low $P\text{O}_2$) or hyperoxic (high $P\text{O}_2$). Samples in children, however, are typically taken from a vein or a capillary sample, in which case $P\text{O}_2$ is likely to be a poor indicator of arterial values. If the $P\text{O}_2$ is low on an arterial sample, the cause for this needs to be urgently identified (see Emergency Paediatrics chapter 23). It is generally possible to increase the value using a non-rebreathe oxygen mask, nasal cannulae or head box and adjusting the inspired oxygen to keep the $P\text{O}_2$ in the normal range (normoxic). Transcutaneous oxygen saturation monitoring is now widely used for continuous oxygen assessment.

$P\text{CO}_2$

A high partial pressure of carbon dioxide ($P\text{CO}_2$) indicates underventilation. This is due to central hypoventilation (such as is in coma) or can be caused by intrinsic airway or respiratory

disease such as severe asthma or respiratory distress syndrome (p. 445). A high $P\text{CO}_2$ causes respiratory acidosis (see Table 7.7).

A low $P\text{CO}_2$ in a mechanically ventilated child indicates that the machine's settings are too high for the state of the child's lungs. It also occurs when a child hyperventilates and excessively 'blows off' carbon dioxide, as can sometimes occur with anxiety. A low $P\text{CO}_2$ causes respiratory alkalosis (see Table 7.7).

In an asthmatic attack the $P\text{CO}_2$ will typically be low due to hyperventilation. Normalization of the $P\text{CO}_2$ suggests that the child may be tiring, and may be a sign of deterioration.

Bicarbonate

This anion varies with acid–base status and this is the most important buffer for hydrogen ion. In metabolic acidosis the serum bicarbonate is low. Examples of situations where this occurs are neonatal asphyxia (p. 429) and diabetic ketoacidosis (p. 302).

In acute respiratory acidosis the bicarbonate may initially be normal, but eventually rises in an attempt to compensate and normalise the pH.

One cause of high bicarbonate in infants is excessive vomiting due to pyloric stenosis (see below and p. 203).

A simple approach to interpreting blood gases

Blood gases are not difficult to interpret if you take a systematic approach (see Figure 7.4).

First look at the pH and decide if the child is acidotic (pH < 7.35) or alkalotic (pH > 7.45).

- *If the child is acidotic*, decide if the cause is respiratory or metabolic. To do this, you need to look at the $P\text{CO}_2$ and the serum bicarbonate. If the $P\text{CO}_2$ is high, it means the child is in respiratory distress and is not able to blow off carbon dioxide adequately, thus causing a respiratory acidosis. If the cause of the respiratory distress is long-standing, the bicarbonate is likely to be high, as the body tries to compensate for the acidosis by retaining bicarbonate. The $P\text{O}_2$ may be low if the respiratory condition means that the child is unable to take in enough oxygen.

If the child is acidotic but the $P\text{CO}_2$ is normal or low, retention of carbon dioxide is obviously not the cause of the acidosis – so now turn to the bicarbonate. It will be low, indicating that the acidosis is metabolic. This occurs, for example, in neonatal asphyxia, gastroenteritis, diabetic ketoacidosis or shock,

Table 7.6 Causes of acidosis and alkalosis

	Causes
Metabolic acidosis	Severe dehydration
	Renal failure and renal tubular disease
	Neonatal asphyxia
	Shock
	Diabetic ketoacidosis and inborn errors of metabolism
Metabolic alkalosis	Pyloric stenosis
Respiratory acidosis	Respiratory failure of any cause
Respiratory alkalosis	Overventilation
	Overbreathing e.g. asthma

Table 7.7 Changes in acid–base and blood gas values according to type of alkalosis or acidosis

	Metabolic acidosis	Metabolic alkalosis	Respiratory acidosis	Respiratory alkalosis
pH	Low	High	Low	High
$P\text{O}_2$	Normal	Normal	Normal or low	Normal
$P\text{CO}_2$	Normal (or low*)	Normal (or high*)	High	Low
Bicarbonate	Low	High	Normal (or high*)	Normal (or low*)

*Compensated state.

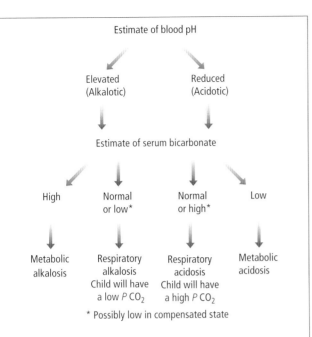

Estimate of blood pH

Elevated (Alkalotic) — Reduced (Acidotic)

Estimate of serum bicarbonate

High — Normal or low* — Normal or high* — Low

Metabolic alkalosis — Respiratory alkalosis Child will have a low $P\text{CO}_2$ — Respiratory acidosis Child will have a high $P\text{CO}_2$ — Metabolic acidosis

* Possibly low in compensated state

Figure 7.4 Flow diagram to guide the interpretation of blood gas results.

when the body tissues accumulate acid due to poor tissue perfusion. The $P\text{CO}_2$ may also be low in an attempt to raise the pH by blowing off carbon dioxide.

The *anion gap* can be calculated to consider the cause of metabolic acidosis. It incorporates the measured anions (negatively charged ions; primarily bicarbonate and chloride) and cations (positively charged ions; usually sodium). If the difference between these electrolytes is increased it implies the presence of an unmeasured acid (e.g. lactic acids or ketoacids).

- *If the child is alkalotic*, the cause again will be respiratory or metabolic. Once again, look at the $P\text{CO}_2$. If it is low, it means the child is hyperventilating (or being overventilated) and is blowing off too much carbon dioxide, thus making the pH rise and causing a respiratory alkalosis. You may find a low bicarbonate level as the body tries to compensate metabolically.

If the $P\text{CO}_2$ is normal or high, the alkalosis is not respiratory, and you will find the source is a high bicarbonate causing a metabolic alkalosis. Since the body is naturally an acid-producing machine, this situation is rare and essentially only occurs in pyloric stenosis when H+ ions are lost through vomiting.

Examples of pathology

Dehydration

Three types of dehydration occur: hyper-, iso- and hyponatraemic (see p. 416):

- *Isotonic dehydration*. In this form of dehydration, there are equal losses of sodium and water, so the serum sodium is normal. This is the commonest form, and children show physical signs commensurate with the degree of fluid loss.
- *Hyponatraemic dehydration*. In this type of dehydration, the serum sodium is less than 130 mmol/L. This is a result of

Na+ loss in excess of fluid loss. The cause is usually replacement of fluid losses, such as sweat or diarrhoea, with hypotonic solutions such as water or fizzy drinks. The child is lethargic, and the skin is dry and inelastic.

- *Hypernatraemic dehydration*. In this type of dehydration the serum Na+ is above 150 mmol/L. It may be caused by severe and acute water loss, such as in babies in whom there are difficulties establishing breast-feeding or in massive watery diarrhoea and vomiting. It can occur when a parent gives over-concentrated formula feeds by incorrectly measuring out scoops of powdered milk. Metabolic acidosis is a common feature of this condition. The child characteristically appears to be very hungry, but has fewer clinical signs of dehydration. The skin feels doughy.

Diabetic ketoacidosis (DKA) (p. 302)

The major metabolic and electrolyte abnormalities in DKA occur as a result of hyperglycaemia and ketoacidosis. The blood pH falls as a result of accumulation of ketoacids. As a consequence of the metabolic acidosis, the child attempts to compensate by hyperventilation (Kussmaul breathing, p. 410) which reduces the $P\text{CO}_2$. The high blood sugar causes an osmotic diuresis which leads to progressive dehydration with increased creatinine/urea levels. The 'corrected sodium' (taking into account the glucose level) should rise as the glucose slowly falls. A failure of this to occur increases the risk of cerebral oedema. Electrolytes need to be frequently monitored during the acute phase of therapy as there will be a shift of electrolytes in and out of the cells during the rehydration phase and as insulin is commenced. The main biochemical abnormalities are therefore summarized as:

- pH — low
- $P\text{CO}_2$ — low
- bicarbonate — low
- sodium — normal, high or low
- potassium — normal or high
- creatinine/urea — high
- glucose — high

Pyloric stenosis (p. 203)

In this condition vomiting causes excessive loss of hydrogen and chloride ions with increasing alkalosis. Because of the obstruction between stomach and duodenum, there is little sodium and potassium loss in the vomitus. Bicarbonate is increased and potassium is lost through the kidney in exchange for conserving hydrogen ions. The abnormalities seen in pyloric stenosis are:

- pH — high
- bicarbonate — low
- chloride — low
- potassium — low
- sodium — normal or low
- creatinine/urea — normal or high

Cerebrospinal fluid

Meningitis can only be diagnosed by examining the cerebrospinal fluid (CSF) at lumbar puncture. This should not be performed if there are signs of raised intracranial pressure as coning may occur (p. 235).

- The *pressure* of the CSF can be measured by connecting a calibrated plastic tube (manometer) to the needle and waiting for the fluid level to stabilize. The child must be quiet when the pressure is measured as crying causes an artefactually high pressure. Normal CSF pressure is <20-28 cmH$_2$O. A raised CSF opening pressure with a history of chronic headache or papilloedema may indicate idiopathic intracranial hypertension (pseudo-tumour cerebri) (see p. 245).
- The *colour* of the CSF should be described. It is normally absolutely clear, and cloudiness suggests infection. Bloodstained CSF may occur as a result of intracranial bleeding or as the result of a traumatic tap. A traumatic tap occurs if a blood vessel is penetrated by the needle on passage into the subarachnoid space. Intracranial bleeding can be differentiated from a traumatic tap by allowing the bloodstained fluid to drip into three successive containers. If the blood staining becomes less in successive containers, the tap was traumatic, but if the blood staining remains uniform throughout the three containers, it is likely to be because of intracranial haemorrhage. Old blood from a previous haemorrhage gives a yellow 'xanthochromic' appearance.

The CSF should be sent to the laboratory for the following analyses:

- *Microscopy.* No cells should be seen; more than five white cells in a non-bloody tap is indicative of meningitis, although up to 20 is normal in the neonatal period. In bacterial meningitis there are a large number of polymorphs, whereas in viral meningitis there are more lymphocytes. Organisms may be seen on Gram stain.
- *Chemistry.* A blood sugar should be taken at the same time as the lumbar puncture to compare the plasma and CSF glucose ratio, with the CSF glucose being at least 60% of the plasma glucose. In bacterial meningitis the CSF glucose is generally reduced to <50% of the plasma glucose. The chemistry results obtained from CSF contaminated by blood reflect serum rather than CSF levels and are therefore unreliable.

- *Culture.*
- *PCR.* If the case is a partially treated bacterial meningitis or herpes infection is possible, the sample can be sent for polymerase chain reaction analysis, which may also include enterovirus and other viral meningitides.

Normal CSF findings and abnormalities found as a result of viral and bacterial meningitis are shown in Table 7.8.

Urinalysis

It is important that you are able to examine urine, carry out urinalysis using commercially available dipsticks and interpret laboratory results. Fresh urine should be collected into a sterile container from a midstream specimen if possible. If a clean-catch urine is unobtainable, a urine bag applied over the genitalia can be used in babies, or a urine collection pad used, but the risk of contamination is high. If the child is ill, and cannot produce urine, the specimen needs to be obtained by suprapubic aspiration or catheterisation.

Observation

- *Clarity.* Is the urine cloudy? (suggests infection).
- *Colour.* Red or brown urine suggests the presence of blood. A red or pink colour suggests the bleeding is from the lower urinary tract. Cola-coloured urine suggests the blood has come from the kidneys.
- *Odour.* A smell of acetone indicates the presence of ketone bodies.

Dipstick testing

Dipsticks contain a number of reagent blocks, each one about 5 mm^2. Depending on the type of stick, there may be up to 10 reagent squares on the stick. The tests are all at best

Table 7.8 Interpretation of CSF analysis			
	Normal	**Bacterial meningitis**	**Viral meningitis**
Appearance	Clear	Turbid	Clear
Gram stain	No organisms	Organisms identified	No organisms
White cells	<5/mm³	+++Polymorphs (in early stages cells may be absent)	+ Lymphocytes (in early stages cells may be absent)
Protein	0.15–0.4 g/L	High	Normal or raised
Glucose	<50% of blood glucose	Low	Normal
Culture	No growth	Positive growth (unless partially treated)	No growth

semiquantitative (expressed as +, ++, etc.), so if quantitative information is required, the urine should be sent to the laboratory.

The procedure for dipsticking is illustrated in Figure 7.5.

1. Immerse the entire dipstick area (all the reagent squares) in the urine and remove the stick immediately.
2. Shake off excess urine from the stick.
3. Hold the strip in a horizontal position and compare the test areas with the colour chart label on the container.

Many of the reagent squares require the result to be read at an exact time after the exposure to urine. This information is on the colour chart and is summarized in Table 7.9. Colour changes that occur after 2 minutes are unreliable and should be discarded. Increasingly these dipsticks are placed into a point-of-care automated analyser which produces a printed report of the dipstick result. It is important, however, to be able to test manually and to be able to instruct parents and carers how to do this at home, if needed.

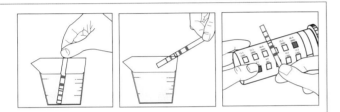

Figure 7.5 Testing urine using dipsticks. This is now often performed using a machine.

Urinalysis and culture

The only way to diagnose a urinary tract infection is by culture. A pure growth of >10^5 colony-forming units (CFU) of a single organism is indicative of a urinary tract infection. There will often also be >50 white cells. Contamination is often a problem, except when a specimen has been obtained by catheter or suprapubic aspiration. You should suspect contamination if more than one type of organism is grown, and if bacteria are found but unaccompanied by large numbers of white cells on microscopy. The laboratory will provide information on the sensitivity of the organism to a number of antibiotics.

If significant haematuria, proteinuria, nitrites or leucocytes (more than +) are found on the dipstick, the sample should be sent for microscopy in the laboratory, although in infants under 3 months it should always be sent, as dipstick testing is unreliable. NICE gives advice on when to diagnose UTI depending on the age of the child, the urine dipstick and the symptoms.

 See NICE guideline: Urinary tract infection in under 16s
https://www.nice.org.uk/guidance/cg84

Examples of pathology

Haematuria

The most common causes of haematuria are urinary tract infection, acute glomerulonephritis, stone, tumour, or a congenital malformation. The approach to diagnosing the cause of haematuria is discussed in detail on pp. 324–5.

Table 7.9 Timing and interpretation of dipstick urinalysis		
Substance in urine	**Time for block to be read**	**Comments**
Glucose	30 s	This test is specific for glucose, not other reducing substances. Glycosuria is indicative of diabetes mellitus or renal glycosuria
Bilirubin	30 s	Bilirubin in the urine suggests hepato-biliary disease
Ketones	40 s	Elevated with fasting and is always present in DKA
Specific gravity	45 s	Assesses how concentrated or dilute the urine is, particularly useful in the diagnosis of diabetes insipidus or the syndrome of inappropriate anti-diuretic hormone (SIADH)
Blood	60 s	This is a very sensitive test and may be positive in clear urine. Quantification of haematuria by urine microscopy should be carried out if positive. For diagnosis of haematuria see pp. 324–5
pH	60 s	Urinary pH can be altered by diet and serum pH
Protein	60 s	This is very sensitive and a trace or a '+' is usually not significant. If there is significant proteinuria, send a protein:creatinine ratio on an early morning specimen
Urobilinogen	60 s	High levels may be seen in jaundice
Nitrites	60 s	A positive result suggests bacterial infection. A false negative can occur when the urine has not been resident in the bladder for over 4 hours and is therefore an unreliable test in infants
Leucocytes	120 s	A positive result suggests bacterial infection, especially if nitrites also positive; however, it can also be raised by systemic infection. Confirm by sending urine for microscopy and culture

DKA, diabetic ketoacidosis.

Proteinuria

Proteinuria is an important sign of renal disease. The standard way of quantifying it is through analysis of urine protein:creatinine ratio (ideally from an early morning sample). An important paediatric cause is nephrotic syndrome, where the child presents with generalised oedema (see p. 332).

Urinary tract infection

A typical example of urine findings is as follows:

- Dipstick   Positive for blood, protein, nitrite and leucocytes (+, ++, etc.)
- Urinalysis   White cells $>50 \times 10^6$
  Red cells $1–10 \times 10^6$
- Urine culture $>10^5$ cfu/mL coliform species
  Trimethoprim sensitive
  Nitrofurantoin sensitive

Reading a chest X-ray

In most cooperative children a posterior–anterior (PA) film is taken in inspiration. This means that the child stands with his or her chest against the X-ray plate and the X-ray beam is directed from the back through the chest to the plate. In sick children or neonates the image is usually anterior–posterior (AP), when the baby lies supine on the plate with the X-ray beam above. If the X-ray is AP this should be indicated, and may alter the size of organs, such as the heart.

It is only rarely justified to increase radiation exposure in order to perform a lateral chest X-ray. The normal appearances and the anatomical landmarks are shown in Figure 7.6, and abnormal findings in Figures 7.7 and 7.8.

It is important to approach reading a chest X-ray in a systematic manner (see Box 7.1). You are not necessarily expected to make a correct diagnosis, but you are expected to describe your findings clearly. The following approach is recommended:

- *Identification*. Check the patient's name and date of birth on the film, the date that the radiograph was taken and the orientation (right and left).
- *Quality of the film*. Check that important anatomical landmarks have not been excluded, including the costophrenic angles, the ribs and soft tissues into the root of the neck. Comment on attached lines, endotracheal tube, drains, etc.
- Look at whether the *penetration* is good, under- or overexposed. An underexposed film will appear more white with less contrast and an overexposed film will be blacker with the bones clear but little distinction between the heart and the lung fields. Penetration is ideal if the vertebrae can just be seen through the heart shadow. With modern digital imaging the penetration of most radiographs can be subsequently optimized.
- Check the *positioning*. Is the patient standing square to the plane of the X-ray beam? You can see this by checking if the vertebral bodies and transverse processes are symmetrical. The clavicles and ribs should also be symmetrical. If there is

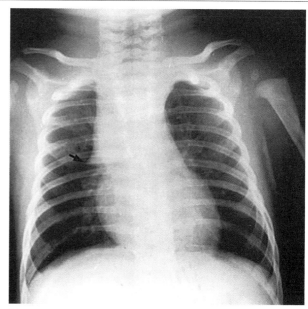

(a)

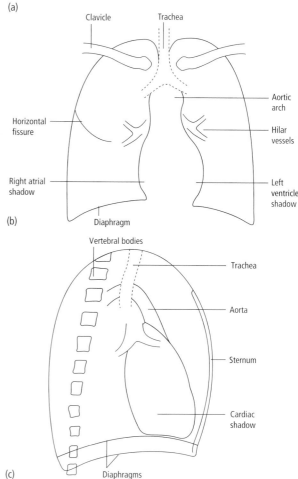

(b)

(c)

Figure 7.6 (a) A normal PA chest X-ray. The thymus gland is seen as a 'sail-shaped' shadow (indicated by the arrow); (b) anatomical landmarks of a PA chest X-ray; (c) anatomical landmarks of a lateral chest X-ray.

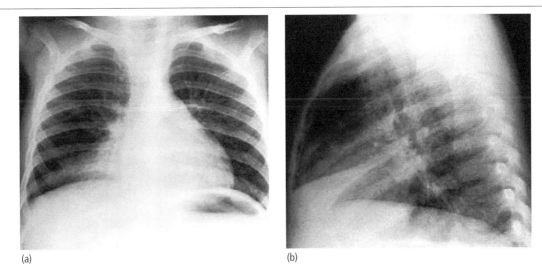

(a)   (b)

Figure 7.7 Chest X-ray. (a) PA film showing collapse of right middle lobe with loss of definition of the right heart border; (b) the collapsed right middle lobe is seen as a wedge-shaped shadow on the lateral film.

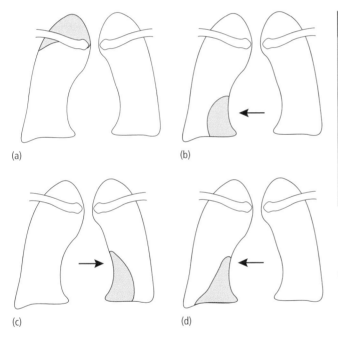

(a)   (b)

(c)   (d)

Figure 7.8 Some commonly seen abnormal features of a chest X-ray film. The arrow represents possible deviation of the heart shadow which occurs with collapse rather than consolidation. (a) Right upper lobe collapse; (b) right middle lobe collapse with loss of the right cardiac outline; (c) left lower lobe collapse; (d) right lower lobe collapse with loss of right diaphragm shadow.

rotation, the clavicles look asymmetrical. Estimating heart size or lung fields is unreliable in a rotated film.

- *Bony structures.* Look at the ribs, clavicles and vertebral bodies, and comment on any asymmetry or congenital abnormality. Count the ribs on both sides (12 pairs should be apparent). Missing ribs may occur as the result of cardiothoracic surgery

Box 7.1 Approach to reading a chest X-ray

- Identify the image with patient's name, date of birth, date and laterality
- Comment on quality of the film (penetration and rotation)
- Examine bony landmarks and count ribs
- Examine the diaphragms
- Examine heart border. Comment on cardiomegaly and any lack of clarity of the heart outline
- Examine lung fields. Comment on symmetry, clarity and any opacity. Comment on hilar regions

or represent a congenital abnormality. Look for incidental fractures, suggestive of physical abuse.

- *Diaphragms.* Both diaphragms should be clear, and the right is normally higher than the left because of the liver position. Examine the costophrenic angles, which should be clear and sharply defined. If they are not, a small pleural effusion may be the cause. Look for air below the diaphragm, which is always abnormal.

- *Cardiac outline.* Measure the cardiac outline at its widest point and compare it to the widest diameter of the ribs to determine if there is cardiomegaly. In infants the normal ratio of cardiac to widest chest wall diameter is 0.6, and in older children a ratio of up to 0.5 is normal. Comment on the clarity of the cardiac outline. If the right border of the heart is obscured, this suggests right middle lobe collapse/consolidation (Figures 7.7 and 7.8b). If the left is indistinct the lingula is involved.

- *Lung fields.* The lung fields should be symmetrical and of uniform radiolucency. The only markings within the lung fields should be pulmonary blood vessels. Comment on the hilar shadows. It requires considerable experience to decide whether there is excessive or normal hilar shadowing. Identify the horizontal fissure on the PA film (see Figure 7.6b).

- *Lateral chest X-ray.* A lateral film is occasionally indicated. Interpretation of lateral chest X-rays requires some experience, but the various normal landmarks should be recognised (see Figure 7.6c).

Examples of pathology

Collapse and consolidation

Collapse and/or consolidation of a lung lobe can usually be seen by an area of focal opacity (see Figures 7.7a and 7.8). The right middle lobe is a common site, which causes loss of definition of the right heart border. It is also seen as a wedge-shaped shadow if a lateral film is done. Right lower lobe collapse causes loss of the right diaphragm shadow.

If there is deviation of the mediastinal shadow with lung field opacity, this suggests collapse rather than consolidation.

Pleural effusion

Small pleural effusions blunt the costophrenic angles and large effusions cause extensive radio-opacity in the affected lung field, often with the mediastinal shadow pushed to the opposite side.

Electrocardiograph (ECG)

The ECG in children and infants follows the same electrode landmark positioning as that in adults. The only exception to this in the smaller infant where, due to space constrictions, the lead V4 can be switched to the same position but on the right chest wall, and it is labelled V4R.

Each electrical sequence (which usually correlates to one heart beat) of the ECG is made up of five waves (see Figure 7.9):

- *P wave* – this is created by the depolarization of the atria; therefore abnormalities are often associated with atrial pathology. The presence of a P wave before each sequence indicates sinus rhythm. In children it is more common to find *sinus arrhythmia*, which is where sinus rhythm is present, but the heart rate is irregular. The irregularity in sinus arrhythmia is exacerbated by breathing and can therefore be quickly checked clinically by asking the child to hold their breath.
- *QRS complex.* The *Q wave* is a downward deflection prior to the R wave. Q waves are often normally found in children, especially in the chest leads and inferior leads. The *R wave* is an upward deflection, and the *S wave* another downward wave. The QRS complex is caused by the depolarization of the ventricles and therefore abnormalities in the width of the complex are associated with conduction defects. The amplitude of the QRS wave, assuming that the ECG is set up with a standard gain, can indicate ventricular hypertrophy, if excessive.
- *T wave* – this wave results from repolarization of the ventricles and it is usually an upward wave. In children and infants, however, T waves in V1-3 should be inverted (therefore a

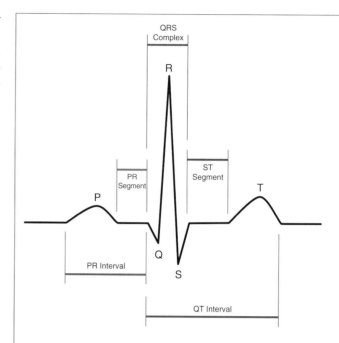

Figure 7.9 The electrical sequence of waves that make up the ECG.

downward wave) and gradually flip during childhood (starting with V3, and finishing with V1). If an upward T wave is seen in V1 in a young child, this suggests atrial hypertrophy.

ECG interpretation in paediatrics

Standard ECG interpretation follows a typical approach:

Check the details	Check patient demographics, date and time of ECG
Rate	Check the heart rate, remembering that the normal heart rate in children is usually much faster than in adults
Rhythm	Look at the rhythm and check each wave to ensure that a P wave precedes it
Axis	There are various different techniques to measure the axis. These techniques involve assessing the R and S waves, usually in leads aVF and lead I. If R>S in both aVF and lead I (both positive) this is a 'normal axis'; however, most children have a slight right axis deviation, therefore aVF is positive but lead I is negative
Wave forms and intervals	Assess the wave forms, detailed above, as well as the intervals between the waves, specifically PR interval, ST interval and QT interval (see below)

In *infants* the right ventricle is relatively large given the in utero environment. This results in an ECG suggestive of right ventricular hypertrophy with dominant R wave in the V1 lead; right axis deviation; and T wave inversion in leads V1-V3.

Long QT syndrome is a cardiac conduction abnormality which can cause sudden cardiac death. It is therefore important to be vigilant for the electrocardiac signs. The calculated QT (QTc) is used in children due to the increase in sinus arrhythmia (as above) and takes into account the heart rate (using the RR interval). QT is measured from the beginning of the Q wave to the end of the T wave. A QTc of over 450ms is considered abnormal.

Peak Expiratory Flow Rate (PEFR)

This is a common, and important, bedside test in children, and it is important that you fully understand in order to explain to children and families how to check it at home. PEFR (or 'peak flow') is a monitoring technique for children with asthma, when a reduction in usual flow suggests an exacerbation. It can usually be taught to children over 4–5 years old.

The peak flow is the maximal flow generated by one forceful expiration, and should be checked three times in order to find the best result. Reference charts can be used to compare the expected flow rate for the child's age, gender and height. A peak flow diary is often provided for families to record the values over time, looking for diurnal variation and pre- and post-inhaler.

1. Stand the child up and explain the process. Check that the moveable tab, which displays the reading, has been reset to zero.
2. The child will need to take a deep breath in, and then place the device in the mouth, making a tight seal with the lips around the mouthpiece. The device should be horizontal and fingers should not obstruct the channel.
3. The child must then blow, strongly and quickly, to push the tab away from the mouth.
4. Take a note of the score and then repeat two more times (with recovery time in between) in order to find the best of the three scores.

Ultrasound

Ultrasound is a frequently used investigation in children. It is generally well tolerated and safe, and unlike X-rays it does not involve exposure to ionizing radiation. Common indications for ultrasound include assessing the size and texture of abdominal and pelvic organs (Figure 7.10), assessing fluid collections within the chest, and imaging the brain of an infant via the anterior fontanelle (Figure 7.11).

CT scan

Computed tomography (CT) scans generate detailed views of any region of the body as apparent 'slices'. The technique is particularly useful for rapidly detecting large masses or bleeds within the head (Figure 7.12), and for detecting bronchiectasis and other lung disease (Figure 7.13). The child needs to lie still for 1–2 minutes, so toddlers may require sedation. Unfortunately, CT scans involve a relatively high dose of ionizing radiation, and this needs to be balanced against the value of the information the scan may provide. For cranial imaging which is less urgent, or where the child requires sedation, an MRI is usually preferable.

MRI scan

Magnetic resonance imaging (MRI) uses electromagnetic fields, rather than ionizing radiation, to produce very detailed 'slice' images. MRI is particularly good at imaging the brain and spinal cord, giving much more detail than CT scanning, particularly in terms of differentiating between white matter and grey matter (Figures 7.14, 7.15, 7.16). To get clear images the child needs to lie still for many minutes, and the scanner can be noisy, so sedation is usually required.

Sweat test

The sweat test is the common physiological test for cystic fibrosis (CF) (p. 175). It is performed by stimulating a small part of the arm to sweat by pilocarpine iontophoresis.

Collection and analysis of sweat

Sweat is collected from the skin using pilocarpine applied to the skin and a painless electrical current, to stimulate the sweat glands. The sweat is then collected over the next 30 minutes

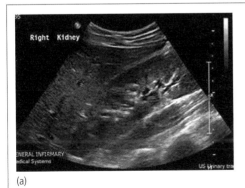
(a)

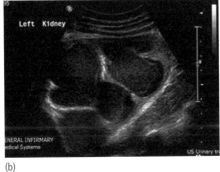
(b)

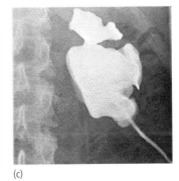
(c)

Figure 7.10 (a) Ultrasound of normal right kidney. (b) Ultrasound of hydronephrotic left kidney, with dilated renal pelvis showing up as echo-poor area: contrast with normal right kidney seen in (a). (c) Contrast study via nephrostomy, showing massive dilation of hydronephrotic renal pelvis and obstructed ureter (same patient as a and b). *Source:* Images courtesy of Dr Rosemary Arthur.

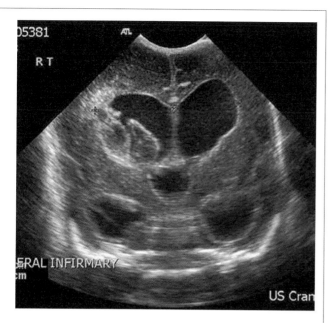

Figure 7.11 Cranial ultrasound of a preterm neonate, showing a coronal view of dilated lateral ventricles. Intraventricular haemorrhage is visible on the right, with some surrounding venous infarction.

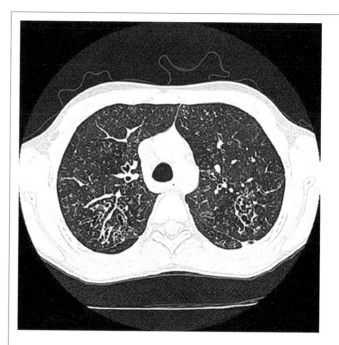

Figure 7.13 High-resolution CT scan of the lungs, showing bronchiectasis affecting both upper lobes. This child has cystic fibrosis.

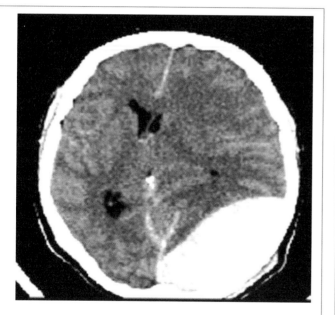

Figure 7.12 Head CT scan showing a severe extradural haematoma on the left with compression of the left lateral ventricle and midline shift towards the right.

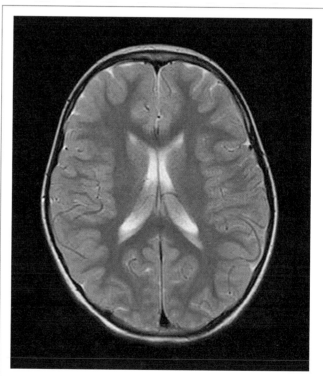

Figure 7.14 MRI scan of a normal 6-year-old. On this T_2-weighted image, cerebrospinal fluid in the lateral ventricles appears white. The dark grey areas show areas rich in myelin.

using a plastic coil, gauze or filter paper and analysed in the laboratory. A specific volume of sweat needs to be collected, but this is usually possible in children older than 2 weeks of age. Children with cystic fibrosis have more chloride in their sweat than normal, with chloride levels of 60 mmol/L suggestive of CF.

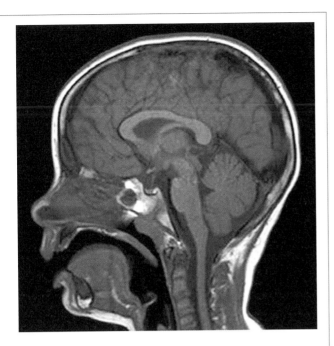

Figure 7.15 Sagittal T$_1$-weighted MRI scan of a normal 6-year-old. Note the midline structures, including corpus callosum, brainstem and cerebellum. Note that cerebrospinal fluid appears black on T$_1$-weighted images.

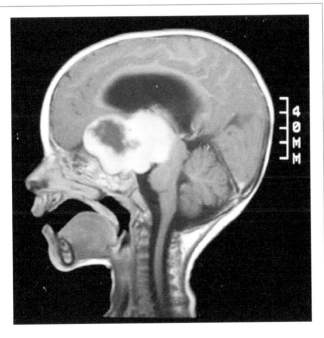

Figure 7.16 Sagittal T$_1$-weighted MRI scan showing large white optic glioma, with some darker cystic change within it.

Genetic testing

Genetic testing is being used much more frequently to diagnose illnesses in children, and is a rapidly developing field. During the course of your medical career it is likely that further huge advances will continue in clinical genetics and that genetic testing, and 'personalized medicine', will be standard. From a cost of $100m to sequence the complete human genome in 2001, the price had reduced to around $1000 by 2017, and it is increasingly being used in paediatric conditions.

Examples of genetic tests:

- *Karyotype.* The karyotype is a rapid assessment in which all the 22 pairs of chromosomes, plus the sex chromosomes (labelled as X or Y) are identified. It can be used to detect trisomy (more than two pairs of a chromosome), or very large deletions.
- *FISH.* For rapid assessment of possible trisomy or specific genetic abnormalities associated with an identifiable genetic location, the FISH (fluorescence in situ hybridization) test is used. This uses a radio-labelled marker specific for a certain region of DNA and promptly indicates whether the area is present or not. It is used for initial identification of trisomy 21, 18, or Prader-Willi syndrome, but cannot be used for syndromes where multiple genetic causes are implicated.
- *CGH array.* Many units are using CGH array 'microarray' testing (comparative genomic hybridization) as a replacement for karyotype. This procedure compares the patient's DNA to control specimens and can be used to detect much smaller deletions or duplications. It will not detect balanced chromosome rearrangements, such as translocation. It is frequently used in children with neurodevelopmental problems. As it is a non-specific test it can detect wholly unrelated problems (e.g. risk of developing breast cancer) and families need to be counselled regarding this.
- *Gene panels.* Specific gene panels are also being used more frequently for specific diseases such as epilepsy, with now around 100-gene panels being offered for children with complex epilepsies. As with all genetic testing, detailed medical information is needed in order for the geneticists to interpret the significance of any 'abnormal' findings and parental gene tests are often required in order to help determine whether the 'abnormality' is pathological or not.
- *Whole exome and whole genome sequencing* are becoming increasingly used for complicated cases. One drawback is the finding of many variations whose significance is unknown (VUS). The interpretation of these techniques requires special expertise.

To test your knowledge on this part of the book, please see Chapter 26

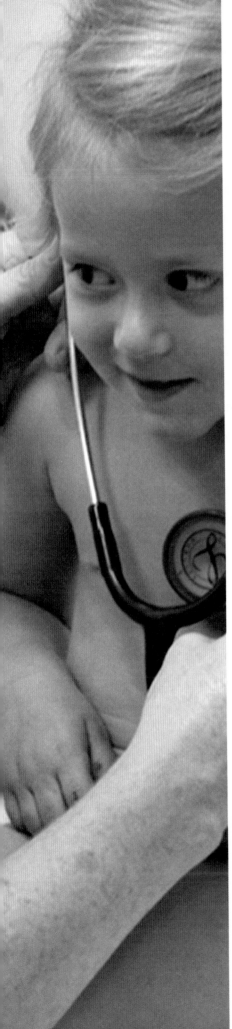

CHAPTER 8
Prescribing for children

She found a little bottle….., and tied round the neck of the bottle was a paper label, with the words "DRINK ME" beautifully printed on it in large letters.

Alice in Wonderland, Lewis Caroll

KEY COMPETENCES

YOU MUST...

Know and understand

- The principles underpinning drug development in children
- The differences, physiological and other, between children and adults that affect prescribing
- The principles of prescribing safely and effectively for children
- The routes available for drug administration and their relative advantages and disadvantages

Be able to

- Find reliable information for safe prescribing
- Write a legible, safe and legal prescription for IV fluids (bolus and maintenance), oral rehydration solution, common analgesics, antibiotics, asthma medications and emergency medications, e.g. adrenaline for anaphylaxis
- Calculate dosage according to weight and surface area
- Understand common prescribing errors in children

Appreciate that

- Prescribing errors are the commonest cause of preventable adverse drug events
- Compliance issues are very frequent causes of treatment failure
- Allergy to drugs can be life-threatening but is greatly over-diagnosed

Essential Paediatrics and Child Health, Fourth Edition. Mary Rudolf, Anthony Luder and Kerry Jeavons.
© 2020 John Wiley & Sons Ltd. Published 2020 by John Wiley & Sons Ltd.
Companion website: www.wiley.com/go/rudolf/paediatrics

In this chapter we will examine how prescribing for children is different from adults and how it presents special challenges and problems.

Why prescribing for children is important

Children are not little adults in many fundamental biological respects. Their bodies are different as is their behaviour, and they are highly dynamic in growth and development. This makes extrapolation of adult pharmacotherapeutics into the paediatric age group very difficult. The result is that prescribing errors are common in children and that these can sometimes lead to serious injury or death. Many clinical incidents in paediatrics are the results of drug errors. Drugs administered to pregnant or breast-feeding mothers may also have serious impacts on the child, unborn or born.

Knowledge in paediatric pharmacotherapeutics has in many ways trailed behind that which is known in adults, and some of the reasons for this will be examined at the end of this chapter. However better information and guidance have been produced in recent years. A key resource is the *British National Formulary for Children©* which provides essential practical information for healthcare professionals involved in prescribing, dispensing, monitoring and administration of medicines to children.

Pharmacology, physiology and paediatrics

In order to understand how drugs interact with children, three areas of pharmacological science are particularly important:

1. Pharmacodynamics. This deals with mechanism of action of drugs, at a cellular, systemic and biochemical level. 'What drugs do to us'.
2. Pharmacokinetics. This is the study of how drugs behave over time. The principal areas of interest are absorption, bioavailability, distribution, metabolism and excretion. 'What we do to drugs'.
3. Pharmacogenetics. This discipline is still relatively young and studies the relationship between genes and drugs. 'Different people, different drugs'.

Generally the mechanisms of action of many drugs are similar in children and adults although their consequences may be very different, both in desired and adverse effects. For example, there are some conditions which are primarily paediatric such as growth hormone deficiency, certain kinds of epilepsy or specific malignancies such as neuroblastoma. Drugs used in these disorders have effects not therefore seen in adults. On the other hand, many drugs have adverse side effects in children that are not applicable in adults.

Antibiotics provide excellent examples, for example the 'grey baby syndrome' with chloramphenicol, neonatal jaundice with sulphonamides, cartilage damage by quinolones and permanent tooth enamel staining by tetracyclines. Another important example is dystonia induced by the antiemetic metoclopramide.

Many differences exist between fetuses, infants, toddlers, older children, adolescents and adults in the way they handle pharmacological agents. It is important to understand aspects of physiology which are the main determinants of this heterogeneity in order to be able to prescribe for children in a professional and competent manner.

1. *Body size and constitution.* The first and most obvious variable is body weight (see next paragraph), which influences the dose of a drug that will be safe and effective. In addition, however, babies' bodies are considerably different in composition from adults. In young infants, the proportion of body fat is low (approximately 10-20% of body weight), while the total body water content is relatively high (80-90% of the body weight) compared with adults (50-60%). The distribution of water between the intra- and extracellular compartments is also different, with the proportion of extracellular water falling from around 50% in infancy to 20% in adulthood. These facts affect dose relative to body weight. For example, water-soluble drugs such as penicillin or beta-blockers have a higher volume of distribution relative to weight compared to adults, while the opposite is true for a lipid-soluble drug such as diazepam. In addition, drugs which are soluble in fat or specific tissues (such as digoxin in heart muscle) are likely to be cleared, excreted or metabolized more slowly in adults and therefore have shorter half-lives in children.

2. *Calculation of body size.* The size of the body can be most conveniently evaluated by weight or more accurately by body surface area (BSA). In practice most paediatric drugs are prescribed relative to weight. In some cases in which therapeutic ranges are relatively wide, the age of the child is a sufficient guide to dosing without reference to weight. An example is paracetamol administration in infants. Some drugs that are poorly absorbed like mebendazole, can be given in a standard dose. However, care must be taken not to use weight indiscriminately as a guide, particularly in older children in whom a maximum adult dose may be approached and should not be exceeded. It must be also borne in mind that drugs that penetrate the blood–brain–barrier (BBB) well will have a relatively large volume of distribution in children since the CNS reaches 90% of adult size by 6 years of age, a full decade before somatic growth reaches the same ratio. In addition, the BBB is relatively porous in infants and

drugs penetrate it better leading to possible toxicity (e.g. amphotericin).

3. *Drug metabolism and clearance.* The liver is the prime site of drug metabolism and biliary clearance, while the kidney clears drugs in the urine. Both organs are immature and relatively inefficient in neonates and infants. The liver is especially important if a drug is administered orally, and the absorbed drug undergoes first-pass metabolism. Drug metabolism in the liver consists of oxidation, reduction and hydrolysis reactions primarily dependent on the cytochrome P450 system, which is present at about 30–40% of adult levels in infants and which reaches maturity at the end of the first decade. The effects of this are complex, tending to extend drug half-life in many cases and reducing it in other cases. The efficacy of drugs which are administered in the form of a pro-drug and which require metabolism to become active may be affected by age. Conjugation with gluconate or sulphate may also alter behaviour, so that in the case of paracetamol this actually protects the young child from toxicity. There are also examples of drugs that produce metabolites in children that are not normally present in adults. These metabolites may be responsible for some of the desired or side effects seen in children. An example is theophylline in very young infants which produces caffeine, a product not usually seen in adults.

The kidney also has different age-dependent mechanisms for excretion of drugs related to the glomerular filtration rate, which may be as low as 2–4 mL per minute per 1.73 m² in neonates rising to around 90 mL/min/1.73 m² in adults. Tubular absorption and secretion add to the complexity.

4. *Gastrointestinal function.* Gastrointestinal function is important for the oral administration of drugs to children, as well as biliary excretion (which affects, e.g., cephalosporins in the treatment of cholangitis). The potential obstacles begin with the mouth, and getting drugs into it! Compliance and drug refusal are important everyday issues requiring skill and experience. Assuming the child takes a drug, swallows it and does not vomit, the journey has just begun. Many anatomical and physiological parameters are important for drug action in children. Among the important variables are gastric emptying time, gastric pH, pancreatic maturity, bowel motility, mucosal surface area, function and integrity, and biliopancreatic function. Increasing interest has also been paid in recent years to the gut microbiome as an important determinant of biological function. All these functions change and develop with age, not always in a linear fashion, and they all affect the ways drugs are given and work in children.

5. *Binding proteins.* Many drugs are mostly present in the plasma in a bound form, either to albumin or globulins. Common important examples include ibuprofen, furosemide, diazepam, digoxin, ceftriaxone and montelukast. The binding proteins may be found at reduced levels in neonates and infants. Physiological changes in infants, such as increases in bilirubin or free fatty acids, or indeed other drugs, can compete with drugs for binding sites and displace them from protein binders. This can increase the risk of toxicity and requires adjustment in drug dosage accordingly.

6. *Skin permeability.* Skin permeability is maximal in premature infants steadily falling as the child ages. Permeable skin allows a high insensible fluid loss requiring replacement, while drugs may be absorbed from patches by this route in selected cases. A permeable skin also puts the child at risk of absorbing drugs from topical medications such as creams and lotions. An example is the unwanted systemic action of steroids or antiseptics absorbed form creams widely applied in an infant.

Genetic disorders often present in childhood and therefore a knowledge of those that impact drug therapy is important in paediatrics. The science of personalized prescribing dependent on genetic polymorphism is in its infancy and is currently most developed in the field of oncology. A child with a malignant disease will undergo thorough genetic evaluation including panels of genetic mutations which may affect prognosis and importantly, the efficiency and toxicity of drug therapy. An important monogenetic disorder which affects drug tolerance is Glucose-6-Phosphate Dehydrogenase Deficiency (G6PDD). This is relatively common in natives of the Mediterranean countries as well as black Africans. Exposure to forbidden substances in these patients may cause severe and sudden haemolysis and jaundice. Remember that moth balls and fava beans are also forbidden for these patients.

Prescribing fluids for children

This is a special area of prescribing since the administration of fluids is so common. In general, dehydration is best treated with oral rehydration solutions (ORS) (see Chapter 23, pp 416–419), even if the child has mild to moderate vomiting. ORS has been shown to be safe and effective and has undoubtedly saved millions of lives. The principle of ORS is to provide a solution of cations for replacement of losses (especially sodium and potassium), anions (usually chloride and citrate) and glucose (usually about 2 g per 100 mL). The glucose is necessary for the efficient absorption of cations via glucose-dependent channels in the bowel mucosa. When intravenous fluids are necessary it is important to provide the correct amount of the correct fluid at the correct rate. Further details of prescribing fluids are given in Chapter 23.

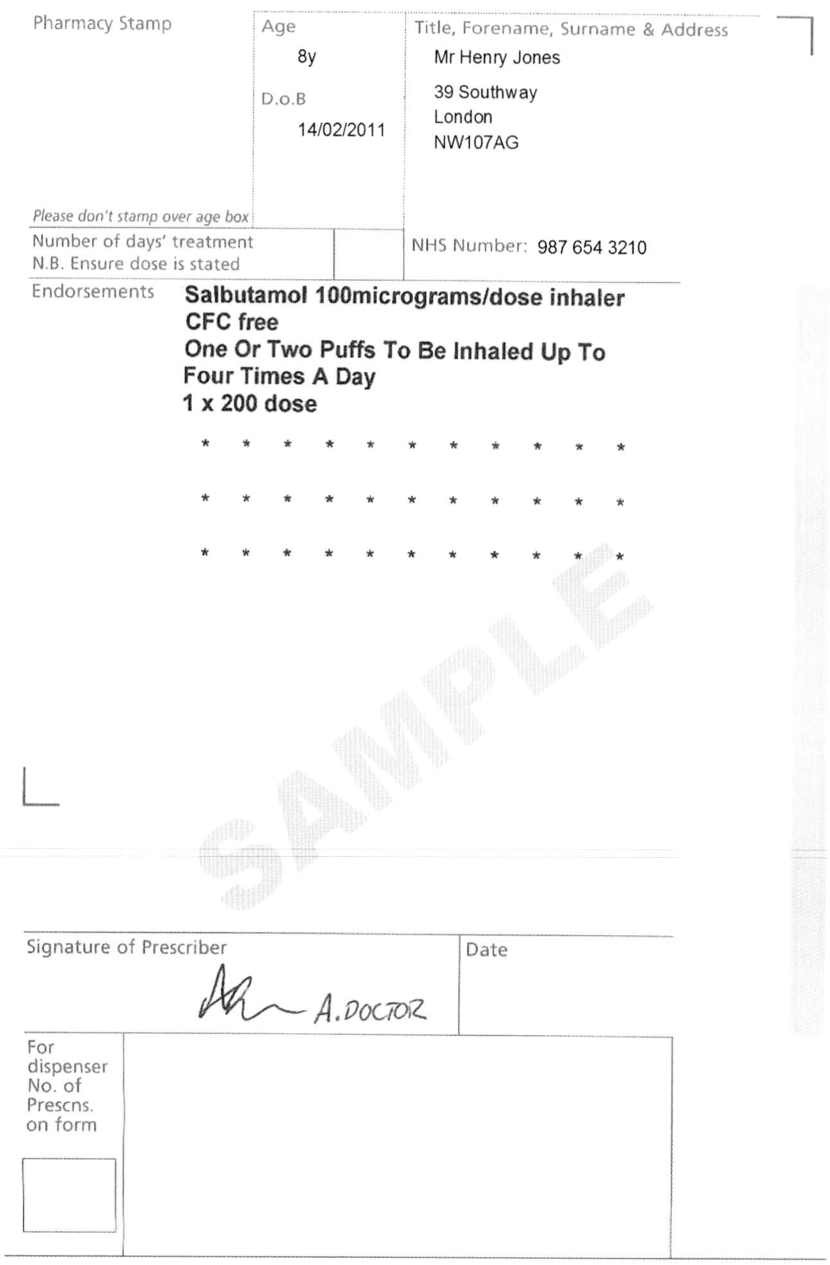

Pharmacy Stamp	Age	Title, Forename, Surname & Address
	8y	Mr Henry Jones
	D.o.B	39 Southway
	14/02/2011	London
		NW107AG

Please don't stamp over age box

Number of days' treatment N.B. Ensure dose is stated		NHS Number: 987 654 3210

Endorsements

Salbutamol 100micrograms/dose inhaler
CFC free
One Or Two Puffs To Be Inhaled Up To
Four Times A Day
1 x 200 dose

* * * * * * * * * *

* * * * * * * * * *

* * * * * * * * * *

Signature of Prescriber	Date
A.DOCTOR	

For dispenser No. of Prescns. on form

Figure 8.1 Prescription for salbutamol by inhaler for an 8-year-old boy.

Principles of formulations and writing a prescription

Medications for children may be prescribed in many different formulations and via different routes. Giving medications orally successfully to children requires care, patience, experience and sometimes ingenuity! Many medications for children come in liquid form, either as syrups or as concentrated drops. It is vital to check in every case the concentration of the syrup as many come in different concentrations (e.g. paracetamol, amoxicillin) and size of a drop (e.g. many dropper bottles provide 25 drops/mL). Because of the many possibilities for con-

fusion and error, it is safer and more appropriate to prescribe drugs as milligram (mg) doses rather than volumes or numbers of drops. Some drugs may be prescribed in micrograms (note that the word 'micrograms' should not be abbreviated, see Box 8.1 below) rather than milligrams (e.g. adrenaline). Surprisingly many children find swallowing tablets, mini-tablets, granules or capsules easier than fluids, since the latter often have nasty tastes. When this is the case, the prescription may need to be given in a rounded up or down dose. If a child vomits a dose within 15–30 minutes of administration, it is usually advisable to repeat the dose; the danger of overdose is small. If a child is recalcitrant (and even some adolescents are

Box 8.1 *BNF Children*© Dose Writing Guidelines

- The unnecessary use of decimal points should be avoided, e.g. 3 mg, not 3.0 mg.
- Quantities of 1 gram or more should be written as 1 g, etc.
- Quantities less than 1 gram should be written in milligrams, e.g. 500 mg, not 0.5 g.
- Quantities less than 1 mg should be written in micrograms, e.g. 100 micrograms, not 0.1 g.
- When decimals are unavoidable, a zero should be written in front of the decimal point where there is no other figure, e.g. 0.5 mL, not .5 mL.
- Use of the decimal point is acceptable to express a range, e.g. 0.5 to 1 g.
- 'Micrograms' and 'nanograms' should not be abbreviated. Similarly 'units' should not be abbreviated.
- The term 'millilitre' (mL) is used in medicine and pharmacy, and cubic centimetre, c.c., or cm³ should not be used.
- Dose and dose frequency should be stated; in the case of preparations to be taken 'as required', a minimum dose interval should be specified. Care should be taken to ensure the child receives the correct dose of the active drug. Therefore, the dose should normally be stated in terms of the mass of the active drug (e.g. '125 mg three times daily'); terms such as '5 mL' or '1 tablet' should be avoided except for compound preparations.

unwilling to take oral medications) some drugs may be given as rectal suppositories or nasal drops. These are often not conveniently dosed, however. Recently sub-lingual 'melts' and dissolvable oral films have extended the options available.

Another important route for paediatric prescription is the nebulizer or the metered-dose inhaler (MDI). These are frequently used in respiratory disorders such as asthma (see p. 169). The physician needs to specify the dose of an inhaled drug and diluent, as well the frequency of administration. An MDI is used with a spacer-device for young children as they cannot coordinate the spray operation, inhalation and holding breath. Careful technique teaching and instruction is vital for the efficient use of these excellent methods of treatment. (see p. 169).

Sometimes parenteral therapy at home is needed, such as subcutaneous insulin injections for diabetes or growth hormone for growth hormone deficiency. In recent years infusion-pumps for insulin have become increasingly popular (see Chapter 15). Children and their families can be taught to manage these injections, and children at a surprisingly young age can learn to auto-inject. Intramuscular injections need to be given by trained nurses; they are often painful although local anaesthetics may ameliorate discomfort. Intravenous medications and continuously infused medications are the province of the hospital ward, or intravenous outreach services. Special calculators are available for the calculation of continuous infusions which are weight- and rate-dependent.

Drugs should always be prescribed after careful consideration as to the necessity and appropriateness of the medication; its route, dose, frequency and duration of administration; careful explanation to the family about desired and undesired effects and what to do if they arise (including possible allergic or intolerance reactions). Doses must be accurate and clearly written (see Box 8.1 and Figures 8.2 and 8.3). The prescription will usually be in the form of the amount to be given at each administration and the number in 24 hours. The total amount to be prescribed should be noted. Although equal

A. PRN (as needed) prescriptions

Medication	Paracetamol
Dose	500mg
Route	PO
Indication	Pain
Max dose in 24 hours	2g
Minimal dosing interval	4 hours
Print name and contact	
Sign	

Medication	Adrenaline
Dose	300 micrograms
Route	IM
Indication	Anaphylaxis
Max dose in 24 hours	N/A
Minimal dosing interval	5 minutes
Print name and contact	
Sign	

B. IV fluid prescriptions

	Route	Additives	Volume	Rate	Print name and contact	Sign
0.9% sodium chloride/5% glucose	IV	20 mmol potassium chloride	500ml	56ml/hr		
0.9% sodium chloride bolus	IV	N/A	340ml	Bolus over 20 minutes		

Figure 8.2 Examples of prescriptions written in the hospital setting.

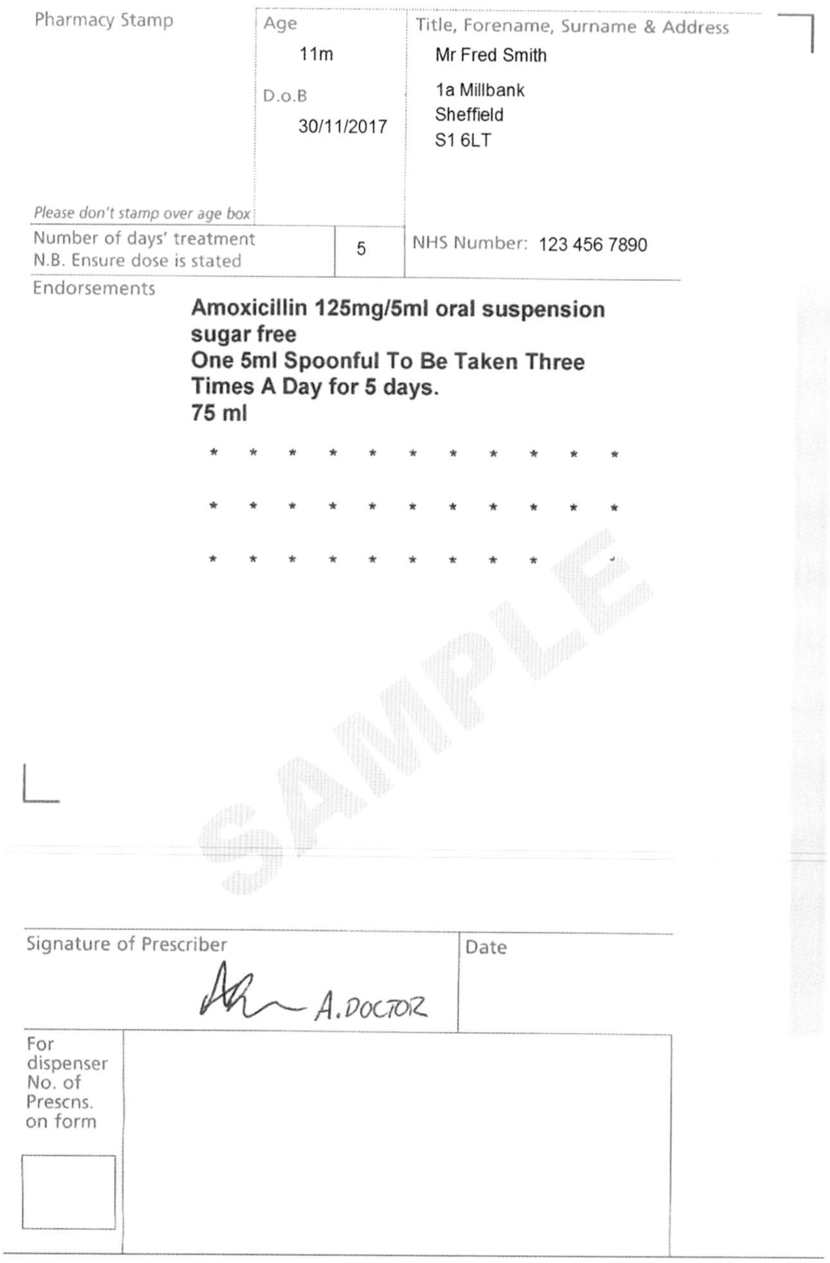

Pharmacy Stamp	Age		Title, Forename, Surname & Address
	11m		Mr Fred Smith
	D.o.B		1a Millbank
	30/11/2017		Sheffield
			S1 6LT

Please don't stamp over age box

Number of days' treatment N.B. Ensure dose is stated	5	NHS Number: 123 456 7890

Endorsements

Amoxicillin 125mg/5ml oral suspension
sugar free
One 5ml Spoonful To Be Taken Three
Times A Day for 5 days.
75 ml

```
*  *  *  *  *  *  *  *  *  *  *

*  *  *  *  *  *  *  *  *  *  *

*  *  *  *  *  *  *  *  *
```

Signature of Prescriber	Date
A. DOCTOR	

For dispenser No. of Prescns. on form	

Figure 8.3 Prescription for amoxicillin for an 11-month-old baby.

spacing of administration is desirable, some flexibility due to child care constraints, sleep, meals, etc. may be necessary and is rarely harmful. If a dose is forgotten, it is often better to give an extra dose rather than risk under treatment. Some drugs require frequent drug-level monitoring for efficacy (e.g. anti-convulsants) or to avoid toxicity (gentamicin, digoxin).

The prescription should clearly state the identity of the patient, his/her age, date of birth, weight (or BSA if appropriate), the date and the total amount of the drug to be prescribed as well as dose, route, frequency and duration. Drug names should be written in capital letters and in their generic form (unless prescribing a standard proprietary combination formulation). Lastly, the prescription must be written indelibly, legibly, be signed by the doctor and his name and address and phone number appended.

When prescribing, the use of abbreviations should be kept to a minimum and then only use those which have reached wide acceptance as a result of long and traditional use (see Boxes 8.2 and 8.3 below).

Box 8.2 Some commonly used abbreviations in prescribing

Formulation		Route of administration		Frequency		Dose	
amp	Ampule	im	Intramuscular	Bd/bid	Twice daily	g or gm	Gram
cap	Capsule	io	Intraosseus	nocte	At night	Kg	Kilogram
crm	Cream	ip	Intraperitoneal	od	Once daily	mg	Milligram
drp	Drops	inh	Inhalation	prn	As required	mL	Millilitre
sup	Suppository	iv	Intravenous	q	Every		
syr	Syrup	po	Per os (orally)	qid/qds	4 times daily		
tab	Tablet	pr	Per rectum	tid/tds	3 times daily		
ung	Ointment	pv	Per vagina	x	Times		
		sc	Subcutaneous				
		sl	Sublingual				

Rx, R, R$_x$ Take as prescribed
PN Parenteral nutrition

Box 8.3 Safe prescribing for children

A. Check Patient Information
- Name and address of patient and or ID number
- Date and time (for hospitals)
- Age, date of birth, weight, medical and drug history
- Are there known allergies?
- Is renal function compromised?

B. Check Drug Information
- Use a reliable source if unsure about the drug, its dose or administration route
- Are there potential drug interactions?

C. If you are requested verbally to write a prescription
- Ensure instructions are complete
- Repeat back the verbal request
- Check allergy status

D. Check your prescription for
- Dose calculation
- Appropriate route
- Completeness
- Indications for a PRN drug
- Legible indelible writing
- Any errors
- Dangerous abbreviations
- Generic and approved names only without abbreviation

Compliance

The commonest cause of drug failure in paediatrics is poor compliance. There are many causes for this and they include poor patient education or communication, misunderstanding, patient resistance or refusal, and a disorganized family. It is important to check compliance at each follow-up visit, usually by asking 'how often do you forget to give the medicines?', as this will lead to a more realistic response than assuming compliance. Prescribing a different formulation of a drug or one that requires less frequent administration during the day may help compliance. Handy memory aids such as charts and daily pill-boxes may also be helpful.

Off-label prescribing

This is the use of a drug in a dose, indication, route or at an age other than that recommended by the manufacturer. Unlicensed drug use refers to the use of an unregistered drug, an untested formulation of a registered drug or the use of a non-pharmacopoeial substance. Historically, many drugs have not been developed for children or their efficacy and safety investigated in children. This is because doses and markets may be small, making the development of a drug uneconomic, as well as logistical and ethical problems in drug testing in children. There are several consequences of off-label prescribing, including an increased potential for adverse drug reactions (ADRs), possible financial disadvantages for families and fear of litigation by practitioners. However, off-label prescribing is not illegal and in practice is often unavoidable in order to give best-practice treatment. The educated physician must ultimately use his best judgement in his patients' best interests. In recent years, developments in medical ethics as well as legislative and regulatory reform have contributed to a significant improvement in paediatric drug development and testing in clinical trials.

Prescribing for pregnant and breast-feeding mothers

The advantages of breast-feeding over formula-feeding babies outweigh, in almost all cases, any concerns there may be regarding prescribed medicine use by the mother. Nevertheless, every effort should be made to reduce drugs prescribed to the minimum. In the case of drugs with short half-lives it is better to feed the baby before ingesting the drug. Accurate and current information on drugs should be obtained in every case. Any effect on a baby will depend on the same principles of pharmacodynamics and pharmacokinetics that were discussed at the beginning of this chapter, with the extra variable of drug excretion into the milk. Drugs enter breast milk mostly by passive diffusion and therefore reflect the free (not protein-bound) maternal plasma drug levels. Highly protein-bound drugs like ibuprofen or warfarin, therefore, enter milk in very small amounts. High molecular-weight drugs like insulin and heparin also enter in small amounts. Breast milk is slightly more acidic then plasma (pH 7.2 v. 7.4), which tends to attract some drugs like opiates and repel others such as penicillin. Some drugs can increase or decrease the supply of breast milk.

All babies breast-feeding from a medicated mother should be carefully monitored for any untoward effects. Babies younger than 2 months, small and premature infants, and ill or jaundiced infants may be at increased risk for toxicity. Few drugs are actually contraindicated during breast-feeding, and include radiopharmaceuticals, lithium, cytotoxics, amiodarone, retinoids, iodine and gold salts.

Social drugs should be discouraged. Smoking is associated with a higher rate of SUDIC (sudden, unexplained death in infants and children), and cannabis may cause delayed development, drowsiness and irritability. Excess caffeine ingestion may also affect sleep patterns. Alcohol should only be ingested in moderate amounts, 2–3 hours before feeding and after feeding the baby, if possible. Pregnancy carries with it the extra hazards of teratogenicity and drugs should only be prescribed when absolutely necessary for maternal health and then only by an expert knowledgeable in obstetrics and maternal–fetal health.

To test your knowledge on this part of the book, please see Chapter 26

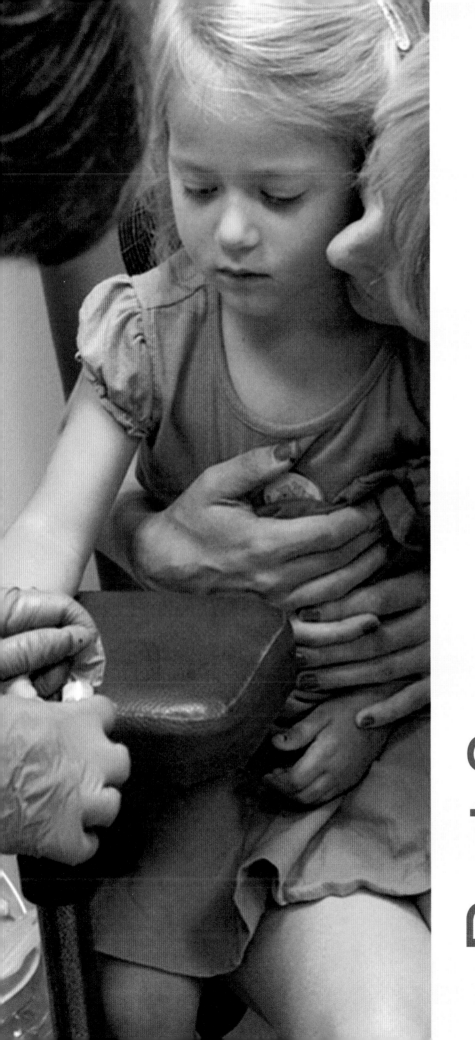

Part 3
An approach to problem-based paediatrics

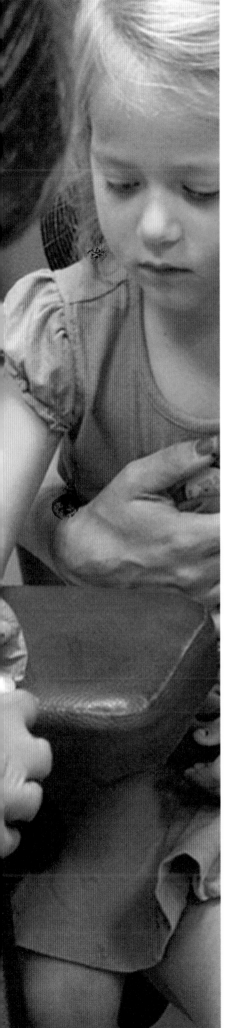

CHAPTER 9
The febrile child

The Doctor came round and examined
his chest,
And ordered him Nourishment, Tonics, and Rest,
'How very effective,' he said as he shook
The thermometer ......
The Doctor next morning was rubbing
his hands,
And saying, 'There's nobody quite understands
These cases as I do. ....'
The Dormouse and the Doctor, AA Milne

KEY COMPETENCES
YOU MUST...

Know and understand

- The differential diagnosis of children presenting with fever with and without rash, fever and neck swellings, PUO and recurrent fever and infections
- How to diagnose and manage serious and common infections of childhood
- The features and management of common infectious exanthems
- How to approach the management of a high temperature
- The definition of PUO

Be able to

- Take a temperature accurately
- Take a history directed toward diagnosing the cause of fever
- Recognise when a child has a serious infection or signs of shock
- Recognise investigative features that suggest bacterial infection
- Distinguish clinically between swellings in the neck

Appreciate that

- Fever and hyperthermia are different conditions
- Fever can be a very worrying symptom for parents
- Most children with fever have self-limiting and mild disease
- Fever reduction is usually of no medical benefit
- Fever or hypothermia can be serious signs in very young babies
- Cervical lymphadenopathy should prompt a search for generalised lymphadenopathy and hepatosplenomegaly

Essential Paediatrics and Child Health, Fourth Edition. Mary Rudolf, Anthony Luder and Kerry Jeavons.
© 2020 John Wiley & Sons Ltd. Published 2020 by John Wiley & Sons Ltd.
Companion website: www.wiley.com/go/rudolf/paediatrics

Fever as symptom and sign

Finding your way around ...

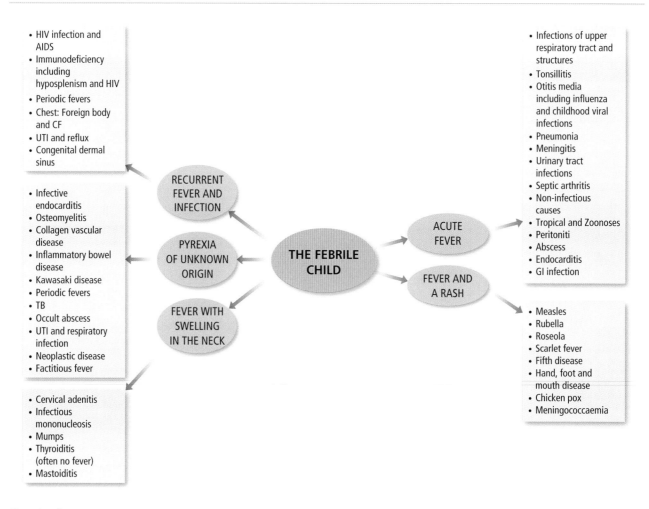

- HIV infection and AIDS
- Immunodeficiency including hyposplenism and HIV
- Periodic fevers
- Chest: Foreign body and CF
- UTI and reflux
- Congenital dermal sinus

- Infective endocarditis
- Osteomyelitis
- Collagen vascular disease
- Inflammatory bowel disease
- Kawasaki disease
- Periodic fevers
- TB
- Occult abscess
- UTI and respiratory infection
- Neoplastic disease
- Factitious fever

- Cervical adenitis
- Infectious mononucleosis
- Mumps
- Thyroiditis (often no fever)
- Mastoiditis

RECURRENT FEVER AND INFECTION

PYREXIA OF UNKNOWN ORIGIN

FEVER WITH SWELLING IN THE NECK

THE FEBRILE CHILD

ACUTE FEVER

FEVER AND A RASH

- Infections of upper respiratory tract and structures
- Tonsillitis
- Otitis media including influenza and childhood viral infections
- Pneumonia
- Meningitis
- Urinary tract infections
- Septic arthritis
- Non-infectious causes
- Tropical and Zoonoses
- Peritoniti
- Abscess
- Endocarditis
- GI infection

- Measles
- Rubella
- Roseola
- Scarlet fever
- Fifth disease
- Hand, foot and mouth disease
- Chicken pox
- Meningococcaemia

Acute fever

Common and important causes of acute pyrexia in childhood

Upper respiratory tract	Other infections	Other causes of fever
Viral upper respiratory tract infection	Viral syndromes	Factitious: taking oral temperature after a hot drink; deliberate manipulation of the thermometer (see p. 142)
Otitis media	Gastroenteritis	
Tonsillitis and pharyngitis	Common viral exanthems—enteroviruses, HHV 6 and 7, parvoviruses, EBV*	
Cervical adenitis	Influenza	
Mastoiditis	Lower respiratory tract infections	Excessive crying or exertion
Sinusitis	Urinary tract infection	Hyperthermia due to excessive swaddling, hot environments, sunstroke.
Mumps (non-immunised child)	Meningitis	
Infectious mononucleosis	Endocarditis	
	Septic arthritis	
	Abscess	
	Peritonitis	
	Tropical infections and Zoonoses	

Non-infectious causes of acute, recurrent or prolonged fever

Kawasaki disease, Still disease, PFAPA, Familial Mediterranean Fever, Malignancy, 'Malignant hyperthermia'

* In non-immunised children measles, chicken pox and rubella are also important

Fever is a very common symptom in children. High fever occurs in many non-serious conditions and is the body's response to pyrogens, which have an effect on the nuclei of the brain responsible for temperature control. Fever usually occurs as a result of infection, but may result from chronic inflammation or an immune response. The body's response to fever is to lose heat by skin vasodilatation, which causes the flush that is often seen in feverish children. Alternatively, when the temperature is rising the body tries to conserve heat by peripheral vasoconstriction which leads to dusky and cold mottled skin in the peripheries with a hot trunk and head.

A fever is a temperature above 37° C orally although it is rarely troubling below 38° C. One of the most important skills you will require as a doctor is to assess the child with a fever, decide on the likely cause, and treat appropriately. Babies under the age of 4 weeks are particularly difficult to assess, and may deteriorate rapidly. They should be admitted. For the older baby and child your clinical evaluation should lead you to the likely cause of the fever and a decision as to how ill the child is. Contrary to common belief, neither the height of the fever nor the response to antipyretics correlate with serious or bacterial infection.

The temperature should generally be taken using an electronic or mercury thermometer. In young and unconscious children, the rectal route is most reliable and closest to core temperature. A chemical dot thermometer placed in the axilla, or an infrared tympanic thermometer in the ear can be used for older and mildly ill children. Oral temperatures are routine for cooperative children. The correct technique for taking a temperature is described in Box 9.1.

History – must ask!

- *Height of fever*. A fever below 38° C is unlikely to be significant.
- *Character of fever*. Ask how long the fever has been present and whether it occurs at particular times of the day.
- *General features*. Poor appetite and malaise are non-specific features in any febrile child. Headache, diarrhoea, and vomiting may also be non-specific. Rigors (shivering) may indicate rapid increases in temperature and are common in bacterial infections and influenza.

Box 9.1 Taking the temperature

Place the thermometer in the axilla and hold the arm down by the child's side until the electronic beep, or 3–5 minutes for a mercury thermometer. Axillary temperatures are 0.5–1.0° C lower than oral or rectal temperatures. If using an infrared tympanic thermometer, place the tip in the external auditory meatus, pointing anteromedially towards the tympanic membrane. Press the measurement button, and after a few seconds a reading will be obtained. Core body temperature is normally 37.5° C and is measured by inserting a thermometer in the rectum. This is the most convenient method in infants or unconscious children

- *Pain*. Has there been local pain or pain referable to a specific body system or part, which may give a clue to the cause? Excessive crying in a baby may be a feature of pain.
- *Specific symptoms*. Vomiting, diarrhoea, coryza, cough, stridor, wheeze and rash are examples of specific clues to a diagnosis.
- *Animal contacts or foreign travel*. Diseases rare in the UK may be imported or caught from animals. Appropriate history may be a clue to Malaria, Rickettsial disease, Typhoid fever, Brucellosis, Chlamydia, Tuberculosis, Legionnaire disease, Q fever, cat-scratch fever, Borreliosis, Lyme disease, or other insect-borne tropical disease. These diseases may also have a rash (see below – Fever and rash).

Physical examination – must check!

- *General*. Does the child look seriously ill? Is the child dehydrated? Is there tachycardia or tachypnoea? Is conscious level normal? Is there excessive apathy or irritability?
- *Skin*. Is there a rash? Purpuric and ecchymotic lesions in a febrile child are hallmarks of meningococcaemia, whereas fine symmetric petechiae are often seen in viral infections. Exanthemata are common in viral infections and drug reactions. (See Chapter 19 for how to diagnose exanthematous diseases.)
- *Respiratory system*. Are there signs of upper or lower respiratory disease? Examine carefully for signs of serious disease such as bronchiolitis or pneumonia.
- *Cardiac*. Is there a murmur, tachycardia, muffled heart sounds or pericardial rub?
- *Abdomen*. Is there tenderness (including rectal examination) or organomegaly?
- *Central nervous system*. Is the child orientated? Is the child floppy? In older children assess for the presence of neck stiffness or Kernig's sign.
- *Nose and Ears*. Examine the tympanic membranes. Are they immobile, oedematous and/or bulging? Is there nasal discharge?
- *Throat*. Are the tonsils inflamed or is there an exudate? Is there lymphadenopathy?
- *Urine*. No physical examination of a febrile child is complete without examination of the urine to exclude urinary tract infection.

Note: Leave the examination of throat and ears to the end as this often upsets young children.

Investigations

In general, if the child does not look toxic, and a focus of infection is evident, the child does not need to be investigated. The investigations in Table 9.1 are only required in seriously ill-appearing children. In neonates there may be few or no localizing signs of infection and so they must all be investigated. At any age urinary tract infection (UTI) should be suspected as the cause of fever.

Table 9.1 Investigations that may be indicated in a child with fever (these are always required in an infant <4 weeks old)

Investigation	What you are looking for
Full blood count	Elevated white cell count with increased neutrophil count suggests a bacterial infection
Inflammatory markers	Raised CRP and procalcitonin in babies are linked to a higher chance of invasive bacterial infection
Throat swab	Culture of *beta-haemolytic Streptococcus* (after 2 years of age)
Blood cultures	Culture of a single organism on two separate cultures indicates bacteraemia Multiple organisms suggest contamination
Stool culture	*Shigella, Salmonella* or *Campylobacter*
Lumbar puncture	See Table 7.8, p. 114
Chest X-ray	Consolidation (generalised or focal) indicates pneumonia
Urine analysis and culture	Pure growth of >10^5 cell colonies from a mid-stream or clean catch* indicates infection (p. 326)*. Stick examination showing nitrites, >50 white cells, red cells and protein are indicators of UTI.

* Fewer colonies from a catheter or SPA urine are also indicative of UTI.

Managing fever as a symptom

Fever is often an unpleasant symptom, and can be treated but only if the child is irritable or uncomfortable. It should be noted that except in some specific cases, reduction of temperature is of no medical benefit and indeed may be harmful. Temperature can be brought down by a number of methods:

- Dress the child in loose clothing. Many parents' reaction to a fever is to wrap the child with blankets. This must be discouraged.

- Antipyretics reduce pyrexia centrally. Paracetamol (Calpol) and ibuprofen are most widely used. Aspirin is rarely given to children because of its possible association with Reye syndrome.
- Sponging or tepid baths. These cool the body but do not reduce pyrexia. Heat loss is encouraged by sponging with lukewarm water to allow vasodilatation and evaporative heat loss. Cold water causes vasoconstriction and may increase body temperature. Alcohol sponges and cold wet flannels on the head or face should never be used. Physical cooling does not affect the brain's thermostat and a rapid rise in temperature may therefore occur.
- Fluid administration. A febrile child loses heat by sweating, breathing fast, and passing warm urine. All of these require copious fluid administration.

Note that there is no evidence that reducing fever stops or prevents recurrence of febrile seizures (p. 422).

Key points: The child presenting with fever

- Confirm the presence of fever by recording the temperature
- Assess whether the child requires hospital admission, but remember that the height of the fever does not relate to severity of illness
- In babies less than 1 month old localizing signs may not be present
- Take measures to reduce temperature only to improve subjective wellbeing, and do not become obsessive.
- Examine for focal signs of infection
- If a child looks ill, re-evaluate when the fever settles
- Admit and investigate babies below 4 weeks of age
- Antibiotics are not fever-reducing agents.
- In a child who appears septic or shocked, intravenous broad-spectrum antibiotics are given early, before results of investigations become available

Clues to the differential diagnosis of acute fever in children

	Symptoms	Signs	Investigations
Tonsillitis	Sore throat	Tonsillar redness ± exudate Cervical lymphadenopathy	Throat swab
Otitis media	Ear pain, irritability	Bulging and immobile tympanic membrane	
Pneumonia	Cough Dyspnoea	Tachypnoea, use of accessory muscles, grunting Reduced air entry, dullness to percussion, crepitations	Chest X-ray

(Continued)

Clues to the differential diagnosis of acute fever in children (*Continued*)

	Symptoms	Signs	Investigations
Meningitis	Headache, irritability, drowsiness, vomiting	Neck stiffness* ± change in conscious level	Lumbar puncture
Urinary tract infection	Dysuria, frequency, abdominal pain, jaundice (babies)		Urine microscopy and culture
Meningococcal disease	Malaise	Shock, purpura	Blood cultures
Septic arthritis	Joint pain, limp, refusal to walk	Swollen joint, limited movement of joint	Aspiration of joint
Dysentery	Diarrhoea with blood or mucus	Abdominal discomfort	Stool culture
Exanthemata	Rash and fever	Maculo-papular, vesicular or petechial rash	Serology or PCR

* This sign is usually not present in young infants.

 See NICE guideline: Fever in under 5s: assessment and initial management https://www.nice.org.uk/guidance/cg160

Fever with a rash

Common infectious causes of fever and a rash

Macular and maculopapular	Measles
	Rubella
	Roseola
	Scarlet fever (erythroderma)
	Fifth disease and parvovirus
	Enterovirus
Vesicular	Chicken pox
	Hand, foot and mouth disease
Purpuric	Meningococcaemia

Most children presenting with fever and a rash have one of the common infectious diseases of childhood. Most of these exanthematous conditions require only supportive treatment and so a specific diagnosis is often not critical. However, the exception is meningococcaemia, which presents with a purpuric rash. It is life-threatening and must be identified promptly. The other reason for accurately diagnosing exanthematous conditions is for public health purposes so that epidemics can be recognised. A description of the characteristics of different rashes is given on p. 347.

History – must ask!

- *Is the child ill?* Most of the exanthematous diseases are accompanied by fever and malaise. In measles and meningococcaemia the child is often very ill; in rubella, fifth disease, and enteroviral exanthema the child often appears remarkably well; measles is suspected if the three 'Cs' (coryza, cough and conjunctivitis) are present; in roseola the rash appears once the fever falls after 3–5 days; scarlet fever is preceded by tonsillitis.

- *Is the rash itchy?* Itchiness suggests chicken pox (if the rash is vesicular) or an allergic response (possibly due to antibiotics given for the underlying illness).

- *Past medical history.* A history of a previous attack of an infectious disease makes a further attack unlikely, but there is a high incidence of inaccurate diagnoses, particularly with maculopapular rashes. It is obviously relevant to ask about the child's immunisation history. An atypical rash commonly follows some 10 days after measles, mumps and rubella (MMR) vaccination.

- *Contact with anyone ill.* Enquire whether anyone else in the family, or at school or nursery has been diagnosed as having an infectious disease.

- *Animal contacts or foreign travel.* This may be a clue to rickettsial disease, Typhoid fever, Brucellosis, Legionnaire disease, Lyme disease or other insect-borne tropical disease.

Physical examination – must check!

The rash

You need to describe the rash carefully, focusing on the following:

- *Characteristics.* Is the rash macular, papular, maculopapular, vesicular, purpuric or petechial? An important part of the examination is to test the rash for blanching, as purpuric and petechial rashes do not blanch on pressure whereas maculopapular rashes do. (Note that fever is usually absent in purpuric rash from other causes, namely Henoch–Schönlein purpura and idiopathic thrombocytopenic purpura). Peripheral centripetal rash if polymorphic may be a clue to rickettsial disease.

- *Distribution.* Measles and rubella both start on the face and work their way down the body. Roseola and chicken pox are mostly on the trunk. Fifth disease is mostly confined to the cheeks.

- *The presence of an enanthem.* Look in the mouth for an enanthem. In chicken pox, the vesicles rapidly break down so that shallow ulcers are seen. In measles, Koplik spots (appearing like grains of salt on a red background) are seen during the prodromal period only.

General examination

Carry out a complete physical examination, although other than finding fever and possibly lymphadenopathy it rarely contributes to the diagnostic process. Complications like pneumonia, encephalitis and otitis may be diagnosed.

Investigations

In general, the viral diseases including exanthems do not need a serological confirmation of the diagnosis, unless for public health reasons. An exception is when Rubella is suspected in a pregnant girl. If a sample is taken for viral titres, a second convalescent sample is required 10 days later, without which a diagnosis cannot be confidently made. Outbreaks of some diseases like measles and mumps in an otherwise immunised population are serious developments and serological diagnosis may be required. In the influenza season, sentinel sites are chosed for epidemiological serological diagnosis and for severely ill patients.

Blood culture and meningococcal polymerase chain reaction (PCR) are required in meningococcaemia. Cultures may prove negative if penicillin has been given prior to testing.

If the rash is petechial, a platelet count is required, as fever could be an incidental symptom in a child who was thrombocytopenic.

Management

Before the advent of immunisation, childhood infectious diseases were common and regular epidemics occurred. There was little difficulty in recognizing these diseases then, but these clinical skills have now diminished. It is, however, still important to recognise the various diseases so that appropriate advice about incubation periods and recommendations for isolation can be made (Table 9.2). in general, children are infective during much of the incubation period and before the specific rash emerges.

If meningococcaemia (see p. 154) is suspected, the child should immediately be given intramuscular penicillin, as rapid deterioration can occur, and urgent admission to hospital must be arranged.

Table 9.2 Diagnostic patterns - The course of some childhood infectious diseases

Disease	Incubation	Duration of rash	Recommended isolation
Measles*	10–14 days	5 days	From onset of catarrhal stage to day 5 of rash
Rubella*	14–21 days	2–3 days	None, except from non-immune women in first trimester of pregnancy
Roseola	Probably 10 days	1 day	None
Scarlet fever	2–4 days	5 days	1 day after start of treatment
Fifth disease	4–14 days	Weeks	None
Chicken pox*	14–17 days	6–10 days	Until all lesions are crusted (usually 5–6 days)
Mumps*†	16–21 days	None	Until swelling subsides (usually 5–10 days)
Pertussis*†	7 days	None	4 weeks or until cough has ceased

* Immunisations against these diseases are routinely given (see p. 36).
† Mumps and pertussis are included for completeness although there is no associated rash.

Clues to diagnosing a febrile illness with a rash

	Type of rash	Characteristics of the rash	Other features
Measles	Maculopapular	Begins on the face and spreads downwards	Koplik spots, coryza, cough and conjunctivitis, ill child
Rubella	Macular	Tiny pink macules on the face and trunk, works downwards	Well child, lymphadenopathy sometimes
Roseola	Macular	Faint pink rash on the trunk	Rash occurs after fever defervesces
Scarlet fever	Maculopapular	Fine punctate red rash with sandpapery feel, followed by peeling	Strawberry tongue, perioral pallor, tonsillitis
Fifth disease	Maculopapular	'Slapped cheek' appearance; lace-like rash on the arms, trunk and thighs	Well child, lasts up to weeks
Chicken pox	Vesicular	Occurs in crops on face and trunk. Papules, vesicles and crusts are present	Shallow ulcers of the mucous membranes
Meningococcaemia	Purpuric	Morbilliform (resembling measles), petechial or purpuric	May progress rapidly to shock and coma
Rickettsia	Polymorphic	Centripetal (peripheral)	Maybe be fatal if untreated

Online
Interactive Q1

🔑 Key points: Fever with a rash

- Decide if the rash is macular, maculopapular, vesicular or purpuric
- Determine if the child is septic or shocked
- If the rash is petechial or purpuric and the child is unwell, treat with penicillin IM and admit for investigation
- Specific serologic or PCR diagnosis may be required for pregnant patients and epidemiological purposes

Fever with neck swelling

Causes of fever and a swelling in the neck

Cervical lymph nodes	Upper respiratory tract infection
	Tonsillitis and retro-pharyngeal abscess
	Cervical adenitis
	Infectious mononucleosis
	Neoplastic processes (Table 3.5, p. 53)
Parotid gland	Mumps
Thyroid gland	Thyroiditis (generally no fever)
Mastoid	Mastoiditis

The commonest glands to enlarge in the neck are the anterior cervical nodes, which drain the tonsils and pharynx.

This may occur with any upper respiratory tract infection (URTI) and, if the child is not ill and the glands not obviously tender, is of little significance. Acute enlargement with fever is usually a result of streptococcal infection, with the differential diagnosis including infectious mononucleosis. Cytomegalovirus, toxoplasmosis and rubella are also causes which are often accompanied by generalised lymphadenopathy. Leukaemia and lymphoma are sometimes accompanied by striking degrees of lymph node enlargement, and other malignant tumours occasionally metastasize to lymph nodes.

Mumps used to be the commonest cause of parotid swelling, which can be unilateral or bilateral. Nowadays in the era of MMR vaccination, EBV and adenoviruses are commoner causes. Swelling of the mastoid process is included here, although it is not strictly part of the neck. Infection can spread from the adjacent ear and cause serious morbidity.

Goitre (swelling of the thyroid gland) is not usually accompanied by fever, although occasionally sore throat and fever can occur at the onset of auto-immune thyroiditis. Late-onset congenital hypothyroidism is sometimes identified when the child presents with an unrelated febrile illness. Since the iodisation of salt, goitre secondary to iodine deficiency no longer exists in children brought up in Britain or most of the industrialized world.

The first aspect of the clinical evaluation is to identify the site of origin of the enlarged gland(s). You can usually achieve this on your clinical examination.

🔍 Clues to diagnosing enlarged glands in the neck

	Features of the gland	Conditions causing enlargement of the gland
Cervical lymph nodes	May swell unilaterally or bilaterally along the anterior cervical chain	Upper respiratory tract infection
Parotid glands	Overlie the angle of the jaw. When enlarged they may be distinguished from the cervical lymph glands as they obscure the bony angle of the jaw and displace the ear upwards and outwards	Mumps

(Continued)

	Clues to diagnosing enlarged glands in the neck (*Continued*)	
	Features of the gland	**Conditions causing enlargement of the gland**
Mastoid process 	When enlarged is seen as a tender, inflamed swelling behind the ear which pushes the ear outwards	Mastoiditis
Thyroid gland 	Midline anterior structure overlying the trachea at the level of the thyroid cartilage. Best palpated by standing behind the child with hands encircling the neck (Figure 15.8). Fever is not usually a feature. Examination is helped by asking the child to drink water–on swallowing, the gland can be seen and felt to move	Thyroiditis Congenital hypothyroidism (Cancer very rare)

History and physical examination – must ask and check!

The history and physical examination depend on the gland involved. Ask about malaise and pain if you suspect infection of the lymph glands, parotids or mastoid. Focus your physical examination on identifying other sites of infection such as tonsillitis and otitis media. If you find generalised cervical lymphadenopathy, you must examine the axillae, groins, liver and spleen to see if the lymphadenopathy is generalised.

If you diagnose a goitre you need to decide if the child is euthyroid, hypothyroid or hyperthyroid (see p. 295).

Investigations

See Table 9.3. In the primary care setting it is usually acceptable to treat cervical adenitis without laboratory confirmation of an organism. If you suspect infectious mononucleosis, a full blood count and Epstein–Barr virus screen are advisable. Mumps does not require investigation, but an ultrasound examination or serum or urine amylase is helpful if it is not clear if the swelling is sited in the parotid or lymph glands. Thyroid function tests and antibodies are indicated in a child with goitre.

> **Key points: Fever and swelling in the neck**
>
> - Identify the structure involved
> - If the process is thought to be infective, assess how sick the child is
> - If cervical lymphadenopathy is identified, look for generalised lymphadenopathy and hepatosplenomegaly
> - If a goitre is found, assess if the child is clinically hypothyroid, hyperthyroid or euthyroid
> - If mastoiditis is found, admit the child as an ENT emergency

Table 9.3 Investigations which may be indicated for a swelling in the neck

	Investigation	**Significance**
Cervical lymph nodes	Full blood count	Elevated white cell count and shift to the left in bacterial infection, atypical lymphocytes in infectious mononucleosis
	Epstein–Barr virus screen	Positive in infectious mononucleosis
	Throat culture	Group A haemolytic streptococcal infection
Parotid glands	Serum or urine amylase, ultrasound	Elevated in mumps
Mastoid process	Tympanocentesis	To identify responsible organism and drain infection
Thyroid gland	Thyroxine, thyroid-stimulating hormone	To confirm whether the child is hypo-, hyper- or euthyroid
	Thyroid antibodies	Often positive in thyroiditis

Pyrexia of unknown origin

Causes of pyrexia of unknown origin		
Bacterial infection	**Viral infection**	**Other causes**
Urinary tract infection	Infectious mononucleosis	Collagen vascular disease including Still disease
Pneumonia	Hepatitis	Inflammatory bowel disease
Endocarditis	HIV infection	Neoplastic disease
Occult abscesses (NB dental)		Factitious fever
Tuberculosis		Kawasaki disease
Osteomyelitis		Periodic fevers

In most children presenting initially with fever and no apparent site of infection, the diagnosis becomes apparent or the fever resolves within a short period of time. Pyrexia of unknown origin (PUO) refers to prolonged fever, which is defined as more than 1 week in young children and 2–3 weeks in the adolescent.

The underlying cause in most cases of PUO is infection. Usually it is an atypical presentation of one of the common illnesses such as UTI or pneumonia, although endocarditis is an important consideration in a child with cyanotic or post-surgical congenital heart disease. Other significant causes include the collagen vascular diseases, malignancy and inflammatory bowel disease in the adolescent. In young children Kawasaki disease is a very important consideration because it may lead to coronary arteritis and is treatable. Systemic juvenile chronic arthritis (Still disease), which often presents as a remitting fever (see p. 316), may present an initial diagnostic challenge. Both Crohn disease and ulcerative colitis may present as PUO alone, although often a careful history reveals abnormalities in bowel patterns, which have been accepted by the child as being normal. After foreign travel, Malaria, Typhoid, Lyme disease, Legionella, Tuberculosis Rickettsial, Borreliosis and other insect-borne viral diseases must all be considered. Animal exposure may lead to Brucellosis, Q fever, and Chlamydial disease. Leukaemia may present as PUO, but it is less usual for other malignancies to do so.

A thorough history and repeated physical examinations are particularly important as clues may emerge which can lead to a diagnosis.

History – must ask!

- *Review of systems.* A thorough review of all organ systems is imperative as symptoms may be elicited which provide a lead to the aetiology.
- *Contact with infectious diseases.* Clues may be found on identifying someone in the family or school who is ill. Ingestion of infected food and drink should be excluded.
- *Travel.* Ask about any history of travel reaching back to birth, as re-emergence of disease may occur years after visiting an endemic area. Many infections are common abroad even if rare at home.
- *Exposure to insects and animals.* Zoonotic infections can be acquired from pets or wild animals, and insect-borne disease can be very dangerous abroad.
- *Genetic and ethnic background.* Some rare genetic disorders can cause PUO. Tuberculosis is still prevalent in Asian communities.

Physical examination – must check!

A meticulous physical examination, including all organ systems, may lead to diagnostic clues and so save the child from unnecessary of investigations. The physical examination may need to be repeated a number of times to look for the emergence of new signs.

- *Temperature chart* (see Figure 9.9). Repetitive chills and temperature spikes are common in children with septicaemia from any cause, but particularly suggest an abscess, pyelonephritis, malaria (after foreign travel) or endocarditis. Factitious fever should be suspected if there is an absence of tachycardia and sweating associated with peaks of fever.
- *The mouth and sinuses.* Look for tenderness to tapping over the sinuses and teeth and transilluminate the sinuses. Finding candida in the mouth may be a clue to a disorder of the immune system. Hyperaemia of the pharynx may suggest infectious mononucleosis.
- *Muscles and bones.* Palpate the muscles and bones. Point tenderness suggests either osteomyelitis or bone marrow invasion from neoplastic disease. Generalised muscle tenderness occurs in collagen vascular disease.
- *Heart.* A new or changed murmur suggests infective endocarditis.
- *Skin.* Rashes may be fleeting in Still disease, typhoid, endocarditis and connective tissue disease. Encourage the patient to photograph any rash.

Investigations

The number of investigations that can and often are performed are legion (see Table 9.4). You should only order investigations, beyond those commonly available, cautiously. It is important to obtain blood cultures and thick blood smears for parasites at fever peaks as the yield at that time is much higher, and at least three specimens should be taken.

Table 9.4 Examples of investigations and their relevance in pyrexia of unknown origin

Investigation	Relevance
Full blood count	Elevated white cell count and shift to the left in bacterial infection. Very high white cell count in leukaemia
Urine analysis and culture	Occult urinary tract infection
Examination of blood smear	Parasitic infections, e.g. malaria, Borrelia
ESR, CRP, ferritin	Elevated in bacterial infection. Highly elevated in collagen vascular disease and malignancy
Blood cultures (aerobic and anaerobic)	Bacterial infection. Repeated samples needed to diagnose endocarditis, osteomyelitis and occult abscesses
Liver function tests	Hepatitis
TB skin test	Tuberculosis
X-rays: chest, bones, sinuses,	Characteristic findings with bacterial infection
Gastrointestinal tract	Stool cultures
Bone marrow aspirate	Leukaemia, metastatic neoplasms, rare infections
Serological tests	Infectious mononucleosis, many infections, rarely helpful in collagen vascular disease
Radioactive scans	Helpful in detecting osteomyelitis and abdominal masses, tumours, abscesses
Echocardiography	In endocarditis, vegetations can be seen on the leaflets of heart valves
Ultrasonography	Identification of intra-abdominal abscesses
Total body CT or MRI scanning	Detection of neoplasms and abscesses

In general, radiological tests should be guided by clues obtained on the clinical evaluation. Ultrasound, CT or MRI can be used to guide aspiration or biopsy of suspicious lesions.

Managing the child with a PUO

In general, the child should be hospitalized for careful observation as much as for investigation. This may also provide relief of parental anxiety. Antipyretics should not at first be given as they obscure the pattern of fever. Antibiotics should never be used as antipyretics, and empirical trials should in general be avoided, as they are dangerous and can obscure the diagnosis of infections such as endocarditis and osteomyelitis.

It is helpful to know that the child with PUO has a better prognosis than that reported for adults, and that the cause is usually an atypical presentation of a common childhood illness. In many cases no diagnosis is established but the fever abates spontaneously.

Vary rarely, factitious fever – caused by the patient (often adolescent) or parent manipulating the thermometer – is the cause of a PUO. If this is in any way suspected, temperatures must be documented in hospital by an individual who stays with the patient while the temperature is being taken.

Key points: Pyrexia of unknown origin

- A thorough history and repeated physical examinations are required and may save the child from multiple, unpleasant investigations
- Hospitalization is needed to confirm and observe the pattern of the fever
- The characteristics of the fever may give a clue to diagnosis
- Samples for blood culture should be taken at the peak of fever

Recurrent infections

Causes of recurrent serious infections

Defective white cell function
Immunoglobulin deficiency
    Congenital deficiency
    HIV
Splenectomy
Chest
    Foreign bodies
    Cystic fibrosis
Urinary tract
    Reflux
Meningitis
    Congenital dermal sinus
    Complement deficiency

Most children experience recurrent minor infections. These are commonly respiratory infections, colds and tonsillitis, which peak when the child starts school or nursery or when an older sibling brings infections home. Poor nutrition, poverty, poor housing and inadequate hygiene may be contributing factors. Breast-feeding provides some protection during infancy, at least from otitis media and gastroenteritis.

The common recurrent minor infections of childhood may cause great parental concern, but should not initiate a diagnostic exploration. However, the child who experiences recurrent infections of a serious nature needs to be thoroughly evaluated for the underlying cause. Details of the investigation of immune deficiency states are beyond the scope of this book.

Periodic fevers

Online
Interactive Q8

Not every child with periodic fever has periodic or recurrent infections. A well-defined group of auto-inflammatory conditions is known which may cause repeated episodes of fever, sometimes very regular and stereotypical. These disorders can sometimes be challenging to diagnose and manage. Details of the diseases are beyond the scope of this book but some of the more important ones are shown in Table 9.5.

Table 9.5 Some conditions causing repeated episodes of fever

	FMF	HIDS	TRAPS	MWS FCU NOMID	PFAPA
Onset	Early childhood	<12 months	<20 years	infancy	~5 years
Ethnicity	Seph. Jews Turks, Arabs, Armenians, etc.	Dutch, French, Other Europeans	Irish, North Europeans, etc.	North Europeans, etc.	none
Duration	1–4 days	3–7 days	>1 week (up to 3 w)	2–3 days	3–6 days (q 4–6 weeks)
Abd. pain	+++	++ diarrhoea, N/V	+++ N/V	rare	+
Arthritis	++ (mono/oligo)	++ (polyart)	rare	++(chronic in NOMID)	+/-
Myalgia	+	+	+++ (migratory)	++	?
Chest pain	++	rare	++	none	?
Rash	+	+++	++ (migratory)	+++ (erythema urticaria)	rare
Other	pericarditis, HSP, scrotal inv	l. nodes, HSM, HA	conjuctivitis, periorb. edema	hearing loss, papillitis	exud. tonsillitis aphthae
Therapy	colchicine anti-TNF?	sympt. etanercept simvastatin	steroids etanercept	sympt. anakinra etanercept	single dose of steroids

FMF=Familial Mediterranean Fever; HIDS=Hyper IgD Syndrome (mevalonic aciduria); TRAPS=TNF-receptor associated periodic fever; MWS=Muckle Wells syndrome, FCU=Familial Cold Urticaria, NOMID/CINCA=Neonatal Onset Multi-system inflammatory disease/Chronic Infantile Neurological Cutaneous and Articular Disease (MWS, FCU and NOMID are all Cryopyrin associated auto-inflammatory diseases); PFAPA=Periodic fever, aphthous stomatitis, pharyngitis, adenitis.

Febrile illnesses

Upper respiratory tract infection

Upper respiratory tract infection (URTI) is very common in young children, particularly when they first start playgroup and school, as they become exposed to a number of viral organisms for the first time to which they have no immunity. The mother often describes her child as having 'one cold after another', but mothers (and doctors) need to understand that frequent mild infections in these young children are common, benign and even helpful for the maturing of the immune system.

Clinical features   The child often has coryza (runny nose) and sneezing or acute pharyngitis associated with fever. After a few days the child's nose becomes blocked, with consequent mouth breathing. This leads to a dry scratchy throat. A cough is often present, for which the child may unnecessarily receive repeated courses of antibiotics. On physical examination purulent mucus is visible in the nares or running down the upper lip. The tympanic membranes may be red but not purulent, and in acute pharyngitis the pharynx, the soft palate and the tonsillar fauces are red and swollen, often accompanied by cervical lymphadenopathy. Investigation is unnecessary.

Management   This is a mild self-limiting condition and treatment is symptomatic. In infants, nasal obstruction may be a particular problem as young babies are obligate nose breathers, and saline nasal drops with gentle suction immediately before feeds may be helpful. Fever in older children is treated with antipyretics and nasal obstruction may be relieved by a decongestant, but ephedrine should not be used for more than a few days because of the risk of mucosal hypertrophy. Antibiotics are *not* indicated for uncomplicated URTI. There is no evidence for the use of cough suppressants, mucolytics, herbal or homeopathic medications or vitamins especially vitamin C. If there is no improvement within 2–3 days, complications such as otitis, sinusitis and pneumonia should be excluded.

Tonsillitis

Tonsillitis is usually caused by a viral infection, particularly in young children. In children over 5 years, the commonest bacterial organism is the group A beta-haemolytic Streptococcus.

Clinical features   The child is feverish and usually complains of a sore throat, although younger children may experience abdominal pain due to mesenteric adenitis. On examination the tonsils are enlarged and inflamed (Figure 9.1), although it is important to remember that tonsils normally

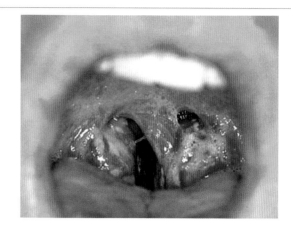

Figure 9.1 Acute tonsillitis in an 8-year-old child presenting with fever and a sore throat.

enlarge to a maximum size by 4–5 years. This normal enlargement should not be confused with infection. A white exudate and tender enlarged cervical lymph glands, in the absence of viral URTI symptoms, suggest bacterial infection. Exudates can also occur in infectious mononucleosis and diphtheria (now very rare due to immunisation). A throat swab should be taken where bacterial infection is suspected.

Management   Symptomatic treatment with lozenges, saline gargles and paracetamol is helpful. Most cases of tonsillitis in young children do not require antibiotics. Streptococcal tonsillitis should be treated with penicillin for 10 days. Recent evidence has shown that a single-dose of a steroid can reduce pain and time to resolution in non-EBV pharyngitis. Tonsillectomy is only rarely indicated even in recurrent tonsillitis.

Prognosis   The prognosis is good. Complications include:
- Otitis media.
- Scarlet fever.
- Cervical adenitis
- Chronic or recurrent tonsillitis. Upper airway obstruction and sleep apnoea is an important complication of chronically enlarged adenoids and this requires adenoidectomy and or tonsillectomy.
- Peritonsillar abscess (quinsy) and retro-pharyngeal abscess
- Post-streptococcal allergic disorders, e.g. acute rheumatic fever and acute glomerulonephritis (p. 331).

Tonsillitis at a glance

Epidemiology
Common over the age of 2 years

Aetiology
Beta-haemolytic strep, group A
Viral

History
Sore throat, dysphagia
Fever
Abdominal pain

Physical examination
Large inflamed tonsils with exudate
Cervical lymphadenopathy

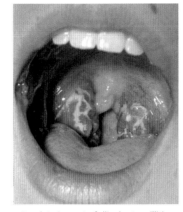

Exudate in acute follicular tonsillitis.

Confirmatory investigations
Throat swab grows beta-haemolytic strep, group A

Differential diagnosis
Viral pharyngitis
Infectious mononucleosis

Management
Antipyretics for fever
Gargles
Penicillin for 10 days

Prognosis/complications
Recurrent tonsillitis ⎤ Most
Otitis media ⎦ common
Peritonsillar abscess (rare but serious)
Rheumatic fever; scarlet fever
Acute glomerulonephritis (certain strains of strep only)

Otitis media

This is an extremely common childhood disorder and occurs most frequently in the first 5 years of life. It may also occur in the neonate. The commonest infecting organisms are viruses, *Streptococcus pneumoniae* and *Haemophilus influenzae*. Otitis media is especially common in conditions associated with eustachian tube dysfunction because fluid cannot drain from the middle ear. Eustachian tube dysfunction commonly occurs following the common cold, in adenoidal hypertrophy, cleft palate, in children with lysosomal storage disease (Hurler and Hunter syndromes) and Down syndrome.

Clinical features   Otitis media usually presents with fever, a painful ear, and hearing loss, and is usually preceded by an URTI. In younger children, anorexia, vomiting, and diarrhoea may be the presenting features alone. For this reason, it is important to examine the ears (p. 34) in all febrile children. It is best to use a pneumatic otoscope so that drum mobility can be assessed. In otitis media the tympanic membrane is inflamed and bulging, with loss of landmarks, mobility and the light reflex (Figure 9.2). Perforation of the tympanic membrane may occur spontaneously, in which case the ear canal will be obscured by pus. The diagnosis is made on otoscopic findings, and culture of pus is generally unhelpful due to ear canal flora contamination.

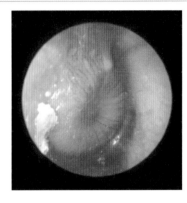

Figure 9.2 Bulging tympanic membrane seen on otoscopy of a child with otitis media. Note the inflammation and loss of landmarks.

Management   Many cases are caused by viruses and resolve spontaneously, and hence in children over 6 months of age antibiotics are only given for symptoms that have persisted for at least 48 hours. Amoxicillin is the recommended first-line drug in non-penicillin allergic children for persistent or bilateral cases, and younger infants.

Prognosis   Most cases of otitis media resolve satisfactorily even if perforation has occurred. Complications may occur and include secretory otitis media, conductive deafness (p. 272), mastoiditis (p. 149) and, rarely, cholesteatoma.

Secretory otitis media and glue ear

In secretory otitis media, recurrent acute infections lead to a thick glue-like exudate building up in the middle ear, and conductive hearing impairment (p. 272). On examination the tympanic membrane appears thickened and retracted with an absent light reflex. If there is significant hearing loss, ventilation tubes (grommets) may be inserted through the tympanic membrane to allow aeration of the middle ear. These are particularly indicated if there is language delay due to the conductive deafness associated with glue ear.

 Otitis media at a glance

Epidemiology
Common, especially as a
  complication of URTI

Aetiology
Viral
Haemophilus influenzae
Streptococcus pneumonia

History
Ear pain and hearing loss
  (older child)
Irritability (younger child)
Fever*
URTI symptoms

Physical examination
Bulging inflamed tympanic
  membrane

NB *Signs and symptoms are
variable

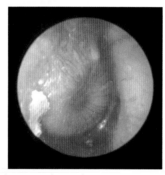
Bulging tympanic membrane seen on otoscopy.

Confirmatory investigations
None

Differential diagnosis
URTI
Secretory otitis media

Management
Oral antibiotics reduces
  duration of symptoms
Uncomplicated unilateral cases
  over 6 months of age
  managed symptomatically

Complications
Perforated ear drum with
  discharge (generally
  heals well)
Chronic secretory otitis media
  with or without conductive
  hearing loss
Mastoiditis

Other viral infections

Febrile illnesses of a flu-like nature are caused by a number of viruses of which the influenza virus is one. Other common viruses include adenoviruses, rhinoviruses, metapneumoviruses, respiratory syncytial virus (in infants), parainfluenza and enteroviruses. These viruses are spread by droplets from the upper respiratory tract of affected children and adults.

Clinical features   Children usually present with a brief but acute illness with fever, and varying degrees of malaise, chills, headache, cough and myalgia. A non-specific erythematous rash is a relatively common symptom. The term 'flu' is often used to describe these symptoms. There are no specific physical signs on examination, and it is unnecessary to investigate for a specific viral cause unless there are epidemiologic considerations.

Management   Treatment is symptomatic with antipyretics. Antibiotics are only necessary if there is evidence of secondary bacterial infection. Recovery should be followed as rarely complications such as myocarditis, pneumonia and encephalitis can occur even in otherwise healthy children. Routine influenza vaccination is recommended every year for all chronically ill or susceptible children and all others from 6 months to 5 years.

Prognosis   Some children are particularly susceptible to viral infections, such as those who have cystic fibrosis or congenital heart disease or those who are immunosuppressed.

Cervical adenitis

Bacterial cervical adenitis usually results from infection by the group A beta-haemolytic Streptococcus, or sometimes staphylococcus. The child presents as acutely unwell with tender swollen cervical lymph glands, with or without signs of tonsillitis. Bacterial infection is indicated by an elevated white cell count with a shift to the left, and the organism confirmed by positive throat or blood culture. In the primary care setting it is acceptable to prescribe penicillin or cephalosporin on a clinical basis without laboratory confirmation.

Infectious mononucleosis (glandular fever)

The Epstein–Barr virus (EBV) is the commonest cause of this infection. When tonsillitis is prominent the differential diagnosis includes streptococcal infection and diphtheria in an unimmunised child.

Clinical features   Infectious mononucleosis usually presents in the child, as in the adult, with marked cervical lymphadenopathy, fever, sore throat and enlarged purulent tonsils. Generalised lymphadenopathy and splenomegaly are commonly found, and a macular rash occurs in 10–20% of cases, especially if ampicillin is inadvertently given. Hepatitis sometimes occurs, occasionally with jaundice.

Investigations   The diagnosis is supported by the presence of lymphocytosis with large unstained cells (LUC) and atypical lymphocytes in the blood film which may account for 10–25% of the total white cell count. The test for heterophile antibodies is positive in 60% of cases in the first week of the illness and anti-EBV IgM is present in the early stages. Liver function tests may be abnormal. Sometimes other viruses like CMV or toxoplasmosis can cause a similar syndrome.

Management and prognosis   Infectious mononucleosis is a self-limiting disease. The course of the condition is variable. The throat may be so inflamed as to preclude drinking, and if so the young child may need intravenous fluids. Children often recover from infectious mononucleosis without the prolonged fatigue and depression which characterize adolescent and adult infection.

👁 Infectious mononucleosis at a glance

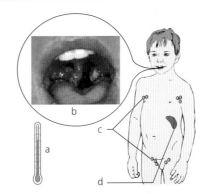

Aetiology
Epstein–Barr virus
Cytomegalovirus

History
Fever (**a**)
Sore throat

Physical examination
Large purulent tonsils (**b**)
Generalised lymphadenopathy,
  particularly cervical (**c**)
Splenomegaly (**d**)
Hepatomegaly*
Macular rash*

Confirmatory investigations
Atypical lymphocytes (10–25%
  of white cell count) on blood
  smear
Epstein–Barr virus serology
  IgM-positive early
Abnormal liver function tests

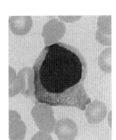

NB *Signs and symptoms are variable

Differential diagnosis
Streptococcal tonsillitis
(Diphtheria now rare)
Leukaemia
Lymphoma
Toxoplasmosis
Hepatitis

Management
Supportive
Consider steroids if symptoms
  very severe

Prognosis/complications
Self-limiting disease
Splenic rupture rarely EBV
  associated malignancy
Dehydration may develop in the
  young child
Fatigue/depression are rare in
  children

Parotitis and mumps

Mumps remains a concern as a cause of parotitis despite the introduction of immunisation (see p. 39). Other causes such as EBV, adenovirus, sialectasis, parotid stone, Sjogren and staphylococcal parotitis should all be considered. Mumps itself is, in general, a mild illness in childhood. The child is contagious until the swelling has resolved.

Clinical features   After an incubation period of 16–21 days, the child presents with fever and malaise, and enlargement of the parotid glands, which may be bilateral or unilateral (Figure 9.3). The swelling lasts for 5–10 days.

Management   The diagnosis is clinical and confirmed by raised serum or urinary amylase, and serology.

Complications   Deafness and meningoencephalitis are the major complications. The incidence of post-mumps sensorineural deafness is one in 15 000. It is usually severe and unilateral. Meningoencephalitis is very common, but is usually mild and characterised by headache, neck stiffness and photophobia. Orchitis does occur, but very rarely in the prepubertal boy. Mumps has been implicated in the development of diabetes.

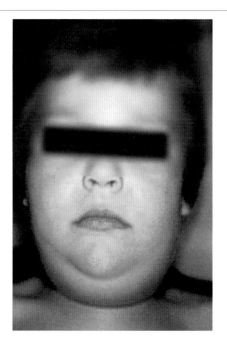

Figure 9.3 An 11-year-old child with mumps. Note the swelling of the parotid gland obscuring the angle of the jaw. *Source*: CDC/ Patricia Smith; Barbara Rice.

Mumps at a glance

Immunisation
Live attenuated virus given at 12–18 months

Aetiology
Mumps virus

History
Fever (**a**)
Malaise
Neck swelling
Pain on swallowing sweet/ sour liquids

Physical examination
Unilateral or bilateral parotid swelling (**b**)
10% Meningoencephalitis (**c**)

Confirmatory investigations
Clinical diagnosis often sufficient PCR or serology (Serum/urinary amylase raised)

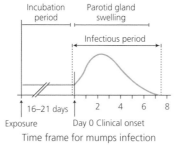

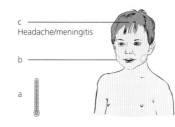

Time frame for mumps infection

Differential diagnosis
Cervical lymphadenopathy
Adenovirus
EBV
Other viruses
Bacterial parotitis
Sialectasis and stone
Tumour (Lymphoma)

Management
Supportive

Course
Incubation period 16–21 days
Contagious until swelling subsides

Complications
Sensorineural deafness
Meningoencephalitis
Orchitis rare in prepubertal boy

Mastoiditis

Mastoiditis is now a rare but serious infection of childhood, which demands urgent treatment. The infection usually extends from the middle ear, and the responsible bacteriae include streptococci, staphylococci, pneumococci and *Haemophilus influenzae*. Treatment is by surgical drainage and intravenous antibiotics.

Measles

Despite widespread use of the MMR immunisation, measles is still occasionally seen. It is a miserable and very infectious viral illness characterised by a distinctive maculopapular rash (see Figure 9.4a) in conjunction with the three 'Cs' (cough, coryza and conjunctivitis). Immunisation with a live attenuated vaccine is given at about 13 months and 3–5 years (see p. 39).

Clinical features   After an incubation period of 10–14 days there is a prodromal illness with fever and upper respiratory symptoms, followed by onset of the rash on the 3rd or 4th day. The rash begins on the face and behind the ears and spreads downwards to cover the whole body. In contrast to some of the other childhood infectious diseases, the child is ill and irritable. The rash begins to fade after 3 or 4 days and becomes blotchy. During the prodromal period a distinctive exanthem can be visualized. Koplik spots (see Figure 9.4b), looking like grains of salt on a red background, appear on the buccal mucosa of the cheeks. In developing countries there is a high morbidity and mortality and diarrhoea is a common feature.

Complications   Acute otitis media and bronchopneumonia are common complications. The serious complication of post-measles encephalitis occurs in one in 5000 cases and causes drowsiness, vomiting, headache and convulsions. The prognosis for normal neurological survival in these cases is poor. It generally occurs a week after the measles is diagnosed and is probably caused by an immunological cross-reactivity between measles virus and neural tissue. Subacute sclerosing encephalitis (SSPE) is a very rare complication, which occurs some 4–10 years after an attack and is characterised by slow progressive neurological degeneration.

Management   Treatment of measles is supportive. Antibiotics are required if otitis media or bronchopneumonia develop. The child is contagious from before the onset of the rash to the 5th day of the rash.

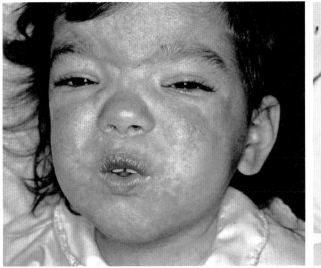
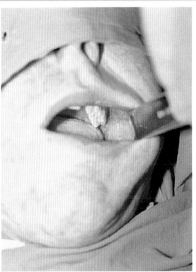

(a)   (b)

Figure 9.4 (a) A 2-year-old child with measles, demonstrating the typical maculopapular rash, conjunctivitis and miserable appearance. (b) Koplik spots.

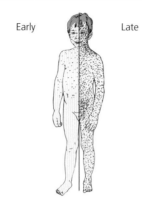

Measles at a glance

Immunisation
Live attenuated vaccine at age
  15–18 months
Very rare in immunised individuals

History
Cough
Coryza
Fever

Physical examination
Conjunctivitis
Rash on face, behind ears
  spreading down to trunk
Ill, irritable
Koplick spots during prodrome
Lymphadenopathy

Confirmatory investigations
Clinical diagnosis
Rise in antibody titre
PCR urine or blood

Early   Late

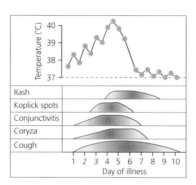

Differential diagnosis
Non-specific viral exanthem
Rubella
Scarlet fever
EBV
Drug rash

Management
Supportive
Antibiotics for otitis media and
  pneumonia
Child is contagious of rash
  until day 5
Course
Incubation period 10–14 days
Rash lasts 5 days

Complications
Otitis media and pneumonia
  common
Post-measles encephalitis rare
  but serious
Subacute sclerosing
  encephalitis (SSPE) very rare
High morbidity and mortality in
  developing countries

Rubella (German measles)

Rubella is usually a mild illness and the rash may not even be noticed. The importance of the condition does not lie with the effect on the child, but on the devastating teratogenic effects if rubella is contracted by a pregnant woman during the first trimester of pregnancy. The fetus may die or develop congenital heart disease, mental retardation, deafness and cataracts. In order to reduce exposure of young mothers to the virus, and to protect girls before they reach childbearing age, rubella immunisation is given in early childhood (p. 39), usually together with mumps and measles vaccine (MMR). If a rash occurs during pregnancy, rubella titres should be measured immediately and again after 10 days to determine whether recent infection has occurred.

Clinical features   After an incubation period of 14–21 days, the rash appears as tiny pink macules on the face and trunk and works its way down the body (Figure 9.5). The suboccipital lymph nodes are enlarged and there may be generalised lymphadenopathy. Thrombocytopenia, encephalitis (particularly cerebellitis) and arthritis are rare complications, although reactive arthralgia is common. The rash is quite non-specific, and the diagnosis of rubella is often made erroneously and overconfidently on clinical grounds.

Management   No specific management is required.

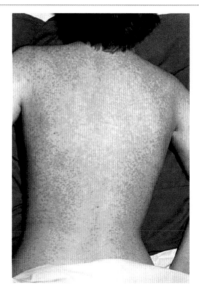

Figure 9.5 Rubella. A 10-year-old girl with rubella – small pink macules shown on the back.

👁 Rubella at a glance

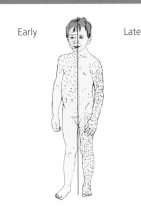

Early   Late

Immunisation
Live attenuated vaccine at age
  15–18 months
Very rare in immunised individuals

History
Generally well
Fever*

Physical examination
Tiny pink macules on face and
  trunk rapidly working
  downwards
Not ill
Enlarged suboccipital nodes*
Generalised lymphadenopathy

Confirmatory investigations
Rise in rubella antibody titre

NB *Signs and symptoms are
variable

Differential diagnosis
Non-specific viral exanthem
Drug rash

Management
None required

Course
Incubation period 14–21 days
Rash lasts 2–3 days

Complications
If pregnant, devastating effects
  on fetus possible
Thrombocytopenia
Encephalitis
Arthritis rare

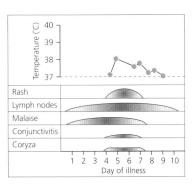

Roseola

Roseola affects children under the age of 2 years and has a very characteristic course. The cause is Human Herpes Virus (HHV) type 6 and 7.

Clinical features   The child has a pronounced fever reaching to 39 or 40 °C lasting for 3–4 days. In general, despite the height of the temperature the child does not seem to be particularly unwell, although febrile convulsions may occur on the first day. Occipital lymph nodes are often enlarged. On the 4th day the temperature drops and a faint pink macular rash appears on the trunk, lasting for only a few hours or a day or so. The child then makes an uneventful recovery.

Management   The fever needs to be controlled. There are no recommendations to isolate the child.

Scarlet fever

Scarlet fever, which is now uncommon, is the only childhood erythematous or maculopapular exanthem caused by a bacterium and therefore requiring antibiotic treatment (although children with measles may need antibiotics for complications). It is caused by a strain of group A haemolytic streptococci.

Clinical features   After an incubation period of 2–4 days, fever, headache and tonsillitis appear. The rash (Figure 9.6) develops within 12 hours and spreads rapidly over the trunk and neck, with increased density in the

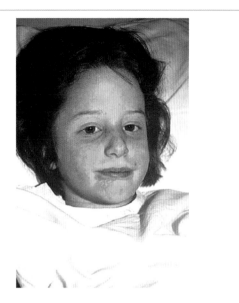

Figure 9.6 Scarlet fever. Note the fine punctate maculopapular rash and perioral pallor.

neck, axillae and groins, but spares the circumoral area It has a fine punctate erythematous appearance, a 'sandpapery' feel and blanches on pressure. The tongue initially has a white coating, which desquamates leaving a sore 'red strawberry' appearance. The rash lasts about 6 days and is followed by peeling, which is useful in making a retrospective diagnosis.

Investigations Throat swab may show group A Streptococcus, and anti-streptolysin O (ASO) titre is usually elevated.

Management A 10-day course of penicillin or 5 days of azithromycin eradicates the organism and may prevent other children from being infected.

Complications Sequelae such as rheumatic fever and acute glomerulonephritis (see p. 331) are now less common but still seen in developed societies.

👁 Scarlet fever at a glance

Aetiology
Group A haemolytic
 Streptococcus pyogenes

History
Fever
Headache
Sore throat

Physical examination
Fine punctate rash with
 sandpapery feel, blanches on
 pressure
Particularly dense in neck,
 axillae and groins
In later stages, rash peels and
 coalesces
White-coated tongue, changing
 to 'red strawberry'
 appearance
Tonsillitis

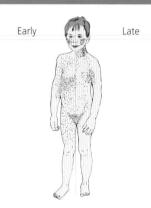

Early   Late

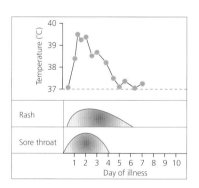

Confirmatory investigations
Group A streptococcus on
 throat culture
Rise in antistreptolysin O (ASO)
 titre

Differential diagnosis
Non-specific viral exanthem
Measles

Management
Penicillin or azithromycin or
 amoxicillin for 10 days

Course/complications
Rash lasts 5 days
Rheumatic fever and acute
 glomerulonephritis now less
 common in Western societies

Fifth disease (erythema infectiosum)

This condition is caused by human parvovirus B19. It is called fifth disease for arcane historical reasons. (The other four were rubella, measles, scarlet fever and Filatov–Dukes disease – a mild, atypical form of scarlet fever.)

Clinical features   The illness usually begins with the sudden appearance of livid erythema of the cheeks, giving the child a 'slapped cheek' appearance. There are usually no prodromal symptoms, and fever is absent or low grade. A symmetrical maculopapular lace-like rash (Figure 9.7) then appears on the arms, trunks, buttocks and thighs. The rash can last up to 6 weeks and may be pruritic. Recrudescences may appear with temperature, exercise and emotional upset. Arthralgia and arthritis occur infrequently.

Management   Isolation is not required, and as the illness is mild and the duration of the rash may be prolonged, children should be allowed to attend school.

Chicken pox (varicella)

Chicken pox is a common and highly contagious disease of childhood which, luckily, is usually mild in this age group. It may be contracted from a patient with shingles. Children who are immunocompromised (such as those on corticosteroids or being treated for leukaemia) are at risk for severe, often fatal chicken pox. If such a child comes into contact with chicken pox, prophylaxis with zoster immunoglobulin should be considered. A vaccine against chicken pox is part of routine immunisation in the United States, but currently is only given to those in high-risk groups in the United Kingdom.

Clinical features   After an incubation period of 14–17 days, the rash (Figure 9.8) appears on the trunk and face. The spots appear in crops, passing rapidly through the stages of macule to papule and then vesicle. The appearance of the vesicles has been likened to 'dewdrops' on an erythematous base. The vesicles rapidly turn into pustules and then crust over. At the height of the illness the lesions simultaneously consist of papules, vesicles and crusts. Itching is constant and annoying. Vesicles in the mucous membranes, particularly in the mouth, rapidly become macerated and form shallow ulcers. The severity of the disease varies from a few lesions in a well child to many hundreds of lesions with severe toxicity. Eczematous children may develop severe rash and impetigo.

Complications   The commonest complication is secondary infection of the lesions and scarring. A more severe complication is encephalitis, which produces cerebellar signs with ataxia. Thrombocytopenia with haemorrhage into the skin can occur. Varicella pneumonia is uncommon in children.

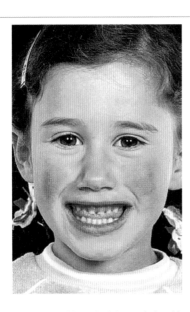

Figure 9.7 Fifth disease. Note the 'slapped cheek' rash in a well looking child.

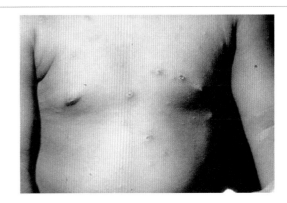

Figure 9.8 Chicken pox. Note the characteristic vesicular rash at various stages of development, although few have reached the pustular or crusted stage.

Management   Itching can be alleviated to some extent by cool baths and application of calamine lotion. If the child is very distressed, promethazine syrup can be helpful. Cutting fingernails short and keeping them clean can reduce second-ary infection. The child is contagious until all the lesions have crusted over. If the disease develops in an immunocompromised child, urgent admission for intravenous acyclovir is indicated.

 Chicken pox at a glance

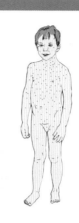

Aetiology
Varicella-Zoster virus (contracted
    from chicken pox or shingles)

Immunisation
Vaccine for high-risk and routine in
infancy groups
Immunoglobulin
    indicated for immunocompromised
    child exposed to chicken pox

History
Fever
Itching lesions
Irritability*

Physical examination
Lesions: a mixture of papules,
    vesicles, pustules and crusts
    over the trunk and face lesions
    emerge in crops over a few days
Ulcers in mouth
May look toxic if severely
    affected*

Confirmatory investigations
Clinical diagnosis

NB *Signs and symptoms are
variable

Differential diagnosis
Usually unequivocal

Management
Relieve itching by cool baths,
    calamine lotion±
    promethazine syrup
Child contagious until all lesions
    crusted
If child is immunocompromised,
    give IV acyclovir

Course
Incubation period 14–17 days
Lesions last 6–10 days

Complications
Secondary infection of lesions
Encephalitis (cerebellar signs
    with ataxia pneumonia)
Thrombocytopenia with skin
    haemorrhages
Chicken pox is severe or even
    fatal for the
    immunocompromised child

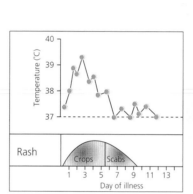

Hand, foot and mouth disease

Hand, foot and mouth disease is caused by a Coxsackie virus. It occurs in epidemics affecting young children. Vesicular lesions appear on the palms of the hands and fingers, the soles of the feet and in the mouth. The vesicles clear by absorption of the fluid in about a week. There may be a low-grade fever.

Meningococcal septicaemia

Meningococcal septicaemia often starts insidiously and then may rapidly become severe and life-threatening. The underlying organism, *Neisseria meningitidis*, most commonly causes meningitis, but in some cases septicaemia is the predominant presenting condition.

Clinical features   There is often a short coryzal prodrome, followed by fever (Figure 9.9), malaise and the development of a petechial/purpuric rash. The hallmark of meningococcaemia is petechial, purpuric skin or ecchymotic lesions that do not blanch on pressure. The purpura may enlarge rapidly as the child deteriorates (Figure 9.10), leading to necrosis. Signs of meningitis may be present. Meningococcal septicaemia is often fulminant with rapid deterioration, disseminated intravascular coagulopathy and shock. Death may occur within a few hours of presentation, caused by shock and adrenal failure (Waterhouse–Friderichsen syndrome).

Management (see Box 9.2)   As the course so often is fulminant, treatment must be started on the basis of strong clinical suspicion rather than awaiting the result of investigations.

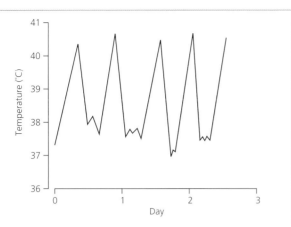

Figure 9.9 A temperature chart showing swings suggestive of septicaemia.

Box 9.2 Managing the child with meningococcal septicaemia

- Give IM or IV penicillin as soon as diagnosis suspected
- Arrange rapid admission to hospital and give regular IV cefotaxime
- Treat shock with intravenous fluids
- Treat all close contacts with rifampicin

Any seriously ill child seen at home with petechial or purpuric lesions should be given penicillin immediately by the family doctor. This should preferably be given intravenously, but intramuscular injection is acceptable. If it is possible to take blood cultures prior to giving antibiotics this is preferable, but it may not be feasible. The child must be rushed to hospital as quickly as possible.

Management in hospital consists of antibiotics (intravenous cefotaxime) and intensive care directed towards supporting the circulation. Shock is a common and severe feature, and massive volumes of plasma may be necessary to reverse this. Mortality is high.

The meningococcus colonizes the upper respiratory tract of asymptomatic children, and close contacts of children with meningococcal infection are at increased risk of infection. Such contacts should be given a 2-day course of prophylactic rifampicin. Anti-meningococcal vaccine is now being introduced for some strains of this bacteria.

Prognosis   Mortality is high in children who present with meningococcal septicaemia; some die before reaching hospital. Even with rapid antibiotic treatment, death may occur as a result of irreversible shock. If the child survives, the prognosis for intact recovery is good. Only a relatively small proportion of those who survive meningococcal septicaemia will have long-term sequelae.

👁 Meningococcal septicaemia at a glance

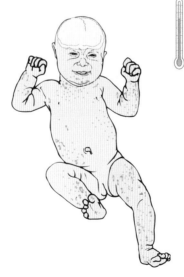

Epidemiology
5 in 10 000 children <10 years
Immunisation becoming available

Aetiology
Neisseria meningitidis

History
Fever
Malaise rash

Physical examination
Ill child shock
Petechial/purpuric rash
Meningeal signs*

NB *Signs and symptoms are variable

Confirmatory investigations
Immediate parenteral penicillin must be given on suspicion of diagnosis even if cultures not taken
Organism grown from blood, CSF or petechiae

Differential diagnosis
Septicaemia/meningitis caused by other organisms
Other causes of shock

Management
See Box 9.2

Prognosis/complications
High mortality in meningococcal septicaemia with shock
Good prognosis for meningococcal meningitis ± septicaemia

HIV infection and AIDS

Paediatric acquired immunodeficiency syndrome (AIDS) is caused by human immunodeficiency virus (HIV) type 1. The two paediatric populations at risk are:

1. infants born to infected mothers;
2. adolescents who acquire infection sexually or by the intravenous use of drugs.

There is essentially no risk of being infected by casual contact with an HIV-infected child in the family, at nursery or at school. Most children with HIV are diagnosed before the age of 3 years.

Clinical features   Infected infants are usually diagnosed because they have features of immunodeficiency – namely, failure to thrive, rash, fevers, diarrhoea, candidiasis or hepatosplenomegaly – or because they develop severe bacterial infections. Severe life-threatening infections include pneumonia, septicaemia, persistent pulmonary infiltrates, *Pneumocystis jiroveci* pneumonia (PCP), tuberculosis and systemic candida.

Diagnosis   Diagnosis is made by the detection of HIV antibody, which is very specific and sensitive or PCR. However, passive maternal transplacental IgG obscures the diagnosis in young infants, as the antibody may still be measurable up to the age of 18 months in uninfected clinically well infants. Hence, in children under 2 years of age, detection of HIV antigen or PCR is required to confirm the diagnosis.

Management   At present the goals of intervention in HIV-infected patients focus on the use of antiviral drugs, prophylactic antibiotics, viral vaccines and, where necessary, immune serum globulin. The psychosocial and emotional needs of the family must also be addressed.

Prognosis   Of babies born to HIV-positive mothers 20–30% become HIV positive themselves, although this rate can be dramatically reduced by preventive measures. In children with clinical HIV infection the prognosis is very variable, but in general, the earlier and more severe the presentation, the worse the prognosis.

 HIV infection and AIDS at a glance

Epidemiology
Infants born to infected mothers
Adolescents: acquired sexually
 or by IV drug use

Aetiology
Human immunodeficiency virus
 type 1

Prevention
Perinatal management:
• zidovudine to HIV-positive
 pregnant women
• delivery by caesarean section
• zidovudine at birth
• avoidance of breast-feeding
 (Western countries)
Other ages:
• universal precautions for body
 fluids
• safe sex

History
Severe bacterial infections
Poor weight gain
Diarrhoea*
Loss of developmental
 milestones*

NB *Signs and symptoms are
variable

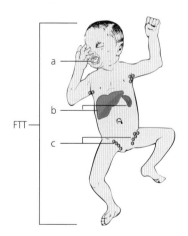

Physical examination
Failure to thrive (FTT)
Candidiasis (**a**)
Hepatosplenomegaly (**b**)
Lymphadenopathy (**c**)
Chest signs*
Other specific signs relating to
 organs involved*

Confirmatory investigations
HIV antibody detection (but in
 infants this may have been
 passively acquired and is not
 necessarily a sign of infection)
HIV PCR in blood for viraemia
Immunological testing

Differential diagnosis
Depends on organ systems
 involved
Other immunodeficiency
 disorders

Management
Lifelong antiviral drugs
Prophylactic antibiotics
Immune serum globulin
Psychosocial/emotional support

Prognosis/complications
20–30% babies born to
 HIV-positive mothers become
 infected
High risk for pneumonia,
 septicaemia, persistent
 pulmonary infiltrates,
 *Pneumocystis jiroveci
 pneumonia*, tuberculosis,
 systemic candida
Variable prognosis: earlier and
 more severe presentations
 have worse prognosis

Prevention   The administration of combination antiretroviral therapy including zidovudine to HIV-infected pregnant women, and delivery by caesarean section, reduces the transmission of the virus to infants. At birth the infant should also receive zidovudine for 4 weeks. In developed countries where the risks of bottle-feeding are low, HIV-positive mothers should not breast-feed, as the virus may be transmitted in breast milk. For the adolescent and adult, prevention of HIV includes precautions in coming into contact with bodily fluids and the practice of safe sex, with the use of condoms.

Kawasaki disease

Also known as mucocutaneous lymph node syndrome, this is a severe febrile illness of young children of unknown cause. The incidence is unknown but is probably between 10-50/100 000 children below the age of 5 years, and is more common in Japan. It is a non-contagious and non-genetic disorder. Some have postulated that abnormal immune responses to antigen or 'super-antigen' may be causative. Pathologically necrotizing microvasculitis with fibrinoid necrosis is found.

Clinical features   The hallmark feature is high fever for more than 5 days, poorly responsive to antipyretics, non-responsive to antibiotics and associated with marked irritability. Non-suppurative bulbar conjunctivitis is frequent sometimes complicated by uveitis or keratitis. In the mouth, dry red cracked lips are found, together with stomatitis, pharyngitis and a raw red 'strawberry tongue'. See Figure 9.10. Cervical lymphadenopathy of greater than 1.5 cm, often unilateral, is found in the majority of patients. It is minimally painful, not fluctuant but erythema of the overlying skin may occur. Other skin manifestations include polymorphic (but non-vesicular) and maculopapular rashes of the face, limbs, trunk and peri-genitalia areas. The palms and feet may be oedematous and erythematous with sharp demarcation. In the convalescent phase of the disease marked skin desquamation around the nails and fingers may become prominent. A variety of other manifestations may occur, including arthralgia or arthritis, diarrhoea, aseptic meningitis, optic neuritis, pneumonitis, hepatitis and a large number of rarer manifestations. The most dangerous complications are cardiac, including myopericarditis, cardiac valvulitis and coronary artery aneurysms. If left undiagnosed or untreated, there is a distinct danger of myocardial infarction or cardiac failure. The acute febrile phase lasts 1–2 weeks, the sub-acute desquamative and coronary aneurysmal phase lasts up to a month and the convalescent phase lasts up to 8 weeks.

Diagnosis   is clinical and based on fever and the presence of the common features listed above. Many cases particularly in young infants may be atypical and require experience and acumen to diagnose. There are no specific laboratory tests but

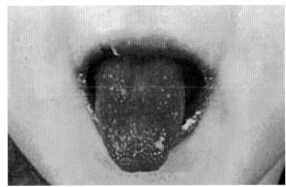
Dry cracked lips, strawberry tongue

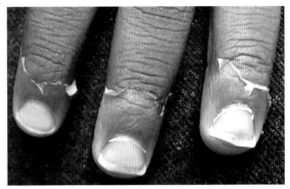
Peri-ungular desquamation

Figure 9.10 Kawasaki disease: note the cracked lips, strawberry tongue and desquamation of the skin in the fingers.

raised inflammatory markers, neutrophilia and thrombocytosis (after the first week), abnormal liver functions and proteinuria are all characteristic findings. An echocardiogram should be done as early as possible in order to diagnose cardiac complications. Differential diagnoses include sepsis, juvenile rheumatoid arthritis, vasculitis, scarlet fever and toxic shock syndrome.

Management   is based on exclusion of infection and the administration of intravenous immunoglobulins. To this is added high-dose, then tapering doses of acetyl-salicylic acid (aspirin). Steroids may be used in some refractory cases as are cyclophosphamide and plasma-exchange.

Prognosis   is generally good if the disease is diagnosed and treated early. Overall mortality from cardiac complications in treated patients is less than 2%. Refractory cases and recurrence are rare.

Prevention   There is no known prevention for Kawasaki disease.

Kawasaki disease at a glance

Epidemiology
10-50 in 100000 children

Aetiology
Super antigen implicated

History
5 days or more high fever
Non-response to antibiotics
Poor response to antipyretics
Marked irritability

Physical examination
- Bulbar conjunctivitis
- Pharyngitis, stomatitis, dry cracked red lips, 'strawberry tongue'
- Cervical lymphadenopathy
- Polymorphic rash
- Limb oedema and skin desquamation (convalescent phase)
- Cardiac involvement: especially coronary artery aneurysms

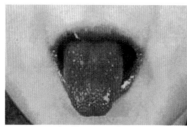
Dry cracked lips, strawberry tongue

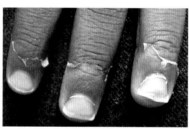
Peri-ungular desquamation

Diagnosis
5 days fever and 4–5 major features
Exclusion of other diagnoses

Suggestive investigations
Raised inflammatory markers and neutrophilia
Thrombocytosis (after the first week)
ECG and echocardiogram (to exclude coronary disease)

Differential diagnosis
Viral exanthemata
Juvenile rheumatoid arthritis (Still disease)
Scarlet fever

Management
Intravenous immunoglobulins
Aspirin

Prognosis/complications
Good
Cardiac failure/infarction <2% treated cases

To test your knowledge on this part of the book, please see Chapter 26

CHAPTER 10
Respiratory disorders

Christopher Robin
Had wheezles
And sneezles,
They bundled him
Into
His bed.
They gave him what goes
With a cold in the nose,
And some more for a cold
In the head.
'Now We are Six', AA Milne

KEY COMPETENCES

YOU MUST...

Know and understand

- The differential diagnosis of children presenting with cough, wheeze, stridor, breathing difficulty and chest pain
- How to diagnose and manage serious and common respiratory conditions
- The key preventer strategies and reliever medications used in asthma and how to administer them to children of different ages

Be able to

- Examine the respiratory system competently
- Recognise the signs of respiratory distress
- Carry out peak flow measurements (see p. 119)
- Manage the choking child
- Show a family how to use an inhaler and assess inhaler technique
- Recognise when a child with asthma is in severe respiratory distress
- Take a systematic approach to reading a chest X-ray (p. 116)

Appreciate

- The impact that asthma or cystic fibrosis has on the child and family
- The principles involved in managing chronic respiratory disorders

Essential Paediatrics and Child Health, Fourth Edition. Mary Rudolf, Anthony Luder and Kerry Jeavons.
© 2020 John Wiley & Sons Ltd. Published 2020 by John Wiley & Sons Ltd.
Companion website: www.wiley.com/go/rudolf/paediatrics

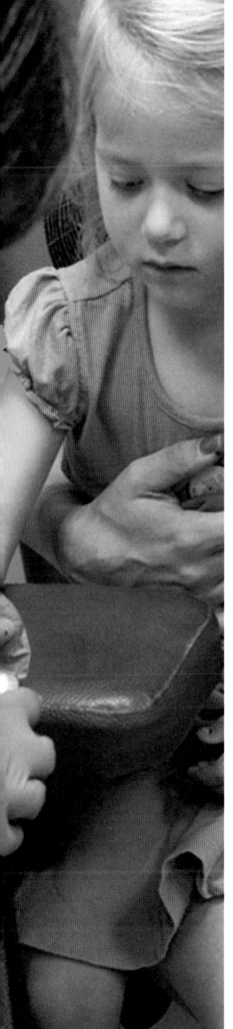

Respiratory symptoms and signs

Finding your way around ...

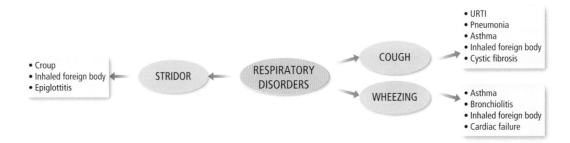

Cough

Causes of cough by age		
Infancy	**Preschool**	**School age to adolescence**
Infections	Infections	Asthma
upper respiratory tract	upper respiratory tract	Infections
bronchiolitis	croup	upper respiratory tract
pneumonia	acute bronchitis	Cigarette smoking
pertussis (whooping cough)	pneumonia	Postnasal drip
Congenital malformations of the	foreign body	Psychogenic
airway	Asthma	Cystic fibrosis
Gastro-oesophageal reflux	Cystic fibrosis	
Cystic fibrosis	Passive smoking	

Cough is a common symptom occurring with fever in an acutely ill child or as a troublesome and persistent problem. It generally results from a simple viral infection but may be an indicator of a serious infection or a chronic condition such as asthma (see Red Flag box).

> **Evidence of serious chronic lower respiratory tract disease in children**
>
> - Productive cough which improves with antibiotics but quickly recurs
> - Restriction of activity
> - Failure to grow or gain weight
> - Nail clubbing
> - Persistent tachypnoea

Illnesses causing cough vary with age, although the commonest cause of cough for all ages is infection affecting the upper or lower respiratory tract. A cough may persist and perpetuate itself after any illness, as coughing can injure the tracheal mucosa, making it more susceptible to irritation. Passive exposure to smoking exacerbates coughing and respiratory disease.

In infancy, upper respiratory tract infections (URTIs) can be particularly troublesome as the infant's ability to feed can be affected. Bronchiolitis, which affects the small airways (see p. 179), is a disease specific to this age group. If cough is chronic in infancy, serious causes such as congenital anomalies of the airways or aspiration of stomach contents should be considered.

In the preschool years, exposure to respiratory illnesses increases and cough is very common. Bronchitis is a rather non-specific term used either in relation to a productive cough (acute bronchitis) or bronchospasm. It is important to appreciate, however, that chronic bronchitis is not a paediatric disease. Asthma (see p. 168) often presents for the first time in the preschool years, and it may be manifested by cough as well as wheeze. Foreign bodies are also common, and the cough may occur some time after the episode of choking has been forgotten.

In older children, asthma and minor infections are the commonest causes of cough. Smoking must be considered as a possible cause of cough in adolescence.

History – must ask!

- *What does the cough sound like?* The sound of the cough can give a clue to the aetiology (Table 10.1). The rattling sound of mucus in the tracheobronchial tree is quite distinctive from either a dry laryngeal cough or the wheezy cough of asthma.
- *What is the sputum like?* Young children swallow sputum, rather than expectorate, so asking about the sputum is of limited value. Older children, however, may be able to cooperate. Persistent purulent sputum suggests suppurative lung disease such as cystic fibrosis or bronchiectasis. In asthma, sputum is clear and tenacious. Bloody sputum, if not from nasopharyngeal irritation, suggests a foreign body.
- *When is the coughing worst?* A non-productive nocturnal cough suggests bronchospasm, postnasal secretions or gastro-oesophageal reflux. A productive cough on getting up suggests bronchiectasis or cystic fibrosis. Paroxysms of coughing suggest either a foreign body or pertussis, and coughing related to eating points to aspiration.
- *Is the cough acute, persistent or recurrent?* Coughing may persist for weeks even after a mild respiratory infection. However, persistent cough in conjunction with other signs may indicate a chronic lung condition. Recurrent coughing, particularly at night, suggests asthma. Diaries kept by parents are valuable if the cough is persistent or chronic.
- *Is the child ill?* Fever indicates infection, but does not differentiate between upper and lower respiratory tract infection. If the child is ill, lower respiratory tract infection must be considered (see pneumonia, p. 177).
- *Are there associated symptoms or precipitating factors?* Coughing with wheezing strongly points to asthma, and other atopic manifestations in the child or the family helps in the diagnosis. Exacerbations during the spring and summer suggest an allergic aetiology. An episode of choking might be recalled, suggesting inhalation of a foreign body. Chronic symptoms of oily diarrhoea suggest cystic fibrosis.
- *Does anyone smoke in the family?* Passive smoking has an irritant effect on the young airway and can cause coughing in itself. It also predisposes to asthma and infections. Adolescents may not confess to smoking, particularly if accompanied by a parent.
- *Past medical history.* A history of previous chest infections, particularly if confirmed radiologically, should suggest chronic lung disease. Chronic sinusitis or middle ear effusions, in the presence of chronic respiratory infections, may suggest ciliary dyskinesia.

Physical examination – must check!

- *Growth.* Measure height and weight in all children, as poor growth occurs in chronic conditions such as cystic fibrosis, bronchiectasis, immunodeficiency or severe asthma.
- *Signs of respiratory distress.* Tachypnoea, subcostal and intercostal retractions (Fig. 5.14, p. 79) and nasal alar flaring indicate respiratory distress and in childhood are often more significant than auscultation findings. In an infant, an expiratory grunting sound suggests severe respiratory distress. Tachypnoea may be the only sign of serious respiratory pathology.
- *Examination of the chest.* Examination of the chest is obviously important, however, interpret your findings on auscultation cautiously. Transmitted sounds from the upper airways are commonly heard in the child with a cold, and must be differentiated from crepitations. Focal chest signs are less reliable than in adults in indicating the site of infection. Expiratory wheezing suggests the diagnosis of asthma, but may not be present between attacks unless the asthma is severe. Decreased air entry indicates bronchial obstruction from any cause.
- *Other signs.* Clubbing in a child with a cough suggests the possibility of suppurative lung disease or associated cardiac pathology. Signs of atopy such as eczema or allergic-appearing eyes point towards a diagnosis of asthma.

Investigations (see Table 10.2)

Investigations are required if a child has evidence of pneumonia or chronic lung disease (see Red Flag box and Table 10.2). The interpretation of chest X-rays is covered on p. 116. X-rays are too often repeatedly obtained in children with asthma.

If a foreign body is suspected, chest fluoroscopy is required to look for mediastinal shift on inspiration. Bronchoscopy is needed to confirm the diagnosis and remove the foreign body.

A sweat test for cystic fibrosis is indicated for recurrent productive cough, particularly if accompanied by poor

Table 10.1 Characteristics of coughs

Loose, productive	Bronchitis, wheezy bronchitis, cystic fibrosis, bronchiectasis
Wheezy	Asthma, wheezy bronchitis
Barking	Croup
Paroxysmal (with or without vomiting)	Cystic fibrosis, pertussis, foreign body, asthma
Nocturnal	Asthma, sinusitis
Most severe on waking	Cystic fibrosis, bronchiectasis
With vigorous exercise	Exercise-induced asthma, cystic fibrosis, bronchiectasis
Disappears with sleep	Habitual cough

Table 10.2 Investigations and their relevance in a coughing child

Investigation	What you are looking for
Full blood count	Raised white count and shift to the left with bacterial infection
	Possible eosinophilia in asthma/atopy
Blood culture	Lower respiratory tract infection
Pernasal swab	To identify pertussis
Chest X-ray	Congenital anomalies of the lungs
	Lower respiratory tract infection
Sweat test	Cystic fibrosis
Videofluoroscopy and bronchoscopy	Aspirated foreign body
Trial of bronchodilators ± peak flow measurements	Asthma

growth or abnormal stools. As asthma is a common cause of recurrent cough, diagnosis using tests of peak flow and spirometry are desirable when the child is old enough to cooperate.

Managing cough as a symptom

Antibiotics have no place in the management of URTIs, and should only be given if there is good evidence of infection of the lower tract. A good trial of bronchodilators, delivered by a technique appropriate for age, is required when asthma is suspected or diagnosed (see p. 168).

Psychogenic cough is a diagnosis of exclusion. Characteristically, an early-school-age child will have a recurrent loud 'brassy' barking dry cough that never occurs when the child is asleep. The family is often very anxious about the cough. If there is no suggestion of serious pathology in the history or examination, the child and family should be reassured. The cough will often resolve if ignored by the family for several weeks; if it persists, further investigation may be necessary.

Smoking is an important cause and exacerbator of cough. Every effort must be made to discourage exposure, whether passive or active.

Key points: A coughing child

- Transmitted sounds from the upper airways are commonly heard and should not be confused with crepitations or wheeze
- Observation of tachypnoea, intercostal or subcostal retractions and alar flaring are often more important signs than findings on auscultation
- Asthma commonly presents with cough in young children as well as wheezing
- High fever in itself does not indicate lower respiratory tract infection
- In a child with chronic or persistent cough, look for evidence of chronic lung disease

Clues to the differential diagnosis of the coughing child

	Fever	Features of cough	Respiratory signs
Upper respiratory tract infection (URTI)	+/−	Non-productive	None, other than transmitted sounds
Pneumonia	+	Productive	Alar flaring, intercostal, subcostal recessions, +/−/? dullness to percussion, diminished breath sounds
Asthma	− or +/− if URTI present	Wheezy, often nocturnal or on exercise	Alar flaring, intercostal, subcostal recessions, expiratory wheeze (but may be absent at time of examination)
Foreign body	− (until infection develops)	Often preceded by choking episode	Wheeze, diminished breath sounds on right

Wheezing

Commoner causes of wheezing

Asthma
Bronchiolitis and other viral agents
Aspiration of food or a foreign body
Sequelae of neonatal lung disease (bronchopulmonary dysplasia)
Cardiac failure

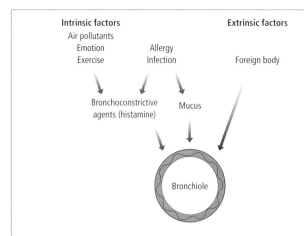

Figure 10.1 Intrinsic and extrinsic factors causing wheeze in childhood.

Noisy breathing is a common symptom in children which may be caused by partial obstruction of either the upper or lower airway. The upper airway comprises the nose, pharynx, larynx and extrathoracic portion of the trachea. The lower airway comprises intrathoracic trachea, bronchi and bronchioles. Partial obstruction of the upper airway causes an inspiratory noise (*stridor*) and partial obstruction of the lower airway an expiratory *wheeze*. In many cases noises can be heard on both inspiration and expiration, and it requires concentration to determine the phase of breathing in which the predominant noise occurs.

A wheeze is a prolonged musical note heard mainly on expiration and is very common in childhood. It may also be referred to as a *rhonchus* on auscultation. It is fairly easily distinguished from stridor (p. 165), which is an inspiratory upper airway noise. Transmitted noises from the upper airway are often heard when auscultating the young child's chest. This may make interpretation of intrathoracic noises more difficult. It may be helpful to hold the bell of the stethoscope to the child's throat and listen to the upper airway noise. These noises can then be mentally subtracted from the noises heard when listening for lower airway signs.

Wheezing is caused by partial obstruction of the intrathoracic airways and is a result of intrinsic or extrinsic factors (Figure 10.1). Bronchi have a layer of smooth muscle within the wall of the tube. Various factors may cause the muscle to spasm thereby narrowing the tube. Intrinsic factors are mediated through histamine release as part of the inflammatory response which causes acute narrowing of the bronchi and bronchioles. The commonest causes are allergy and infection. Extrinsic causes of airway narrowing include the presence of a foreign body and mucus oversecretion as a result of infection. Therefore, viral infection may cause wheeze from both constriction of the tube's muscle wall as the result of intrinsic release of vasoconstrictive substances and from the production of mucus as a result of the infectious agent.

Viral wheeze   It is estimated that 20% of all children will wheeze at some time in the first 5 years of life. Children (particularly under 3 years of age) are prone to wheezing with viral infections because bronchospasm, mucosal oedema, and secretions have a greater impact in narrowing their relatively smaller airways. Other risk factors which predispose to preschool wheeze are premature birth, exposure to cigarette smoke, environmental pollutants, previous exposure to Respiratory Syncytial Virus (RSV) and genetic associations.

The presence of wheeze in preschool children does not necessarily equate that the toddler will develop asthma (a chronic atopic illness) in older childhood. Children may have viral wheeze (associated exclusively with episodes of upper respiratory viral infections) or multi-trigger wheeze. Multi-trigger wheeze is frequently associated with change in weather (especially humidity) or exertion, and signals that the airways are hyper-responsive.

History – must ask!

Take the history from the parents if the child is young or acutely distressed. It is important to determine from the history the effect that the wheeze is having on the child, symptoms which may suggest a specific cause (e.g. inhaled foreign body) and the chronic history of recurrence.

- *The acute episode.* Was there a triggering event? Asthma is often triggered by exposure to allergens such as house-dust mite, pet hair, grass pollens and irritants such as tobacco smoke. It is also precipitated by acute emotion, physical exercise or going out on a cold morning. Viral infection can be an important trigger for asthma, but may be a cause of wheezing in its own right, for example in bronchiolitis or viral wheeze.
- *Severity of the episode.* Find out how incapacitated the child is. Ask if he or she is able to feed normally and if the wheezing interferes with play and activity. Severe wheeze and breathlessness may affect the child's ability to talk.
- *Family history.* Asthma is suggested by a family history of *atopy*, including asthma, eczema or hay fever.

- *History of choking*. Aspiration of food or a foreign body is most likely in toddlers who are mobile and put everything they find into their mouths.
- *Apnoea*. Bronchiolitis and other viral infections cause wheezing in infants and may be associated with apnoea and quite severe respiratory distress.

Physical examination – must check!

- *Assessment of growth*. Plot the child's height and weight on a growth chart. Growth failure does not occur unless the asthma is very severe; poor growth suggests a condition such as cystic fibrosis.
- *Signs of respiratory distress*. Signs of respiratory distress include shortness of breath (dyspnoea), tachypnoea, alar flaring, intercostal and subcostal recession (see p. 406) and the use of accessory muscles for breathing. Features of severe respiratory distress include an inability to talk (in the older child), cyanosis, confusion, restlessness and drowsiness, and any of these symptoms demands rapid assessment and investigation.
- *Chest signs*. In contrast to adults, chest signs in young children are often not localized and may not relate to X-ray findings. Listen for hyper-resonance and dullness on percussion. On auscultation, widespread crepitations with wheezing suggest infection, particularly bronchiolitis in infants, whereas unilateral wheeze suggests aspiration of a foreign body. Wheezing may also be a sign of cardiac failure in a child with congenital heart disease, in which case listen for murmurs, assess the heart size and examine the upper abdomen for hepatomegaly.
- *Other signs*. Look for signs of chronic lung disease such as barrel chest and clubbing. Clubbing is suggestive of chronic suppurative lung disease and rarely occurs in chronic asthma.
- *Peak flow*. This should be part of the assessment of any wheezing or breathless child who is old enough to cooperate (see p. 171).

Investigations

Most children with acute wheeze require only a careful history and examination. Further investigation is, however, required in an acute onset of wheeze in a very young child, asymmetrical signs on examination or failure to thrive. The seriously ill child needs a full blood count and may require a chest X-ray. Repeated chest X-rays in a child with recurrent episodes of acute wheeze from asthma are not warranted.

The child who shows severe signs of respiratory distress will also need careful assessment for respiratory failure. Oxygen therapy is monitored by transcutaneous oxygen measurement and oxygen titrated against oxygen saturation. Arterial or capillary blood gas measurement may help determine the need for respiratory support (see p. 111).

Managing wheezing

Children with acute onset of wheeze and their parents may be very frightened by the symptom, and reassurance is necessary after appropriate assessment. Immediate management is directed towards assessing whether the child is in actual or incipient respiratory failure, when respiratory support may be required. The need for oxygen therapy is assessed by transcutaneous pulse oximetry.

- *Preschool children* - An acute exacerbation of viral wheeze in a preschool child is likely to respond to inhaled bronchodilators and families should have a plan for home on how and when to give these. Evidence has shown that oral corticosteroids are not generally beneficial in this age group and should be avoided. Preschool children with atopy and a severe episode of multi-trigger wheeze requiring admission hospital may, however, benefit. Preventative therapy in preschool children with recurrent wheeze may be considered, specifically a trial of inhaled corticosteroid, and a small subgroup have been shown to benefit from leukotriene receptor antagonists (montelukast).
- *Older children* - Asthma is the commonest cause of recurrent wheezing in older children and, provided there is no indication of other conditions on history or physical examination, you should give a trial of a bronchodilator to confirm the diagnosis. Clinical improvement in wheezing indicates that the bronchospasm is reversible, and a diagnosis of asthma can be made. In the older, cooperative child, peak flow measurements before and after the trial are useful.
- *Infants* - Some babies wheeze very persistently. If the wheeze is not affecting eating, temperament and growth, this need not arouse too much concern. Such children have been called 'happy wheezers' historically, and the symptoms subside as they grow. Milk allergy is often implicated, but withdrawal of cow's milk protein is only rarely effective. A more important intervention is to stop exposure to cigarette smoke.

🔑 Key points: The wheezing child

- Asthma is by definition *recurrent* wheezing
- Preschool children may have wheeze from viral infections or multi-trigger wheeze.
- Oral corticosteroids should be avoided in preschool children
- Tachypnoea, alar flaring and intercostal/subcostal recessions are signs of respiratory distress
- Unilateral wheeze in a toddler is suggestive of a foreign body
- Children with asthma in general do not need a chest X-ray at each attack
- Localized chest findings often do not correlate with those on the X-ray

Clues to the differential diagnosis of wheezing in children

	Age	Percussion	Auscultation	Chest X-ray	Specific features
Asthma	Any age but diagnosed with caution in a child <2 years	Increased percussion note	Widespread wheeze. Variable crepitations	Overinflated	Recurrent wheezing. Triggered by URTI or allergens. Responsive to bronchodilators. Family history of atopy
Foreign body	Toddlers	Focal dullness with increased resonance if compensatory emphysema	Unilateral wheezing and crepitations, or focal reduced air entry	Segmental collapse or emphysema	Unilateral wheezing. May be preceded by choking episode
Bronchiolitis	Babies	Variable	Widespread wheeze and crepitations	Overinflation, consolidation	Apnoea may be a feature in infants. Often RSV+. Increased lymphocytes on FBC. Wheeze is often unresponsive to bronchodilators
Viral-induced wheeze/ wheezy bronchitis	Toddlers	Normal	Wheeze and crepitations	Normal	Wheezing with URTI
Cardiac failure	Any age	Normal	Wheeze	Enlarged heart	Child with congenital heart disease. Hepatomegaly also a feature

RSV, respiratory syncytial virus; FBC, full blood count.

Stridor

Causes of stridor

Acute causes
Croup (acute laryngotracheobronchitis)
Acute epiglottitis
Foreign body

Chronic causes
Laryngomalacia
Subglottic stenosis

Stridor is a noise heard on inspiration and is caused by narrowing of the extrathoracic upper airway. Stridor is most likely to arise from the larynx and is usually a sign of croup, a non-severe, self-limiting viral illness which is very common in young children, particularly in the winter. The challenge of the condition is to recognise those children with an acute but non-severe self-limiting illness who can be observed at home and those who, if untreated, may develop life-threatening upper airway obstruction.

History – must ask!

- *Coryza and fever.* The commonest cause of stridor is croup (acute laryngotracheobronchitis), when the stridor coincides with a barking cough. It is often preceded by coryzal symptoms and fever. The main differential diagnosis is epiglottitis (a life-threatening illness which is rarely seen since the introduction of the *Haemophilus influenza* B (HiB) immunisation). In epiglottitis the child is severely ill.
- *Nature of the stridor.* The degree of stridor depends on the effort of the inspiratory breath. The stridulous noise is usually louder when the child cries and is softer during sleep.
- *Aspiration.* Aspiration of a foreign body should always be considered in acute stridor. If a foreign body is a cause of upper airway obstruction the stridor is usually very severe and the child is dramatically ill.
- *Features of onset.* Laryngomalacia (floppy larynx) is a congenital condition which resolves with age. Laryngomalacia is usually worse on lying the infant prone. Subglottic stenosis can develop after a previous intubation, particularly in children who were born prematurely.

Physical examination – must check!

- *Chest signs*. Signs in the chest, including crepitations and wheeze, are strongly suggestive of croup and are very uncommon with acute epiglottitis or upper airway foreign body obstruction.
- *Airway obstruction*. Stridor is an important sign because it may proceed to acute airway obstruction, a potentially fatal condition. Never examine the throat of a child with severe stridor, as acute airway obstruction may occur; this examination should only be undertaken in the presence of an anaesthetist who can intubate the child if necessary. Signs of increasing airway obstruction include:
  - cyanosis;
  - confusion;
  - reduction in stridor with exhaustion;
  - drooling with increasing dysphagia.

Investigations

If the child is suspected of having impending respiratory failure or acute epiglottitis, a full blood count and blood culture should be done, and blood gases measured. Care must be taken to avoid precipitating acute airway obstruction, and if this is considered to be a risk, prior intubation is necessary.

Managing stridor

Stridor caused by croup (see p. 181) is usually a self-limiting condition, but in a few cases progressive airway obstruc-

tion occurs. Mild croup (without stridor and with only a barking cough) is best managed at home with no specific treatment, and the parents counselled on features of deterioration. If the condition worsens, hospital assessment is necessary. A team approach involving paediatric anaesthetics and ENT is usually advised and intubation by an experienced doctor is needed if there are signs of impending airway obstruction.

If acute epiglottitis is suspected, urgent senior paediatric assessment, antibiotic treatment and intubation is essential as airway obstruction is very likely to develop.

Complete upper airway obstruction caused by a foreign body is a medical emergency and if untreated will rapidly lead to death (pp. 407–8).

 Key points: The child with stridor

- Assess how severe the airway obstruction is and observe any progression
- Assess the likelihood of foreign body aspiration
- Look for the systemic features of acute epiglottitis, and hospitalize as an emergency
- Do not examine the throat or upset the child if stridor is present without anaesthetic presence

---

Clues to the differential diagnosis of stridor

	Age	Clinical features
Croup	6–24 months	Coryzal prodrome
		Barking cough
Epiglottitis	2–7 years	Toxicity and high fever
		Drooling
Foreign body	9–18 months	History and sudden onset
Laryngomalacia	Newborn	Presents at birth and persists
		Worse on crying
		Improves with age
Subglottic stenosis	0–6 months	Previous history of intubation
		Exacerbations with URTI

Breathing difficulty

Most cases of breathing difficulty are also associated with cough, stridor or wheeze as above.

History – must ask!

- *Fever.* The presence of a fever indicates an infective cause. This may be viral wheeze, an infective exacerbation of asthma or a chest infection. The fever in croup is likely to be mild, but a high-grade fever and a septic appearance are seen with epiglottitis. Infants with bronchiolitis would not be expected to have a fever.
- *Diabetes or acidosis.* Children with diabetic ketoacidosis (often as a new presentation of diabetes mellitus), or those with metabolic acidosis, have 'Kussmaul breathing', which are large sighing respirations. These can be mistaken for tachypnoea.
- *Shortness of breath on exertion.* This may indicate severe anaemia or heart failure, as well as asthma.
- *Snoring.* Children can present with sleep apnoea and a history of snoring with pauses in breathing at night would require sleep studies.

Physical examination – must check!

- *Chest examination.* A full chest examination, including expansion, assessment of chest shape and auscultation to assess for air entry, wheeze or crepitations.
- *Cardiac examination.* The presence of a heart murmur with cardiomegaly, and possibly hepatomegaly, would suggest cardiac failure. Dependent oedema (which will be sacral in small children, rather than to ankles) may also be seen.
- *Neurological assessment.* Neuromuscular disorders, such as Guillain-Barré, are associated with respiratory compromise, but there is usually a history of preceding motor difficulties.
- *Anaemia.* Severe anaemia will lead to respiratory compromise due to reduced oxygen-carrying capacity. Conjunctival pallor is seen in children with anaemia. This is especially important to check in children with dark skin, where skin pallor may be harder to detect.
- *Systemic examination.* Occasionally, a respiratory presentation may be seen in children with large tumours, particularly those involving the mediastinum.

Investigations

- *Full blood count.* This may reveal anaemia, which if present, may prompt checks on ferritin levels and haemoglobinopathy screen.
- *Blood gas.* This would reveal if metabolic acidosis were present, as well as reveal the P_{CO_2} to indicate the respiratory efficacy.

- *Blood glucose.* Raised blood glucose with glycosuria and raised ketones (blood or urine) indicates diabetic ketoacidosis.

Chest pain

> **Causes of chest pain**
>
> Idiopathic
> Psychogenic
> Stitch
> Musculoskeletal
> Oesophagitis/gastro-oesophageal reflux
> Cardiovascular (very rare)

Chest pain is a relatively common complaint which is usually benign and self-limited, but generates a lot of anxiety because of the connotations that chest pain has for adults. Musculoskeletal pain can occur as a result of muscle strain, cough, trauma and stress fracture. Pain at the costochondral junctions due to costochondritis is not uncommon and is often preceded by an URTI or exercise. A stitch is a familiar type of pain thought to be caused by peritoneal ligament stress occurring when exercising in the upright posture. Oesophagitis (see p. 202) can present as pain in older children.

History – must ask!

The history is important as there are rarely any physical signs. Ask about the duration, frequency, quality and location of the pain, and whether there is any exacerbation or relief with position, exertion, eating, coughing or stress.

Physical examination – must check!

Your examination should focus on the presence of fever or weight loss, signs of trauma and altered breathing patterns, as well as inspection of the chest and spine and a good respiratory and cardiac assessment. Localized tenderness over the costal cartilages, adjacent to the sternum, is typically found in costochondritis.

Investigations

Investigations such as blood counts, sedimentation rate, chest X-ray and electrocardiogram (ECG) are rarely required but may provide extra reassurance.

Managing chest pain

You should acknowledge the pain, provide relief for the symptoms in terms of rest and simple analgesics, and reassure the family of the benign nature of the problem.

Respiratory disorders

Asthma

Definition and pathophysiology

The definition of asthma is episodic, reversible, intrathoracic airway obstruction. Reversibility may occur spontaneously or as a result of therapy. The symptoms of asthma, cough and wheeze are caused by narrowing of the bronchi and bronchioles as a result of bronchoconstriction, mucosal swelling and viscid secretion obstructing the lumen. Various allergic and non-specific stimuli may initiate this process in the susceptible individual by triggering the release of histamine and other mediators. These stimuli include dust mites, air pollutants, cigarette smoke, cold air, viral infections, stress and exercise.

Prevalence

Asthma is the commonest chronic condition of childhood, affecting up to 20% of children. There is clustering of cases in children living near motorways or in urban environments.

Initial presentation of asthma

Most children with asthma become symptomatic in infancy or the preschool years; however, most preschool children with wheeze do not go on to develop asthma. The diagnosis of asthma is usually made clinically on the basis of a persistent or recurrent cough or wheeze, which is responsive to medication. A family or past medical history of atopy contributes to the diagnosis. Children over 5 years old with asthma are advised in NICE Guideline (NG80) "Asthma: diagnosis, monitoring and chronic asthma management" to have objective tests for asthma including spirometry with evidence of bronchodilator reversibility testing and fractional exhaled nitric oxide levels. These investigations may not be readily obtainable, however, and a good clinical history is usually sufficient in the absence of diagnostic uncertainty.

Wheeze in infancy

Many babies have episodes of wheezing, in part as a result of their relatively narrow airways, which readily become obstructed. These episodes may be related to infection by the respiratory syncytial virus (RSV). The majority of wheezing babies do not persist in having troublesome symptoms, and there is therefore no advantage to labelling them as having a chronic medical condition, particularly as the treatment of the wheezy baby is the same whether he or she has a diagnosis of asthma or not (see p. 163). If the baby has another atopic condition or there is a family history of atopy and asthma, however, the wheezing is more likely to be a manifestation of asthma. In infancy, as the airways are so narrow, the contribution of secretions and mucosal oedema to the obstruction is greater, and there is often a poor response to bronchodilator treatment.

Diagnosis of asthma in childhood

Recurrent episodes of coughing and wheezing, especially if aggravated or triggered by exercise, viral infection or inhaled antigens, are highly suggestive of asthma. The diagnosis is made on the basis of the response to bronchodilator treatment. In the younger child this response is judged clinically by the reduction in respiratory distress and wheeze. In the older child, reversibility of airway obstruction can be demonstrated by peak flow measurements. Although X-rays are not often indicated in the child with asthma, a chest X-ray should be considered at the first episode to exclude a foreign body in the lung or oesophagus.

Allergy testing

Allergy tests are not usually carried out, but may be useful after diagnosis to aid in identifying triggers. Skin testing is not usually helpful, as false positives and false negatives are common and a skin response may not reflect airway hypersensitivity. Radioallergosorbent tests (RAST) may identify allergens to be avoided.

Management of asthma

The goals of management include those for any chronic condition of childhood (see p. 47). The principal goal is the prevention and relief of symptoms of wheeze and cough, both night and day (see Box 10.1). The child and the parents must be educated so that they can manage a large part of the disease themselves. Good management should promote normal growth and development and allow the child to become involved and participate in all types of exercise and sport.

Medication

The principles of management are shown in Box 10.2. Most asthma medications are delivered by inhalation, where possible, as this ensures delivery of the drug direct to the target organ, the bronchioles.

Box 10.1 Goals in managing asthma

- Rapid relief of symptoms
- Prevention of symptoms both night and day
- Normal levels of activity, including sport
- Normal growth and development
- Self-management

Box 10.2 Management of asthma

- Use inhaled beta-agonists to relieve symptoms
- If used frequently, introduce inhaled steroids
- Treat acute attacks promptly with high-dose inhaled bronchodilator; consider short course of prednisolone
- If attack persists, admit for nebulizer treatment, intravenous steroids +/– IV therapies (magnesium sulphate, salbutamol, aminophylline).
- In severe cases ventilation may be required
- In poorly controlled asthma, refer to a respiratory paediatrician

The recommended step-by-step plan to control symptoms is shown in Table 10.3. The child needs to be regularly reviewed to see if gradual step-down is possible, or if step-up is required. If long-term oral or high-dose inhaled steroids are needed, the side effects of adrenal suppression and poor growth may occur. Children with frequent wheeze under the age of 2 years would usually require referral to a paediatric respiratory physician.

The drugs used for treating asthma may be classified into 'relievers' and 'preventers'. All children require 'relievers', which are usually beta-agonists such as salbutamol or terbutaline, although the antimuscarinic ipratropium bromide is sometimes used. If the child needs to use 'reliever' treatment frequently (if using three doses a week or more), the condition warrants prophylactic management with 'preventer' medication in the form of inhaled steroids or leukotriene receptor antagonist.

Metered dose inhalers (MDIs) are preferred over dry-powder inhalers (DPI) in children of all ages.

Spacer device

Infants and toddlers can usually use an MDI by using a spacer device with a valve system (Figures 10.2 and 10.3). An MDI dispenses the dose into the chamber and the child inhales the medication over six or seven inhalations. The device ensures that the medication reaches the lungs rather than landing in the mouth or throat. Even young infants can use a spacer device if a closely fitting mask is attached.

Nebulizer

For severe asthma attacks when constant additional oxygen is required, a nebulizer is needed to provide an aerosol which is

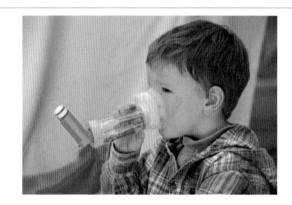

Figure 10.2 Child using a spacer device.

Table 10.3 The medical management of asthma in children*

<5 years	5 years and over
Step 1 Mild intermittent asthma	
Inhaled short-acting β_2-agonist prn	Inhaled short-acting β_2-agonist as required
Step 2 Regular preventative therapy	
Add very low dose ICS 100–200 µg/day or LTRA	Add ICS 100–200 µg/day
Step 3 Add-on therapy	
	1. Add LABA and assess response
Add LTRA	2. Consider adding LTRA
	3. Consider increasing ICS to 200–400 µg/day
Step 4 Persistent poor control	
Refer to respiratory paediatrician	Refer to respiratory paediatrician and consider increasing ICS to medium dose (800 µg/day) or adding theophylline
Step 5 Continuous or frequent use of steroids	
Not used	Add oral low-dose daily steroids
	Refer to respiratory paediatrician

* Adapted from the Asthma Guidelines of the British Thoracic Society and the Scottish Intercollegiate Guidelines, September 2016. ICS – Inhaled corticosteroids; LTRA – leukotriene receptor antagonist; LABA – Long-acting β_2-agonist.

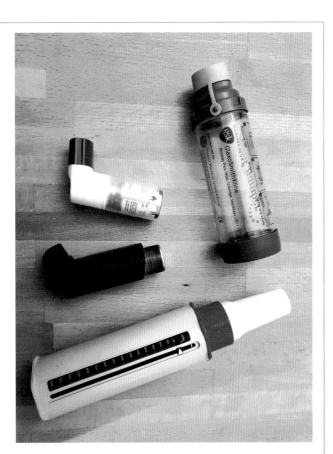

Figure 10.3 Inhalers and older child (blue) spacer with peak flow meter.

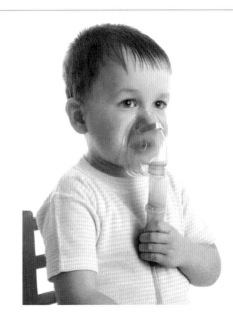

Figure 10.4 Child using a nebulizer.

then delivered by a face mask held close to the child's face (Figure 10.4).

Management of an acute attack

An acute episode of asthma may be precipitated by allergens, viral infection or exercise. The child experiences cough, wheeze and breathlessness, and on examination the chest is generally hyper-resonant and widespread rhonchi are heard. Signs of severe respiratory distress include dyspnoea, cyanosis and recession of the subcostal and intercostal muscles. A chest X-ray is not usually required but may show an overinflated chest with no other abnormalities. Peak flow is reduced.

If the attack does not respond quickly to the child's usual treatment at home, he or she will need urgent treatment by multiple puffs of bronchodilator via spacer or nebulizer attached to an air compressor or compressed oxygen supply. This may be given by the GP, but if a doctor is not immediately available the child must be taken to hospital for treatment. This may require escalation to IV treatments such as aminophylline, salbutamol or magnesium sulphate. If the episode is severe or recurrent, a short course of oral or IV steroids may be required. Prednisolone given for only 3–4 days does not require tapering off and will not cause adrenal suppression or affect growth.

If there is inadequate improvement from the high-dose bronchodilator, the child must be admitted for further high-dose inhaled or nebulized bronchodilator and, if required, intravenous steroid, aminophylline or beta-agonist infusion. Most severe attacks respond rapidly to this treatment, but occasionally intubation and ventilation is required.

In general, children with asthma are often subjected to a large number of unnecessary chest X-rays. Beyond the initial episode at diagnosis, X-rays are only indicated if another problem such as pneumonia, pneumothorax or foreign body is suspected. This is best assessed after the bronchospasm has been relieved.

Environmental control

Symptoms and drug requirements may be minimized by reducing exposure to allergens and irritants. Particularly critical is protection from exposure to cigarette smoke. Smoking in the home, at least in the child's presence or bedroom, must be avoided. The teenager must be warned about the undesirability of smoking.

House dust, house-dust mites, grass pollens and pets are the commonest allergens. Complete avoidance of house dust is impossible, but feather pillows, duvets and fitted carpets can be avoided. Mattresses should be covered with plastic and the child's room cleaned regularly. Pets, especially cats, may present a problem, and while it is hard to remove a family pet, acquiring new pets can be discouraged.

It is commonly believed that certain foods can cause asthma. Exclusion diets are not generally indicated, but occasionally certain foods or fizzy drinks are identified as causing attacks. It seems reasonable to avoid these, but care must be taken to make sure the diet remains balanced.

Monitoring the condition

Asthma is monitored by keeping a diary of symptoms, where wheezing, cough and activity levels are recorded along with medications given. In the child old enough to cooperate, peak flow monitoring can form part of the record.

Peak flow monitoring (see p. 119)

The majority of children do not need sophisticated lung function tests; however, the peak flow rate is a useful measure of asthmatic control. See Figures 10.5 and 10.6.

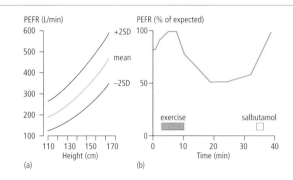

Figure 10.6 Peak flow chart: how exercise can affect peak flow. (a) The peak flow rate must be related to the child's height to interpret whether it is low. (b) Fall in peak flow rate with exercise in an asthmatic child. Peak flow rate recovers on administration of salbutamol.

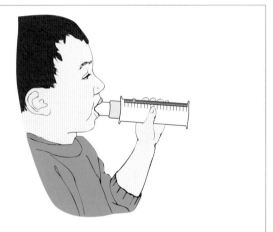

Figure 10.5 Child using a simple meter to measure peak flow rate.

The diary

An example is shown in Figure 10.7. The diary serves two functions. It allows the physician to review the child's course and in conjunction with regular clinical reviews to advise on changes in medication requirements. It also may alert the physician to other factors affecting the child, such as stress, compliance or environmental triggers. The diary's second function is to help the family follow the course of the condition, make sensible decisions about the need for medication and alert them when to obtain medical advice.

Routine follow-up of the child with asthma

Regular follow-up (see Checklist) is required for all children with asthma. The frequency of visits depends on the severity of the condition and how capable and confident the family is on managing symptoms.

✓ Checklist for review of a child with asthma

If the child is new to you or the clinic, check:
- [ ] The family's understanding of asthma and their ability to make adjustments in medications
- [ ] Inhaler technique
- [ ] Environmental control, especially smoking
- [ ] Accessibility of inhaler at school

Physical examination
- [ ] Height and weight
- [ ] Examination of chest
- [ ] Consider checking inhaler technique

Investigations
- [ ] Peak flow measurement

At routine follow-up, review:
History
- [ ] Diary, or if unavailable ask about symptoms of cough and wheeze
- [ ] Frequency of reliever treatment
- [ ] Number of severe attacks
- [ ] Number of absences from school as a result of asthma
- [ ] Any activities restricted because of asthma

Action:
- [ ] Advise on increasing or decreasing preventer treatment
- [ ] Consider changing device as child matures
- [ ] Counsel about particular issues such as lifestyle and independence

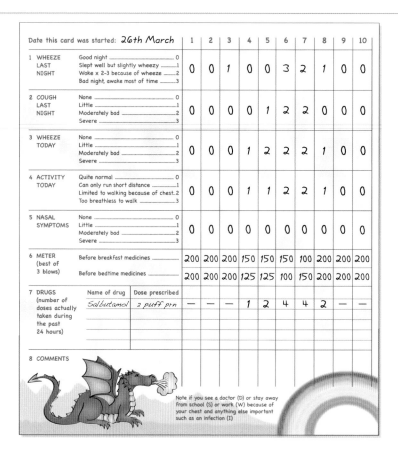

Date this card was started: **26th March**	1	2	3	4	5	6	7	8	9	10
1 WHEEZE LAST NIGHT — Good night ....0 / Slept well but slightly wheezy ....1 / Woke x 2-3 because of wheeze ....2 / Bad night, awake most of time 3	0	0	1	0	0	3	2	1	0	0
2 COUGH LAST NIGHT — None ....0 / Little ....1 / Moderately bad ....2 / Severe 3	0	0	0	0	1	2	2	0	0	0
3 WHEEZE TODAY — None ....0 / Little ....1 / Moderately bad ....2 / Severe 3	0	0	0	1	2	2	2	1	0	0
4 ACTIVITY TODAY — Quite normal ....0 / Can only run short distance ....1 / Limited to walking because of chest ..2 / Too breathless to walk 3	0	0	0	1	1	2	2	1	0	0
5 NASAL SYMPTOMS — None ....0 / Little ....1 / Moderately bad ....2 / Severe 3	0	0	0	0	0	0	0	0	0	0
6 METER (best of 3 blows) — Before breakfast medicines	200	200	200	150	150	150	100	200	200	200
Before bedtime medicines	200	200	200	125	125	100	150	200	200	200

7 DRUGS (number of doses actually taken during the past 24 hours)	Name of drug	Dose prescribed	1	2	3	4	5	6	7	8	9	10
	Salbutamol	2 puff prn	—	—	—	1	2	4	4	2	—	—

8 COMMENTS

Note if you see a doctor (D) or stay away from school (S) or work (W) because of your chest and anything else important such as an infection (I)

Figure 10.7 Diary kept by a 9-year-old boy showing good control of his asthma until days 6 and 7.

History   It is important to find out how often the child is coughing or wheezing, and the degree to which everyday activities are affected. It is also important to ascertain whether there have been any severe attacks in the interim or absences from school, and whether the child is experiencing any psychosocial difficulties as a result. A diary can be helpful in monitoring asthma (see Figure 10.7).

Physical examination   At routine appointments, more often than not there is no evidence of asthma on physical examination. In the child with chronic severe asthma the chest may take on a barrel shape and Harrison's sulcus (an anterolateral depression of the thorax at the insertion of the diaphragm) may be present (Figure 5.15). Clubbing of the fingers is rare even in severe asthma and suggests other causes of chronic obstructive lung disease.

Investigations   Pulmonary function tests other than peak flow measurements are rarely indicated. Newer techniques such as fraction of exhaled nitrous oxide are becoming more widely used in the diagnosis of asthma, but the long-term management of asthma is essentially clinically based.

Issues for the family

Education

The family has to be taught how to recognise the symptoms and signs of asthma, and how the medications differ in their action. They need to know how to use the various inhalation devices and to identify when the child is too distressed to take the medication by the usual route. They must also learn the technicalities of peak flow monitoring and, if the child is severely affected, the importance of keeping an effective diary and utilizing it to make changes in treatment. Parents may need to adapt the home environment, and smoking is likely to be the most important and difficult issue to tackle. As the child grows, he or she needs to take responsibility, and must learn how and when to use an inhaler independently, particularly at school.

It does not seem that there is any particular advice to give the family regarding the prognosis for subsequent children being affected other than avoiding smoking antenatally as well as postnatally. Although breast-feeding protects against the development of eczema in susceptible infants, no such clear connection has been established for asthma.

Psychosocial

Asthma too often is responsible for absences from school and interferes in full participation in both school and extracurricular activities. Even when symptoms are controlled during the day, children perform poorly following disturbed nights. A particularly difficult period may be during adolescence, when poor compliance or smoking may complicate the picture.

Asthma is a condition which can be frightening for the child and the family. This may lead to a tendency to overprotect the child. As emotional factors can trigger symptoms, this too can affect the functioning of the family. The role of the health professional is important not only in managing the physical symptoms of asthma, but also in addressing these issues and maximizing the child's chance of leading a full and normal life.

Issues at school

Given the prevalence of asthma, there are likely to be two or three children with asthma in any class. It is important, therefore, that all teachers have an understanding of the condition. In the young child the teacher must be able to recognise symptoms and help the child in administering his or her therapy.

It is critical that all asthmatic children have ready access to their inhalers. Older primary school children should be allowed to carry the inhaler around at all times, and certainly should have it with them for sports activities. Younger children should have the inhaler accessible in their tray–it will do no good locked in the teacher's drawer or the school office. Teaching staff need to understand that inadvertent use by the child or friends will cause no harm. A spare inhaler should be prescribed to be kept in school.

Staff at school can also be helpful in reporting symptoms to the parents or school nurse. This may be of particular value at secondary school, when poor compliance can be a particular issue.

Prognosis

Most children with asthma improve as they grow older. Preschool children who wheeze only with colds are likely to grow out of it in the early school years. The prognosis varies with the severity of the condition. Only 5% of those with mild asthma progress to develop severe disease. In contrast, 95% of those with severe disease continue to suffer as adults. After remission, asthma may recur in adulthood.

 See NICE guideline: Asthma: diagnosis, monitoring and chronic asthma management
https://www.nice.org.uk/guidance/ng80

◉ Asthma at a glance

Epidemiology
Commonest chronic respiratory condition. Some 10% of children are affected

Aetiology/pathophysiology
Environmental factors cause bronchoconstriction, mucosal oedema and excessive mucus production in a genetically predisposed child

How the diagnosis is made
Diagnosis is clinical, based on recurrent or persistent cough/ wheeze which is reversed by bronchodilators

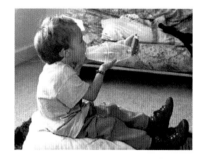

Clinical features
History
• Recurrent episodes of cough/ wheeze
• Nocturnal cough
• Dyspnoea
• History of atopy*
• Family history of atopic disease*

Physical examination
• Expiratory wheeze
• Normal chest exam between attacks
• Acute, often severe respiratory distress during attack
• Barrel-shaped chest if long-standing asthma*
• Poor growth, delayed puberty if severe disease*

Investigations
• Reduced peak flow rate, improved by bronchodilators
• Hyperinflation on chest X-ray

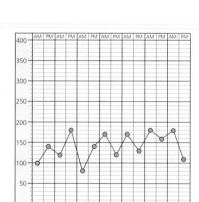

Peak flow chart

General management
Medication
involves 'preventers' and 'relievers' by delivery system appropriate for age

Environmental control
• No smoking in child's presence
• Dust/mite-free environment

Monitoring of asthma
• Home diary of symptoms and treatment
• Peak flow meter

Education
• Understanding asthma
• Competent use of inhalers
• Environmental control
• Self-management

School
• Education of staff
• Inhalers must be accessible
• Monitoring of school perform- ance, absences and compliance

Management of acute problems
Acute attacks need prompt treatment, often by nebulizer and short course of steroids

Points for routine follow-up
Monitor
• symptoms of cough/wheeze
• activity levels
• school absence
• acute attacks
• growth
• chest exam
• peak flow rate

Prognosis
Asthma resolves over time for most children unless severe. Deaths still occur from asthma in the UK

NB *Signs and symptoms are variable

Cystic fibrosis

Prevalence and pathophysiology

Cystic fibrosis is the commonest cause of suppurative lung disease in children in the UK. It is inherited as an autosomal recessive condition, one in 25 of the population being carriers. In northern Europe the commonest gene mutation is Δ*F508*.

This gene codes for a protein which controls sodium and chloride transport across the membrane of secretory epithelial cells. The mutation leads to a high salt content of sweat, and thick secretions produced by the epithelial cells of some organs. Clinically, in the lungs, the thick mucus obstructs the small airways and predisposes to infection. In the pancreas, the ducts become obstructed and fibrosis develops. Similarly, biliary cirrhosis and obstruction of the vas deferens with male infertility may occur.

Initial presentation of the child with cystic fibrosis

Approximately 20% of patients present with meconium ileus (obstruction of the bowel by thick meconium, p. 444) at birth. Most of the remainder will present through newborn screening performed on the newborn blood spot screening programme performed throughout the United Kingdom since 2007 (see p. 32). The sweat test (see p. 120) can be used to investigate children with suspected cystic fibrosis, as the neonatal screening test will occasionally have false negative results.

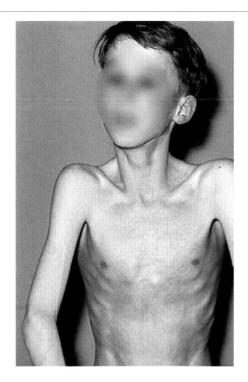

Figure 10.8 A boy severely affected by cystic fibrosis, with barrel chest and reduced muscle mass.

Clinical features of cystic fibrosis

Respiratory tract

The lungs are normal at birth, but the child later develops a tendency to frequent and prolonged infections. Unless treatment is rigorous, the cough becomes chronic and productive. In severe cases there may be digital clubbing, chest deformity and growth retardation (see Figure 10.8). The rate of progression of lung disease is very dependent on the intensity of treatment.

The chest X-ray in advanced cystic fibrosis shows patchy collapse, consolidation, cystic and linear shadows, and hyperinflation (Figure 10.9). Sputum typically cultures *Haemophilus* species, *Staphylococcus aureus* or *Pseudomonas aeruginosa*. Bronchiectasis is best evaluated by performing a CT scan of the chest (Figure 10.10).

Intestinal tract

Most children show evidence of malabsorption caused by exocrine pancreatic insufficiency. Symptoms include frequent, bulky, greasy stools and failure to gain weight even when food intake appears large. A protuberant abdomen, decreased muscle mass and poor growth are typical signs.

Fat globules and a low chymotrypsin level are found in the stool. A sweat test is required to make the diagnosis (see p. 120). A chest X-ray is usually normal in the early stages.

Management of the child with cystic fibrosis

The principles involved in the follow-up of any child with a chronic medical condition (pp. 47–8) are important for the child with cystic fibrosis. Medical management must focus on both the respiratory and gastrointestinal tracts. Children with cystic fibrosis should avoid contact with other children with cystic fibrosis, as there is a risk of cross-contamination with difficult to treat commensals, particularly pseudomonas. In contrast to usual paediatric out patients, in CF clinics each family will usually wait in a room, with health professionals moving between the rooms.

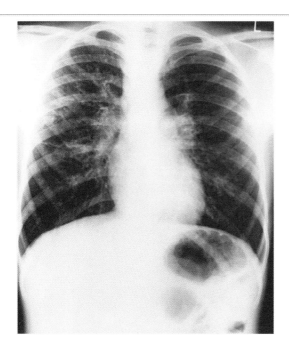

Figure 10.9 Chest X-ray of a boy with cystic fibrosis. There is gross overinflation of the lungs with hilar enlargement and ring shadows caused by bronchial wall thickening and bronchiectatic change.

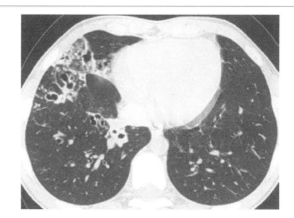

Figure 10.10 High-resolution chest CT scan image of a child with severe bronchiectasis caused by cystic fibrosis.

Respiratory tract

The aim of treatment is to clear secretions, prevent infections and treat them promptly and effectively when they occur. Parents are taught how to carry out regular chest physiotherapy. Antibiotic therapy is often required, intravenously or orally, at high dosage for prolonged periods. Some new therapies are in development which target the molecular and genetic defects causing cystic fibrosis.

Malabsorption and diet

Children require dietary adjustment, pancreatic enzyme replacement and supplementary vitamins to correct their loss of pancreatic function and inadequate digestion of fat and protein.

Pancreatic enzyme supplements have to be taken with all meals and snacks.

The diet needs to be high in energy and protein, and there is no need to restrict fat. Dietary supplements are often needed at times of illness or if there is anorexia, and all patients require supplements of the fat-soluble vitamins A, D and E. Extra salt is also needed in hot weather or if the child is febrile to replace losses in sweat.

Prognosis

Cystic fibrosis remains a life-limiting condition although the outlook has improved greatly in recent years so that average life expectancy is now 40–50 years. In general, with good treatment, most individuals can lead relatively normal lives in the childhood years. Growth may slow down in later childhood and puberty may be delayed. In adulthood, the slow progression of lung disease may eventually become disabling. Lung transplantation is considered in severe cases.

Cystic fibrosis may affect other systems. Diabetes develops in some children during adolescence. Most males are azoospermic, but have unimpaired sexual function.

Cystic fibrosis at a glance

Epidemiology
Commonest cause of suppurative lung disease in UK children
One in 25 individuals are carriers

Aetiology
Gene mutation affects sodium and chloride transport across secretory epithelial cells → airway obstruction and pancreatic insufficiency

History
Chronic cough +/– wheezing (**a**)
Frequent chest infections
Failure to thrive (FTT)
Frequent, bulky, greasy stools (**b**)
History of meconium ileus*
Family history of cystic fibrosis*

Physical examination
Poor growth (**1**)
Chest deformity
Wheezing and crepitations (**2**)
Clubbing (**3**)
Protuberant abdomen (**4**)

NB *Signs and symptoms are variable

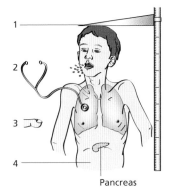

Pancreas

Confirmatory investigations
Elevated sodium (>60 mmol/L) and chloride on sweat test
Screening at birth can detect up to 90% of cases
Chronic changes on chest X-ray
Decreased stool chymotrypsin

Differential diagnosis
Other causes of chronic lung disease
Other causes of malabsorption

Management
Lungs:
• physiotherapy
• frequent and prolonged courses of antibiotics, often needed IV
Nutrition:
• pancreatic enzyme supplements
• high protein, high calorie diet
• fat soluble vitamins and salt
• dietary supplements at times

Prognosis/complications
Chronic deteriorating lung disease
Life expectancy now 40–50 years
Usually reasonable quality of life in childhood

Non-respiratory problems:
• diabetes
• delayed puberty
• biliary atresia
• male infertility

Pneumonia

Pneumonia is caused by a wide range of viral and bacterial organisms as shown in Table 10.4. *Streptococcus pneumoniae* often causes lobar pneumonia.

Predisposing factors to acute pneumonia should always be considered in children who present with pneumonia. These include:

■ congenital abnormality of the tracheo-bronchial tree;
■ inhaled foreign body;
■ persistent lobar collapse;
■ chronic aspiration;
■ large left to right intracardiac shunt;
■ immunocompromise.

Clinical features   The child with acute pneumonia presents with a short history of fever, cough and respiratory distress. Meningismus may be present, and shoulder tip or abdominal pain can divert attention from the correct diagnosis. Signs of respiratory distress include tachypnoea, nasal

Table 10.4 The commoner organisms causing pneumonia

Bacterial

Streptococcus pneumoniae (especially in younger children)

Mycoplasma pneumoniae (more insidious onset)

Haemophilus influenzae (uncommon in Britain)

Group B beta-haemolytic *Streptococcus* (only in the newborn)

Viral

Respiratory syncytial virus

Influenza viruses

Parainfluenza

Adenovirus

Coxsackie viruses

flaring, and intercostal and subcostal recession (Fig. 5.14, p. 79). Grunting is also a common feature in severely affected infants. Dullness to percussion indicates underlying consolidation, and crepitations are commonly heard. Focal signs in young children (in contrast to adults) may not correlate with the anatomical site of infection seen on the X-ray. Diagnosis is made clinically but an X-ray may show focal (confined to a lobe) or diffuse changes (Figure 10.11). Radiological changes may not be apparent in the early stages. Sputum (obtained in older, cooperative children) and blood cultures may be taken, which may isolate the infecting organism. Cold agglutinins are present in the serum in cases of *Mycoplasma pneumoniae*.

Management   Antibiotics should be used in all cases of pneumonia. If the child is acutely ill, intravenous penicillin is given, but oral amoxicillin is appropriate in a less ill child.

Prognosis   Complications of pneumonia include:

- lung abscess (rare, but may follow staphylococcus infection);
- empyema (infected pleural effusion);
- pneumothorax;
- septicaemia with infective foci elsewhere;
- bronchiectasis (following pertussis or measles in malnourished children);
- Syndrome of Inappropriate Anti-Diuretic Hormone (SIADH);
- pleural effusion.

👁 Pneumonia at a glance

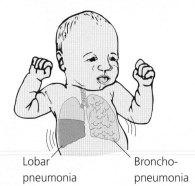

Lobar pneumonia   Broncho-pneumonia

Aetiology
Viral (particularly respiratory syncytial virus in infants)
Strep. pneumoniae at all ages
Mycoplasma pneumoniae at school age
Staphylococcus aureus and *Haemophilus influenzae* uncommon

History
Fever
Cough
Respiratory distress
Shoulder tip/abdominal pain*
Sputum production in older child*

Physical examination
Tachypnoea
Nasal flaring
Intercostal/subcostal regression
Grunting in infants
Meningism*

Confirmatory investigations
Chest X-ray: focal consolidation suggests bacterial cause; diffuse consolidation suggests viral
Blood count: leucocytosis and shift to left if bacterial
Blood culture
Cold agglutinins in older child for mycoplasma

Differential diagnosis
URTI
Bronchiolitis
Acute bronchitis
Asthma
Non-specific viral infection
Inhaled foreign body

Management
Appropriate antibiotic (based on appearance of chest X-ray); often amoxicillin or IV penicillin if acutely ill
Antipyretics
A repeat chest X-ray to ensure resolution may be needed
Cough syrup unnecessary

Prognosis/complications
Complete recovery usual
Rare complications include:
- lung abscess
- empyema
- pneumothorax
- septicaemia
- bronchiectasis

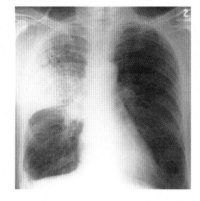

NB *Signs and symptoms are variable

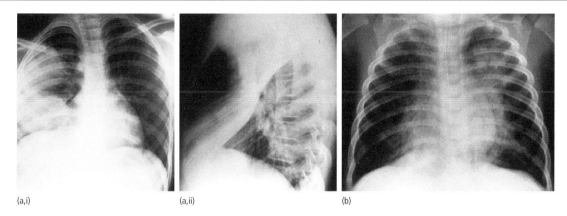

Figure 10.11 (a,i) Chest X-ray of a boy presenting with fever and cough. Consolidation of the right upper and middle lobes are seen. (a,ii) The lateral film shows the consolidation clearly delineated posteriorly by the oblique fissure. (b) X-ray of a child with viral pneumonia. Diffuse shadowing is seen throughout the lung fields.

Bronchiolitis

Bronchiolitis is an acute viral infection which causes respiratory distress and wheezing in infants less than 18 months, due to obstruction of the small airways. It is usually caused by respiratory syncytial virus (RSV), and occurs in epidemics in the winter months. Parainfluenza, rhinovirus and adenovirus can also cause bronchiolitis. Infants with congenital heart disease or underlying chronic lung disease may be very severely affected by bronchiolitis.

Clinical features   The illness starts with coryza, followed by signs of respiratory distress, including wheeze and cough. Some babies have difficulty feeding and may develop apnoea. On examination there is overexpansion of the chest, and wheeze and crepitations on auscultation.

Diagnosis   A chest X-ray is not necessary in the diagnosis, but if performed shows overinflated lungs, and collapse or consolidation may be seen (Figure 10.12). Nasal swabs can be taken to look for RSV and other viruses, which can help in cohorting infants with the same pathogens.

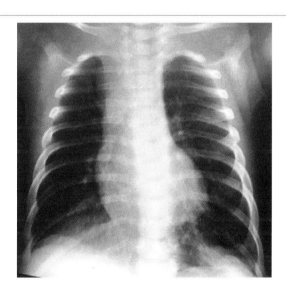

Figure 10.12 Chest X-ray of an 8-week-old baby with bronchiolitis. The X-ray shows gross overinflation of the lungs, clearly seen by the level of the diaphragm and the intercostal spaces. There is also some bronchial wall thickening.

Management   Most babies are not ill and, provided they take feeds well (at least 50% of usual volumes) and do not require oxygen, they can be managed at home. At discharge it is important to counsel families on the features of concern, and if the child presents within the first few days of infection, explain that they are likely to deteriorate on, or around, day 3. Admission is required if there is cyanosis, increasing respiratory distress, apnoea or poor feeding. Treatment is largely supportive, with oxygen given to maintain adequate saturations at or above 92%, and feeds may need to be given nasogastrically. Ventilatory support may be necessary in severely affected babies.

Prognosis   Most babies recover uneventfully from this condition within 7–10 days. Immunity is short-lived and recurrent bronchiolitis is not uncommon. Many babies who suffer from bronchiolitis show a predisposition to recurrence of wheeze through infancy. Death is rare, but can occur in babies who have severe underlying chronic lung disease. A monoclonal antibody (palivizumab) against RSV can be given prophylactically to high-risk infants throughout the winter months to provide passive immunity against infection.

Online Interactive Q5

Bronchiolitis at a glance

Aetiology
Respiratory syncytial virus
(RSV), occasionally other
viruses
Only infants and babies affected

History
Coryza
Difficulty breathing
Feeding difficulty
Rarely, a brief fever*

Physical examination
Widespread wheezing and
crepitations
Tachypnoea
Subcostal/intercostal retractions
Nasal flaring
Overinflated chest

NB *Signs and symptoms are
variable

Confirmatory investigations
RSV confirmed by
immunofluorescence of
nasopharyngeal secretions
Chest X-ray shows overinflation
of lungs and patchy areas of
collapse

Differential diagnosis
Asthma (see text)
Pneumonia

Management
Supportive

Prognosis/complications
Usually good, but mortality
1–2%
High proportion go on to have
recurrent wheeze through
infancy

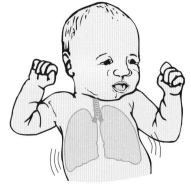
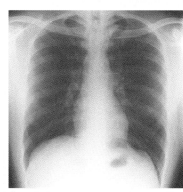

Aspirated foreign body (see also pp. 407–8)

Foreign bodies are usually aspirated by toddlers who are mobile and put small objects into their mouths. Small plastic or wooden beads and peanuts are most likely to be aspirated. Peanuts are particularly dangerous as they swell in the airway, become firmly lodged and are difficult to remove because they tend to fragment. Children, particularly toddlers, may aspirate a foreign body without the parent realizing that this has occurred.

Clinical features   Usually there is an immediate episode of coughing or choking, or a history of such an episode days or weeks earlier, but the child may present with cough alone. The main symptoms are respiratory distress and wheeze, with cough as a prominent feature. The chest may appear asymmetrical, with a localized dull percussion note if collapse has occurred distal to the obstruction. As the commonest place for a foreign body to lodge is the right main bronchus (Figure 10.13), there may be signs of right lung collapse and unilateral wheezing. Compensatory emphysema may occur around the collapsed lobe, producing a percussion note of increased resonance. Ideally an inspiratory and expiratory chest X-ray is required, where segmental collapse or hyperinflation is seen.

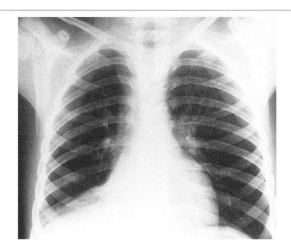

Figure 10.13 X-ray of a child admitted with fever and cough which failed to respond to treatment. At bronchoscopy a Dinky car steering wheel was found in the right intermediate bronchus. The chest X-ray shows collapse of the right middle and lower lobe with loss of definition of the right hemidiaphragm and right heart border.

Management If aspiration of a foreign body is suspected, bronchoscopy should be performed. Removal of the foreign body is curative. Complete airway obstruction is a medical emergency (pp. 407–8).

Prognosis If there is delay in diagnosis, bronchiectasis may occur in the lung distal to the obstruction, causing destruction of bronchial architecture. This leaves dilated air sacs which become chronically infected and eventually require surgical removal.

👁 Aspirated foreign body at a glance

Epidemiology
Toddlers most at risk

Aetiology
Peanuts are a particular
  problem
Foreign body commonly sited in
  right main bronchus

History
History of choking*
Cough

Physical examination
Wheeze (may be unilateral)
Asymmetric chest signs

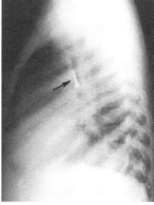
(a) Note foreign body at the carina

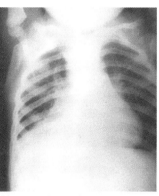
(b) Note collapse of right lower lobe

Confirmatory investigations
Chest X-ray in inspiration and
  expiration may show
  segmental collapse
Bronchoscopy

Differential diagnosis
URTI
Pneumonia
Asthma
Acute bronchitis

Management
Manage choking with emergency
  manoeuvres
Bronchoscopy to remove
  foreign body

Prognosis
Usually good, but risk of
  bronchiectasis if diagnosis
  is delayed

NB *Signs and symptoms are
variable

Croup (acute laryngotracheobronchitis)

This common condition is caused by a parainfluenza virus. It most commonly affects children aged 6 months to 2 years and causes symptoms initially in the larynx (stridor), and then in the trachea and bronchi (cough and wheeze), hence the term laryngotracheobronchitis. It occurs in the winter months and children may have repeated episodes.

Clinical features Croup starts with coryzal symptoms and fever and proceeds to stridor and barking cough. Hoarseness, particularly on crying, is a common feature. The stridor may appear to become acutely worse as a result of associated laryngeal spasm. Further progression down the respiratory tract may cause wheezing and tachypnoea. Although usually mild, it may progress rapidly in young children to become very severe. Signs of deterioration include increased work of breathing, cyanosis and restlessness. Severe deterioration is often accompanied by a reduction in the stridulous noise.

Management Most cases resolve spontaneously. There is no evidence that humidity shortens the duration or severity of the stridor. However, adequate fluids are essential to prevent dehydration. If the child worsens, hospital assessment is required. Oral dexamethasone is used to reduce the airway inflammation and often results in a dramatic clinical improvement. In cases that remain severe, hospital admission is required, and, rarely, nebulized therapy such as adrenaline or even early intubation by an experienced anaesthetist may be needed.

👁 Croup at a glance

Epidemiology
Commonly affects children
   aged 6 months to 2 years

Aetiology
Parainfluenza virus

History
Stridor and barking cough
Coryza
Fever
Hoarseness*

Physical examination
Stridor
Wheezing*
Tachypnoea*
Cyanosis if severe

Confirmatory investigations
Nil

Differential diagnosis
Acute epiglottitis
Foreign body

Management
Oral corticosteroids if stridor
Avoid distressing the child
Intubation if exhaustion or
   imminent obstruction

Prognosis
Good

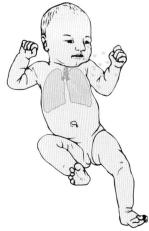

NB *Signs and symptoms are variable

Acute epiglottitis

Acute epiglottitis is a life-threatening condition caused by infection with *Haemophilus influenzae*. It is now very rare since *Haemophilus influenzae* B (HiB) immunisation was introduced. It presents with signs of toxicity, fever, drooling and inability to swallow. If the condition is suspected, examination of the mouth must not be attempted as acute and total airway obstruction may occur. Protection of the airway is the first aim, and investigations need to be done after intubation. Blood cultures grow *Haemophilus influenzae* and treatment is with intravenous cephalosporins. With airway protection and appropriate antibiotics, the prognosis is excellent, but death or severe brain injury were seen when acute airway obstruction occurred.

To test your knowledge on this part of the book, please see Chapter 26.

CHAPTER 11
Gastrointestinal disorders

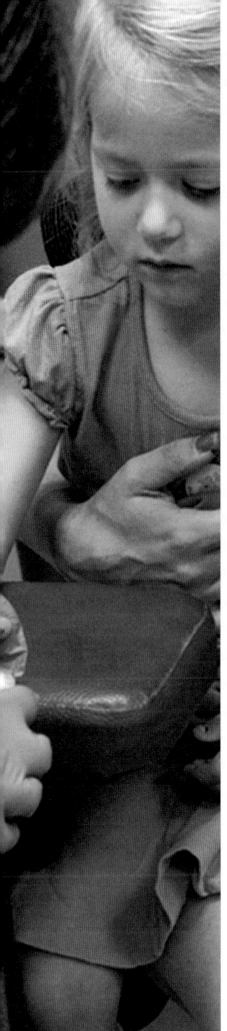

*The churning inside me
never stops;
Days of suffering
confront me.*
Job 30: 27

Essential Paediatrics and Child Health, Fourth Edition. Mary Rudolf, Anthony Luder and Kerry Jeavons.
© 2020 John Wiley & Sons Ltd. Published 2020 by John Wiley & Sons Ltd.
Companion website: www.wiley.com/go/rudolf/paediatrics

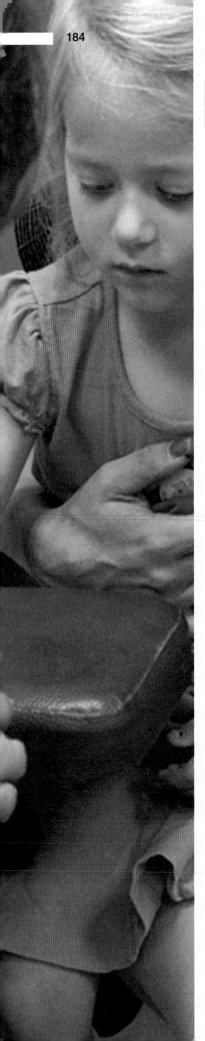

KEY COMPETENCES
YOU MUST...

Know and understand

- The differential diagnosis of children with vomiting, diarrhoea, abdominal pain, constipation, blood in the stool and jaundice
- How to diagnose and manage serious and common gastrointestinal conditions
- Babies' normal stool pattern in the first year
- The difference between vomiting and posseting
- Fluid and dietary management of acute gastroenteritis
- The signs and symptoms that suggest the presence of a chronic disease in a child with gastrointestinal symptoms
- The management of a child who is jaundiced
- The characteristic features of colic

Be able to

- Take an age-appropriate gastrointestinal and nutritional history and perform a focused physical examination
- Assess for dehydration in infants and toddlers with gastrointestinal symptoms
- Advise a parent about oral rehydration and diet for a child with gastroenteritis
- Differentiate non-organic from organic recurrent abdominal pain and provide appropriate guidance

Appreciate that

- Constipation is not diagnosed on infrequent stools alone
- Antidiarrhoeal agents are generally inappropriate for children
- Most recurrent abdominal pain is non-organic, but children still benefit from appropriate medical input

Gastrointestinal symptoms and signs

Finding your way around ...

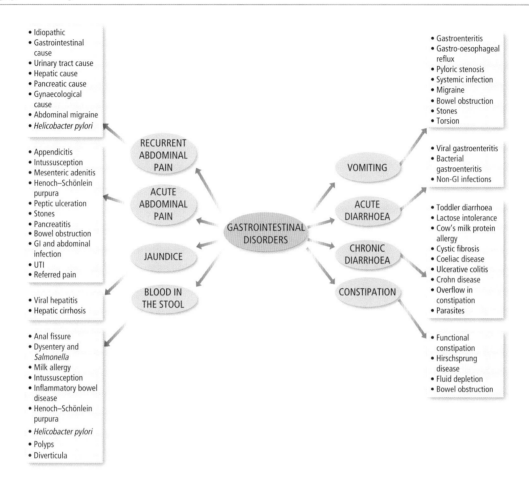

- Idiopathic
- Gastrointestinal cause
- Urinary tract cause
- Hepatic cause
- Pancreatic cause
- Gynaecological cause
- Abdominal migraine
- *Helicobacter pylori*

- Appendicitis
- Intussusception
- Mesenteric adenitis
- Henoch–Schönlein purpura
- Peptic ulceration
- Stones
- Pancreatitis
- Bowel obstruction
- GI and abdominal infection
- UTI
- Referred pain

- Viral hepatitis
- Hepatic cirrhosis

- Anal fissure
- Dysentery and *Salmonella*
- Milk allergy
- Intussusception
- Inflammatory bowel disease
- Henoch–Schönlein purpura
- *Helicobacter pylori*
- Polyps
- Diverticula

- Gastroenteritis
- Gastro-oesophageal reflux
- Pyloric stenosis
- Systemic infection
- Migraine
- Bowel obstruction
- Stones
- Torsion

- Viral gastroenteritis
- Bacterial gastroenteritis
- Non-GI infections

- Toddler diarrhoea
- Lactose intolerance
- Cow's milk protein allergy
- Cystic fibrosis
- Coeliac disease
- Ulcerative colitis
- Crohn disease
- Overflow in constipation
- Parasites

- Functional constipation
- Hirschsprung disease
- Fluid depletion
- Bowel obstruction

RECURRENT ABDOMINAL PAIN

ACUTE ABDOMINAL PAIN

JAUNDICE

BLOOD IN THE STOOL

GASTROINTESTINAL DISORDERS

VOMITING

ACUTE DIARRHOEA

CHRONIC DIARRHOEA

CONSTIPATION

Vomiting

Common and important causes of vomiting

Infancy
Gastroenteritis (pp. 205–6)
Gastro-oesophageal reflux
Overfeeding
Anatomic obstruction
  pyloric stenosis
  intussusception (p. 211)
  bowel obstruction
Systemic infection, particularly meningitis, pyelonephritis, pneumonia
Inborn errors of metabolism

Childhood
Gastroenteritis (pp. 205–6)
Food poisoning
Systemic infection
Toxic ingestion or medications (p. 419)
Whooping cough (p. 38)
Foreign body ingestion

Adolescence
Gastroenteritis (pp. 205–6),
Food poisoning
Systemic infection
Migraine (p. 244)
Raised intracranial pressure
Pregnancy
Bulimia (p. 463)

The return of small amounts of food during or shortly after eating is called *regurgitation*. When this occurs in a baby at or after a milk feed it is known as *posseting* and is seen as effortless, low-volume, frequent 'spills' from the mouth. More complete emptying of the stomach is called *vomiting*. Within limits, regurgitation is normal, especially during the first 6 months or so of life. It can be reduced by winding the baby during and after a feed, by gentle handling, by preventing the baby from becoming upset and swallowing air before feeding, and by propping the baby after a feed. A common cause of apparent vomiting in the bottle-fed infant is overfeeding, as the infant will often continue to suck on a bottle even after the comfortable capacity of the stomach has been achieved. A surprisingly large volume of excess milk can then be regurgitated back as the parent tries to wind the baby. Provided the child is gaining weight and generally contented, the family can be reassured that it is simply a laundry problem, and that the baby will grow out of it by the time he or she is walking at about 1 year. Nowadays 'anti-reflux formulas' which become thicker on contact with the acid pH in the stomach are popular, although of unproven value. 'Rumination' refers to chronic regurgitation, which is often self-induced by the baby. If it occurs with growth failure, psychological factors should be suspected.

Vomiting is one of the commonest symptoms of infancy, if not of childhood. Vomiting may be associated with a variety of disturbances, both trivial and serious. It is most commonly associated with gastroenteritis (pp. 205–6) or food poisoning, but may accompany any infection, from minor ailments such as otitis media to more serious illnesses such as pyelonephritis. Vomiting may also be the first symptom of a potentially lethal disease such as meningitis, metabolic disease, poisoning, and intracranial causes such as the 'shaken baby syndrome' or serious intra-abdominal disease such as pyloric stenosis, pancreatitis, obstruction, intussusception or peritonitis. In infants, the first step is to differentiate simple regurgitation from vomiting. If vomiting is truly the problem, the underlying diagnosis can usually be suspected by a thorough history and physical examination. Worrying features are shown in the Red Flag box.

♿ Worrying features in a vomiting child

- Bile-stained vomitus*
- Blood in the vomitus
- Drowsiness
- Refusal to feed
- Malnutrition
- Dehydration
- Abdominal tenderness or distension
- Abdominal mass
- Encephalopathy
- Rectal bleeding

*This suggests intestinal obstruction and is always a serious sign which must be investigated urgently.

History – must ask!

- *How well is the child?* The general health of the child, and particularly appetite, is a guide to the severity of the problem. Significant vomiting is likely to be accompanied by weight loss and, if long term, poor weight gain. Fever suggests an infective cause.
- *What is the vomiting like?* Decide whether a baby is vomiting, posseting or regurgitating. Vomiting from infectious causes tends to be non-projectile, whereas in pyloric stenosis it can be dramatically projected over a distance. Paroxysms of coughing (as occur in whooping cough) can precipitate vomiting. Blood-stained vomiting indicates inflammation in the upper gastrointestinal tract. Bile-stained vomitus is a serious sign, suggesting intestinal obstruction; it must be investigated urgently.
- *Are there associated symptoms?* Gastroenteritis and other infections are usually accompanied by diarrhoea. Constipation suggests intestinal obstruction. Irritability or pain may accompany infection or reflux. Aspiration and apnoea are worrying signs of gastrooesophageal reflux. Behavioural changes and abdominal pain or distension are red flag indicators
- *Bottle-fed babies.* Ask how much milk the baby is taking. If the baby is taking in excess of 200 mL of milk per kilogram body weight in 24 hours, and is well with no weight loss, then regurgitation secondary to overfeeding is likely.
- *Adolescents.* You need to focus your questions to adolescents differently. Ask about symptoms of migraine, and consider gynaecological causes. Bulimia rarely presents as vomiting as the adolescent is careful to hide this symptom. Headache indicates migraine or raised ICP. Vomiting may be cyclic or related to periods or lack of them (pregnancy).

Physical examination – must check!

- *General examination.* Carry out a full examination to exclude infection in sites other than the gastrointestinal tract, particularly if there is fever. Severe infection such as meningitis or pyelonephritis can present with vomiting. Poor weight gain indicates dehydration in the short term, and malnutrition in the longer term. Exclude hypertension. A careful neurological exam is important including retinal examination ('shaken baby') and signs of trauma.
- *Signs of dehydration.* Persistent vomiting leads to dehydration. The signs of dehydration are described on pp. 416–19.
- *The abdomen.* The abdomen may be tender in gastroenteritis, with increased bowel sounds. In the rare event of intestinal obstruction, the bowel sounds are tinkling or absent. If pyloric stenosis is present an 'olive' can be palpated (Figure 11.1). Severe tenderness may suggest appendicitis, particularly if the onset of the pain preceded the vomiting. Organomegaly, mass or distension should be carefully sought. Rectal examination is important to exclude foecal impaction, perianal disease or pelvic abscess. Never forget the groins (incarcerated hernia) and testes in a male (torsion, orchitis)

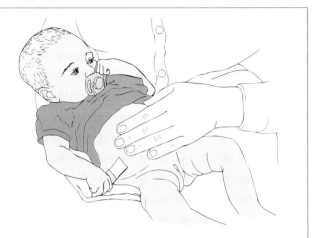

Figure 11.1 Palpation of the abdomen for pyloric stenosis.

Investigations

Depending on the clinical picture, psychiatric, neurological, metabolic, infectious and surgical investigations may be warranted, and include electrolytes, renal and liver function tests. In suspected pyloric stenosis and intussusception an ultrasound scan may be definitive. Other imaging techniques may be required.

Management of the vomiting

Antiemetics have no place in the management of vomiting in young children (other than rare specific circumstances such as during chemotherapy for childhood cancer, or in migraine or cyclical vomiting). The child needs to be maintained in a well-hydrated state, by offering water or oral hydration fluids in small amounts frequently. If the child develops signs of significant dehydration, intravenous fluids are required (see p. 418).

🔑 Key points: The vomiting child

- In infants – differentiate posseting from vomiting
- Look for evidence of infection, whether gastroenteritis or extra-gastrointestinal
- Determine whether the child is dehydrated
- In the infant with projectile vomiting, palpate the abdomen carefully for pyloric stenosis
- Suspect reflux in the infant or child with physical disability, failure to thrive, blood-stained vomitus, irritability, aspiration or apnoea
- Bright green bile-stained vomiting should be referred straight to the surgeons as the child may need an emergency laparotomy for bowel obstruction
- Exclude hypertension as a cause
- Rare disease occurs rarely but is often potentially serious, and therefore must be considered

---

Acute diarrhoea

Causes of acute diarrhoea

Viral gastroenteritis
Bacterial gastroenteritis
   Shigella
   Escherichia coli
   Salmonella
   Campylobacter
Giardiasis
Infections outside the gastrointestinal tract
Food intolerance
Antibiotic-induced

Diarrhoea is defined as an increase in the frequency, fluidity and volume of faeces. Children are likely to experience as many as three acute severe episodes in the first 3 years of life. These episodes are almost invariably infectious in aetiology, although the infection may be outside the gastrointestinal tract.

When you assess a child with diarrhoea, you need to focus on whether the child requires treatment for dehydration or has an infection outside the gastrointestinal tract that has precipitated the diarrhoea. A search for an underlying organism is generally unimportant unless you suspect dysentery.

Any form of infection can cause acute diarrhoea, particularly in the young child. These commonly include URTIs, chest infections, otitis media and urinary tract infections (UTI). Non-infective causes of diarrhoea include food intolerance and intussusception, a serious condition that may present with bloody (characteristically 'red currant jelly') stools (see p. 211). Antibiotic therapy in itself commonly causes diarrhoea.

History – must ask!

- *What is the illness like?* Get a good description of the illness, and whether the increase is in frequency, volume or liquidity of the stools. This provides a guide to whether the child is likely to be dehydrated. Blood, mucus, abdominal pain and fever suggest a bacterial cause – important to recognise for public health reasons.
- *Is the child likely to be dehydrated?* Apart from frequency of stools, there are other clues as to whether the child is dehydrated. If he or she is urinating infrequently (less than three times in 24 hours is a guide) some degree of dehydration is likely. A history of weight loss is also important.
- *Are there other symptoms?* Symptoms such as earache, dysuria or coryza suggest an infection outside the gastrointestinal tract. Convulsions and pain are characteristic of Shigella.

Blood or mucus in the stool are suggestive of dysentery or intussusception, if there is no fever. Nappy rash suggests severe diarrhoea or lactose intolerance.

- *Is anyone else affected?* If others in the family or at child care are affected, consider a cause such as food contamination – useful epidemiological information.
- *Immunisations* – Has the child been immunised against rotavirus?

Physical examination – must check!

- *Assessment of hydration.* This is covered in detail on p. 417. You need to assess the state of alertness, moistness of mucous membranes, presence of tears, skin turgor, sunken fontanelle and eyes, and pulse rate.
- *Signs of any extra-gastrointestinal infection.* Otitis media, tonsillitis and chest infections commonly cause diarrhoea.
- *Weight.* Always weigh the child. If a recent weight is available, weight loss provides important evidence of dehydration. In any event, the weight is a valuable baseline if the child deteriorates.

Investigations

If the child is not dehydrated, nor the stools bloody, investigations are not generally necessary unless the child is hospitalized or has been exposed to others with proven bacterial gastroenteritis. Stool microscopy and culture is needed if there is blood and mucus in the diarrhoea. Rotavirus can be detected by stool immunoassay. If extra-gastrointestinal infection is suspected, confirmation may be required from blood and urine cultures or X-ray. Investigations to be considered are shown in Table 11.1.

Managing acute diarrhoea

Fluids and nutrition

The management of dehydration is covered on p. 417. If signs of dehydration are mild or absent, the child can be managed at home. There is no evidence that exclusion or special diets alter the course of acute gastroenteritis. Milk feeds are usually continued, and solid foods are re-introduced when the child has an appetite and has ceased vomiting. Probiotic containing foods like some natural yoghurts may shorten the period of diarrhoea. If diarrhoea persists, you need to recheck the state of hydration to see if more aggressive management is required.

Use of antiemetics and antidiarrhoeal agents

These agents have no place in the management of diarrhoea in young children. They are ineffective and have a high incidence of side effects. Probiotics as foods (yoghurts and biodrinks) or as preparations may reduce the symptom severity and duration in older infants and children.

 Key points: Acute diarrhoea

- Assess the degree of hydration (see Table 23.7)
- Look for evidence of infection outside the gastrointestinal tract
- Identify features suggestive of bacterial gastroenteritis

Table 11.1 Investigations to be considered in acute diarrhoea

Investigation	Indication	What you are looking for
Stool microscopy and culture	Blood and mucus in the stool	Bacterial gastroenteritis Parasites
Stool immunoassay	Hospitalized child	Rotavirus Cryptococcus *Clostridium difficile* toxin
Blood count	High fever	Possible bacterial infection
Blood and urine culture, chest X-ray	Suggestion of extra-gastrointestinal infection in clinical evaluation	Bacterial infection

Clues to the differential diagnosis of acute diarrhoea

	Rotavirus	*Shigella*	*Escherichia coli*	*Salmonella*	*Campylobacter*
Age	<2 years non-vaccinated	1–5 years	<2 years	Any	Any
Stool	Watery	Watery, blood, mucus, pus	Loose	Loose and slimy, blood	Watery, blood, mucus
Pain	Occasional	Common	Common	Common	Common
Fits	Rare	10%	Rare	Rare	Rare
Vomiting	Common	Uncommon	Common	Common	Rare
High fever	Common	Common	Rare	Common	Common
Season	Winter	Usually late summer	Usually late summer	Usually late summer	Usually late summer

 See NICE guideline: Diarrhoea and vomiting in under 5s: assessment and initial management
https://www.nice.org.uk/guidance/cg84

Chronic diarrhoea

Common causes of chronic or recurrent diarrhoea

Watery
Non-specific diarrhoea
Toddler diarrhoea
Lactose intolerance
Parasites – *Giardia lamblia*
Cow's milk protein allergy
Overflow diarrhoea in constipation

Fatty
Cystic fibrosis
Coeliac disease

Bloody
Ulcerative colitis
Crohn disease

Chronic diarrhoea is a common complaint, particularly in infants and young children. However, there is a large variation in normal bowel patterns (Table 11.2) at this age and, before

Table 11.2 Normal stool patterns

0–4 months	Breast-fed	2–4 per day (range 1–7), yellow to golden, porridgy consistency, pH 5. Infrequency of stools is also normal (up to once per week)
0–4 months	Bottle-fed	2–3 per day, pale yellow to light brown, firm, pH 7
4 months–1 year		1–3 per day, darker yellow, firmer
After 1 year		Formed, like adult stool in odour and colour

launching into any form of assessment, a good description of the stool pattern should be obtained in order to be sure that diarrhoea is really a problem. Broadly speaking, the diarrhoeal illnesses of childhood can be divided into malabsorption, inflammation and infections. However, when working through a differential diagnosis it may be more helpful to think in terms of the characteristics of the stool.

In your clinical evaluation, you must differentiate the healthy child who has loose frequent stools from the child with a medical problem. You should identify any worrying features suggesting a pathological process, and then request appropriate investigations so that a definitive diagnosis can be made.

Infants with cystic fibrosis (see p. 175) often present with diarrhoea and failure to thrive as a result of pancreatic insufficiency, rather than with the respiratory symptoms seen in older children. Inflammatory bowel disease is a cause of chronic diarrhoea in late childhood and adolescence; both Crohn disease (p. 208) and ulcerative colitis (p. 208) are characterised by unpredictable exacerbations and remissions. The soiling that results from constipation is sometimes interpreted as being diarrhoea. A careful bowel history is required along with evidence of constipation on examination.

History – must ask!

- *What are the stools like?* You should ask about the bowel pattern, including any increase in frequency, volume and fluidity of the stools, so you can decide whether the pattern is abnormal or not. The stools' appearance, consistency and presence of blood or mucus are helpful in coming to a diagnosis, but odour and 'flushability' are usually not.
- *What precipitated the diarrhoea?* The problem may have been precipitated by an episode of acute infective diarrhoea, or you may identify troublesome foods. There may be other affected individuals in the family or at child care.
- *Are there associated symptoms?* It is important to determine whether the diarrhoea is an isolated problem in an otherwise healthy child or whether there are concomitant symptoms. Weight loss or abdominal pain are particularly significant.
- *Review of symptoms.* As many diseases can cause failure to thrive with rather non-specific bowel symptoms, a complete review of symptoms is required.
- *A symptom diary.* As for most recurrent and chronic problems, asking the family to keep a diary is helpful to assess the severity and pattern of the symptom.

Physical examination – must check!

- *Growth measures.* Height, weight and head circumference must be recorded and compared with earlier measurements (if available). Poor weight gain suggests a process that needs further evaluation. Height and weight also serve as a critical baseline if the diarrhoea persists for any length of time.
- *Other features.* Your examination should include an evaluation of hydration, pallor, abdominal distension, tenderness and finger clubbing.
- *General examination.* As diseases of many different organ systems can cause failure to thrive, a complete examination is required.
- *Anorectal examination.* Any significant degree of diarrhoea causes perianal irritation, particularly if the child is still in nappies. Rectal examination is not routinely indicated, but it should be considered to rule out impaction

(if soiling is considered as the diagnosis) and to obtain a sample of the stool.

Laboratory investigations

See Table 11.3. If a child is thriving and there are no accompanying symptoms or signs of disease or nutritional derangement, laboratory investigations are rarely necessary. However, if you are concerned that a pathological process is present, investigations are required and should help you differentiate the three types of chronic and persistent diarrhoea – malabsorption, inflammatory and infection.

Malabsorption

The commonest causes of malabsorption in childhood result from pancreatic insufficiency, protein intolerance and lactose intolerance.

- *Pancreatic insufficiency.* In pancreatic insufficiency (as occurs in cystic fibrosis), low faecal elastase levels are found in the stool, and on microscopic inspection fat globules are seen.
- *Protein intolerance.* The commonest form of protein intolerance is coeliac disease. Coeliac antibodies (TTG, IgA and IgG) are useful as a screening test. If positive, or there are other concerns that malabsorption is present, jejunal biopsy is needed to confirm the diagnosis.
- *Sugar malabsorption.* Sugar malabsorption (secondary lactose intolerance is the commonest) is suggested by the presence of reducing substances in the stool and a low pH. The low pH results from bacterial production of organic acids from the unabsorbed sugar.

Inflammation

Faecal blood loss suggests inflammatory bowel disease, food sensitivity, polyps, Meckel diverticulum, or an ulcer. High levels of inflammatory markers: CRP, ferritin, fibrinogen plasma viscosity, or ESR support a diagnosis of inflammatory bowel disease. The diagnosis is made by MRE, CT and endoscopy.

Infection

Repeated examination of at least three stool specimens should identify parasitic infection, of which *Giardia lamblia* is the commonest. Urine culture excludes chronic UTI as a cause for diarrhoea.

Managing diarrhoea as a symptom

Many children have episodes of loose, frequent stools for which no cause is found. These may follow on from an acute episode

Table 11.3 Common laboratory investigations in the assessment of chronic diarrhoea

Investigation	Finding	Significance
Blood		
Full blood count	Anaemia	Blood loss, malabsorption or poor diet
	Eosinophilia	Parasites or atopy
Serum immunoglobulins	High or low	Both findings may indicate immune deficiency
Plasma viscosity or sedimentation rate	High	Non-specific finding. If very high, suggestive of inflammatory bowel disease
Coeliac antibodies (Anti-TTG)	Present	Screening test for coeliac disease
p-ANCA antibodies	Positive	Inflammatory bowel disease esp. UC
ASCA antibodies	Positive	Inflammatory bowel disease esp. Crohn
Electrolytes and acid base	Low K, high or low Na, metabolic acidosis/ alkalosis	Potential consequences of chronic diarrhoea
Serum alkaline phosphatase	Low	Zinc deficiency (malabsorption)
Serum alkaline phosphatase	High	Hypocalcaemia, Vitamin D deficiency (malabsorption)
Serum proteins and albumin	Low	Protein-losing enteropathy, malnutrition, catabolic state
Iron and folate	Low	Jejunal dysfunction
Fat soluble vitamins ('ADEK') and PT	Low	Fat malabsorption
B12	Low	Terminal ileal and gastric dysfunction
Stool		
Occult blood	Positive	Cow's milk intolerance, inflammatory bowel disease
White blood cells	Positive	Infectious and inflammatory colitis
Calprotectin	Positive	Inflammatory bowel diseases
Alpha-1 antitrypsin	Positive	Protein-losing enteropathy
Clostridium toxins	Positive	Pseudo-membranous colitis
Ova and parasites	Positive	Parasite identified
Reducing substances and pH*	Positive and low pH	Sugar intolerance (usually lactose)
Stool anion gap**	>100	Osmotic diarrhoea (<100, secretory)
Chymotrypsin	Low	Pancreatic insufficiency
Microscopy for fat globules	Globules seen	Fat malabsorption (usually pancreatic insufficiency)
Other		
Urine culture and sensitivity	Positive	Urinary tract infection
Sweat test	Elevated sweat Na+ and Cl- concentration	Cystic fibrosis
Breath hydrogen test	High H_2	Sugar intolerance
Jejunal biopsy	Flattened villi	Coeliac disease
Endoscopy	Characteristic lesions	Inflammatory bowel disease

* This is performed by mixing stool with water and testing it with Clinitest tablets (as for urinary glucose).
** $290 - [(Na^+ + K^+) \times 2]$

of gastroenteritis. If the child is well and thriving, reassurance is all that is required, with monitoring of growth for the duration of symptoms.

Antidiarrhoeal medication has no place in the management of acute diarrhoea in children. Food intolerance is often a concern, and omission of suspected foods may be tried, although care must be taken to ensure that the child's nutritional intake is not compromised.

Key points: Chronic diarrhoea

- Check that the stool pattern is really abnormal for age
- Attempt to classify the character of the stool – watery, fatty or bloody
- Identify any features suggestive of significant pathology, e.g. weight loss or poor weight gain, abdominal pain

Clues to the differential diagnosis of chronic diarrhoea

	Characteristics of diarrhoea	Associated features	Age of child
Non-specific diarrhoea	Loose watery stools	Thriving child, may follow episode of acute gastroenteritis	Any age
Toddler diarrhoea	Loose with undigested food in stool	Thriving child, may have large fluid intake	Toddler
Lactose intolerance	Watery, low pH, reducing substances in stool	Follows acute gastroenteritis	Baby and toddler
Giardiasis	Watery	Weight loss and abdominal pain variable	Any age, common in nurseries
Cow's milk protein allergy	Watery, may be bloody	May have urticaria, stridor or bronchospasm	Babies
Functional constipation	Soiling rather than diarrhoea	Constipated stool palpable per abdomen or per rectum	Any age
Cystic fibrosis	Fatty	Failure to thrive, respiratory symptoms	Usually infancy
Coeliac disease	Fatty	Failure to thrive, irritability, muscle wasting, abdominal distension, iron deficiency anaemia	Usually late infancy, but can be any age
Inflammatory bowel disease	Bloody in ulcerative colitis and Crohn	Weight loss, exacerbations and remissions, abdominal pain and anorexia in Crohn disease	Late childhood and adolescence

Recurrent abdominal pain

The more common causes of recurrent abdominal pain

Idiopathic
Functional
Gastrointestinal
  Irritable bowel syndrome
  Oesophagitis
  H. pylori gastroduodenitis
  Lactose intolerance
  Inflammatory bowel disease
  Acute constipation
  Malabsorption
  Giardiasis

Urinary tract
  Infections
  Stones
Hepatic
  Hepatitis
  Bile stones

Pancreas
  Pancreatitis

Gynaecological
  Dysmenorrhoea
  Pelvic inflammatory disease
  Haematocolpos
  Ovarian cyst

Other
  Abdominal migraine
  Lead poisoning
  Testicular torsion

Table 11.4 Features differentiating organic and non-organic causes of abdominal pain

	Organic	Non-organic
Characteristics	Day and night	Periodic pain with intervening good health. Nocturnal pain is unusual
	Character depends on underlying cause	Often periumbilical
		If psychosomatic, may be related to school hours
History	Weight loss and/or reduced appetite	Otherwise healthy child
	Lack of energy	
	Recurrent fever	
	Organ-specific symptoms, e.g. change in bowel habit, polyuria, menstrual problems, vomiting	
	Relationship to food, especially lactose containing	
	Occult or frank bleeding from any orifice	
	Family history of gastrointestinal problems	
Physical exam	Ill appearance, growth failure, other signs of systemic disease, swollen joints	
	Localized abdominal tenderness, organomegaly	
Preliminary investigations	Anaemia leucocytosis, raised sedimentation rate or eosinophilia on blood count	Normal, thriving child
	Abnormal urinalysis and/or culture	Normal

Recurrent abdominal pain is one of the commonest symptoms presenting in children, with 10–15% of school-age children at some point experiencing it. Of these, only 1 in 10 are found to have an organic problem, the majority having no identifiable cause for the pain. Rarely, abdominal pain can be a manifestation of a more serious chronic childhood disorder relating to the gastrointestinal, urinary or gynaecological systems.

The purpose of your clinical evaluation is to decide as rapidly as possible whether there is an organic or non-organic cause for the pain. Table 11.4 summarizes the features that will help you come to that decision. If there is no indication of an organic cause then appropriate reassurance and support is needed, rather than letting anxiety linger that there might be a serious problem that you have not identified.

History – must ask!

Take a complete history, reviewing the child's lifestyle and habits as well as focusing on symptoms related to each organ system.

- *What is the pain like?* The character of the pain can help you identify the cause. The child may be able to describe whether the pain is colicky or constant, and how it is related to daily activities, bowel habit or diet. Even if the child cannot describe the pain, the site can often be located.

Non-organic pain is classically periumbilical, and it has been said that the further the pain is from the umbilicus, the greater the chances that an aetiology can be identified. A diary kept by the family can be quite helpful in clarifying the frequency of episodes and their relation to other events.

- *What is the timing?* Is there a temporal relationship between the onset of abdominal pain, meals and school? Is it less at weekends or at night?
- *Are there other abdominal symptoms?* Symptoms related to specific organ systems may give clues to an organic cause. Constipation, diarrhoea, or vomiting suggest a gastrointestinal cause, and frequency and dysuria suggest a cause in the urinary tract. Do not forget to enquire about gynaecological symptoms in teenage girls.
- *A full dietary history* focusing on cow's milk, gluten, fats, lactose
- *Are there general constitutional symptoms?* General constitutional symptoms such as anorexia, weight loss and fever are important indicators that there is a serious underlying cause.
- *Are there emotional or family difficulties?* You should always enquire about emotional and family problems, as they are commonly associated with abdominal pain. Try to establish how much the symptoms interfere with life at home and at school.

■ *Family history*. A family history of gastrointestinal disease, especially peptic ulcers, *H. pylori,* and stones may be relevant.

Physical examination – must check!

You should always carry out a complete physical examination. Don't limit it to the region below the diaphragm and above the pelvis!

■ *Growth*. Height and weight measurements are particularly important, as weight loss indicates serious pathology. If the problem is long-standing, fall-off in growth may also occur.

■ *General examination*. Look for signs of pallor, jaundice and clubbing.

■ *Abdominal examination*. Examine the abdomen for localized tenderness, hepatomegaly, splenomegaly, enlarged kidneys or a distended bladder.

■ *Anorectal examination*. Inspection of the anus and a rectal examination are not routine in children, but need to be carried out if there is any suspicion of sexual abuse, and at times for constipation.

Investigations

See Table 11.5. The diagnosis of non-organic pain can be made in many children on the basis of the history and examination. If in doubt, a full blood count, sedimentation rate, stools for ova and parasites, and urinalysis and culture can be helpful as inflammatory bowel disease, chronic UTI and gastrointestinal

Table 11.5 Useful investigations in assessing the child with recurrent abdominal pain

Investigation	What are you looking for?
Blood tests	
Full blood count	Anaemia, eosinophilia, infection
Sedimentation rate or plasma viscosity	Elevated in inflammatory bowel disease
Liver function tests	Liver dysfunction
Urea and electrolytes	Renal failure
Amylase	Pancreatitis
Urine test	
Urinalysis and culture	Urine infection
Stool	
Ova and parasites (x3 samples)	Gastrointestinal parasites, e.g. giardiasis
Occult blood	Gastrointestinal blood loss, e.g. inflammatory bowel disease or peptic ulcer
Urease breath test	*Helicobacter pylori* (see* below)
Ultrasound	
Abdominal and pelvic	Urinary obstruction at all levels, organomegaly, abscesses, cysts, ascites, pregnancy, gonadal cyst and torsion, mesenteric lymphadenopathy, biliary and urinary stones
Other	
Plain abdominal	Constipation, renal calculi if radiopaque, lead poisoning
Ultrasound	Renal and biliary stones, cysts, abscesses, tumours, pregnancy
Barium swallow	Tracheo-oesophageal fistula, hiatus hernia, malrotation
Barium enema	Hirschsprung disease, polyps, diverticula
Abdominal CT or MRE	Inflammatory bowel disease, malformations, vasculitis, renal calculi
Endoscopy	Peptic ulceration, *Helicobacter pylori* disease, enteritis, coeliac disease

Note: Some uncommon causes of recurrent abdominal pain are typically negative in routine testing. They include nerve entrapment syndromes, internal hernias, metabolic disorders (e.g. lead poisoning and porphyria), and genetic disease (familial Mediterranean fever).

parasites may present with abdominal pain alone. You should only consider further investigations if there are findings suggestive of a particular disease process.

Managing abdominal pain

The management of abdominal pain obviously depends on the aetiology. Analgesics are often prescribed, but are in fact usually unhelpful in relieving the pain. If you have come to the conclusion that an organic cause is unlikely, the family still require care. The approach described in Box 11.1 may be helpful. Abdominal pain in children is a very common symptom. Acute and chronic or recurrent abdominal pain are discussed separately, as the presentation and causes are quite different.

 Key points: Recurrent abdominal pain

- Obtain a full picture of the pattern of episodes of pain
- Identify symptoms related to the various abdominal organs
- Determine whether there are any constitutional symptoms
- Decide if the pain is likely to be organic or functional in origin
- Obtain a picture of the psychosocial circumstances and the effect the pain has on the child's activities

---

Box 11.1 Managing the child with non-organic recurrent pain

- Assure the parents and child that no major illness appears to be present. In particular, rule out and focus on diagnoses which concern the family
- A diagnosis of psychosomatic pain should not be made simply by exclusion of pathology. Positive emotional and psychological causes must be identified
- In the child where neither an organic nor a psychosomatic cause is found, it can be helpful to label the diagnosis, such as 'tension headache' or 'growing pains', while qualifying this with an explanation that the aetiology is unknown
- Identify those symptoms and signs which the parents should watch for and which would suggest the need for a re-evaluation
- Do not communicate to the parents that the child is malingering; the pain is real
- Develop a system of return visits to monitor the symptom. Having the family keep a diary of pain episodes and related symptoms can be helpful
- During return visits, allow time for both the child and parent to uncover stresses and concerns
- Make every effort to normalise the life of the child, encouraging attendance at school and participation in regular activities

---

Clues to the diagnosis of recurrent abdominal pain

	Features of the pain	Associated symptoms
Idiopathic (functional) recurrent abdominal pain	Periodic	Well between episodes
	Periumbilical	
Psychogenic pain	Periodic	Psychosomatic symptoms
Irritable bowel syndrome	Non-specific	Flatus and variable bowel pattern
Helicobacter related gastritis	Epigastric	In children <6 years pain is often exacerbated by food (opposite to adult pattern)
	Relieved by food and antacids	
	Family history	
Gastro-oesophageal reflux	May be chest pain	Vomiting
		Failure to thrive
		Heart burn, hiccoughs
Inflammatory bowel disease	Colicky (Crohn)	Anorexia
		Diarrhoea +/− blood and mucus
		Weight loss
Constipation	Colicky	Hard, infrequent stools

(Continued)

🔍 Clues to the diagnosis of recurrent abdominal pain (*Continued*)

	Features of the pain	Associated symptoms
Parasitic infection (e.g. giardiasis)	Variable	Variable
Urinary tract infection	Back or loin pain	Dysuria, frequency, enuresis
Dysmenorrhoea	Varies with menstrual cycle	
Pelvic inflammatory disease	Low abdominal pain	Vaginal discharge
Lead poisoning	Variable, generalised	Anorexia and irritability
		Pica
		Hypochromic microcytic anaemia
Abdominal migraine	Recurrent, may be severe	Nausea and vomiting
		Family history of migraine
		Travel sickness

Acute abdominal pain

Commoner causes of acute abdominal pain in children

Bowel	Renal	Other
Acute appendicitis	Urinary tract pneumonia	Lower lobe pneumonia
Intussusception	Hydronephrosis	Torsion of gonad
Mesenteric adenitis	Renal calculus	Genitourinary problems in girls
Henoch–Schönlein purpura		
H. pylori associated gastro-duodenitis		
Inflammatory bowel disease		
Intestinal obstruction		
Pancreatitis		
Constipation		
Gastroenteritis		

When a child presents with acute and severe abdominal pain, the differential diagnosis includes a number of important conditions which require surgical intervention.

In some children, pain presents acutely and settles spontaneously, only to recur some time later. There may be a gradual merging of episodes of acute abdominal pain with more chronic pain, and this can make the categorization of acute and chronic abdominal pain difficult. Acute intra-abdominal pathology may occur in very small babies when a clear history of pain cannot be given by the patient.

History – must ask!

It is often hard to elicit a good description of the intensity, duration and position of the pain, as this will depend on the child's age and verbal skills. In younger children, there is very often no clear history of pain.

- *Pain.* The features of pain in young children include intermittent spasms of screaming for no obvious cause. In older children, the child may be able to point to the area of pain or rub the affected part of the abdomen. Children are not good at localizing the point of maximum pain and often refer to pain all over the abdomen. Ask specifically whether the pain wakes the child at night and whether it is related to eating particular foods. Pallor during a bout of screaming is an important feature. In older children, a description of the pain migrating from the periumbilical area to the right iliac fossa is very suggestive of acute appendicitis.
- *Blood in stool.* A history of blood in the stool should always be treated seriously. In children with intussusception, the classical description is 'red currant jelly' stools consisting of blood and mucus.
- *Associated features.* Ask about any other features such as anorexia (a particular feature of acute appendicitis); vomiting

and diarrhoea; fever; whether there has been any joint pain or swelling; symptoms referable to other systems (tonsillitis, adenitis, cough, urinary and genitourinary).

Physical examination – must check!

The physical examination must be undertaken very carefully and with great sensitivity, as the child may anticipate additional pain when the examiner's hand is placed on the abdomen. It may be most appropriate to examine young children while they are lying on their mother's lap, and sometimes the child's confidence can be gained by placing the examiner's hand on the child's and lightly palpating the abdomen in that manner. This makes the child feel more in control. It is most important to watch the child's face during palpation of the abdomen because this will give a very useful clue as to whether palpation elicits pain. It is obvious that as little additional pain should be inflicted on the child as possible, although it may be inevitable in the elucidation of signs, and maximum diagnostic use should be made of any pain observed.

- *General observation.* If the pain is a result of a condition causing peritoneal irritation (peritonism), the child lies very still, and movement causes severe pain. Spontaneous movement of the child is an important feature in elucidating the severity of the pain. However, renal colic can cause writhing pain.
- *General examination.* Conditions remote from the abdomen may cause abdominal pain, including tonsillitis and mesenteric adenitis, or basal pneumonia causing pain referred to the abdomen. The child may have tachycardia and an increase in blood pressure in association with pain.
- *Abdomen.* Examination of the acute abdomen may cause extreme agitation in a child who anticipates that the examining doctor will make the pain worse. It is extremely important to reassure the child first, but not to say that 'it will not hurt', as this may be untrue. It is best to precede the examination with an explanation of what will be done and a promise to be as gentle as possible.

  The signs of peritonism include great reluctance to move spontaneously, rebound tenderness, guarding and rigidity.
- *Genital examination and examination of the groin, hips and lumbar spine* are all part of the abdominal examination.
- *Rectal examination.* Although rectal examination may be a considerable intrusion on the child's person, it is an important part of the physical examination in the child who may have an acute appendicitis. It should not, however, be a routine part of all abdominal examinations.

Investigations

If the child has been vomiting, assessment of serum electrolytes and urea is essential to assess the state of hydration. Important investigations in the child with acute abdominal pain are shown in Table 11.6.

Table 11.6 Basic investigations in children with acute abdominal pain and their significance

Investigation	Significance
Full blood count	Leucocytosis found in acute appendicitis and urinary tract infection
Amylase	Pancreatitis
Urine microscopy and culture	Pyuria and organisms indicate infection
Plain abdominal X-ray	Intussusception (Figure 11.7), obstruction
Ultrasound scan	May be particularly helpful in intussusception, and to exclude renal and biliary pathology
Air enema	For diagnosis and treatment of intussusception, see p. 211

Managing acute abdominal pain

The most important question to ask yourself when assessing a child with an acute abdomen is whether the child requires a laparotomy. If the child has signs of peritonism (guarding or rigidity, rebound tenderness or severe tenderness on rectal examination), the answer is likely to be 'yes' and a surgical opinion is urgently required. Bowel rupture will rapidly progress to peritonitis and shock. Although acute appendicitis is by far the most likely cause of peritonism, there are other rare conditions that can cause this condition. Establishing the precise diagnosis is not important because this will be discovered at operation.

Expectant management is appropriate if the child does not have signs of peritonism. Repeated, regular examination of the child's abdomen will determine whether the condition is resolving or getting worse. If there is any doubt as to whether the child has peritonism, a surgical opinion may be very valuable.

For non-operative causes of abdominal pain, treatment depends on the underlying condition.

Key points: Abdominal pain

- The child with peritonitis lies very still, reluctant to move
- Signs of peritonism include rebound tenderness, guarding and rigidity
- Pallor and intermittent bouts of screaming suggest intussusception

Clues to the diagnosis of acute abdominal pain

Diagnosis	Clinical features
Acute appendicitis	Tachycardia
	Anorexia
	Peritonism
Intussusception	Intermittent screaming or apathy
	Pallor
	'Red currant jelly' stool
Mesenteric adenitis	Recent viral infection
	No peritonism, nocturnal pain
Henoch–Schönlein purpura	Joint pain or swelling
	Blood in stool
	Purpura on extensor surfaces
Urinary tract infection	Dysuria
	Frequency
	Enuresis
Peptic ulceration	Nocturnal pain
	Relief or exacerbation by food

Constipation and encopresis

Causes of constipation

Acute
Functional constipation
Bowel obstruction

Chronic
Functional constipation
Dairy protein intolerance
Hirschsprung disease
Hypothyroidism, hypercalcaemia, hyperkalaemia (breast-fed babies)
Coeliac disease

Causes of encopresis:
Functional faecal retention/witholding
Psychological and behavioral causes – uncommon

Constipation In normal children, there is a wide range in frequency of bowel movements. You should therefore base your diagnosis of constipation on hardness of stools and painful defaecation rather than infrequency of bowel movements alone. This is particularly relevant in the exclusively breast-fed, healthy infant, where it can be normal to pass only one stool in 7 days and reassurance is all that is required.

Constipation is common, and is nearly always functional in nature. It is usually due to faecal retention as a result of tightening anal sphincters on defaecation instead of relaxing them (anismus). Stool is therefore partially withheld and accumulates in the rectal ampulla where it may harden. Inadequate propulsion of stool is rare.

Organic causes of constipation or encopresis are rare. Hirschsprung disease (see p. 450) causes constipation virtually from birth, and there is a history of delayed passage of meconium beyond 24 hours after birth. It may be accompanied by failure to thrive and marked abdominal distension, but it does not cause encopresis.

There is surprisingly little evidence supporting the role of diets low in fibre or fruit as the cause of constipation or encopresis and this has probably been overemphasised. The link between constipation and inadequate intake of water is spurious.

Dairy protein intolerance, once thought to only cause diarrhoea, is now recognised as a cause of constipation in infancy and beyond, especially if accompanied by blood or mucus in stool, eczema, a family history of atopy, or perianal fissures or redness. Similarly, constipation is now recognised as a possible presentation of coeliac disease.

Bowel obstruction is rare and results from congenital malformations of the gut. The presentation is usually an acute abdomen (see p. 196) rather than constipation.

Encopresis Encopresis is the inappropriate passage of faeces of any size and consistency. In the vast majority it is involuntary, and is associated with functional faecal retention due to paradoxical tightening of anal sphincters with defaecation. A minority of children with encopresis (2–15%) do not have faecal retention (non-retentive encopresis). In this latter group, the mechanism is poorly understood but there is occasionally an association with externalizing disorders (ADHD), conduct disorder and anxiety/depression.

About one-third of encopretic children also have nocturnal enuresis and day wetting with urgency (overactive bladder), although the pathophysiology that links them is unclear.

Pathophysiology of constipation and encopresis The underpinning pathophysiology is the tendency to withhold faeces by tightening the anal sphincter on defaecation (anismus). This is often the result of past painful or frightening defaecation presumably resulting in fear or apprehension about using the anal sphincter. Withheld faeces become hard and subsequently cause painful or uncomfortable defaecation – thus setting up the cyclical pattern of anismus. Retained, hard or pebbly faeces are the hallmark of constipation. However, retained stools can become soft (spurious diarrhoea) or pasty. Chronic distension of the rectal ampulla may result in diminished sensation of the need to defaecate (rectal hyposensitivity). Subsequent periodic involuntary relaxation of the anal sphincter in the presence of the above factors results in leakage of stool (encopresis). The initial painful/frightening event may be an anal fissure, perianal skin inflammation, toilet training issues or any frightening event related to defaecation.

The principal purpose of your evaluation is to assess the severity of the complaint in order to evaluate the need for treatment. You can rule out rare organic causes on the basis of your history and physical examination.

History – must ask!

- *What are the symptoms?* Is the child truly constipated or are the stools infrequent but normal? The hardness of the stool, painful defaecation, crampy abdominal pain and the presence of blood on the stool or toilet paper indicate the former, although long-standing constipation can be painless.
- *Constipation history.* Was the constipation preceded by a painful or frightening defaecation event such as fissure or onset of toilet training?
- Constipation that started virtually at birth, with delayed passage of meconium suggests Hirschsprung disease. Encopresis or late onset constipation rule it out.
- *Are there associated symptoms?* Bowel obstruction results in constipation, but vomiting and abdominal pain are usually present. Soiling is an important symptom to elucidate.
- *What is the diet like?* The role of diet has traditionally been overemphasised. While a high fibre diet may be of some help in treating constipation, a diet low in fibre is rarely the cause of constipation.

Physical examination – must check!

- *Growth.* Review the growth chart, as failure to thrive occurs with Hirschsprung disease and hypothyroidism.
- *General examination.* Hard, indentable faeces are often palpable in the left lower quadrant of the abdomen and above.
- *Digital per rectal (PR) examination.* Inspection of the anus may reveal fissures or signs of sexual abuse. Rectal examination is generally not performed. Specific indications include impaction, suspected Hirschsprung, pelvic abscess, rectal polyp. If it is carried out it should be done with correct attention to dignity and privacy, and if necessary under sedation.

Investigations

Plain X-ray of the abdomen may reveal the amount of faeces in the colon. This investigation is now less frequently recommended because of high inter-observer variability in the interpretation, high radiation dose in the test and little influence of the result on treatment.

The diagnostic test for Hirschsprung disease is rectal biopsy, and is indicated if the history goes back to infancy and the child has shown poor growth.

Key points: Constipation

- Assess the severity of the constipation
- Attempt to identify a precipitating cause which might explain apprehension about defaecation causing withholding of faeces
- Constipation from birth, in conjunction with failure to thrive, suggests Hirschsprung disease
- Is there nocturnal enuresis with symptoms of overactive bladder?

See NICE guideline: Constipation in children and young people: diagnosis and management
https://www.nice.org.uk/guidance/cg99

Blood in the stool

Causes of blood in the stool

Infancy
Anal fissure
Dysentery and *Salmonella*
Milk allergy
Intussusception
Swallowed maternal blood at birth

Older children
Anal fissure
Dysentery and *Salmonella*
Inflammatory bowel disease
Intussusception
Meckel diverticulum
Henoch–Schönlein purpura
Intestinal polyp

The appearance of blood in the stool is usually alarming. The commonest cause is an anal fissure, which may or may not be visualized. This results from the passage of a large hard stool which tears the delicate rectal mucosa. Bloody diarrhoea is a rare manifestation of cow's milk allergy in babies.

History – must ask!

- *What is the stool like?* Constipation and dysentery are easily differentiated on history. The parent or child should be able to describe whether the blood is outside the stool, indicating that the site of bleeding is in the lower bowel (usually constipation), or whether it is mixed in with the stool, which suggests pathology higher up. In intussusception, the blood is characteristically described as being 'like red currant jelly'. Blood from the upper intestinal tract is usually digested and appears as melaena, and has a black, tarry consistency, and a characteristic odour.

- *Is there pain?* Pain is a useful symptom. Constipation severe enough to cause bleeding is usually associated with significant pain on defaecation. In intussusception (p. 211), the baby has rhythmical attacks of screaming from pain. A description of pain in the older child may suggest peptic ulcer or inflammatory bowel disease.
- *Is there bleeding from other sites?* Bleeding from other sites indicates a more generalised bleeding disorder.

Physical examination – must check!

- *General examination.* High fever occurs with dysentery. If significant blood has been lost, the child may appear anaemic. The rash of Henoch–Schönlein purpura is usually characteristic, with purpura on the extensor surfaces (see Figure 19.14a).
- *The abdomen.* In any of the conditions resulting in rectal bleeding the abdomen may be tender. In constipation, you may palpate faecal loading in the left lower quadrant and above.
- *Anal and rectal examination.* Inspect the anus. The commonest finding is an anal fissure (see Figure 11.8), which results from passage of a large hard stool. Signs of more gross trauma indicate abuse. If there is no fissure, a rectal examination may be needed to confirm constipation or to obtain a stool sample for culture or occult blood.

Investigations

Investigations are not required if a diagnosis of functional constipation is made. Bloody diarrhoea requires stool culture to confirm dysentery. If intussusception is suspected, an urgent ultrasound and air enema is required for diagnosis and treatment (see p. 211). Inflammatory bowel disease requires confirmation, radiologically and endoscopically.

The commoner causes of jaundice in childhood	
Predominantly unconjugated	**Predominantly conjugated**
Haemolysis	*Hepatic*
Sickle cell disease (p. 376)	Hepatitis
	Cystic fibrosis
Spherocytosis	Cirrhosis
Thalassaemia	Metabolic and auto-immune disorders
	Drug toxicity (paracetomol)
Hepatic	
Rare	*Obstructive*
	Hepatitis
	Biliary atresia or obstruction (stones)

Jaundice

Jaundice outside the neonatal period is always a significant sign, and the child must be investigated rapidly and fully so that a definite diagnosis can be made. It is the commonest sign of liver disease, but may also occur as the result of non-liver pathology, notably haemolysis. Neonatal jaundice is discussed in Chapter 24.

Jaundice is caused by accumulation in the skin of the yellow pigment bilirubin. Bilirubin metabolism is summarized in Figure 11.2. Bilirubin is produced as a result of the breakdown of haem from haemoglobin. This is insoluble and referred to as unconjugated bilirubin. Unconjugated bilirubin is metabolized by the liver cells to a soluble conjugated form and is excreted via the hepatic and bile ducts into the duodenum. Bilirubin and bile salts in the bowel aid the absorption of fats and fat-soluble vitamins. Approximately one-half of the conjugated bilirubin is reabsorbed from the bowel as urobilinogen in the enterohepatic circulation. Urobilinogen may be excreted in the urine or re-metabolized through the liver. In hepatic and cholestatic jaundice, excessive conjugated (soluble) bilirubin may be excreted in the urine, which causes the urine to be a dark 'tea' colour.

The causes of jaundice can be divided into those that cause either predominantly unconjugated or conjugated hyperbilirubinaemia. Outside the neonatal period, unconjugated hyperbilirubinaemia is usually caused by haemolysis. Conjugated hyperbilirubinaemia can be divided into either hepatic or obstructive causes.

History – must ask!

- *Features of jaundice.* Ask about the duration of the jaundice. The first sign of a more insidious onset is a yellow appearance to the sclerae of the eyes. Onset is rapid in haemolysis.
- *Malaise.* Ask about the duration of malaise, abdominal pain and presence of anorexia.
- *Symptoms of anaemia.* Anaemia occurs as the result of haemolysis. Symptoms such as breathlessness and pallor may be present.

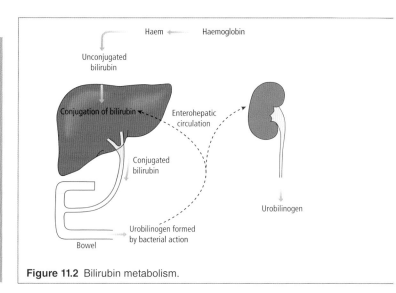

Figure 11.2 Bilirubin metabolism.

Table 11.7 Basic investigations indicated for the child with jaundice

Investigation	What you are looking for
Haemoglobin (Hb)	Low Hb with increased reticulocytes indicates haemolysis, low haptoglobin levels
Bilirubin	Unconjugated excess suggests haemolysis
	Conjugated excess suggests hepatic or post-hepatic disease
Liver enzymes	Elevated in hepatitis
Liver function tests	Albumin and PT low
Alkaline phosphatase	Elevated in cirrhosis or in cases of long-standing jaundice
Serum bile acids	Elevated in cholestasis
Serology	Identification of hepatitis and other viruses
Auto-immune antibodies	Frequently positive in auto-immune hepatitis
Ultrasound	Ascites, hepatomegaly, tumour, gall bladder abnormalities

- *Pruritus.* Pruritus refers to intense skin irritation and occurs as a result of deposition of bile salts in the skin.
- *Urine.* Ask about the colour of the urine (and observe it). Very dark-coloured ('coca-cola') urine strongly suggests a conjugated cause of the jaundice.
- *Stools.* Steatorrhoea refers to frothy, foul-smelling stool which floats in the toilet pan and is commonly seen in children with long-standing cirrhotic liver disease. Pale stools may indicate cholestasis.
- *Family history.* Hereditary causes such as G6PD (drug and fava bean exposure).

Physical examination – must check!

- *Growth.* Failure to thrive or poor growth may occur as the result of any long-standing cause of liver disease.
- *Skin signs.* Scratch marks may be seen on the skin. Signs of long-standing liver disease include spider naevi, clubbing and ascites, bruising, vasculitic rash.
- *Hepatosplenomegaly.* Carefully palpate the liver for enlargement and firmness. A hard liver suggests cirrhosis.

Splenomegaly, if large, may suggest haemolysis, but splenomegaly may also occur as a result of cirrhosis.
- *Eye, CNS and joints examination*

Investigations

The investigations that are indicated in the child with jaundice are shown in Table 11.7.

 Key points: Jaundice

- Jaundice is first seen in the sclerae
- Dark urine and pale faeces indicate conjugated jaundice
- Presence of anaemia and splenomegaly are suggestive of haemolysis
- As part of an initial assessment of jaundice, measure both conjugated and unconjugated components of serum bilirubin

Clues to the differential diagnosis of jaundice

	Haemolysis	Infectious hepatitis	Cirrhosis
Onset of jaundice	Acute	Acute	Insidious
Dark urine	–	+	+++
Anorexia	–	+++	+
Pruritus	–	–	+++
Anaemia	+++	–	+
Hepatosplenomegaly	+++	–	++
Liver tenderness	+	++	–

Gastrointestinal disorders

Dental caries

Dental caries, or tooth decay, is one of the commonest chronic diseases worldwide. The prevalence has decreased markedly in developed countries since the 1970s, in association with increased fluoridation of drinking water and improved oral hygiene.

Clinical features   Dark spots or pits may be seen on the surface of the teeth; there may be associated areas of yellowish dental plaque. 'Baby-bottle tooth decay' classically presents in infants or young toddlers with the upper front teeth severely decayed (Figure 11.3), there is often a history of the child being frequently pacified in their cot for long periods with a sugary drink in a bottle with teat.

Investigations   In developed countries dental caries can be an early marker of neglect, and the child should be clinically assessed for other markers such as failure to thrive. A dietary history should be taken, particularly focusing on intake of sugary drinks and food.

Management   The child should be referred to a dentist, and dietary advice given to the parents. Children with congenital heart disease or who are immunosuppressed are at particular risk from dental caries as the infection may become disseminated, and thus should undergo regular dental surveillance.

Prevention   Dental caries is now considered a major public health concern. Sweet foods and drinks should be limited.

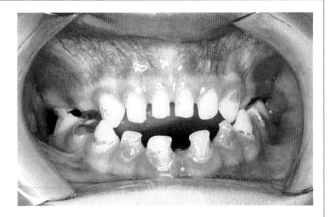

Figure 11.3 Severe dental caries in a 2- year-old child who was given milk and juice by propping the bottle in the cot during night feeds.

Children should brush their teeth at least twice per day from emersion of the first tooth, using age-appropriate toothpaste. Fluoride toothpaste should be used, and children aged 2–4 years old can have fluoride varnish applied to their teeth by a dentist.

Gastro-oesophageal reflux

Gastro-oesophageal reflux is very common in babies and also in children with developmental disabilities, such as severe cerebral palsy. It results from a chronically lax gastro-oesophageal sphincter, or frequent spontaneous decreases in sphincter tone, which allows reflux of stomach contents back up the oesophagus.

Clinical features   The symptoms range from trivial possetting to life-threatening episodes. Common problems are vomiting, oesophagitis, aspiration and, to a lesser extent, apnoea. Vomiting is the commonest complaint and may cause failure to thrive. Oesophagitis causes irritability and anorexia, and should be particularly suspected if there is blood in the vomitus or occult blood in the stools. Opisthotonos (arching of the back) and other head posturing may occur and is possibly an attempt to reduce the pain associated with acid reflux. Aspiration can manifest as episodes of choking and must be suspected in the baby with recurrent episodes of cough, wheezing and pneumonia. Reflux can also cause reflex apnoea and bradycardia. The relationship to acute life-threatening events is controversial.

Investigations   In mild cases, a careful clinical assessment is sufficient, and the diagnosis is confirmed by the response to treatment. The severity and frequency of reflux can be documented by continuous pH and/or impedance monitoring (usually 24 hours) with a probe placed in the lower third of the oesophagus. Oesophagoscopy with biopsy is the best technique for demonstrating oesophagitis, which may also be suspected if a ragged mucosal outline is seen on the barium meal.

Management   In mild uncomplicated cases, propping the child, using an AR (acid reflux) formula and attending to burping may resolve the problem. In infancy a prokinetic may be helpful in increasing gastric emptying. If oesophagitis is present, drugs may be prescribed to reduce gastric acid production (ranitidine, omeprazole). If symptoms do not respond to a good trial of medical agents, or if recurrent aspiration and apnoea are major problems, surgery is indicated, with the commonest procedure being Nissen fundoplication.

◉ Gastro-oesophageal reflux at a glance

Epidemiology
Common in babies, and
children with
Down syndrome and severe
cerebral palsy

Aetiology
Lax gastro-oesophageal
sphincter

History
May be asymptomatic
Vomiting*
Irritability and anorexia*
Pseudo-seizures (Sandifer syndrome)
Choking*
Apnoea*
History of pneumonia*

Physical examination
Normal
Chest signs if aspirating*
Failure to thrive*
Opisthotonos*

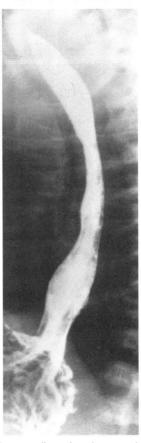

Barium swallow showing massive
retrograde gastric-oesophageal
reflux

NB *Signs and symptoms are variable

Confirmatory investigations
Barium swallow: reflux
visualized
pH monitoring: increased
acidity in oesophagus
Oesophagoscopy: oesophagitis

Differential diagnosis
Normal posseting
Colic in young babies
Other causes of vomiting
(pp. 185-6)
Other causes of recurrent
pneumonia
Other causes of apnoea
(p. 441)

Management
Thickened feeds and
propping
Most babies need only
re-assurance and follow-up
Trial of anti-reflux formula
Medication: drugs to reduce
gastric acid production
(ranitidine, omeprazole)
Surgery: Nissen fundoplication
required if aspirating, apnoea
or poor response to
medication (rare)

Prognosis/complications
Reflux resolves in most normal
children by the time they are
eating solids/walking

Pyloric stenosis

Pyloric stenosis is caused by hypertrophy and hyperplasia of the pylorus muscle. It usually develops in the first 4–6 weeks of life, and is commonest in firstborn male children.

Clinical features   The vomiting is characteristically projectile and generally occurs during or immediately after feeding (although not necessarily at every feed). The vomit may be blood-tinged but is not bile-stained. The infant is hungry and is prepared to take another feed immediately. Weight loss is seen on examination, with varying degrees of dehydration. In advanced cases, the infant may be moribund. Visible peristalsis from the left upper quadrant to the right is most prominent immediately after a feed or just prior to vomiting. Careful palpation should reveal a hard

mobile tumour (the pylorus), which feels like an acorn or an olive just to the right of the epigastrium. Once the tumour has been palpated there is no need for barium studies or ultrasound. However, if the diagnosis is suspected, but the tumour not palpable, the diagnosis can be confirmed by ultrasound (Figure 11.4). If vomiting is protracted, the loss of acidity from the stomach results in hypochloraemic alkalosis and reduced sodium and potassium levels in the serum (see p. 113).

Management   Treatment is surgical. The Ramstedt procedure consists of splitting the pylorus muscle, without penetrating the mucosa. If the infant is dehydrated, rehydration must take place prior to surgery with replacement of sodium, chloride and potassium (see pp. 417–18). Oral feeds can be gradually given within hours postoperatively.

◉ Pyloric stenosis at a glance

Epidemiology
Age 4–6 weeks
7 boys : 1 girl
Age 1–10 weeks

Aetiology
Hypertrophy and hyperplasia of
the pylorus muscle

History
Projectile vomiting during or just
after feed (**a**)
Infant hungry immediately after
vomit
May be constipated

Physical examination
Many babies are now diagnosed
early with ultrasound before
the classic signs and symptoms
are evident
Weight loss +/– dehydration
Visible peristalsis from left
upper quadrant to right upper
quadrant (**b**)
Mobile olive-sized tumour
palpable to right of
epigastrium during feed (**c**)

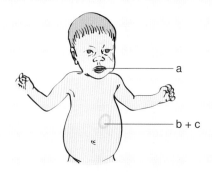

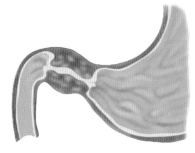

Illustration of thickened and
prolonged pyloric sphincter

Confirmatory investigations
Abdominal ultrasound (not
needed if 'olive' felt)
Hypochloraemic alkalosis
(see p. 113)
Low serum sodium and
potassium

Differential diagnosis
Posseting
Gastro-oesophageal reflux
Gastritis
Systemic infection

Management
Rehydration
Surgical correction: Ramstedt
procedure

Prognosis/complications
Excellent following surgery

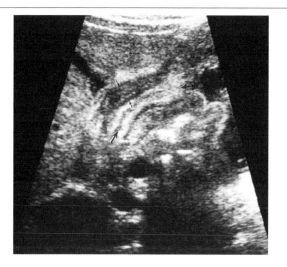

Figure 11.4 Ultrasound of a baby with pyloric stenosis. Arrows
indicate the elongated pyloric canal (thick arrow) and thickened
pyloric muscle (thinner arrow).

Colic

The term 'colic' describes a common symptom of paroxysmal
crying which occurs in babies principally under 3 months of
age, and which is now primarily thought to be of behavioural/
developmental origin, although it is widely believed to be of
intestinal origin. Certain infants are particularly susceptible to
colic. It may be associated with hunger and swallowed air, or
discomfort and distension caused by overfeeding.

Clinical features   The clinical pattern is characteristic. The
attack usually begins suddenly, with crying which often lasts
more or less continuously for several hours. The face may be
flushed, the abdomen distended and tense, the legs drawn up
and the hands clenched. The attack may end when the infant is
completely exhausted, but often there is relief when faeces or
flatus are passed. Attacks commonly occur late in the afternoon
or evening. Careful physical examination is important to eliminate the possibility of intussusception, strangulated hernia or
other disorders.

Management Holding or rocking the baby, carrying him or her in a sling close to the parent, and travel in a car seat can soothe, and secure swaddling occasionally helps. No effective remedies have been found, although recent research suggests that sucrose may be effective. Changes of infant formula, although commonly tried, are rarely helpful. Support and sympathy are important in successful management of the problem, which resolves spontaneously over a few months.

⊙ Colic at a glance

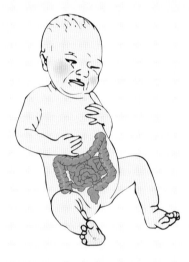

Epidemiology
Babies under 3 months old

Aetiology
Presumed to be intestinal in
  origin
Recent evidence suggests a
  behavioural-developmental basis

History
Crying for several hours, often
  late in the day
Face flushed, legs drawn up*
Abdomen distended *
Relief on passing flatus or
  faeces*

NB * Signs and symptoms are variable

Physical examination
Normal

Confirmatory investigations
None

Differential diagnosis
Discomfort and stress
Reflux oesophagitis
Acute onset:
• intussusception
• otitis media
• milk allergy

Management
Reassurance and support

Prognosis/complications
Usually resolves by 3
  months old

Viral gastroenteritis

Viral infection is the commonest cause of gastroenteritis in young children, although since immunisation has been introduced, rotavirus is no longer responsible for winter epidemics.

Clinical features Diarrhoea usually begins after 1–2 days of low-grade fever, vomiting, and anorexia, although in the younger child the onset is often more rapid.

Management and prognosis Management is discussed on pp. 187–8. Antibiotics should not be given as they encourage gut superinfection with other organisms. The diarrhoea usually resolves within a week. Probiotics may shorten symptoms.

Bacterial gastroenteritis

Bacterial gastroenteritis presents a similar picture to viral gastroenteritis. The commonest pathogens are *Escherichia coli*, *Shigella*, *Salmonella* and *Campylobacter*.

Clinical features The clinical features are described in the *Clues to the differential diagnosis of acute diarrhoea* (p. 189). Particularly noteworthy is the fact that meningismus and febrile fits occur with shigella infection, and that bloody stools are characteristic of *Shigella*, *Salmonella* or *Campylobacter*.

Management and prognosis Antibiotics should not be used in uncomplicated gastroenteritis caused by *Salmonella* as they tend to prolong the carrier state. *Campylobacter* infections are also often self-limiting but can be treated with oral azithromycin. If there is a clinical suspicion of septicaemia in association with gastroenteritis, the child should be admitted to hospital and treated with appropriate antibiotics intrave-

nously. About 10% of children with *E. coli* 0157 gastroenteritis will develop renal failure (haemolytic uraemic syndrome, HUS). The general management of dehydration is covered on pp. 417–18.

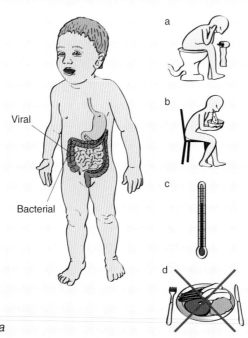

Acute gastroenteritis at a glance

Epidemiology
Common in all ages

Aetiology
Viral, particularly rotavirus
Shigella
E.coli
Salmonella
Campylobacter

History
Diarrhoea (**a**)
Abdominal pain
Malaise
Vomiting (**b**)
Fever (**c**)
Anorexia (**d**)
Febrile fits in *Shigella*
Bloody stools in *Shigella*,
Campylobacter, Salmonella
– called dysentery

Physical examination
Tender abdomen
Sore anus
Dehydration

Viral

Bacterial

N.B. Prevent and treat dehydration

Confirmatory investigations
Usually none in primary care setting
Stool culture if prolonged course, bloody stools or hospitalized

Differential diagnosis
Infections outside the gastrointestinal tract
Antibiotic-induced diarrhoea

Management
Fluid management of dehydration
Antibiotics not usually indicated, even for bacterial causes
Antidiarrhoeal agents should not be prescribed

Course/complications
Usually resolves spontaneously, although may take days to weeks
Carrier state may follow *Salmonella*
Temporary lactose intolerance may develop
About 10% of children with *E. coli* 0157 gastroenteritis will develop renal failure (HUS)

Toddler diarrhoea

Non-specific diarrhoea is very common in the toddler age group. It is likely to be caused by a rapid gastrocolic reflex.

Clinical features Parents commonly describe the appearance of particles of food, particularly meat fibres, peas and beans, in the stool. The child may have a large fluid intake, particularly of fruit juices. The diagnosis should only be made if the child is thriving.

Management and prognosis In some instances, a reduction in fluid intake can be helpful, but usually, if the toddler is

thriving, reassurance is all that is required. In some cases of frequent stooling with severe parental anxiety, loperamide may be used to slow bowel transit time. As the child matures the symptoms resolve.

Lactose intolerance

Secondary lactose intolerance is common in the baby and young child. During an acute episode of gastroenteritis, the superficial mucosal cells containing lactase are stripped off, resulting in high levels of poorly absorbed lactose in the bowel, which prolongs the diarrhoea. Congenital lactose intolerance is extremely rare.

Clinical features   The diarrhoea, which is watery in nature, follows an acute episode of gastroenteritis. The diagnosis is suspected if the gastroenteritis persists for several days, particularly if the temperature has resolved and there is excoriation in the peri-anal area. Laboratory evidence is found in a low stool pH (<6.0) and the presence of reducing substances (lactose) in the stool (>0.5%). It is rarely necessary to perform lactose challenge or breath hydrogen tests.

Management and prognosis   In the bottle-fed baby, an empirical change of infant formula to a lactose-free milk can be tried. Soya milk formulas can be used in infants greater than 6 months of age, but contain oestrogens, and thus in younger infants specially formulated lactose-free milks should be used. The baby should revert to cow's milk formula once symptoms are resolved. The breast-fed baby needs no change of milk, and symptoms should eventually resolve.

Coeliac disease

Coeliac disease (see Figure 11.5) results from a permanent inability to tolerate gluten, a substance found in wheat, rye, barley and other cereals. Oats are usually tolerated in small amounts.

Clinical features   Most children present before the age of 2 years with failure to thrive, irritability, anorexia, vomiting, diarrhea and anaemia, although some have few symptoms. Examination classically shows abdominal distension, wasted buttocks, irritability and pallor. The stools are pale and foul. Additional physical signs may include mouth sores, a smooth tongue, excessive bruising, finger clubbing and peripheral oedema.

The range of clinical features is very wide, and some persons affected have such mild symptoms that the diagnosis is only made in adulthood. The most constant features are decrease in weight gain and linear growth.

Investigations   Anaemia is common, usually with an iron-deficient picture, but folate too may be low. Most children eating significant amounts of fat will have steatorrhoea and the faecal smear will demonstrate fat globules. Detection of coeliac antibodies (anti-tissue transglutaminase (TTG) IgA and IgG) can be used as a screening test, but a definitive diagnosis must be made by jejunal biopsy. The characteristic finding is subtotal villous atrophy (Figure 11.6).

Management   Response to a gluten-free diet, which consists of eliminating all wheat, rye and barley products, is usually prompt, with an improvement in mood, resolution of diarrhoea and good growth. The diet is quite constricting, but special gluten-free products are now widely available. Children with coeliac crises may be given steroids. Vitamin and mineral supplements are often needed initially. As the intolerance to gluten is permanent, the diet has to be continued indefinitely.

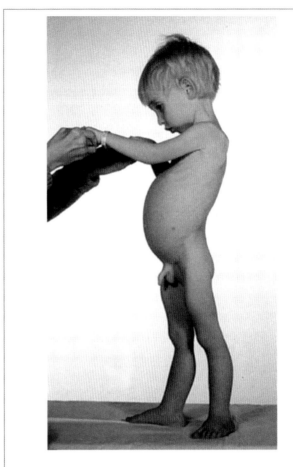

Figure 11.5 A 2-year-old child with coeliac disease, showing marked abdominal distension and wasted buttocks.

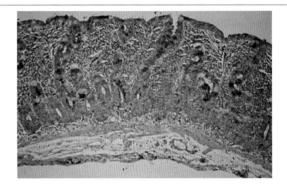

Figure 11.6 Histology of a jejunal biopsy taken from a child with coeliac disease, showing atrophy of the villi.

Until recently, children were rechallenged with gluten after 2 years of the diet and the biopsy repeated before they were consigned to life-long dietary restriction. Guidelines now suggest that there is no need for a second biopsy if TTG levels fall and the clinical picture resolves.

Prognosis   The prognosis is excellent provided the child adheres to the diet.

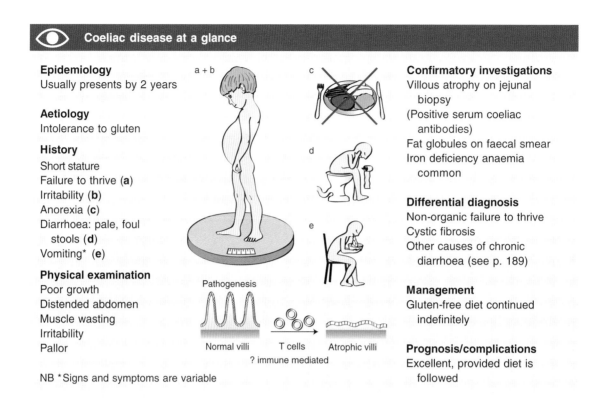

Coeliac disease at a glance

Epidemiology
Usually presents by 2 years

Aetiology
Intolerance to gluten

History
Short stature
Failure to thrive (**a**)
Irritability (**b**)
Anorexia (**c**)
Diarrhoea: pale, foul
stools (**d**)
Vomiting* (**e**)

Physical examination
Poor growth
Distended abdomen
Muscle wasting
Irritability
Pallor

NB *Signs and symptoms are variable

Pathogenesis
Normal villi   T cells   Atrophic villi
? immune mediated

Confirmatory investigations
Villous atrophy on jejunal
biopsy
(Positive serum coeliac
antibodies)
Fat globules on faecal smear
Iron deficiency anaemia
common

Differential diagnosis
Non-organic failure to thrive
Cystic fibrosis
Other causes of chronic
diarrhoea (see p. 189)

Management
Gluten-free diet continued
indefinitely

Prognosis/complications
Excellent, provided diet is
followed

Cow's milk protein intolerance

Allergy to cow's milk protein is rare and often overdiagnosed.

Clinical features   Cow's milk protein intolerance is a cause of chronic diarrhoea and vomiting. Classically, the diarrhoea is bloody, and urticaria, stridor and bronchospasm may occur. Very rarely, the sensitivity can be life-threatening. The condition is less common in babies who have been breast-fed.

The diagnosis is clinical. Symptoms should subside within one week of withdrawing cow's milk from the diet. The child should be rechallenged after a period of time (in hospital if the original symptoms were severe), and observed for recurrence of symptoms.

Management and prognosis   Treatment consists of removing cow's milk from the diet. Soya milk infant formulas provide adequate nutrition from 6 months of age. Younger infants require a special cow's milk protein free formula, hypoallergenic formula, hydrolysed protein or dipeptide amino acid-based formula. In most cases, the intolerance is transitory, usually resolving in 1–2 years. Prolonged breast-feeding reduces the likelihood of cow's milk intolerance.

Crohn disease

Crohn disease is a cause of chronic diarrhoea in late childhood and adolescence. The underlying cause of this chronic inflammatory condition is unknown. Both Crohn disease and ulcerative colitis are characterised by unpredictable exacerbations and remissions.

Clinical features   Crohn disease presents with recurrent abdominal pain, anorexia, growth failure, fever, diarrhea which may be bloody, oral and perianal ulcers and arthritis.

Investigations   Anaemia is almost universal, ASCA antibodies are specific and p-ANCA may be positive. Inflammatory markers such as (C-reactive protein) CRP and ESR are persistently elevated. The diagnosis is confirmed by CT or MRE and endoscopy.

Management   Remission can be induced by nutritional programmes based on elemental diets. This approach is as effective as steroids and avoids the hazard of growth impairment. Surgical resection may be indicated in localized disease, obstruction and fistulization. Antibiotics are used if abscesses develop. Chronic management today involves a range of drugs including systemic or local steroids, antibiotics, immunomodulators, aminosalicylates and biological agents such as TNF inhibitors. Surgery is occasionally required.

Prognosis   The inflammatory activity continues to remit and exacerbate throughout life.

Ulcerative colitis

Like Crohn disease, ulcerative colitis is a chronic inflammatory condition with unpredictable exacerbations and remissions.

Clinical features   Ulcerative colitis presents with diarrhoea containing blood and mucus. Early on, these episodes may be short-lived and thought to be simply infective in nature. Systemic upset in terms of pain, weight loss, arthritis and liver disturbance may occur.

Management   Treatment is by corticosteroid enemas or suppositories. Sulphasalazine may be given orally, and steroids, immunosuppressive therapy and even colectomy may be required in severe cases.

Prognosis   Most cases starting in childhood are severe in terms of activity and extent of involvement. There is a high risk of colonic cancer developing later in life.

Idiopathic recurrent abdominal pain

There is no identifiable organic cause for the majority of children presenting with recurrent abdominal pain. In this circumstance, the expression 'recurrent abdominal pain' is often used as a diagnostic term, in itself implying that the pain is functional rather than organic. In some children, the abdominal pain is truly psychosomatic and related to stress at home or at school.

Clinical features   Children with recurrent abdominal pain suffer very real pain, which can be severe. The periodicity of the complaint and intervening good health are characteristic of the syndrome. The children are often described as being sensitive, highly strung and high-achieving individuals, although this is by no means always true.

Management and prognosis   Management must be directed towards reassurance, maximizing a normal lifestyle and minimizing school absence. Nutritional changes such as withdrawal of lactose for a period may help. The approach described for children with any form of nonorganic pain in the 'At a glance' guide is generally helpful. If there are psychosocial causes, these need to be addressed. In most cases, simply indicating the link and explaining that children tend to experience tummy aches in a similar way to which adults experience headache is enough to reassure the parents and child. Some children utilize the pain, whether real or fictitious, to their own ends, so missing school or unpleasant events. In this circumstance, confrontation is not usually helpful. An understanding attitude, while maintaining that absence from school is unnecessary, is a good approach. In the majority of children, the pain resolves over time.

 Idiopathic recurrent abdominal pain at a glance

Epidemiology
10–15% of school children

Aetiology
None identified
May be psychosomatic

History
Periodic pain, healthy between
   attacks
Nocturnal pain unusual
Often periumbilical site
Stress at home or at school*
Stools may vary from pellets to
   unformed*
Colic as a baby*

NB *Signs and symptoms are variable

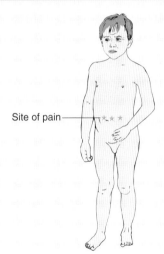

Site of pain

Physical examination
Normal

Confirmatory investigations
None

Differential diagnosis
See p. 195

Management
Reassurance
Minimizing school absence

Prognosis/complications
Resolves over time in the
   majority of cases

Irritable bowel syndrome

The term 'irritable bowel syndrome' is sometimes used instead of 'recurrent abdominal pain', particularly if there are minor gastrointestinal symptoms and no psychological stresses identified. It has been suggested that the discomfort results from a dysfunction of the autonomic system of the gut.

Clinical features   The bowel pattern may be described as varying from pellets to unformed stool. Flatus can also be a feature, and many of these children have a history of colic as babies.

Management and prognosis   Using the term 'irritable bowel syndrome' often gives families the reassurance that a diagnosis has been made. A high fibre and low lactose or fat diet may be helpful as may be probiotics. The symptoms usually resolve over time, but relapses are common.

Helicobacter pylori gastritis

Peptic ulcer and duodenitis-gastritis is now being recognised as an important cause of abdominal pain in childhood. As in the adult, the organism *Helicobacter pylori* is implicated as a cause of gastritis and ulcers in childhood.

Clinical features   The pain may have the classic features of adult peptic ulcer, being epigastric in site and relieved by food. In contrast, in young children under 6 years of age the pain often appears to occur immediately after eating. There may be a family history of peptic ulceration.

Management   If the diagnosis is suspected, a trial of antacids, H_2-receptor antagonists or proton-pump inhibitors may be used empirically; but if symptoms are persistent, confirmation of the diagnosis is required by urea breath test. Gastroscopy and biopsy should be done before eradication therapy of *H. pylori* with antibiotics (usually amoxicillin and clarithromycin) and PPI inhibitors.

Acute appendicitis

Appendicitis is the commonest cause of an acute abdomen in childhood and occurs in three to four per 1000 children. It can occur at any age including very young infants, but is most common over 5 years of age. It presents most difficulties in diagnosis when it occurs in very young children.

There is no such condition as the 'grumbling appendix'. The child either does have acute appendicitis or does not.

Clinical features   In older children, the presentation may be classical, with the description of pain initially in the periumbilical area, moving after a few hours into the right iliac fossa. In young children, a history of pain will not be given, although the mother will often report that she thinks her child is in pain. The two most important features of acute appendicitis are anorexia and great reluctance to move. Abdominal distension and signs of sepsis may develop rapidly in young children. Rectal examination must be performed on all children where acute appendicitis is suspected. If there is doubt as to whether the child has acute appendicitis, regular re-examination is very important to determine whether the symptoms and signs are getting better or worse.

Investigations   Full blood count, electrolytes and urea are essential. The bedrock of diagnosis is an abdominal ultrasound where a non-pliable and engorged appendix is seen. CT may be needed in equivocal cases.

Management   Management is usually surgical in acute appendicitis, but there is a growing interest in antibiotic treatment which may be effective in selected cases. A surgical opinion should be obtained when the diagnosis is suspected.

Prognosis   This is very good with skilled surgery. Peritonitis may cause severe illness, requiring many weeks for full recovery. If intraperitoneal adhesions occur as a result of peritonitis, later bowel obstruction may occur.

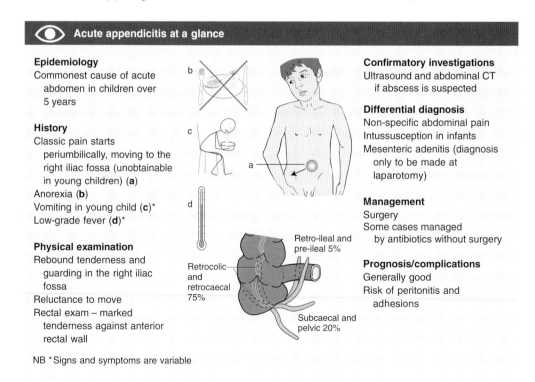

Acute appendicitis at a glance

Epidemiology
Commonest cause of acute abdomen in children over 5 years

History
Classic pain starts periumbilically, moving to the right iliac fossa (unobtainable in young children) (**a**)
Anorexia (**b**)
Vomiting in young child (**c**)*
Low-grade fever (**d**)*

Physical examination
Rebound tenderness and guarding in the right iliac fossa
Reluctance to move
Rectal exam – marked tenderness against anterior rectal wall

NB *Signs and symptoms are variable

Retro-ileal and pre-ileal 5%
Retrocolic and retrocaecal 75%
Subcaecal and pelvic 20%

Confirmatory investigations
Ultrasound and abdominal CT if abscess is suspected

Differential diagnosis
Non-specific abdominal pain
Intussusception in infants
Mesenteric adenitis (diagnosis only to be made at laparotomy)

Management
Surgery
Some cases managed by antibiotics without surgery

Prognosis/complications
Generally good
Risk of peritonitis and adhesions

Mesenteric adenitis

This condition is often diagnosed where no other cause for acute abdominal pain can be found. It is caused by acute enlargement of intra-abdominal lymph nodes as the result of infection in the upper respiratory tract, chest or abdomen (gastroenteritis). The acutely enlarged lymph nodes cause pain which may be severe.

Clinical features   Children with mesenteric adenitis usually have a recent history of infection and signs may still be present in throat or chest. Peritonism and guarding never occur in this condition, and the pain is characteristically episodic and nocturnal. It is a diagnosis of exclusion, and ultrasound is useful.

Management   After other conditions have been excluded, the management is symptomatic and expectant.

Prognosis   The prognosis is excellent.

Intussusception

Intussusception is caused by invagination of one part of the bowel into another (Figure 11.7). The commonest site is the terminal ileum into the caecum. It occurs most frequently between 3 months and 2 years of age. Enlarged lymphatic tissue in the bowel walls (Peyer's patch) may form the leading edge of the intussusception, and this may occur following a recent viral URTI or gastroenteritis.

Clinical features   Classically, the child presents with episodes of severe screaming associated with pallor. The pain is episodic, and the child may appear well between colicky episodes. Passage of a 'red currant jelly' stool occurs in about 75% of cases, and this is an important specific finding. In a proportion of children with intussusception, the symptoms and signs may be very non-specific. An important presentation may be encephalopathy with apathy, stupor and behavioural changes.

Abdominal examination often reveals a sausage-shaped mass in the right side of the abdomen. Ultrasound examination is useful in making the diagnosis.

Management   Ultrasound examination is diagnostic in many cases. In most children, the intussusception can be relieved by air enema examination. This is both diagnostic and curative, as the pressure when the contrast is inserted can be gradually increased to force back the intussuscepting bowel, which can be seen on fluoroscopy. Care must be taken not to use too high a pressure for fear of bowel perforation. Reduction by contrast enema should only be used if the history is less than 24 hours and there is no evidence of peritonism or severe dehydration. Surgical reduction is used if enema reduction fails or if the child is unsuitable for contrast treatment.

Prognosis   Intussusception may be very non-specific in its presentation and is a condition that must always be considered

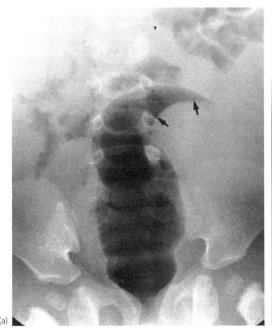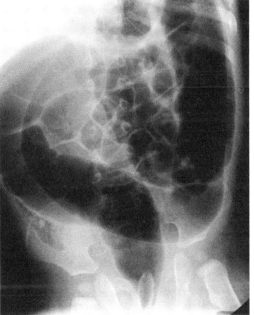

Figure 11.7 Air enema of a child with intussusception. (a) The intussusception is clearly demarcated, indenting the colonic lumen (see arrows). (b) Following reduction, air is now seen in the small bowel.

in a child who is acutely but intermittently unwell. Unfortunately, children still die of this condition because the diagnosis is not considered.

Recurrence of the intussusception is uncommon, but if it occurs the presence of a polyp should be considered as the cause of the repeated bowel invagination.

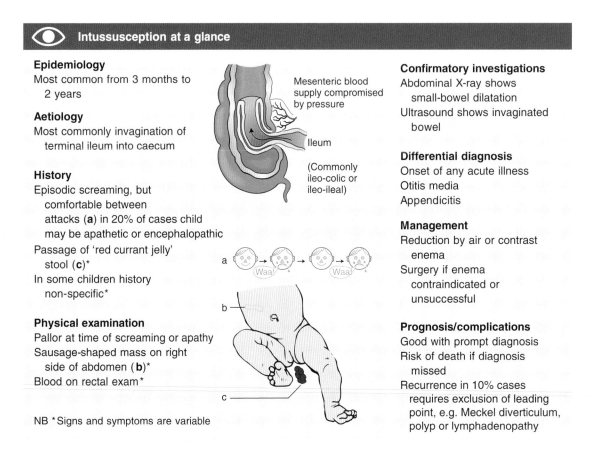

Intussusception at a glance

Epidemiology
Most common from 3 months to 2 years

Aetiology
Most commonly invagination of terminal ileum into caecum

History
Episodic screaming, but comfortable between attacks (**a**) in 20% of cases child may be apathetic or encephalopathic
Passage of 'red currant jelly' stool (**c**)*
In some children history non-specific*

Physical examination
Pallor at time of screaming or apathy
Sausage-shaped mass on right side of abdomen (**b**)*
Blood on rectal exam*

NB *Signs and symptoms are variable

Mesenteric blood supply compromised by pressure

Ileum

(Commonly ileo-colic or ileo-ileal)

Confirmatory investigations
Abdominal X-ray shows small-bowel dilatation
Ultrasound shows invaginated bowel

Differential diagnosis
Onset of any acute illness
Otitis media
Appendicitis

Management
Reduction by air or contrast enema
Surgery if enema contraindicated or unsuccessful

Prognosis/complications
Good with prompt diagnosis
Risk of death if diagnosis missed
Recurrence in 10% cases requires exclusion of leading point, e.g. Meckel diverticulum, polyp or lymphadenopathy

Constipation (functional) and encopresis

Chronic constipation often stems from an episode when passage of a stool is painful or frightening. The child responds by withholding further stools because of apprehension or to avoid pain. The stools remain in the colo-rectum where water is reabsorbed, and the stools become harder and even more painful to pass. Constipation is exacerbated further as the child withholds stool to prevent the severe pain that is experienced on defaecation. Eventually, the cycle becomes self-perpetuating and the rectum so stretched that dilatation of the colon may occur, resulting in megacolon. Constipation is a particular problem in immobile children with physical disabilities.

Constipation may be accompanied by the passage of blood due to an anal fissure caused by hard stool damaging the delicate rectal mucosa (see Figure 11.8). The fissure may or may not be visible.

Encopresis refers to the passage of formed stool in inappropriate places (including underwear) by a child who is mature enough to have acquired bowel continence. It is usually due to functional faecal retention as with constipation. Chronically retained faeces may become hard (constipation) or soft. Chronic stretching of the rectal ampulla causes rectal hyposensitivity, that is the child loses awareness of the withheld stool. Periodic involuntary relaxation of the anal sphincter results in escape of faeces.

Clinical features   It is often not possible to recall the start of the cycle of constipation, and the parent and doctor are simply faced with the chronically constipated child, who may also be soiling (see below). Constipation from birth, absence of soiling and growth failure indicate that the constipation is not functional and Hirschsprung disease or dairy protein intolerance should be considered.

In encopresis, the child often displays avoidance behaviour by hiding, crossing legs or taking on unusual postures during defaecation. This is not true avoidance (as the parents usually think) but rather an attempt by the child to resolve the dilemma of holding the faeces in while knowing that they have to let it go. Understanding the pathophysiology especially the role of rectal hyposensitivity in depriving the child of 'warning' is crucial to demystifying the phenomenon and removing a huge burden of blame heaped on the child (and sometimes the parents). Once the faeces have escaped, the child senses that they have soiled. The child may then bolt to the toilet (as if 'waiting to the last minute'), go and hide, or simply soil themselves.

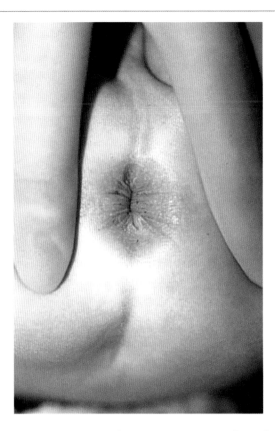

Figure 11.8 An anal fissure (at 6 o'clock) in a child suffering from constipation with rectal bleeding.

Table 11.8 Management of constipation and encopresis	
Stage 1: Evacuation of the bowel	*Diet:* undue emphasis on this is unwarranted Programme of regular sitting and pushing on the toilet with age-appropriate charts and stickers to reinforce sitting and defecating.
	Laxatives: stool softeners such as macrogol 3350 can be used. The dose can safely be increased on a daily basis until the stools become soft.
	Enemas: rarely required and should probably be administered under sedation.
Stage 2: Maintenance	Continue regular sits 2–3 times a day for 4 minutes. Stools should be kept soft. A daily, long-term (3–6 months) maintenance dose of agents such as macrogol 3350, that prevents painful motions is better than treating painful, hard stools only when needed.
Stage 3: Vigilance	Treatment should be started at the first indication of recurrence of hard stools. A regular sit on the toilet each morning is anecdotally helpful. Consideration should be given to long-term, low-dose, stool softener.

Management Explaining the involuntary nature of encopresis to frustrated, angry parents, and a besieged child is revelatory, uplifting and a mandatory first step.

Management can be divided into three stages (Table 11.8):

1. Empty the bowel
2. Keep it empty
3. Vigilance so that the cycle does not recommence.

Emptying the bowel is usually obtained by a routine of regular sitting on the toilet and attempting to push out faeces (despite not sensing the need the do so because of rectal hyposensitivity) for about 4 minutes three times a day. This is often facilitated by using an age-appropriate chart or table whereby the child can put on stickers or ticks with successful defaecation. Material rewards are often unhelpful, and the inflation rate is prohibitive.

Keeping the bowel empty relies on long-term compliance with regular sitting. Stool softeners can often be tapered off after several months. Regular, frequent review with much ongoing encouragement are important.

Vigilance. Rectal hyposensitivity and reaccumulation of faeces can recur for many months and even years after initial remission.

If there is suggestion of hard stool, then stool softeners will help. Agents such as macrogol 3350 (polyethylene glycol, PEG), lactulose or paraffin oil are commonly used, usually for periods of several months on a daily basis. Passing of soft rather than hard stools, repeatedly over many months is thought to be central to the child discarding their ongoing apprehension about defaecation. Bowel stimulants like bisacodyl are not recommended.

Disempaction of severe cases *before* embarking on months of regular toileting and stool softeners, is widely practised but the need for it is unproved. The oral route can be employed using increasing doses of macrogol 3350, until a large expulsion of faeces is achieved (usually within 2–3 days). The rectal route is the alternative using enemas or bowel washouts. Sedation with midazolam should be considered. For manual disempaction a general anaesthetic is required.

Prognosis Constipation often recurs. Long-term use of stool softeners with a programme of regular toileting is recommended. A similar approach is used with encopresis where successful long term remission ranges from 40% to 80% after 6 months of continuing treatment, with some improvement in most of the remainder.

Constipation at a glance

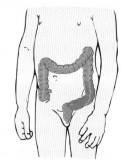

Epidemiology
Any age, but particularly
  problematic in immobile
  disabled children

Aetiology
Cycle of painful defaecation and
  withholding

History
Infrequent hard stools
Painful defaecation
Abdominal pain*
Soiling*

Physical examination
Indentable mass in left lower
  quadrant
Hard stool on rectal examination
  (PR not often indicated)
Anal fissure*

Confirmatory investigations
Faecal loading +/− megacolon
  on plain abdominal X-ray
  (investigation not usually
  indicated)

Differential diagnosis
Hirschsprung disease

Management
Dietary advice
Stool softeners

Prognosis/complications
Problem may recur periodically

NB *Signs and symptoms are variable

**See NICE guideline: Constipation in children
and young people: diagnosis and management**
https://www.nice.org.uk/guidance/cg99

Viral hepatitis

Routine immunisations for hepatitis A and B have made these infections very rare in childhood, as is type C. Other organisms occasionally cause hepatitis, among them viruses such as EBV and CMV which cause mild hepatic dysfunction.

Hepatitis A is transmitted by the faecal-oral route and B by trans-placental, enteral or parenteral routes. Cholestatic type jaundice usually begins after a short flu-like prodrome. Diagnosis is via abnormal liver function tests and specific serological markers. Treatment is supportive, although in recent years, new biological agents have become available for types B and C which may prevent chronic complications such as cirrhosis and hepatocellular carcinoma.

Recent advances in pharmacological treatment provide hope for viral eradication and cure in viral hepatitis.

Viral hepatitis at a glance

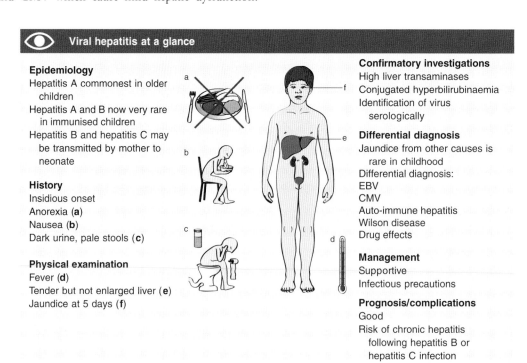

Epidemiology
Hepatitis A commonest in older
  children
Hepatitis A and B now very rare
  in immunised children
Hepatitis B and hepatitis C may
  be transmitted by mother to
  neonate

History
Insidious onset
Anorexia (a)
Nausea (b)
Dark urine, pale stools (c)

Physical examination
Fever (d)
Tender but not enlarged liver (e)
Jaundice at 5 days (f)

Confirmatory investigations
High liver transaminases
Conjugated hyperbilirubinaemia
Identification of virus
  serologically

Differential diagnosis
Jaundice from other causes is
  rare in childhood
Differential diagnosis:
EBV
CMV
Auto-immune hepatitis
Wilson disease
Drug effects

Management
Supportive
Infectious precautions

Prognosis/complications
Good
Risk of chronic hepatitis
  following hepatitis B or
  hepatitis C infection

Hepatic cirrhosis

Hepatic cirrhosis represents the end stage of a number of chronic liver disorders, infectious, metabolic, genetic, malformations and auto-immune. Fatty liver disease (NAFLD) is now one of the more important. Cirrhosis in children most commonly follows biliary atresia (p. 449).

Clinical features   Jaundice may not be prominent. The presenting features may be failure to thrive as a result of steatorrhoea, and vitamin deficiency disorders, such as spontaneous haemorrhages caused by vitamin K deficiency. Clinical examination reveals an enlarged firm liver which may feel knobbly. Other features of chronic liver disease include spider naevi, ascites, palmar erythema and clubbing. Investigations must be pursued to identify the underlying cause.

Management   Management of cirrhosis is highly specialised and needs to be undertaken in a recognised centre regularly dealing with chronic liver disease in children. Particular attention must be paid to appropriate nutrition and correction of fat-soluble vitamin deficiency disorders:

- *Malabsorption.* The lack of bile salts causes steatorrhoea and malabsorption, so the diet needs to be supplemented with medium-chain fatty acids which do not require bile salts for their absorption.
- *Vitamin deficiency.* Fat-soluble vitamin deficiency is common in long-standing conjugated jaundice. Vitamins A, D, E and K should be routinely supplemented to avoid deficiency states.
- *Pruritus.* Itching may be very severe, and may be reduced by cholestyramine.
- *Liver transplantation.* This is increasingly becoming a therapeutic resort in end-stage liver diseases. Surgery is limited to a few national centres.

Parasites

The commonest parasite causing diarrhoea in Britain is *Giardia lamblia*, which commonly causes outbreaks in day-care nurseries. It is endemic in some overseas holiday destinations and infection may be related to travel abroad.

Clinical features   The infected child may either be asymptomatic or have a combination of diarrhoea, weight loss and abdominal pain. The diagnosis is made on microscopic examination of the stool. Three separate specimens are required as excretion of the cysts can be irregular. The blood count may show eosinophilia, and the parasite can be

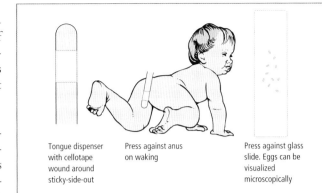

Tongue dispenser with cellotape wound around sticky-side-out

Press against anus on waking

Press against glass slide. Eggs can be visualized microscopically

Figure 11.9 The sticky-tape test for threadworms.

detected in duodenal aspirate (obtained when jejunal biopsy is undertaken for coeliac disease).

Management and prognosis   Treatment is with metronidazole, and in an outbreak, asymptomatic carriers should be treated. Treatment failure is common.

Threadworms or pinworms (enterobiasis)

Threadworm infection causes intense itching of the anus and occasionally the vulval area. It is a common infestation particularly affecting preschool children. The threadworms reside in the gut, and the gravid females migrate by night to the perianal region to deposit their eggs. Scratching transmits the eggs to the fingers and the eggs become disseminated and ingested.

Clinical features   The infestation may be asymptomatic or may be recognised if a child is seen to be scratching or complains of itching or anal pain.

Management   The diagnosis can sometimes be made by examining the anal area during itching, when a tiny (5 mm) white worm may be seen. Alternately, the sticky-tape test can be applied (Figure 11.9). Sticky-tape is applied around the end of a tongue depressor, with the sticky side outermost. This is placed against the child's anus on rising in the morning, and then applied to a glass slide. The threadworm eggs can then be visualized microscopically. Examination of stool specimens does not identify threadworms. Treatment consists of a single dose of mebendazole. The whole family may need to be treated. Reinfection is very common.

To test your knowledge on this part of the book, please see Chapter 26.

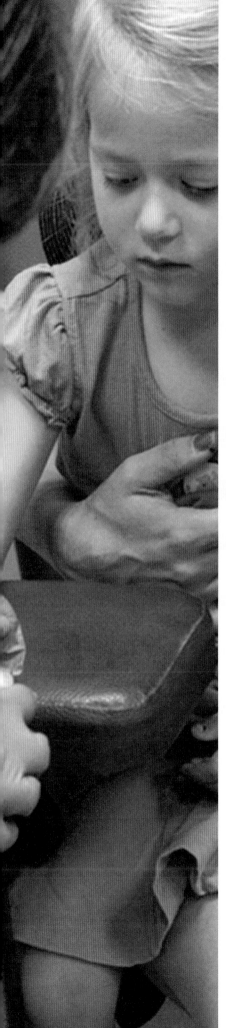

CHAPTER 12

Cardiac disorders

Who could refrain that had a heart to love and in that heart courage to make love known?

Macbeth, William Shakespeare

KEY COMPETENCES

YOU MUST ...

Know and understand

- The clinical features and differential diagnosis of children presenting with heart murmurs, cyanosis and fainting or syncope
- The anatomical and physiological bases of congenital heart disease
- How to diagnose and manage cardiac conditions in children: acquired, congenital, syncope and heart failure

Be able to

- Carry out a good cardiac examination
- Differentiate clinically between innocent and pathological murmurs
- Clinically distinguish between syncope and other fits, faints and funny turns
- Explain the diagnosis of an innocent murmur to a family

Appreciate that

- Most incidental murmurs in childhood are innocent but they may induce parental anxiety
- Most chest pain in children is of non-cardiac origin

Essential Paediatrics and Child Health, Fourth Edition. Mary Rudolf, Anthony Luder and Kerry Jeavons.
© 2020 John Wiley & Sons Ltd. Published 2020 by John Wiley & Sons Ltd.
Companion website: www.wiley.com/go/rudolf/paediatrics

Cardiac symptoms and signs

Finding your way around ...

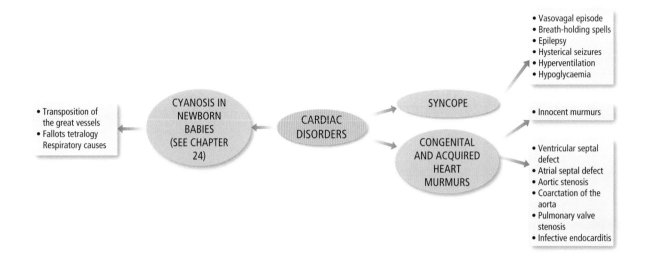

Heart murmurs

Heart murmurs are very common in childhood. About 30% of children have flow related murmurs heard at some time. These are not associated with significant haemodynamic abnormalities and are referred to as normal, insignificant, functional or innocent (preferred). An innocent murmur can be distinguished from a pathological one on clinical grounds and investigations are not normally necessary. It is therefore important to learn to distinguish clinically an innocent murmur from a murmur caused by cardiac malformation or disease (Box 12.1). This can save the child from unnecessary investigations and the family from anxiety. If you suspect that a murmur might be pathological, you should look for signs and symptoms of cyanosis or cardiac failure

Box 12.1 Causes of cardiac murmurs

Innocent murmurs	Commoner pathological murmurs
Systolic ejection	Ventricular septal defect
Venous hum	Atrial septal defect
Vibratory murmur	Aortic stenosis
	Coarctation of the aorta
	Pulmonary valve stenosis
	Patent ductus arteriosus
	Fallot tetralogy
	Mitral valve incompetence

Ventricular septal defect (VSD) at a glance

Epidemiology
Commonest congenital heart lesion

Aetiology/pathophysiology
Clinical features depend on the size of the VSD
There is no correlation between loudness of murmur and size of shunt

Presentation
Murmur usually detected at routine examination

History
Most asymptomatic
Breathlessness on feeding and crying*
Failure to thrive*
Recurrent chest infections*

Physical examination
- Harsh pansystolic murmur at lower left sternal border
- Clinically enlarged heart*
- Parasternal thrill*
- Radiation of murmur over whole chest*
- Signs of congestive heart failure*

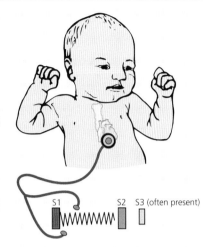

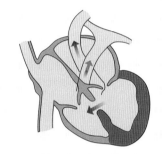

Investigations
Small defect: normal chest X-ray and ECG
Large defect: cardiomegaly and large pulmonary arteries on X-ray, biventricular hypertrophy on ECG
Echocardiography confirms the diagnosis

Differential diagnosis
See Clues box on p. 220
See Table 12.1

Management
Reassurance for small defects
Treatment of cardiac failure if present
Surgery if medical management fails

Prognosis/complications
Small defects tend to close spontaneously
Excellent prognosis for larger defects after surgery
Increased pulmonary blood flow through an uncorrected large VSD causes pulmonary hypertension (cor pulmonale) with reduced life-span

NB *Signs and symptoms are variable

History – must ask!

- *Does the baby or child have symptoms of heart failure?* Fatigue and breathlessness are the most important symptoms of cardiac failure. A baby in heart failure becomes short of breath on sucking and feeds poorly. An older child tires on walking and may become breathless too. A child may have episodes of cold sweats, pallor and unexplained irritability.
- *Have the parents noticed cyanosis?* Peripheral cyanosis may signify poor peripheral flow whereas central cyanosis may be caused by a right-to-left shunt.
- *Is there a family history of congenital heart disease?* There is a higher risk of heart defects in siblings of children with congenital heart disease. Asking about the family history can help you appreciate the level of anxiety about the murmur.

Physical examination – must check!

The cardiac examination is discussed in more detail on pp. 76–9, but the salient points are highlighted here:

- *Neck and precordium.* Check for displaced apex, thrills and parasternal heave. Jugular venous pulse may be visible in older children.
- *The murmur.* Pathological and innocent murmurs are graded for intensity (1–6), and should be classified for location, radiation, quality, type, accentuating or ameliorating features, associated auscultory findings and associated other findings. (Table 12.1). Note that congenital heart disease may have no or very mild murmurs.
- *Growth.* Failure to thrive and poor growth are important signs of cardiac failure in childhood, and are also important in monitoring medical management.

Table 12.1 Characteristics of innocent and pathological murmurs

Innocent	Pathological
Mid-systolic or continuous (venous hum). Normal second sound, no added clicks	Mid or pansystolic, diastolic, continuous (PDA). Often clicks and abnormal second sounds.
Musical, humming or vibratory quality	Harsh or long
Left sternal border, neck, upper chest. No radiation	A thrill, cardiomegaly or cardiac symptoms always indicate a pathological murmur
May vary in intensity with posture, head position or respiration	
Asymptomatic	
Normal peripheral pulses	

- **_Vital signs._** Tachycardia is a sign of cardiac failure. The character of the pulse can also give a clue to cardiac pathology. Palpate the femoral pulses, as in coarctation of the aorta they are absent or weak and delayed compared with the radial pulse. Take the blood pressure, and if you suspect coarctation you need to do this in both arms and legs.
- **_Other signs of heart failure._** Tachypnoea, hepatomegaly and crepitations in the lungs are the major clinical manifestations of cardiac failure in childhood. Peripheral oedema is rare.
- **_Cyanosis._** Cyanosis is unlikely in a child presenting with a cardiac murmur, but if present suggests serious disease.

Key points: Cardiac murmurs

- Describe the murmur
- Describe the heart sounds
- Look for signs and symptoms of heart failure, including failure to thrive
- Examination of the heart is not limited to murmurs!

Clues to the clinical diagnosis of some pathological cardiac murmurs

	Characteristics of the murmur	Associated clinical features
Ventricular septal defect	Loud harsh pansystolic murmur at left sternal border, radiating all over the chest	If severe: heart failure, failure to thrive and recurrent chest infections
Atrial septal defect	Soft systolic murmur in second left intercostal space, wide fixed splitting of the second sound	
Aortic stenosis	Systolic ejection murmur at right upper sternal border, radiating to the neck and down the left sternal border, Often associated with systolic clicks. Pulse pressure may be reduced. Second sound may be single.	Exercise-induced dizziness and loss of consciousness in a minority of older children
Coarctation	Systolic murmur over the left side of the chest, especially at the back	Absent or delayed weak femoral pulses. Hypertension in arms, commonly the right.
Pulmonary stenosis	Systolic ejection murmur over the upper part of left chest anteriorly and conducted to the back, usually preceded by an ejection click. May be heard in axillae. Second sound may be widely split but not fixed.	May be associated with cyanosis if more than mild
Patent ductus arteriosus	Pansystolic murmur in neonates. Continuous murmur after 3 months of age	Collapsing pulse

Investigations

Investigations are only required if the murmur is thought to be pathological. A chest X-ray provides information about cardiac size, laterality and shape as well as pulmonary vascularity. The electrocardiograph (ECG) gives further information about chamber dominance and rhythm disturbances such as heart block. Echocardiography is important in evaluating cardiac structure and performance, gradients across stenotic valves and the direction of flow across a shunt. Cardiac catheterisation is now rarely required for diagnosis, although many lesions can now be treated by catheter without the need for open surgery.

Management of the child with a murmur

If the murmur is thought to be innocent, discuss its lack of significance with the parents. Reassure them fully so that lingering doubts do not generate anxiety and overprotectiveness. It is helpful to describe that the murmur is simply a 'noise' ('like water flowing out of a tap') and does not indicate the presence of a cardiac defect. In general, no investigations are required. If a murmur is considered to be pathological, investigation is required.

Cyanosis

All babies are cyanosed at birth before they take their first breath, but they should rapidly (within minutes) become a healthy pink colour. Many older infants will present with concerns regarding a transient bluish discolouration of the lips or around the mouth, lasting just a few seconds, and often associated with feeding or crying. If the infant is otherwise well, thriving on the centiles, and has a normal examination and oxygen saturations, the parents should be reassured. Mongolian blue spots should be distinguished from cyanosis.

Of greater concern is persistent cyanosis. This is usually most obviously noted in the lips and tongue, but can be difficult to spot, particularly in newborn babies or children with dark skin. Children who have had persistent cyanosis for some time may also have digital clubbing. It is not unusual for babies with congenital cyanotic heart disease to present with oxygen saturations of 60–70%. Administration of oxygen generally makes little or no difference to this saturation, in contrast to cyanosis caused by respiratory problems. Isolated peripheral cyanosis of the hands and feet in a well child (acrocyanosis) is usually of little significance.

Fainting / syncope

Online Interactive Q10

Fainting or syncope is quite a common symptom, particularly in teenage girls. It occurs when there is hypotension and decreased cerebral perfusion. Individuals with poor vasomotor reflexes can faint on standing up rapidly or during prolonged standing (postural hypotension). It is distinguished from other fits, faints and funny turns (see p. 230) by preceding blurring or dimming of vision, light-headedness, sweating and nausea. There are no tonic or clonic movements. Consciousness is rapidly regained on lying flat. Cardiac disease is an uncommon cause of syncope in otherwise well children or adolescents. Clues to the possible existence of a cardiac problem include an abnormal cardiac examination or if the faint occurred during or just after exercise, if the faint occurred in a sitting or lying posture and if there is underlying chronic disease or acute infection, if palpitations or precordial discomfort are reported or if there is a family history of cardiac disease or premature death.

🔍 Clues to the differential diagnosis of syncope

	Characteristic features	Precipitating event	EEG
Vaso-vagal syncopal attacks	Blurred vision, light-headedness, sweating and nausea, resolves on lying down	Painful or emotional stimulus, prolonged standing	Normal*
Postural hypotension	Adolescents; May be associated with dizziness, nausea and seeing 'black'	Frequently after rising from lying, or prolonged standing	Normal*
Hyperventilation	Excessive deep breathing, sometimes tetany. Resolves on breathing into a paper bag	Excitement, fear	Normal*
Breath-holding spells	Toddlers. May appear pale or dusky	Pain, anger, frustration	Normal*
Convulsions	Antegrade and retrograde amnesia; Tachycardia and irregular breathing; tonic, clonic or jerky movements; pre-ictal aura and postictal phase	Uncommonly stress, fatigue, strobe lights or loud noise Mostly spontaneous	Abnormal
Pseudo-seizures	Gradual onset, asynchronous flailing movements, no incontinence or postictal state	Often an emotional stimulus	Normal unless the child has in addition genuine epilepsy

* EEG not required to make the diagnosis.

Cardiac signs and conditions

Innocent (functional) murmurs

These murmurs are commonly heard in children and have no clinical significance. Figure 12.1 shows the sites where they are best heard.

Aortic flow murmur

This is a short systolic murmur occurring during left ventricular ejection and heard along the left sternal edge, second right intercostal space or at the apex. It is musical in character, frequently sounding like the vibration of a tuning fork. It lessens in intensity when the child changes from lying to sitting or standing and is intensified by fever, excitement or exercise. Aortic murmurs that increase in intensity on sitting or standing should be distinguished as they may indicate organic disease such as hypertrophic cardiomyopathy.

Pulmonary flow murmur

This is also a systolic ejection murmur is caused by rapid flow of blood across a normal pulmonary valve. It is a brief, high-pitched, blowing murmur, best heard in the second left intercostal space with the child lying down.

Venous hum

A venous hum is caused by flow through the systemic great veins. It is a blowing, continuous murmur heard at the base of the heart just below the clavicles, sounding like a soft hum during both systole and diastole. It varies with positioning of the head and disappears when the child lies down.

Defects causing a left to right shunt

The commonest defects occur between the two sides of the heart at the level of the ventricles or atria, which permit the shunting of blood from the left to the right side of the heart across a normal pressure gradient. If the hole is large and allows a considerable volume of blood to be shunted, an added burden is imposed on the heart, and hypertrophy, dilatation and failure result. Cardiomegaly with a prominent pulmonary

artery and increased vascular markings on chest X-ray may be seen together with signs of ventricular hypertrophy on the ECG. Echocardiography is diagnostic.

Atrial septal defect (see Figure 12.2)

As the murmur is soft, it may not be detected until the child starts school.

Clinical features   The systolic murmur, which is heard in the second left interspace, is caused by high flow across the normal pulmonary valve and not by flow across the defect. Characteristically the second heart sound is widely split and is 'fixed' (does not vary with respiration). Occasionally the child may experience breathlessness, tiredness on exertion, or recurrent chest infections. These signs may be subtle and easily missed. Irreversible pulmonary hypertension ('Eisenmenger syndrome') may result.

Management   If the defect is moderate or large, closure is carried out using an occluding device placed by cardiac catheterisation, or by open heart surgery.

Prognosis   The prognosis following surgery is good. If untreated, cardiac symptoms often develop in the second decade of life or later.

Ventricular septal defect (see Figure 12.3)

This is the commonest of all congenital heart lesions.

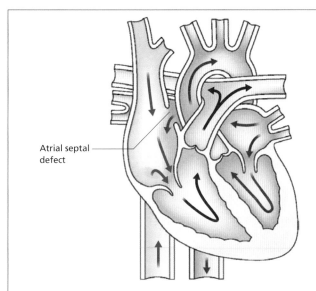

Figure 12.2 Atrial septal defect: high flow through the pulmonary valve causes a systolic murmur. *Source:* © British Heart Foundation 2008.

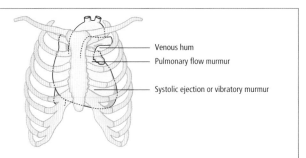

Figure 12.1 Sites of innocent cardiac murmurs.

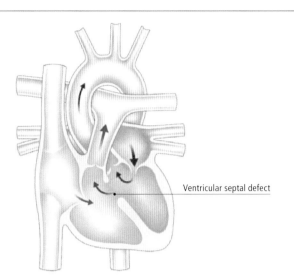

Figure 12.3 Ventricular septal defect: blood flows through the defect to the right side of the heart leading to pulmonary hypertension, cardiomegaly and prominent pulmonary arteries. *Source:* © British Heart Foundation 2008.

Ventricular septal defect

Clinical features   The clinical features depend on the size of the defect. If it is small the child is asymptomatic. A larger defect causes breathlessness on feeding and crying, failure to thrive, and recurrent chest infections. On auscultation a harsh pansystolic murmur is heard at the lower left sternal border. Where there are large defects the heart is enlarged clinically, a thrill is present, and the murmur radiates over the whole chest. The child may have signs of congestive heart failure and be severely ill. Cardiac failure does not occur immediately following birth as the pulmonary vascular resistance is initially high, inhibiting a left to right shunt. A soft murmur may indicate a small or paradoxically very large defect.

Investigations   If the defect is small, the chest X-ray and ECG are normal. The child with a large defect will have cardiomegaly and large pulmonary arteries on X-ray and demonstrate

biventricular hypertrophy on ECG. Echocardiography confirms the diagnosis.

Management   Small defects usually close spontaneously and the parents can be reassured of their benign nature. Initial management of large defects is medical and aimed at control of the cardiac failure. If the child does not respond, surgical treatment is required. Recent guidelines have removed most cardiac lesions from the list of those requiring prophylactic antibiotics before dental and surgical procedures.

Prognosis and complications   Small defects tend to close spontaneously, or may remain the same size but become insignificant as the child grows. For larger defects, the prognosis after surgery is excellent. If a large ventricular septal defect is uncorrected, pulmonary hypertension can result from the increased pulmonary blood flow, making the defect inoperable ('Eisenmenger syndrome') and reducing the child's lifespan (cor pulmonale).

Obstructive lesions

Obstructive lesions occasionally occur at the pulmonary and aortic valves and along the aorta, causing hypertrophy in the chamber of the heart proximal to the lesion. If the obstruction is severe, heart failure may develop.

Aortic stenosis

Aortic stenosis (Figure 12.4) may occur in isolation or in combination with other heart defects. It may be sub-valvular, valvular or supra-valvular. Some bicuspid valves become stenotic with time.

Clinical features   In most cases aortic stenosis is identified by discovery of a heart murmur on routine examination, although in severe cases heart failure may develop in infancy. Some older children may become symptomatic, experiencing faintness or dizziness on exertion. The systolic ejection murmur is heard at the right upper sternal border and radiates to the neck and down the left sternal border. The murmur may be preceded by an ejection click and the aortic second sound is

Congenital heart disease at a glance

Epidemiology
7–8 infants per 1000 live births
Commonest lesion is a
    ventricular septal defect (VSD)

Aetiology/pathophysiology
Genetic and environmental
    factors are implicated

How the diagnosis is made
Most children are identified by
    routine detection of a heart
    murmur
Others present with heart
    failure, cyanosis or on
    antenatal screening
Diagnoses are confirmed by
    CXR, ECG, echocardiography
    and cardiac catheterisation

Clinical features
Heart murmur: distinctive
    features of pathological
    murmurs are described in
    Table 10.1 and box: Clues to
    the clinical diagnosis of
    pathological cardiac murmurs
- **Cyanosis:** central cyanosis is
    seen on the tongue and lips.
    Clubbing, polycythaemia,
    reduced exercise tolerance
    and failure to thrive are seen
    with long-standing cyanosis
- **Heart failure:** breathlessness,
    sweating, poor feeding,
    recurrent chestiness, failure to
    thrive, tachypnoea, tachycar-
    dia, enlarged heart,
    hepatomegaly (not oedema in
    childhood)

NB *Signs and symptoms are variable

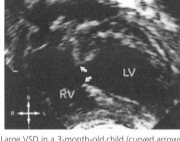
Large VSD in a 3-month-old child (curved arrows)

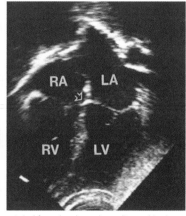
Apical four-chamber echocardiographic view

General management
- Most defects are amenable to
    corrective or palliative surgery
- Heart failure is treated with
    diuretics, ACE inhibitors or
    digoxin
- Prophylaxis against infective
    endocarditis is considered
    especially for cyanotic and
    post-surgical heart disease
- Nutritional supplements if
    child is failing to thrive
- **Education:**
Advise regarding anxiety and
    overprotection
Children with severe disease
    self-restrict activity naturally
Contraceptive advice for
    teenage girls
- **School:**
Need to be aware of any
    limitations in activity
Special arrangements for
    physical education when
    necessary

Points for routine follow-up
- Growth
- Signs or symptoms of cardiac
    failure
- Evidence of infective
    endocarditis

Prognosis
Good after repair of simple
    lesions (e.g. PDA, ASD, PS)
Restricted lifestyle following
    palliative procedures for
    complex heart disease

soft and delayed. The peripheral pulse is of small volume and the blood pressure may be low. A thrill may be palpable at the lower left sternal border and in the suprasternal notch over the carotid arteries.

Investigations   The chest X-ray may show a prominent left ventricle and prominence of the ascending aorta. Left ventricular hypertrophy is found on ECG. Echocardiography is useful in evaluating the exact site and severity of the obstruction.

Management   If the stenosis is severe it is relieved by balloon valvuloplasty – a catheter tip is passed through the aortic valve from the femoral artery and a balloon inflated to widen the stenosed valve. If this is unsuccessful, open heart surgery is required.

Prognosis   Children with aortic stenosis are at risk for sudden death, and so this is the one congenital heart lesion in which strenuous activity should be avoided. If surgery is carried out in childhood, reoperation is often required at a later date.

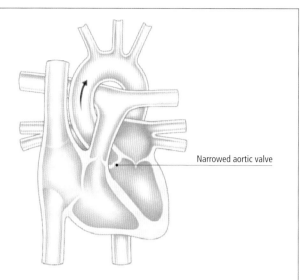

Figure 12.4 Aortic stenosis. The stenosis causes enlargement of the left ventricle and prominence of the ascending aorta. *Source:* © British Heart Foundation 2008.

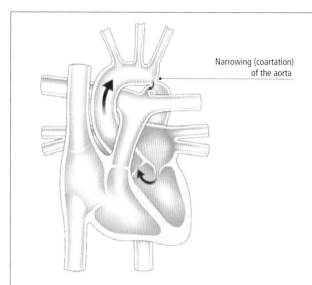

Figure 12.5 Coarctation of the aorta. Blood flow to the lower limbs is maintained through a patent ductus arteriosus. *Source:* © British Heart Foundation 2008.

Coarctation of the aorta

This is a localized constriction of the aorta, usually occurring at the origin of the ductus arteriosus (Figure 12.5). A fraction of the arterial blood bypasses the constriction, reaching the lower half of the body through collateral vessels which enlarge. The left ventricle hypertrophies to overcome the obstruction, and heart failure may result. In severe cases the baby may present with collapse at the end of the first week of life when the ductus arteriosus (through which systemic blood flow has been maintained) closes (p. 449).

Clinical features   The systolic murmur is usually heard over the left side of the chest, especially at the back. The cardinal sign of coarctation is disparity in the pulses and blood pressure of the arms and legs. The right brachial and radial pulses are normal, but the left brachial and femoral pulses are absent or weak and delayed. Hypertension is found in the right arm, but not when measured in the left arm or legs.

Investigations   The left ventricle may be prominent on X-ray, and rib notching may be seen where enlarged intercostal arteries have eroded the underside of the ribs. An ECG may show left ventricular hypertrophy. Echocardiography is diagnostic.

Management   Surgery to resect the narrowed section of the aorta is required as soon as the diagnosis is made.

Prognosis and complications   Following surgery, narrowing may recur at the resected site and surgery is then required again. If the coarctation is left untreated, serious complications related to hypertension develop.

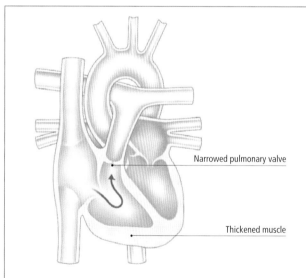

Figure 12.6 Pulmonary stenosis. The right ventricle hypertrophies to overcome the obstruction presented by stenosis of the pulmonary valve. *Source:* © British Heart Foundation 2008.

Pulmonary stenosis

See Figure 12.6. In this condition the pulmonary valve is thickened and stenosed, and the right ventricle hypertrophies to overcome the obstruction.

Clinical features   A short ejection systolic murmur is heard over the upper part of the left chest anteriorly and is conducted to the back. It is usually preceded by an ejection click. With mild or moderate stenosis there are usually no symptoms, and the heart is of a normal size. In more severe stenosis a systolic thrill is palpable in the pulmonary area.

Investigations   On chest X-ray, dilatation of the pulmonary artery is seen beyond the stenosis and, if severe, an enlarged right atrium and ventricle. The ECG shows right axis deviation, and right atrial and ventricular hypertrophy.

Management   The extent of the stenosis can be demonstrated by echocardiography and cardiac catheterisation. If it is severe, balloon valvuloplasty is performed.

Prognosis   Surgery is generally successful and further procedures are rarely required.

Congenital cyanotic heart disease

Transposition of the great vessels

Transposition of the great vessels (Figure 12.7) is the commonest cause of congenital cyanotic heart disease presenting in the neonatal period. In transposition of the great vessels, the aorta arises from the right ventricular outflow tract and the pulmonary artery from the left ventricle. Mixing of venous and arterial blood occurs through the ductus arteriosus and often through a septal defect which may accompany this condition. The less mixing of blood occurs between the two circulations, the more intensely cyanosed the baby appears.

Clinical features   The cyanosis may be difficult to spot, particularly in anaemic babies and those with dark skin, but affected infants often appear pale and there may be difficulty

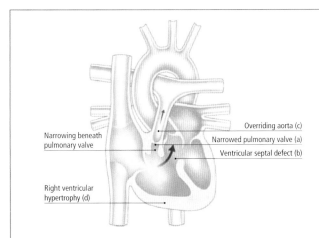

Figure 12.8 Fallot tetralogy. (a) Pulmonary stenosis; (b) ventricular septal defect with shunt; (c) overriding aorta; (d) right ventricular hypertrophy. *Source:* © British Heart Foundation 2008.

establishing feeds. Transcutaneous pulse oximetry should be performed to confirm the cyanosis, and the condition is diagnosed by X-ray (a narrow cardiac pedicle) and by echocardiography.

Management   Surgery offers the opportunity of cure by switching the origins of the pulmonary artery and aorta. Emergency treatment of a severely cyanosed child with poor systemic circulation is by an infusion of prostaglandin to maintain the ductus open, and many babies will also need an emergency balloon septostomy to improve mixing of blood within the heart.

Fallot tetralogy

Fallot tetralogy (Figure 12.8) refers to a cardiac anomaly involving four characteristic features:
- ventricular septal defect;
- overriding of the aorta;
- infundibular pulmonary stenosis;
- right ventricular hypertrophy.

This condition, rarely diagnosed in the newborn, presents with cyanosis at about 3 months of age, often in acute spells. A characteristic sign in older children is 'squatting', a manoeuvre the child learns can reduce cyanosis (by increasing systemic resistance and pressure, thus reducing right-left shunting). The treatment is surgical, and the prognosis is generally good.

Infective endocarditis

Although rare in childhood, infective endocarditis is a serious condition that can have a poor outcome, particularly if the diagnosis is delayed. Children with cyanotic congenital heart disease, artificial valves or devices, or an indwelling central venous catheter are at greatest risk. The usual organisms are streptococci and staphylococci.

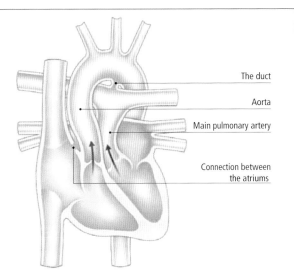

Figure 12.7 Transposition of the great vessels. The pulmonary artery arises from the left ventricle and the aorta from the right. The open ductus allows mixing of the blood. *Source:* © British Heart Foundation 2008.

Clinical features   There is often a gradual onset of malaise and temperatures over a few weeks, although presentation can occur more acutely. On examination fever, a new or changing murmur, petechiae, splinter haemorrhages, and hepatosplenomegaly may be seen. Heart failure may occur, and septic emboli may cause systemic, particularly neurological, complications. The most important investigation is to perform multiple blood cultures before commencing antibiotic treatment, as it is important to determine the causal organism and perform antibiotic susceptibility testing. Echocardiography may show vegetations.

Management   Complete eradication of the infection is required, and appropriate intravenous antibiotics are given for 4–8 weeks. Recent guidelines have redefined the indications for prophylaxis to prevent this condition before dental or certain 'dirty' surgical procedures. Especially important are cyanotic heart disease, a previous history of endocarditis or various post-surgical states.

Syncope (see p.221)

Syncope, or fainting, occurs when there is hypotension and decreased cerebral perfusion. Syncope is quite common, particularly in teenage girls reacting to painful or emotional stimuli. It also occurs in the teenage years in individuals with poor vasomotor reflexes who faint on standing up rapidly or during prolonged standing. Other causes include cardiac dysrhythmia or dysfunction and metabolic upsets.

Clinical features   Blurring of vision, light-headedness, sweating and nausea precede the loss of consciousness which is rapidly regained on lying flat. There may be a history of an unpleasant stimulus or prolonged standing.

Management and prognosis   The evaluation should therefore include a clinical cardiac examination, standing and lying blood pressure and an ECG if there is any doubt as to the cause of the faint. Simple syncope usually becomes less of a problem in adulthood. Syncope occurring with exercise or associated with chest pain is likely to have a cardiac cause and should be urgently referred to a cardiologist.

Heart failure

Heart failure is a syndrome caused by failure of the heart to deliver sufficient oxygen and nutrients to the tissues. The causes are age dependent: in utero severe anaemia (Rhesus incompatibility) and cardiomyopathy; in neonates congenital heart disease, metabolic disorders, systemic infection and respiratory disorders; in toddlers large VSDs, coarctation of aorta, aortic stenosis, dysrhythmias, hypertension and renal disease; in adolescence illicit drugs, cardiomyopathy, myocarditis and ischaemic heart disease (rare).

Clinical features   Tachypnoea, retractions, grunting, sweating, and feeding problems reflect respiratory distress in babies, whereas hepatomegaly and sometimes ascites are the result of systemic venous hypertension. In older children fainting, oedema, and jugular venous distention may be seen. Heart examination will frequently reveal tachycardia and a gallop rhythm (with a third heart sound). Chronic failure may lead to poor growth.

Investigations   Cardiac troponins and muscle enzymes such as CPK and GOT may be abnormal. A blood count may reveal signs of infection and anaemia. Electrolytes, blood gases, and renal function should be evaluated. A chest X-ray will show cardiomegaly and any abnormal heart shadows or location. The ECG reveals rate and rhythm, and signs of chamber dilatation and strain. Myocarditis, ischaemia and pulmonary disease all have specific signs and patterns. Echocardiography shows details of structure and function. Cardiac catheterisation or special diagnostic and genetic tests may be needed.

Management and prognosis   The mainstays of therapy include oxygen, diuretics (to reduce pre-load), inotropic drugs (like dopamine and digoxin) to improve heart muscle contractility, beta-blockers to improve efficiency, and angiotensin-converting-enzyme (ACE) inhibitors and vasodilators to reduce after load. Anti-dysrhythmics, pacing, and cardioversion are used for severe brady- and tachyarrythmias. Other treatment, including surgery and special drugs depend on the cause. Heart failure can often be treated successfully in childhood and, in general, the outlook is optimistic in most cases.

To test your knowledge on this part of the book, please see Chapter 26.

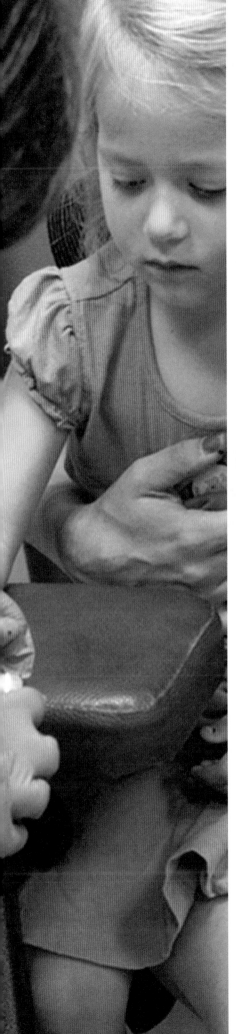

CHAPTER 13
Neurological disorders

> It is thus with regard to the disease called Sacred: it appears to me to be nowise more divine nor more sacred than other diseases, but has a natural cause like other affections …
>
> *Hippocrates, 400BC* (on epilepsy)

KEY COMPETENCES

YOU MUST...

Know and understand

- The differential diagnosis of children presenting with fits, faints and funny turns, headaches, weakness and squint
- The causes and characteristics of cerebral palsy and how it differs from progressive neurological disease
- The range of congenital disorders of the CNS including spina bifida, microcephaly and hydrocephalus
- How epilepsy is managed – both acutely and over the long term, and the principle of a monotherapy approach to anticonvulsants
- The signs and clinical presentation of raised intracranial pressure
- The approach to managing effectively a child with functional headaches
- The principles of managing head injuries in children

Be able to

- Perform and interpret an age –appropriate neurological examination
- Take a full history from a child with epilepsy, including the impact on family and school life
- Place a child who is fitting in the recovery position
- Use DESSCRIBE to summarize the diagnostic process for paroxysmal events
- Recognise indicators of serious pathology when a child presents with headache, weakness or focal signs

Appreciate

- Fits, faints and funny turns, although usually benign, generate great anxiety
- Epilepsy has an impact on the child and family
- Most recurrent headaches in childhood are non-organic, but require medical attention and follow up too
- Head injury and concussion may lead to prolonged and disabling symptoms

Essential Paediatrics and Child Health, Fourth Edition. Mary Rudolf, Anthony Luder and Kerry Jeavons.
© 2020 John Wiley & Sons Ltd. Published 2020 by John Wiley & Sons Ltd.
Companion website: www.wiley.com/go/rudolf/paediatrics

Neurological symptoms and signs

Finding your way around ...

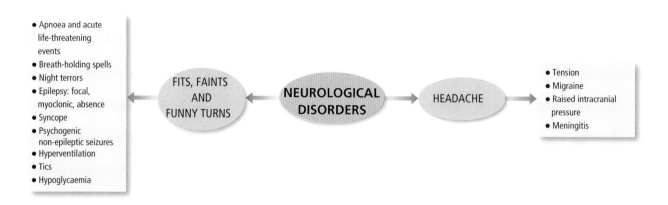

Fits, faints and funny turns

Box 13.1 Types of fits, faints and funny turns at different ages

In infancy	Beyond infancy	School age
Apnoea and brief, resolved, unexplained events (BRUEs)	Febrile seizures	Epilepsies
Febrile seizures	Breath-holding	Syncope
Breath-holding and periodic breathing	• cyanotic spells	Hyperventilation
Epileptic spasms (West Syndrome)	• pallid spells	Psychogenic non-epileptic seizures
Epilepsies	Night terrors	Tics
Hypoglycaemia and metabolic conditions	Epilepsies	
	Benign paroxysmal vertigo	

Children can present with a variety of episodes associated with transient altered consciousness. The term 'fits, faints and funny turns' tends to refer to episodes which present after the event is over and may be recurrent; rather than generalised tonic–clonic seizures or reduced consciousness presenting as a medical emergency (see pp. 410–15). The presentation of these problems varies with different stages of childhood; therefore, it is best to consider them according to age at onset (Box 13.1). Many of these attacks are benign, but they can arouse considerable concern.

Metabolic disorders should be considered in infants and toddlers presenting with paroxysmal episodes, especially when drowsiness is present. A blood glucose should be checked at the acute presentation and further tests may be required (e.g. liver function tests, ammonia, blood gas,

lumbar puncture, lactate, amino and organic acids). Features which may alert you to the possibility of a metabolic disorder would include significant vomiting, developmental impairment, dysmorphic features, hepatosplenomegaly, micro- or macrocephaly or consanguinity.

Young babies not uncommonly present with episodes of having been found limp, choking or twitching – this is labelled as a brief, resolved, unexplained episode (BRUE). The concern lies in whether a cardiac arrhythmia, convulsion or reflux episode has precipitated the event. More often than not, the babies are admitted to hospital for observation and discharged after an uneventful night. If these episodes recur, a serious cause needs to be excluded.

In school-age children parents and teachers commonly raise concerns over 'funny spells' that they have observed in children at home and in the classroom. As the child is rarely observed by the doctor, the history is of paramount importance. You should make every effort to obtain the history from a witness rather than a second-hand version and videos of the episodes from smart phones can be very useful in establishing a diagnosis.

History – must ask!

- *What was the episode like?* When you take the history, it helps to visualize the episodes as they are described and then 'replay' the event back to the witness to make sure that you have obtained an accurate picture. Clarify further details, such as head or eye deviation, whether eyes were open or closed, and other features which the witness may not have mentioned. It is important to establish what the child was doing at the onset, and whether there are any precipitating factors. Other important information includes:
  - the length of the episode;
  - loss of or alteration in consciousness;
  - a description and demonstration of any involuntary movements;
  - change in colour, whether pallor or cyanosis;
  - the reaction of the child to the event;
  - whether the child was sleepy afterwards.
- *Developmental history.* A developmental evaluation is particularly important if you are considering epileptic spasms or metabolic conditions.
- *Family history.* A family history of epilepsy, developmental problems, febrile seizures, consanguinity and metabolic disorders may be relevant.

Physical examination – must check!

The physical examination is rarely helpful in between episodes, which is another reason why the history is so important. You do, however, need to carry out a careful cardiac and neurological examination. Dysmorphic features, micro- or macrocephaly and hepatosplenomegaly are suggestive of a metabolic disorder.

Investigations

The diagnosis of an episode is essentially clinical (see the two Clues boxes on the differential diagnosis of fits, faints and funny turns). Investigations are rarely helpful, although they must be considered if apnoea, cardiac arrhythmia, epilepsy or a metabolic problem is suspected. The appropriate investigations are discussed in the relevant sections. Electroencephalograms (EEGs) should only be used to support a clinical diagnosis of epilepsy. An electrocardiogram (ECG) should be carried out following any motor seizure.

 Key points: Diagnosing fits, faints and funny turns

- Decide on the basis of the history what type of episode has occurred
- Only carry out investigations if merited by the nature of the episode

---

Clues to the differential diagnosis of fits, faints and funny turns in infants and preschool children

	Characteristic features	Precipitating event	Investigations
Apnoea and BRUE	Usually found limp or twitching	None apparent	Depends on cause
Breath-holding spells (cyanotic)	Stops breathing, becomes cyanotic and stiff, may lose consciousness. Then becomes limp and breathes normally	Always precipitated by crying, such as from pain or anger	ECG normal
Reflex anoxic spells (pallid)	Turns pale and collapses. Rapid recovery	Bump on head or other minor injury	ECG normal
Night terrors	Wakes from sleep disorientated and frightened. May be autonomic signs	Sleep	
Benign paroxysmal vertigo	Sudden unsteadiness. Frightened and clings to parent. No postictal state	None	
Epileptic spasms (West Syndrome)	Epileptic spasms occurring in clusters. Developmental arrest or regression	Spasms often occur on waking	Hypsarrhythmia on EEG
Epilepsies	As for the school-age child		Depends on cause

(Continued)

Clues to the differential diagnosis of fits, faints and funny turns in the school-age child

	Characteristic features	Precipitating event	Investigations
Syncope	Blurred vision, light-headedness, pallor, sweating and nausea, resolves on lying down	Painful or emotional stimulus, prolonged standing	ECG normal including QTc
Hyperventilation	Excessive deep breathing, sometimes tetany. Resolves on breathing into a paper bag	Excitement or fear	
Psychogenic non-epileptic seizures	Gradual onset, asynchronous flailing movements, no incontinence or postictal state	Often an emotional stimulus	ECG normal
Tics	Rapid, repetitive, brief, involuntary movements which can be voluntarily controlled	Anxiety and fatigue	
Absence seizures	Fleeting vacant look, may have automatisms	None	EEG shows 3-per-second spike and wave activity
Myoclonic seizures	Shock-like jerks, which can cause sudden falls. Most common in children with known neurological condition	None	EEG abnormal
Focal motor seizures	Twitching or jerking of face, arm or leg	None	EEG and MRI brain may be abnormal
Temporal lobe seizures	Altered or impaired consciousness with strange sensations such as déjà vu, abdominal sensations or hallucinations	None	EEG and MRI brain may be abnormal

Headaches

Causes of headache

Tension headache
Migraine
Cluster headache
Raised intracranial pressure
Hypertension
Dental caries
Infection
Meningitis (acute)
Haemorrhage (rare)
Tumour (rare)
(Eye strain)

Children may present with acute onset of severe headache or, more commonly, a history of recurrent headaches. If the headache is acute and severe and the child ill, the possibility of serious pathology must be considered and intracranial infection (p. 235), haemorrhage (p. 246) or tumour (p. 53) excluded. Meningitis may present with a severe acute headache in a febrile child. Bacterial and viral meningitis is described on p. 235.

An underlying cause for recurrent headaches is rarely found, and the diagnosis of tension headaches can generally be confidently diagnosed on clinical evaluation. They are distinguishable from migraine by their character and lack of associated features. Hypertension is usually asymptomatic in childhood, but headache can be a symptom, and measurement of blood pressure is mandatory in any child presenting with headache.

Headaches often accompany minor systemic infections. Dental caries, sinusitis, and otitis media are all treatable causes of headache, and signs of these problems should be sought on clinical evaluation. Eye strain is often blamed for headaches, although there is little evidence for this. It does no harm, however, to recommend an assessment of visual acuity.

Rarely, headaches can be a sign of an intracranial lesion. Features that should arouse concern are shown in the Red Flag box.

<table>
<tr><td>

Features of concern in a child with headache

- Acute onset of severe pain
- Fever
- Headache intensified by lying down or waking during night
- Associated vomiting
- Diminished school performance or regression of developmental skills
- Consistently unilateral pain
- Cranial bruit
- Hypertension
- Papilloedema
- Fall-off in growth

</td></tr>
</table>

History – must ask!

Find out if the headache is acute, persistent or recurrent. Seek a detailed description of the pain in terms of the character, pattern of attacks and location, although this may be difficult in young children. Try to find out how much school has been lost through headaches. A diary of symptoms kept for a few weeks can be very helpful in demonstrating patterns of attacks and associated symptoms.

- *What are the headaches like?* A constricting or band-like pain suggests tension headache, whereas throbbing suggests migraine. Headaches caused by raised intracranial pressure (ICP) are classically exacerbated by lying down.
- *Is there a pattern to the attacks?* The pattern of attacks is helpful in sorting out the severity of the problem as well as identifying particular events that precipitate an attack. Waking at night, or early morning headaches, suggest raised ICP, particularly if accompanied by vomiting. Tension headaches tend to occur towards the end of the day and psychogenic headaches may be linked to events such as particular lessons. Cluster headaches are severe and sudden in onset.
- *Where are the headaches located?* The location of the pain can be helpful. Tension headaches are rather non-specific, migraine and cluster headaches are classically unilateral, and headaches caused by intracranial pathology are often localized to the site of the lesion.
- *Are there associated symptoms?* Associated symptoms such as nausea and vomiting, travel sickness, a preceding aura and photophobia support a diagnosis of migraine. Autonomic features such as a watering red eye are seen in cluster headaches.
- *What medications are being used?* Sustained, regular use of analgesia for headaches, on more than 2–3 days per week, can cause 'medication overuse headache', for which the management is restricting systemic analgesia and trying topical or distraction techniques.

- *Are there emotional and behavioural problems?* Emotional and behavioural difficulties are a cause of headaches, can also exacerbate them and may affect academic performance. You must be wary, however, of always attributing headaches to these difficulties, as intracranial lesions, although rare, can be the cause of headache and also affect behaviour and intellectual function.
- *Family history.* Ask if there is a family history of headaches and migraine. This can help in making a diagnosis, and it is important in management as children may be suggestible to developing symptoms if headaches are prevalent in the home.

Physical examination – must check!

A careful physical examination is important in order to determine whether there is any evidence of serious pathology. In persistent or recurrent headaches there are usually no signs. Features of concern are shown in the Red Flag box.

It is important to exclude the following:

- *Is the child ill?* Fever, meningeal signs and reduced level of consciousness point to meningitis or meningoencephalitis.
- *Hypertension.*
- *Signs of raised intracranial pressure* – Cushing triad (slow pulse with high blood pressure, irregular bradypnoea) are late signs, papilloedema and, in the preschool child, enlarging head circumference.
- *Focal neurological signs.* The presence of focal signs should always alert the clinician to the possibility of serious underlying pathology, and may help determine the site of a lesion. Cranial nerve palsies and cerebellar signs (nystagmus, ataxia and intention tremor) suggest an infratentorial tumour. Signs of focal spasticity indicate a cerebral lesion, while delayed growth and puberty and visual field defects suggest a pituitary tumour.

Look, too, for evidence of dental caries, sinus tenderness and carotid bruits.

Investigations

Investigations are rarely indicated unless there is evidence of raised intracranial pressure or neurological signs. In this circumstance, a computed tomography (CT) scan or magnetic resonance imaging (MRI) brain is indicated. Sometimes a lumbar puncture with manometry to check the cerebrospinal fluid (CSF) pressure is also required.

Managing headaches as a symptom

Simple analgesia with paracetamol is usually adequate. If the headaches persist, the approach described in Box 11.1 (p. 195) may be helpful.

🔑 **Key points: Headaches**

- A good history usually identifies the headache's aetiology
- Serious pathology can usually be excluded on physical examination
- Signs of raised intracranial pressure include headache exacerbated on lying down, vomiting, papilloedema and in severe cases hypertension with bradycardia and bradypnoea
- Investigations are only indicated if there are physical signs or red flag features

---

🔍 **Clues to diagnosing headaches**

	Character of the headache	Timing of the headache	Associated features	Physical examination
Tension	Constricting, band-like	Towards the end of the day	Nil	Normal
Migraine	Throbbing, may be unilateral	Not specific	Nausea, vomiting, aura, photophobia, family history	Normal
Raised intracranial pressure (ICP)	Worse on lying down, may be localized to site of lesion	Early morning Waking at night	Vomiting without nausea, other features depend on site of lesion	Slow pulse, high blood pressure, irregular breathing, papilloedema, enlarging head circumference, focal signs
Meningitis	Severe, acute	Not specific	Fever, neck stiffness	Drowsiness, irritability, Kernig's sign
Cluster headache	Severe, unilateral	Hyper-acute ('thunderclap') at any time	Tearing, red-eye, autonomic signs	CNS normal

---

Squint (strabismus)

Causes of squint

Non-paralytic strabismus
Failure of binocular alignment
Refractive errors
Ocular abnormalities, e.g. cataracts
Paralytic strabismus

Squints are very common in childhood. They may be convergent, divergent or alternating. Some squints are apparent (manifest), but some may be latent and only appear with fatigue, illness and stress.

Most squints in childhood are caused by a failure of binocular alignment of the eyes, the reason for which is unknown. More rarely a squint may be caused by an underlying ocular or refractive problem. Rarely, squints are a result of paralysis of the extraocular muscles, in which case serious pathology may be the cause.

Irrespective of the cause, the image from the squinting eye is suppressed in the optical cortex so that diplopia is avoided. If the squint is left untreated, the visual pathways from the squinting eye become irreversibly suppressed and a permanent visual defect develops. This is known as amblyopia (see p. 250).

Physical examination – must check!

Evaluation involves simple observation, tests of vision and the application of two relatively simple clinical techniques: the corneal light reflex test and the cover test. The latter is particularly important if a squint is latent. These are described in detail on pp. 96–7.

Management

It is important to confirm the presence of a squint and to refer the child for treatment early before irreversible suppression of visual acuity occurs. All fixed squints, and any squint persisting beyond 5 or 6 months of age, need to be referred for ophthalmological evaluation.

Neurological disorders

Meningitis

Meningitis is a common and serious illness in childhood caused by viral or bacterial infection invading the membranes overlying the brain and spinal cord. Bacterial infections usually remain confined to the meninges, but viruses may invade the underlying brain, causing meningoencephalitis. The causes of meningitis beyond the newborn period are shown in Table 13.1.

Meningitis is more common in the neonatal period than at any other time of life (see p. 447). The neonate shows no focal signs of meningitis in its early phases, so paediatricians must have a high suspicion of this condition and perform a lumbar puncture if any doubt as to the diagnosis.

Clinical features   Viral meningitis is usually preceded by pharyngitis or gastrointestinal upset. The child then develops fever, headache and neck stiffness. The classical feature of head retraction as seen in adults is a late feature of meningitis in children. Neck stiffness is not a reliable sign in infants, and the diagnosis must be considered in any infant with a high-pitched cry suggestive of cerebral irritation. Possible exposure to Herpes Simplex (HSV) also known as the 'cold sore' virus, needs to be considered as this can be fatal in infants.

In bacterial meningitis, drowsiness is an early feature; the infant has a vacant expression with staring eyes and, in severe cases, may present with coma. A reduction in the normal level of consciousness is always a serious sign, but this rarely occurs in viral meningitis. Convulsions are common in infants and may be the presenting feature, although a history of the child being off colour and refusing feeds for a few hours is often obtained.

On examination the child often looks ill, but may have non-specific signs and symptoms, including fever, vomiting and muscle ache. Petechial haemorrhages (a 'non-blanching rash') may be present in the early stages of meningococcal disease (pp. 154, 351). Papilloedema is rarely seen in children, and Brudzinski and Kernig signs, although present in older children, are often absent or late signs in infancy. A bulging, non-pulsatile, fontanelle in infants is a late sign.

The differential diagnosis of meningitis includes:
- septicaemia and other forms of severe infection;
- other causes of raised intracranial pressure (p. 245);
- meningismus – neck stiffness as a result of tonsillitis, otitis media, pneumonia or pyelonephritis.

Diagnosis   Distinction between bacterial and viral meningitis cannot always reliably be made clinically. If meninigitis is suspected, a lumbar puncture must be carried out within 12 hours, as long as there are no contraindications, and the cerebrospinal fluid (CSF) examined (see p. 114). Contraindications to lumbar puncture include deranged clotting, clinical instability and the clinical suspicion of raised intracranial pressure (papilloedema is present), because of the risk of coning (see below).

The appearance of the CSF gives important clues as to the cause of the meningitis. In bacterial meningitis the fluid is often cloudy. Microscopy is essential to count and identify the cells. In some cases of fulminating bacterial meningitis there may be few, or no cells at all, but the fluid is teeming with bacteria. Organisms can be best identified by Gram stain, a routine part of the CSF examination. The fluid must be cultured to confirm the type of infecting organism. Polymerase Chain Reaction (PCR) can rapidly identify viral and bacterial agents and is especially useful in partially treated meningitis. In viral meningitis caused by herpes simplex the liver function tests may be deranged.

The initial CSF findings usually allow the distinction between viral or bacterial meningitis (Table 7.8).

Coning   'Coning' refers to herniation of the brainstem and/or cerebellar structures through the foramen magnum. It can follow a lumbar puncture when the release of spinal fluid results in a pressure differential between the intracranial structures and the intraspinal compartment. The contents of the posterior intracranial fossa are thus squeezed into the upper spinal canal, causing very acute and severe brainstem neurological signs with paralysis and respiratory inhibition which may be irreversible.

Management (see Box 13.2)   Viral meningitis is usually self-limiting and requires no specific treatment. An exception is herpes simplex meningoencephalitis, which can be fatal in infants. It is treated with a prolonged course of intravenous antiviral agent aciclovir.

Table 13.1 Causes of meningitis outside of the neonatal period

Viral causes

Enteroviruses (Coxsackie viruses or echoviruses)

Herpes simplex virus (HSV)

Mumps virus (more common in previous years)

Poliomyelitis (only in developing countries)

Bacterial causes

Neisseria meningitidis (commonest cause in UK)

Streptococcus pneumoniae

Haemophilus influenza type B (now rare)

Tuberculous meningitis (rare in UK)

Treatment of bacterial meningitis is directed towards antimicrobial sterilization of the CSF and avoidance or treatment of complications. A third-generation cephalosporin, such as ceftriaxone, for 7–21 days depending on the organism, along with steroids (dexamethasone) to reduce meningeal inflammation. Meningococcal meningitis is associated with a high carrier rate of *Neisseria meningitidis* in the nasopharynx, and all household contacts should be given prophylactic treatment as guided by Public Health departments to reduce the risk of cross-infection. Intra-muscular benzylpenicillin should only be given in the presence of a petechial or purpuric rash as this is the treatment for meningococcal septicaemia (p. 154).

Complications and prognosis   The prognosis for bacterial meningitis depends on the delay between onset and the start of effective treatment. Important complications of bacterial meningitis include:
- hydrocephalus;
- subdural effusion;
- syndrome of inappropriate antidiuretic hormone (SIADH);
- deafness;
- major deficit (cerebral palsy and/or learning difficulties in 10%).

Neonatal meningitis (p. 447) carries a worse prognosis than bacterial meningitis in older children.

Viral meningitis carries a good prognosis in the majority of cases. Sensorineural hearing impairment should be considered in all children following meningitis and additional hearing screens will need to be arranged, particularly following pneumococcal and mumps meningitis. Herpes meningoencephalitis is associated with high mortality and morbidity rates.

Box 13.2 Managing meningitis

- For non-HSV viral meningitis, no specific treatment is required
- If lumbar puncture suggests a bacterial cause, use appropriate intravenous antibiotics
- If partially treated meningitis, treat as meningitis with a prolonged course of IV antibiotics
- Steroids reduce complication rate in some bacterial meningitis
- Notify public health department and give prophylaxis treatment to all close contacts as advised

---

Meningitis at a glance

Epidemiology
0.5% children <10 years
Neonates are particularly prone to meningitis

Causal factors
Bacterial and viral meningitis are equally common
After the neonatal period the following bacteria are responsible:
- *Neisseria meningitidis*
- *Streptococcus pneumoniae*

Mother first notices child is unwell/irritable   Drowsy/fits/purpuric rash

Level of consciousness (%)
100
80
60
40
20
0
−2 0 2 4 6   16   24
Time (hr)
Coma
RIP

Rapid progression of meningococcal meningitis in a child

Presentation*
Classical symptoms include fever, drowsiness, headaches, bulging fontanelle and convulsions Kernig sign seen in older children. In early stages and in infants symptoms and signs are often non-specific
Neck stiffness is a late sign in infants

Differential diagnosis
Lumbar puncture is essential to make diagnosis in any suspected cases
Viral and bacterial causes distinguished on CSF findings

Management
See Box 13.2

Prognosis
Excellent in viral cases
Deafness is the commonest sequela
In bacterial meningitis, 10% sustain severe neurological damage

NB *Signs and symptoms are variable

See NICE guideline: Meningitis (bacterial) and meningococcal septicaemia in under 16s: recognition, diagnosis and management
https://www.nice.org.uk/guidance/cg102

Epilepsies

Prevalence

The prevalence of epilepsy in school children is in the order of about 4–5 per 1000. The diagnosis is, however, often made erroneously, and it has been estimated that as many as 25% of children referred to specialised clinics do not have epilepsy. Learning difficulties are very common (70% has been cited) in children with epilepsy.

Terminology

Before discussing the problem of epilepsy, it is important to clarify terms. The term 'epilepsies' is preferred to 'epilepsy' as there is a vast array of epilepsy syndromes. A 'seizure' is a manifestation of hypersynchronous and excessive activity in neurons. In an 'epileptic seizure' the event has originated in the neurons. Neurons can also be triggered to seize by metabolic causes, such as hypernatraemia (e.g. from severe gastroenteritis) or hypoglycaemia, but the child or young person would not have epilepsy.

An individual is diagnosed with epilepsy if they have two epileptic seizures, but can be made after one when an epilepsy syndrome is identified.

When considering paroxysmal events, it is important to consider each event separately. This is because people with a correct diagnosis of epilepsy could have a different event such as a faint (syncope), or co-existing psychogenic non-epileptic episodes.

Seizures

A seizure is a discrete paroxysmal episode caused by hypersynchronous neuronal discharges. These discharges could be coming from only one area of the brain ('focal') or effect both halves of the brain ('general'). Sometimes seizures start in one area and then spread more widely. These seizures should be termed 'focal onset bilateral tonic clonic seizures' and the treatment should be tailored to treat focal onset seizures.

Focal seizure

Symptoms of a focal seizure can mimic the usual effects of neurons, for example, motor seizures (movement); autonomic seizures (responses such as flushing, vomiting or nausea); visual seizures (visual hallucinations or temporary blindness); sensory seizures; or more complex sensations such as déjà vu, crying or laughing. A detailed description of the symptoms may help identify where a focal seizure has originated.

Motor (movement) seizures can also be subdivided into 'tonic' (the muscles become tense and stiff); 'clonic' (rhythmical jerking); 'myoclonus' (faster jerks); 'atonic' (loss of muscle tone but consciousness is maintained). An 'epileptic spasm' (previously known as 'infantile spasm') is a type of seizure that is associated with West Syndrome. Spasms can be flexor or extensor, symmetrical or non-symmetrical.

Focal seizures may also impair awareness of the surroundings and the child may be able to subsequently give an account of their experiences. The previous terms 'partial complex' and 'simple complex' are no longer used and it should be stated whether awareness was impaired during the seizure, or not.

Generalised seizures

A generalised tonic clonic seizure starts with a sudden loss of consciousness when the child falls to the ground, the limbs stiff and extend, the back arched and breathing stops. The teeth are tightly clenched, and the tongue may be bitten. This tonic stage is followed by a clonic phase when intermittent jerking movements of the limbs and face occur, with the onset of irregular breathing, and often micturition and salivation. This clonic phase may last only a few minutes, but if prolonged beyond 30 minutes is called status epilepticus (p. 240). At the end of the seizure, the child relaxes and normal respiration resumes. A period of postictal depression follows, where the child may remain sleepy and disorientated for some time.

Absence seizures are seizures associated with a specific EEG finding of regularly occurring spike waves during which the child is staring, is unaware of the surroundings and may have 'automatisms' (automatic movements like scratching the face or finger fiddling). Absence seizures may be triggered by hyperventilation.

After the details of the seizure have been determined the possibility of a recognizable epilepsy syndrome should be considered. This is important for prognosis and appropriate management.

Epilepsy syndromes

Syndromes are typically divided into the age at which they start (see Table 13.2). 'Infantile' onset seizures start in babies; 'childhood' syndromes start in children of around 4–8 years; and 'juvenile' is usually in children over 10 years.

Diagnosing epilepsy

The diagnosis of epilepsy is a clinical one, often based entirely on the history, as the seizures may never be observed by medical professionals. Video filming with smart phones is a recent improvement. It is critical to review the description of the seizures carefully to confirm the diagnosis, and avoid erroneous over-diagnosis. DESSCRIBE (see Box 13.3) provides a useful approach when considering epileptic seizures.

Table 13.2 Characteristics of epilepsy syndromes

Epilepsy syndrome	Seizure types	EEG features	Prognosis
West Syndrome	Epileptic (infantile) spasms	Hypsarrhythmia (high amplitude, chaotic discharges)	Prompt treatment is associated with better neuro-developmental outcome, but some children will develop profound disability
Childhood Absence Epilepsy (CAE)	Absence seizures only	3 per second spike and wave during seizure. No photosensitivity	Excellent, with children likely to outgrow the seizures by puberty
Juvenile Absence Epilepsy (JAE)	Absences, may also have generalised tonic clonic seizures	3.5 per second spike and wave discharges during seizure. May be photosensitivity	Most require life-long medication
Juvenile Myoclonic Epilepsy (JME)	Myoclonic jerks, typically in the morning, generalised tonic clonic seizures, can also have absence seizures	Polyspikes, may be photosensitive	Most require life-long medication
Childhood Epilepsy with Centro-Temporal Spikes (previously 'rolandic epilepsy')	Episodes occurring from sleep of tongue tingling, drool, difficulty speaking and unilateral facial weakness. Some progress to bilateral tonic clonic seizure	Spikes in the 'rolandic' or centro-temporal region	Excellent as children are likely to outgrow these by puberty. Not all children require medicines

Box 13.3 'DESSCRIBE': an acronym to summarize the diagnostic processes for a child with paroxysmal events

Describe the events	Describe what happened during the event paying close attention to the eyes (open, closed, deviated), head turn, whether the seizure started in one area of the body and duration
Epilepsy or not epilepsy?	Is it likely that this episode was an epileptic event or is another cause more likely?
Seizure type	Classify the seizure type
Syndrome type	Identify the syndrome type if possible
Cause	Is there any identifiable cause for the epilepsy? (Genetic, metabolic, structural, infectious, immune, unknown)
Relevant **I**mpairment in **B**ehaviour or **E**ducation	Consider any relevant impairment as there is a higher incidence in children and young people with epilepsies than those with other chronic health conditions

Physical examination is important. Although the majority of epilepsy is idiopathic, the finding of cutaneous or neurological signs may indicate possible underlying pathology.

The cause of most epilepsy syndromes is yet unknown, but increasingly genetic mutations, either de novo or inherited, are being recognised. Other possible causes of epilepsies are 'structural' (e.g. brain tumours or cortical malformations), 'metabolic', 'immune', 'infectious', and 'unknown'. Tuberous sclerosis is a genetic condition which is also a structural cause due to the development of intracranial tubers.

Electroencephalography

The EEG may be characteristic for absence seizures and epileptic spasms, but must be interpreted with caution, as 5% of normal children show epileptiform activity on EEG, and 40–50% of children with established clear-cut epilepsy have normal EEGs on first testing.

Recordings taken over a 24-hour period can be helpful in patients experiencing daily or nightly episodes, and video EEG recordings enable correlation of EEG and seizure appearance (semiology). An example of a generalised seizure on EEG is shown in Figures 13.1 and 13.2.

Radiological investigations

An MRI brain scan is indicated in children who develop epilepsy under 2 years old; have any focal features clinically or on EEG; or who do not respond to an appropriate first-line anticonvulsive medication. A general anaesthetic is usually needed. CT scans may be useful if an acute bleed is suspected.

Management of epilepsy

The goals when managing a child with epilepsy are shown in Box 13.4. First it is important to ensure that the diagnosis is correct. The aim is to control seizures, while minimizing the

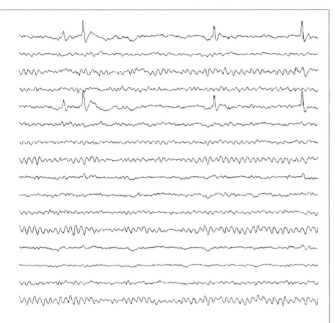

Figure 13.1 Interictal EEG of a child with epilepsy.

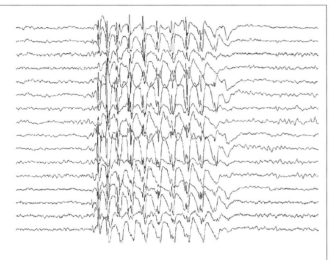

Figure 13.2 EEG capturing absence seizure with 3Hz spike and wave demonstrated.

Box 13.4 Goals in managing epilepsy

- Ensure the diagnosis is correct
- Control seizures
- Minimize drug side effects
- Ensure that any learning and behavioural difficulties are addressed
- Help the child live a normal life with full participation in activities at home and school

Box 13.5 Medical management of epilepsy

- Only treat if seizures are epileptic and recurrent
- Use monotherapy when possible, increasing the drug to maximum therapeutic levels before introducing a second drug
- Check plasma levels if control is inadequate, and discuss why children and young people may not be receiving medication
- For children with prolonged generalised tonic clonic seizures, parents and carers (including school and nursery) should have training in how to administer buccal midazolam for generalised tonic clonic seizures longer than 5 minutes

Table 13.3 Seizure type and drug therapy

Seizure type	Drug options (less preferred options in brackets)
Tonic clonic seizures	Sodium valproate, lamotrigine, (carbamazepine)
Absence seizures	Ethosuximide, sodium valproate, (lamotrigine)
Myoclonic seizures	Sodium valproate, (levetiracetam, topiramate)
Focal, with or without progression to bilateral tonic clonic seizures	Carbamazepine, lamotrigine
Epileptic spasms	Vigabatrin, steroids

- Therapy should be initiated with the most effective drug for the type of seizure and syndrome (Table 13.3), starting at the lowest limit of the therapeutic range.
- A second drug should be substituted if the first is ineffective and the dose increased as before. The first drug should be gradually decreased unless it was partially effective, in which case it may be continued.
- Drugs with sedative effects should be given at night and, if a seizure pattern exists, the peak level timed to coincide with time of seizures.

unwanted side effects of anticonvulsant therapy. Management must also ensure that any learning difficulties are addressed, and the child is encouraged to lead a normal life with full participation in activities at home and in school.

The principles involved in the medical management of epilepsy are shown in Box 13.5.

Medication

The goal of antiepileptic drug therapy is to achieve the greatest control of seizures with minimum side effects. This is best achieved through a monotherapy approach.

Table 13.4 Common side effects of anticonvulsants

Anticonvulsant	Side effects
Sodium valproate	Vomiting, anorexia, lethargy, hair loss, hepatotoxicity
Ethosuximide	Abdominal discomfort, skin rash, liver dysfunction, leucopenia
Clonazepam	Drowsiness, irritability, behavioural abnormalities, excessive salivation
Carbamazepine	Dizziness, drowsiness, diplopia, liver dysfunction, anaemia, leucopenia
Lamotrigine	Drowsiness, vomiting, tremor, headache, visual disturbance
Vigabatrin	Headache, dizziness, arthralgia, weight gain, memory loss
Levetiracetam	Behavioural disturbance, bruising, tingling, chills, fatigue
Topiramate	Diarrhoea, fatigue, weight loss, irritability, coordination problems

N.B. The possible teratogenic effects of anticonvulsants need to be considered in all female patients. All women and girls on sodium valproate are advised to be on a pregnancy prevention programme. The teratogenic effects in newer antiepilepsy medications are not yet known.

Unfortunately, all anticonvulsants have side effects, some of which may be transient or settle on reduction of the dose. Others are life-threatening (Table 13.4).

Other management issues

In cases where seizures persist despite medication, ensure that the diagnosis has been effectively established, discuss medication administration and consider whether medication is being administered properly. It is important to also consider whether each seizure is epileptic or non-epileptic. Watchful waiting, with safety advice and a seizure diary, can be helpful to obtain more evidence about the nature of the events. The mainstay of treatment is medical; however, it is estimated that 0.5% of children with epilepsy would benefit from epilepsy surgery (see Box 13.6). If surgery is not appropriate, other treatments such as a vagal nerve stimulator or the ketogenic diet may be considered.

For most children with epilepsy, restriction of physical activity is unnecessary, other than recommending that the child should be attended by a responsible adult while bathing and swimming. Avoiding cycling in traffic and climbing high gymnastic equipment is prudent. Application for a driving licence can only be made if the young person

Box 13.6 Children who should be referred for epilepsy surgical assessment

Children under 2 years old with focal seizures (irrespective of whether the MRI brain is normal)
Children with focal seizures resistant to two appropriate anticonvulsants
Children with epilepsy who have a lateralized abnormality on MRI brain
Children with tuberous sclerosis or hemiplegia, with seizures not responsive to two anticonvulsants
Children with drop attack seizures

has been seizure-free whilst awake for 12 months, whether on or off medication.

Acute seizures

The management of generalised convulsions is covered in detail in Chapter 23. A child having an acute generalised tonic clonic seizure should be positioned in the recovery position so that patency of the airway is ensured (see p. 412). Seizures lasting longer than 5 minutes should be treated with a benzodiazepine (in the form of buccal midazolam, rectal diazepam, or intravenous lorazepam) (see Box 13.7). Children do not need to be hospitalized each time a seizure occurs. Emergency treatment is not usually required for other types of epileptic seizure.

Status epilepticus

Status epilepticus is defined as a prolonged convulsion lasting 30 minutes or more, or a series of shorter convulsions with failure to regain consciousness between them. Rapid treatment of a prolonged convulsion is necessary. The airway must be maintained, oxygen given, and blood glucose checked.

Box 13.7 Instructions for the use of buccal midazolam (Epilepsy Nurses Association)

- Buccal midazolam is given as a liquid into the side of the mouth between the gums and cheek
- It is absorbed quickly into the bloodstream
- It should be given slowly using a plastic syringe, as the child might choke on it if given too quickly
- If possible, the dose is divided, so half is given to the inside of one cheek, and half to the other
- Watch carefully for any signs of reduced breathing and check to see if seizure is terminated

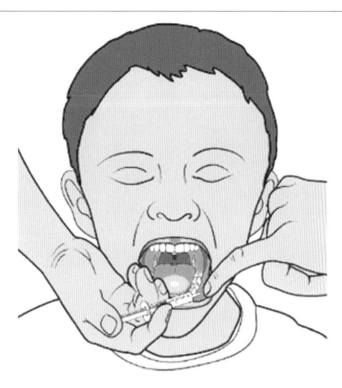

Figure 13.3 Administering buccal midazolam in a child.

A maximum of two doses of benzodiazepine should be administered, as there is a risk of respiratory depression. A phenytoin infusion is usually administered subsequently, although levetiracetam or sodium valproate is sometimes an alternative. If all these have failed, an anaesthetist should be called and the child should undergo rapid sequence induction of anaesthesia with thiopental. Any child with prolonged seizures should be monitored carefully in an intensive care unit.

Monitoring the condition

Routine monitoring of blood levels of anticonvulsants is not required, unless the child's seizures remain uncontrolled or drug toxicity is suspected. Blood levels below the therapeutic range can result from inadequate dosage, poor absorption, rapid drug metabolism, drug interactions, and deliberate or accidental non-compliance.

Routine follow-up of a child with epilepsy (see Checklist)

History   The diary should be reviewed for frequency and types of seizures. Identifying periodicity may be helpful in adjusting drug therapy. A routine part of the history should be to ask how often the medication is omitted in order to discuss drug concordance. Side effects of the drugs must be noted. The family should be encouraged to discuss coping difficulties and the child's progress at school reviewed.

Physical examination   A physical examination is not generally required if all is going well. If there are potential side effects or any deterioration in control, a full physical, neurological and developmental examination is required.

Issues for the family

Education

Most parents are initially frightened by the diagnosis of epilepsy and require support and accurate information about the condition. The child and family need to know about the expected duration of the seizure disorder, side effects of drugs, the dangers of sudden withdrawal of medication, aetiology, and social and academic repercussions. There are often concerns about genetic implications, and in the adolescent girl the teratogenic effects of anticonvulsants and effects of the oral

---

✓ Checklist for review of a child with epilepsy

If the child is new to you or the clinic, check:
- ☐ The diagnosis is substantiated
- ☐ The family's understanding of epilepsy
- ☐ The family's ability to be aware of and manage tonic clonic seizures when relevant
- ☐ Imaging studies have been carried out if seizures developed under 2 years of age; do not respond to appropriate first-line anti convulsive medications or there are any focal features
- ☐ An ECG has been carried out if the child has generalised tonic clonic seizures

At routine follow-up, review:

History
- ☐ Diary, or if unavailable ask about:
  - frequency of seizures
  - side effects of drugs
  - educational and social problems at school
- ☐ Number of absences from school as a result of epilepsy
- ☐ Any activities restricted because of epilepsy

Physical examination
- ☐ Height and weight plus signs of drug side effects – rash, jaundice, hirsutism, etc.
- ☐ Neurological examination if there has been a change in seizures

Investigations
- ☐ Plasma levels of drugs if control is poor

Action
- ☐ Advise on adjusting medication
- ☐ Counsel about psychosocial difficulties
- ☐ Contact school if there are problems there

---

contraceptive pill must be discussed. It is important that the parents learn how to manage an acute seizure safely.

Psychosocial

Epilepsy still carries a stigma and fears may be expressed, not only in the family, but also among teachers and social contacts. Parents should be encouraged to treat the child as normally as possible and not to thwart the child's independence. Issues related to independence are likely to become particularly prevalent in adolescence, when concordance, too, may become a problem. In terms of career guidance, it is important that the adolescent is aware that certain occupations, such as nursing and certain branches of the armed forces, are closed to individuals with epilepsy.

Issues at school

The majority of children with epilepsy attend mainstream schools and it is essential to harness the cooperation of the school staff, as their role can be very important. Their concerns naturally focus around the possibility of tonic clonic seizures occurring at school. They must be taught the correct management of these fits, including how to use buccal midazolam for prolonged seizures, if needed. It is also important that schools are aware of the manifestations of other types of seizure such as absence spells that the child may experience, as well as side effects of drugs, and that these are reported to the parents or school nurse.

Physical exercise is another issue for school. Unless the child is prone to frequent seizures, he or she should not be excluded from any activities including swimming, although a responsible adult must be in attendance and know of the child's epilepsy.

Prognosis

The prognosis for many of the genetic epilepsy syndromes is good with the condition self-resolving during childhood. This includes Childhood Absence Epilepsy (CAE) and Childhood Epilepsy with Centro-Temporal spikes (CECTS). Therapy can be discontinued gradually if a child has been free of fits for 2 years. Other syndrome types, such as Juvenile Myoclonic Epilepsy (JME) or Juvenile Absence Epilepsy (JAE) continue during adult life.

 See NICE guideline: Epilepsies: Diagnosis and management
https://www.nice.org.uk/guidance/cg137

The child with epilepsy at a glance

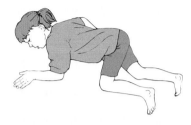

Epidemiology
Approximately 4 per 1000 school children
Learning difficulties are a common association

Aetiology/pathophysiology
Paroxysmal involuntary disturbances of brain function resulting in recurrent seizures

How the diagnosis is made
The diagnosis is clinical, based on history and any video recordings available. The EEG is used to aid in syndrome classification.

Clinical features

Generalised tonic clonic seizures
Tonic phase:
- Sudden loss of consciousness
- Limbs extend, back arches
- Teeth clench, breathing stops
- Tongue may be bitten *

Clonic phase:
- Intermittent jerking movements
- Irregular breathing
- Micturition and salivation *

Postictal phase:
- Child sleepy and disorientated

Absence seizures
Fleeting (5–20 seconds) impairment of consciousness (daydreaming)
No falling or involuntary movements
EEG: characteristic bursts of 3-per-second spike and wave activity

Myoclonic seizures
Shock-like jerks, often causing sudden falls
Usually occur in children with a structural neurological/cerebral degenerative condition

*Signs and symptoms are variable

Clinical features (cont.)

Focal seizures
Twitching or jerking of face, arm or leg
Consciousness usually retained
Jacksonian pattern (starts focally and spreads) *
Temporary weakness of involved part of the body after attack*
May have progession to bilateral tonic clonic seizures

Temporal lobe seizures
Altered or impaired consciousness associated with strange sensations, hallucinations or semipurposeful movements
Chewing, sucking or swallowing movements*
Postictal phase with amnesia *
EEG may show discharges arising from the temporal lobe

Infantile spasms
Onset usually at 3–8 months of age
Flexion spasms ('jack-knife' or 'salaam')
Lasts a few seconds, in clusters lasting up to half an hour
Regression of developmental skills
History of perinatal asphyxia or meningitis*
EEG – characteristic hypsarrhythmic

General management

Medication:
(see Table 13.3 and Box 13.5)

Restriction of activities: none, unless fits are intractable

Education:
Understanding of epilepsy and drugs used
Benzodiazepine e.g. buccal midazolam may be used for prolonged convulsive seizures

Career guidance
Driving restrictions
Teratogenicity of anticonvulsants during pregnancy

School:
Education of staff
Addressing learning difficulties
Supervision in swimming and gymnastics
Monitoring of school performance, absences and compliance

Management of acute problems
Tonic clonic attacks – position child to ensure airway is patent, if >5 mins give benzodiazepine
Only give IV medications in hospital

Points for routine follow-up
Monitor:
Frequency of seizures
Side effects of drugs
Psychosocial and educational problems
Anticonvulsant levels if uncontrolled

Prognosis
Prognosis depends on the syndrome diagnosis, with some types outgrown in childhood

Migraine

Migraine is a common cause of headache in the school-age child, and the pathophysiology is now understood to involve neurological factors as well as neurotransmitter and inflammatory mediators.

Clinical features   Onset is usually in late childhood or early adolescence. Classically, the attack is preceded by an aura, which is often visual in nature, but may consist of other fleeting neurological sensations. Within a few minutes, a throbbing unilateral headache occurs, often accompanied by nausea and vomiting. Sleep usually ends the attack, and the attacks last between 2 and 72 hours. In younger children, the attack is often bilateral with no aura, nausea or vomiting. Rarely, complicated migraine occurs when confusion or focal neurological symptoms and signs are present. The migraine headache always causes some reduction in the child's ability to function normally.

There is often a history of repeated vomiting or travel sickness when the child was younger, and a positive family history is usually present. There is no confirmatory test for migraine and diagnosis is made on the presence of some of the following:

- episodic nature;
- aura;
- visual disturbance;
- nausea (in 90% of cases);
- unilateral headache;
- family history;
- impairment of normal function during an attack.

Management   First-line treatment is rest, with simple analgesia. In some children, attacks are precipitated by certain foods such as chocolate, cheese or nuts, and withdrawal of these items from the diet can be helpful. If attacks are frequent, drug prophylaxis should be considered. Sumatriptan, a 5-hydroxytryptamine agonist, is useful in aborting acute migraine attacks in adolescents. It is not recommended for use in childhood.

Prognosis   Migraine headaches often persist into adulthood, but may undergo remission spontaneously.

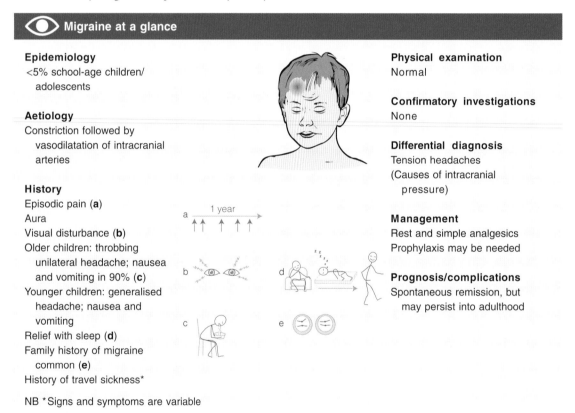

Migraine at a glance

Epidemiology
<5% school-age children/
adolescents

Aetiology
Constriction followed by
vasodilatation of intracranial
arteries

History
Episodic pain (**a**)
Aura
Visual disturbance (**b**)
Older children: throbbing
unilateral headache; nausea
and vomiting in 90% (**c**)
Younger children: generalised
headache; nausea and
vomiting
Relief with sleep (**d**)
Family history of migraine
common (**e**)
History of travel sickness*

NB *Signs and symptoms are variable

Physical examination
Normal

Confirmatory investigations
None

Differential diagnosis
Tension headaches
(Causes of intracranial
pressure)

Management
Rest and simple analgesics
Prophylaxis may be needed

Prognosis/complications
Spontaneous remission, but
may persist into adulthood

a   1 year

Tension headaches

Tension headaches usually develop towards later childhood. They are thought to be caused by persistent contraction of neck and temporal muscles.

Clinical features   Headaches which are constricting or band-like in nature, mild to moderate, symmetric and tend to occur towards the end of the day, but do not interfere with sleep. There may or may not be evidence that the child is under stress. Often, other members of the family suffer from similar headaches. Daily function is usually unimpaired.

Management   The family needs to be reassured that there is no serious underlying pathology. In terms of treatment, rest and sympathy is often all that is required. Simple analgesics such as paracetamol may be given, but should not be used regularly on more than 2 days a week. Any underlying stress and tensions in the child's life need to be addressed. It is important that school absence is kept to a minimum, and the school may have to be approached directly to develop a strategy for when headaches develop in school hours.

If others at home experience headaches, it helps to advise minimizing attention to them as children can be quite susceptible to the symptoms of others.

Prognosis   The headaches often resolve spontaneously or become less frequent.

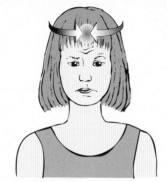

Tension headaches at a glance

Epidemiology
Common in later childhood

Aetiology
Possibly caused by contraction
   of neck and temporal
   muscles

History
Constricting/band-like pain
No interference with sleep
At end of day*
Stress at home or school*
Family history of headaches*

Physical examination
Normal

Confirmatory investigations
None

Differential diagnosis
Migraine
(Causes of raised intracranial
   pressure)

Management
Reassurance
Simple analgesics

Prognosis/complications
Usually spontaneous resolution

NB *Signs and symptoms are variable

Raised intracranial pressure (ICP)

Pseudo-tumour cerebri (idiopathic intracranial hypertension), brain tumours, abscesses and chronic subdural haematomas are rare causes of headache in childhood.

Clinical features   Headaches caused by a rise in ICP are classically exacerbated by lying down, so it is concerning if a child wakes from sleep with headaches. The headache is often accompanied by vomiting with little associated nausea. Raised intracranial pressure may cause papilloedema, altered neurological and visual function, and, as late signs in severe cases, elevated blood pressure, breathing irregularity and bradycardia ('Cushing triad').

The location of the pain is a good localizing sign for the site of the lesion. The commonest tumours are infratentorial in site, causing signs of cerebellar or brainstem dysfunction. Supratentorial tumours may be located in the hypothalamic–pituitary axis, causing endocrine or visual problems, or may be located in the cerebrum, causing epilepsy or spasticity.

Management   MRI or CT scans are reliable in detecting intracranial space-occupying lesions. Treatment depends on the pathology of the lesion. Pseudo-tumour cerebri (idiopathic intracranial hypertension) is treated with diuretics and repeated LPs for decompression.

Hydrocephalus

Hydrocephalus may result from a congenital abnormality of the brain such as aqueductal stenosis, or may be acquired as a result of intracranial haemorrhage, infection, or tumour. Premature babies with severe intracranial haemorrhage are particularly at risk. Hydrocephalus is commonly associated with neural tube anomalies and occurs in 80% of babies with spina bifida (see p. 452).

Clinical features   The clinical features vary with the age of onset and the rate of rise of intracranial pressure. Irritability, lethargy, poor appetite and vomiting are common. In infants, accelerated head growth is the most prominent sign. The anterior fontanelle is wide open and bulging, the sutures separated, and the scalp veins dilated. The forehead is broad, and the eyes deviated down, giving the 'setting sun' sign. Spasticity, clonus and brisk deep tendon reflexes are often demonstrable. In the older child the signs are more subtle, with headache and a deterioration in school performance.

Management   Cranial ultrasound or MRI scans provide information which determines the appropriate neurosurgical procedure. Most cases of hydrocephalus require a ventriculoperitoneal shunt to drain the cerebral fluid into the peritoneal cavity. Shunt complications include blockage and infection, and parents must be taught to

recognise symptoms. They need to seek help urgently if the child becomes lethargic or irritable or there is a change in personality.

Prognosis   Children with hydrocephalus are at increased risk for a variety of developmental disabilities and learning difficulties, particularly those related to performance tasks and memory. Visual problems are also common. For these reasons it is important that they receive long-term follow-up.

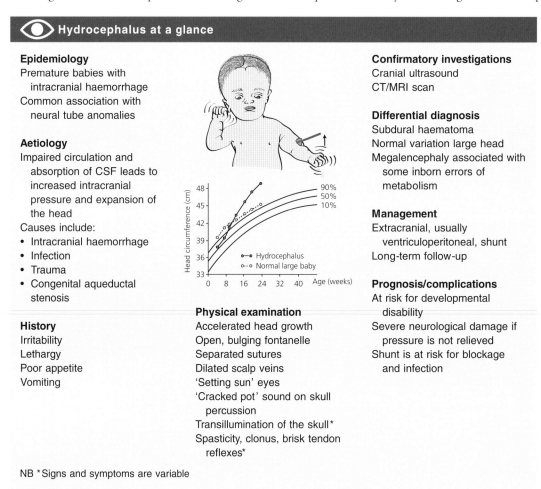

Hydrocephalus at a glance

Epidemiology
Premature babies with
   intracranial haemorrhage
Common association with
   neural tube anomalies

Aetiology
Impaired circulation and
   absorption of CSF leads to
   increased intracranial
   pressure and expansion of
   the head
Causes include:
• Intracranial haemorrhage
• Infection
• Trauma
• Congenital aqueductal
   stenosis

History
Irritability
Lethargy
Poor appetite
Vomiting

Physical examination
Accelerated head growth
Open, bulging fontanelle
Separated sutures
Dilated scalp veins
'Setting sun' eyes
'Cracked pot' sound on skull
   percussion
Transillumination of the skull*
Spasticity, clonus, brisk tendon
   reflexes*

Confirmatory investigations
Cranial ultrasound
CT/MRI scan

Differential diagnosis
Subdural haematoma
Normal variation large head
Megalencephaly associated with
   some inborn errors of
   metabolism

Management
Extracranial, usually
   ventriculoperitoneal, shunt
Long-term follow-up

Prognosis/complications
At risk for developmental
   disability
Severe neurological damage if
   pressure is not relieved
Shunt is at risk for blockage
   and infection

NB *Signs and symptoms are variable

Subdural haematomas

A subdural haematoma is a collection of bloody fluid under the dura. It results from rupture of the bridging veins that drain the cerebral cortex. Although any form of head trauma may produce subdural bleeding, the infant experiencing Abusive Head Trauma (AHT) from physical abuse is particularly susceptible to this injury (see p. 396). Subdural haematomas may be acute or chronic, in which case they may eventually be replaced by a subdural collection of fluid. Subdural haematomas can lead to blockage of cerebrospinal fluid flow and hydrocephalus.

Clinical features   Although an enlarging head is a feature, the infant is more likely to present with seizures, irritability, lethargy, vomiting and failure to thrive. Signs of raised ICP and

retinal haemorrhages are common following AHT (Figure 22.2). Diagnosis of subdural haematoma, from any cause, is made by radiological imaging.

Management   Management is neurosurgical. All cases of subdural haematoma should be evaluated thoroughly for the possibility of abuse.

Prognosis   The prognosis for recovery is variable and depends on the associated cerebral insult.

Breath-holding spells

Breath-holding spells primarily occur in babies and toddlers. They may be cyanotic or pallid in nature.

Cyanotic spells

Clinical features   The description of an episode is characteristic, as the event is always precipitated by crying because of pain or temper. The child takes a deep breath, stops breathing, becomes deeply cyanotic, and the limbs extend. Prolonged attacks of breath-holding can produce transient loss of consciousness and occasionally convulsive jerks of the extremities. The child then becomes limp, resumes respirations and, after a few minutes, returns to full alertness.

The key to the diagnosis is the typical onset with crying and breath-holding. The episodes are more common in children with iron deficiency anaemia.

Management   Reassurance is required. Parents can become quite terrified of these episodes, and as a result may have difficulty in imposing any form of discipline on the child for fear of provoking an attack. An ECG will exclude long QT syndrome. Iron supplementation is an effective treatment.

Prognosis   These attacks are always benign, and disappear before the child reaches school age, although children with this history have a higher incidence of vasovagal attacks later in life.

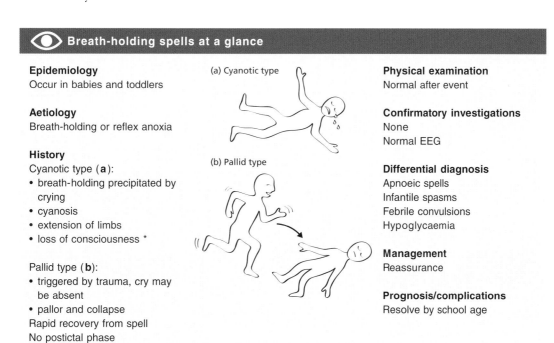

Breath-holding spells at a glance

Epidemiology
Occur in babies and toddlers

Aetiology
Breath-holding or reflex anoxia

History
Cyanotic type (a):
- breath-holding precipitated by crying
- cyanosis
- extension of limbs
- loss of consciousness *

Pallid type (b):
- triggered by trauma, cry may be absent
- pallor and collapse
Rapid recovery from spell
No postictal phase

(a) Cyanotic type

(b) Pallid type

Physical examination
Normal after event

Confirmatory investigations
None
Normal EEG

Differential diagnosis
Apnoeic spells
Infantile spasms
Febrile convulsions
Hypoglycaemia

Management
Reassurance

Prognosis/complications
Resolve by school age

Pallid spells (Reflex anoxic seizures)

Another form of spell is the pallid spell, or reflex anoxic seizure. The spell classically follows a bump on the head or other minor injury, which triggers vagal reflex overactivity, causing transient bradycardia and circulatory impairment.

Clinical features   The child may or may not start to cry, but then turns pale and collapses. There is transient apnoea and limpness, followed by rapid recovery. The typical history can help to distinguish these attacks from epilepsy.

Management   Reassurance is usually all that is required, but cardiac causes should be considered in children with severe, recurrent episodes.

Prognosis   The attacks usually disappear spontaneously prior to school age.

Night terrors

Night terrors usually occur in the preschool years.

Clinical features   The child wakes from sleep, confused and disorientated, does not recognise parents and appears very frightened. Signs of autonomic activity include dilated pupils, sweating, tachypnoea, and tachycardia. The child recovers after a few minutes, and usually has no recall of the event. Night terrors are sometimes mistaken for epilepsy or nightmares.

Management and prognosis   Night terrors require simple reassurance. They are benign and usually self-limited.

Benign paroxysmal vertigo

These episodes are characterised by acute attacks of vertigo in young children aged 1–4 years old, and are thought to be caused by a disturbance of vestibular function. During a typical attack, the child suddenly becomes ataxic, appears frightened, and may clutch at the parent. There is no alteration of consciousness and the child recovers within a few minutes. The condition is often mistaken for epilepsy, the distinguishing feature being the preservation of normal alertness during an attack. The episodes usually resolve within 1–2 years.

Syncope

Syncope, or fainting, occurs when there is hypotension and decreased cerebral perfusion. It can be caused by vaso–vagal stimulation, postural hypotension, metabolic causes, such as hypoglycaemia, and, rarely cardiac causes. Syncope is quite common, particularly in teenage girls reacting to painful or emotional stimuli. It also occurs in the teenage years in individuals with poor vasomotor reflexes after standing up rapidly, after straining or coughing severely or during prolonged standing.

Clinical features Pre-syncopal features of blurring of vision, light-headedness, sweating and nausea often precede the loss of consciousness. There may be a history of an unpleasant stimulus or prolonged standing. It is not uncommon for brief myoclonic jerks to occur during the faint, and these do not indicate epilepsy.

Management and prognosis Syncope can be troublesome and repeated in some adolescents, although it usually becomes less of a problem in adulthood. Good advice includes rising from lying to standing gradually, avoiding standing still for long periods, and 'listening to your body'. The patient should lie down with legs up at the first hint of a faint. Cardiac evaluation is indicated if faints occur during or immediately after exercise, when there are palpitations or chest pain, clinical signs of heart disease or a suspicious family history.

Psychogenic non-epileptic seizures

Psychogenic non-epileptic seizures (sometimes called 'pseudoseizures') are episodes which may mimic epilepsy and not infrequently coexist occur in children with an epileptic condition. The episodes result from a psychological, rather than neurological cause, and patients rarely have control over the episodes.

Clinical features Features suggestive of these seizures are:
- episodes provoked by emotional stimuli;
- gradual rather than abrupt onset;
- unusual aura;
- asynchronous flailing movements;
- eyes closed during a seizure;
- an abrupt change of the episode in response to a stimulus.

Incontinence, bodily injury and postictal drowsiness are usually absent.

Management A normal EEG recording, particularly if taken during an episode, can be helpful in making the diagnosis, but is not required in order to make the diagnosis. A full psychological assessment is required if the diagnosis is suspected.

Hyperventilation

Excitement or fear in some children may precipitate hyperventilation to the point of losing consciousness.

Clinical features The diagnosis is usually evident in that breathing is excessive and deep, and tetany may also occur. A history of tingling lips and pins and needles may be reported.

Management Rebreathing into a paper bag restores the child back to normality. If episodes occur frequently, psychological therapy may be required.

Tics

Tics are rapid, repetitive, brief, involuntary movements such as blinking, jerking or facial grimacing. They are common, particularly in school-age children, and are intensified by anxiety, fatigue, or excitement. They may resemble focal epileptic seizures but can be differentiated by the fact that they can be controlled voluntarily and are not associated with an alteration in consciousness. Severe tics, including vocal tics like grunting and swearing, are indicative of Gilles de la Tourette syndrome.

Refractive errors and disorders of vision

As part of child health surveillance children's eyes are tested periodically to identify the common refractive errors – myopia, hypermetropia and astigmatism (Figure 13.4). Refractive errors,

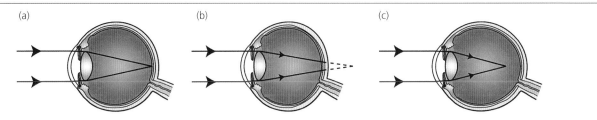

Figure 13.4 Disorders of refraction: (a) normal focusing on the retina; (b) the hypermetropic eye focuses the object beyond the retina; and (c) the myopic eye focuses the object too short – the eye is too long.

if uncorrected, can cause an indifference to schoolwork and have a deleterious effect on educational progress.

Myopia

Myopia is infrequent in infants and preschool children, other than preterm infants and children of myopic parents. There is increased refractive power of the eye, so that light focuses short of the retina. The result is blurred vision for distant objects.

The incidence of myopia increases during the school years, especially during the preteen and teen years. Concave lenses of appropriate strength are required, with changes in prescription required periodically, particularly during adolescence.

Hypermetropia

In hypermetropia refractive power is less than normal, resulting in normal vision over distance, but greater accommodative effort required for close work. This may result in eyestrain, headaches, and fatigue. Convex lenses are required to allow for comfort in focusing on near objects.

Astigmatism

Astigmatism is a distortion of vision that results from irregularities in the curvature of the cornea or irregularity of the lens. Cylindrical or spherocylindrical lenses are used to provide optical correction.

Strabismus (squints)

Squints may be convergent, divergent or alternating. If they are untreated, the visual pathways from the squinting eye become irreversibly suppressed and amblyopia develops. Evaluation involves the corneal light reflex and cover tests (see pp. 96–7).

Paralytic strabismus

Paralytic strabismus is caused by weakness or paralysis of the extraocular muscles. The squint is fixed and characteristically worsens on gazing in the direction of the affected muscle. Paralytic strabismus may be congenital or acquired and, if the latter, is an ominous sign of serious intra-cranial pathology.

Non-paralytic strabismus

Non-paralytic strabismus is the more common type (see Figure 13.5). The problem is one of malalignment of the eyes and no defect is present in the extraocular muscles themselves. The squint may be apparent (manifest) or latent, in which case it is only detected when the child is fatigued or on clinical examination. The underlying causes of non-paralytic strabismus include failure to develop binocular vision at the normal time and, more rarely, underlying ocular defects such as cataracts or high refractive errors.

'False' strabismus

Some children, particularly if they have prominent epicanthal folds and broad, flat nasal bridges, give the appearance of being cross-eyed (Figure 13.6). The corneal light reflex and cover test are, however, normal.

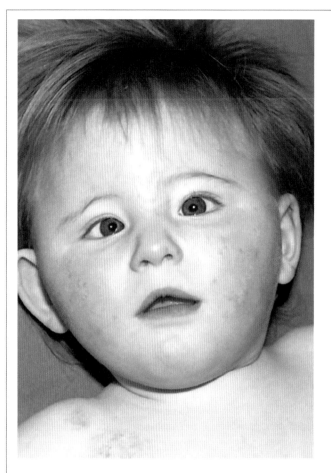

Figure 13.5 A 6-month-old baby with a convergent squint. Note the asymmetrical corneal light reflex which confirms that the visual axes are not parallel and that this child has a squint rather than simply a wide bridge to the nose.

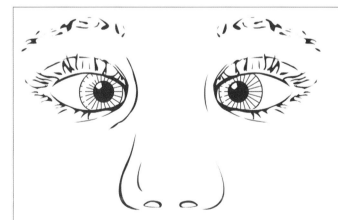

Figure 13.6 Pseudosquint or false strabismus. A wide nasal bridge and epicanthic folds give the appearance of a squint, but the corneal light reflex test is normal.

Management

All fixed squints, and any squint persisting beyond 5 or 6 months of age, need to be referred for ophthalmological evaluation. There are two goals of treatment:

1. To achieve the best possible vision in each eye. This is accomplished by correcting any underlying defect by surgery for a cataract, prescribing glasses for refractive errors and treating amblyopia by occlusion therapy.
2. To achieve the best possible ocular alignment. In many cases surgery is required; it is particularly important in congenital strabismus. Surgery needs to be carried out at the earliest possible age to give the child the best opportunity of developing normal visual pathways.

Amblyopia

Amblyopia can be defined as subnormal visual acuity in one or both eyes despite the correction of any refractive error, and is familiarly known as 'lazy eye'.

Under normal conditions the development of visual acuity proceeds rapidly in infancy. However, if interference in the formation of a clear retinal image occurs during this critical period, irreversible suppression of the visual pathway on that side develops. Examples of interference include cataracts and strabismus, where the child tunes out the image of the deviating eye to avoid diplopia (see above).

Treatment of amblyopia includes:

- Providing the clearest possible retinal image, for example by removing the cataract or by prescribing glasses.
- Stimulation or forced use of the amblyopic eye. This is achieved by occlusion therapy or 'patching' of the normal eye. Covering glasses is not very satisfactory and the best results are obtained by adhesive eye patches. Treatment can be trying and must be closely supervised, or amblyopia can develop in the patched eye.

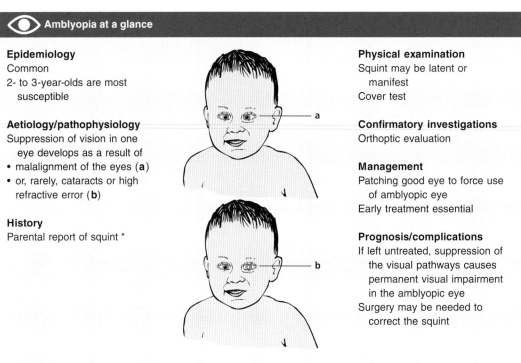

Amblyopia at a glance

Epidemiology
Common
2- to 3-year-olds are most
    susceptible

Aetiology/pathophysiology
Suppression of vision in one
    eye develops as a result of
- malalignment of the eyes (**a**)
- or, rarely, cataracts or high
    refractive error (**b**)

History
Parental report of squint *

Physical examination
Squint may be latent or
    manifest
Cover test

Confirmatory investigations
Orthoptic evaluation

Management
Patching good eye to force use
    of amblyopic eye
Early treatment essential

Prognosis/complications
If left untreated, suppression of
    the visual pathways causes
    permanent visual impairment
    in the amblyopic eye
Surgery may be needed to
    correct the squint

NB *Signs and symptoms are variable

Stroke

Stroke occurs in people of all ages, but the incidence in utero and in the first year of life is especially high.

Clinical features   The presenting features may be a 'thunderclap' severe headache, weakness of the face, arm or leg, or slurred speech.

Management and prognosis   An urgent CT or MRI head scan is indicated, often with carotid artery Doppler studies, and/or angiography. Mild focal weakness may resolve spontaneously, but imaging of the head and cerebral vessels should still occur as a transient ischaemic event may lead to more severe episodes. The aetiology of childhood stroke includes sickle cell disease, primary or secondary hypertension, thrombophilia, and trauma. Stroke is one of the top 10 causes of death in children.

To test your knowledge on this part of the book, please see Chapter 26

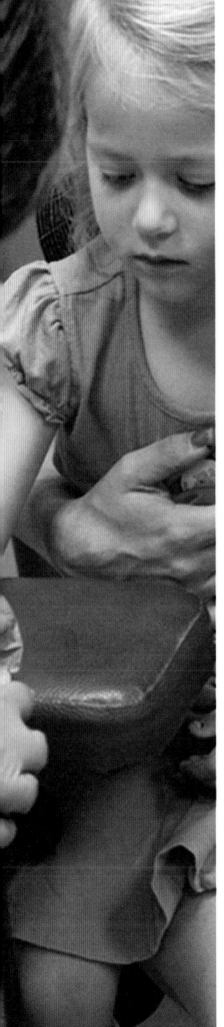

CHAPTER 14

Development and neurodisability

There are some who hear a different drummer
And who march a different pace.
Henry David Thoreau

Developmental concerns

Developmental conditions and disabilities

KEY COMPETENCES

YOU MUST...

Know and understand

- The approach to evaluating developmental delay: global, language and motor
- How serious and common disorders affecting development and causing disability are diagnosed and managed
- The key developmental milestones and developmental warning signs
- How developmental disabilities present
- The cardinal features of autism
- The composition and work of a child development team

Be able to

- Carry out a developmental assessment on babies and toddlers (see Chapter 6)
- Conduct a competent neurological examination on babies and young children (see Chapter 5)
- Recognise when development is following a delayed or unusual pattern

Appreciate that

- Developmental delay in an isolated area with a normal physical and neurological examination is rarely significant
- Delayed or abnormal development causes major parental distress
- Young children may become frustrated when development is delayed or abnormal
- Developmental disorders have a significant impact on children's and their family's lives

Essential Paediatrics and Child Health, Fourth Edition. Mary Rudolf, Anthony Luder and Kerry Jeavons.
© 2020 John Wiley & Sons Ltd. Published 2020 by John Wiley & Sons Ltd.
Companion website: www.wiley.com/go/rudolf/paediatrics

Developmental concerns

Finding your way around ...

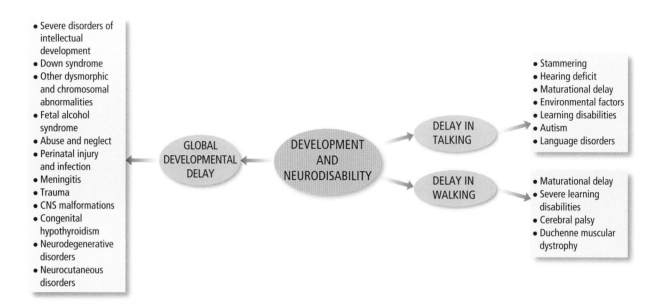

- Severe disorders of intellectual development
- Down syndrome
- Other dysmorphic and chromosomal abnormalities
- Fetal alcohol syndrome
- Abuse and neglect
- Perinatal injury and infection
- Meningitis
- Trauma
- CNS malformations
- Congenital hypothyroidism
- Neurodegenerative disorders
- Neurocutaneous disorders

GLOBAL DEVELOPMENTAL DELAY

DEVELOPMENT AND NEURODISABILITY

DELAY IN TALKING

- Stammering
- Hearing deficit
- Maturational delay
- Environmental factors
- Learning disabilities
- Autism
- Language disorders

DELAY IN WALKING

- Maturational delay
- Severe learning disabilities
- Cerebral palsy
- Duchenne muscular dystrophy

Psychomotor development and growth are issues unique to paediatrics. As in growth, children progress developmentally at different rates and, as in growth, a slower rate of development may be a variation of normal or may be an indicator for serious concern. This chapter discusses the problems of children presenting with delayed or abnormal development and what their care involves.

In order to approach children with possible or proven developmental problems, a good understanding of normal development must be acquired along with skill in evaluating a child's developmental progress (Table 14.1).

Given the wide range of normality that occurs in acquiring developmental milestones, it is important to decide when delays are concerning. In general, if the skills attained are of good quality and the child continues to progress, somewhat delayed or advanced acquisition is unimportant. For guidelines as to when you should become concerned that development is significantly delayed, see the Red Flag box.

⚑ Developmental warning signs

At any age
Maternal concern
Regression in previously acquired skills

At 10 weeks
Not smiling
Failure to fix gaze on face
Failure to startle to sound

At 6 months
Persistent primitive reflexes
Persistent squint
Head lag
Stiff or hypotonic limbs
Hand preference
Little interest in people, toys, noises

At 10–12 months
No sitting
No double-syllable babble
No pincer grasp

At 18 months
Not walking independently
Fewer than six words
Persistent mouthing and drooling

At 2½ years
No two- to three-word sentences

At 4 years
Unintelligible speech

Table 14.1 Skills required in developmental paediatrics
A grasp of normal development (Chapter 6)
Ability to conduct a developmental evaluation (p. 100)
Recognition of delay
Recognition of abnormal patterns of development

Table 14.2 Aetiological factors underlying developmental problems

Factor	Example
Genetic	Chromosomal anomalies
	Mendelian syndromes
	Inborn errors of metabolism
Environmental	Deprivation/neglect
	Lead poisoning
Injury	
Prenatal	Intrauterine infections
	Toxins: alcohol, anticonvulsants, etc.
At birth	Birth trauma/asphyxia
Postnatal	Meningitis
	Head trauma
Complex	Autism

It is important to attempt to identify the factors that underlie a child's delayed or abnormal development, although it is not always possible to do so. Some important factors are shown in Table 14.2 with examples.

Delayed or abnormal development may affect individual areas of development or may be global. Unusual development is commonly identified by the parents or is detected at routine examinations carried out by the health visitor as part of child health surveillance. In certain circumstances, when a child is known to be at high risk of developmental difficulties, such as after neonatal problems, head injury or meningitis, routine medical follow-up is arranged in order to identify any problems early.

Evaluation of a child's development requires time and skill. It is highly dependent on the child's cooperation and often requires evaluation over a period of time. The developmental area in question must be accurately assessed together with a careful neurological examination. All other developmental areas must be evaluated too, so that a complete picture of the child's development is obtained. In addition, it is important to look for an aetiology for the difficulties so that when possible a diagnosis can be reached.

History – must ask!

The history is of paramount importance. Children are quite likely to be uncooperative when relating to an unfamiliar person and in unfamiliar surroundings, and a reliable report by parents can provide much information.

The history should include an assessment of the following:

- current developmental skills;
- history of developmental milestones;
- birth history;
- past medical history;
- family history;
- parental anxieties.

Allowances for prematurity must be made during the first 2 years, but beyond that period catch-up in development rarely occurs. Parents often find it difficult to recall their child's developmental milestones, but in the event of delay they are likely to be more accurate. Of particular importance in taking a history is the identification of any developmental skills that the child previously gained but has subsequently lost (regression). It is important to stress to parents that development is more about quality than simply achieving a certain number of skills by certain ages.

Physical examination – must check!

- *Developmental skills*. You should attempt to evaluate development before carrying out any other part of the physical examination, as undressing the child is likely to arouse some antagonism. Assess each developmental area – gross motor, fine motor/adaptive, language and social skills – in turn, and attempt to evaluate the child's vision and hearing.

  Checklists of developmental skills can be helpful. In addition, you must assess factors such as alertness, responsiveness, interest in surroundings, determination, and concentration, which all can positively influence a child's attainments.

  The child may well not cooperate with particular tasks, particularly if they are tired, shy or at the stage of stranger anxiety. You can gain a great deal of information from simply observing the child at play while taking the history.

- *General examination*. A complete physical examination is needed in order to identify medical problems. Particularly relevant are dysmorphic signs, microcephaly, poor growth, and signs of neglect.

- *Neurological examination*. This needs to be thorough, looking for abnormalities in tone, strength and coordination, deep tendon reflexes, clonus, cranial nerves and primitive reflexes.

Investigations

Investigations may be required, depending on the nature of the problem.

Management

You must address the parents' concerns, whether a particular problem has been identified or not, as ongoing parental anxiety in itself can be damaging to the child. Reassurance may be all that is required, but follow-up is important to ensure that developmental progress is maintained. You may need to refer to an appropriate therapist, either to carry out a more detailed assessment or to provide the child and family with guidance in how to encourage the development of skills. You should always be cautious about developmental predictions, and repeat examinations over time are often needed to predict outcome with any confidence.

When developmental difficulties are complex, the paediatrician alone is unlikely to be able to make a sufficiently detailed assessment of the child's abilities and advise on appropriate management. In this circumstance the child should be referred to a child development team (see p. 49).

> ### 🔑 Key points: Abnormal or delayed development
>
> - Accurately assess the developmental area which is delayed
> - Assess all other developmental areas
> - Attempt to make a diagnosis or identify the aetiology for the difficulties
> - Remember to correct for prematurity in the first 2 years
> - Make sure that the child's developmental skills are not regressing

---

👁 General issues for the child with delayed/abnormal development at a glance

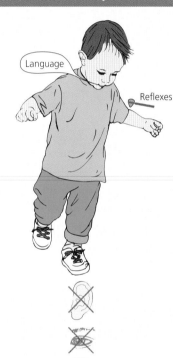

Causes
Often no cause is found, but cerebral insults and genetic and environmental factors should be considered

How the child presents
Delay may be global or affect individual areas of development
Identified by parents, during child health surveillance, or in medical follow-up of high risk problems

Clinical evaluation
Time, skill and cooperation are required
Assess all developmental areas – gross motor, fine motor/adaptive, language and social skills
Correction for prematurity should be made until 2 years of age

History
Current developmental skills
History of developmental milestones
Birth, medical and family history
Parental concerns
Regression in skills

Physical examination
Development
Observation of the child in free play, assessment of specific skills, vision and hearing, and identification of positive features such as alertness, determination and concentration

General examination
Dysmorphic signs, microcephaly or macrocephaly, poor growth, signs of neglect

Neurological examination
Abnormalities in tone, strength and coordination, deep tendon reflexes, clonus, cranial nerves and primitive reflexes

Investigations
Sometimes required

Management
Follow-up and reassurance for simple delay
If a developmental problem is identified:
- full discussion with the parents
- consider referral to a therapist
- referral to a child development team if the problems are complex
Caution is needed in predicting outcome

Delay or difficulty in talking

> **Causes of speech and language difficulties***
>
> *Speech (or articulation) difficulties*
> Stammer
> Cleft lip and palate
>
> *Deafness*
>
> *Developmental*
> Maturational delay (often familial)
> Environmental deprivation and neglect
> Intellectual disabilities (mental retardation)
>
> *Communication difficulties*
> Autism
>
> *Language disorder*
>
> *Speech is not delayed by tongue-tiedness, laziness, or 'everything being done for him'. Children exposed to more than one language may experience confused vocabulary or mild speech delay, but this sorts itself out without intervention.

Language is the most highly developed of all human skills. Not only does it allow us to communicate with others, but it is also a vehicle for thought. Disorders of speech and language are extremely common. In many children the problem is one of unclear speech, or a simple delay so that the child's language resembles that of a younger child. However, in some, delay or difficulty in talking is the presenting feature of more serious disorders such as severe intellectual disabilities, autism and hearing loss which need intervention.

It is important to appreciate the terminology used in developmental paediatrics. The term *language* refers to the whole process whereby we communicate with others, involving both understanding and expressive processes. *Speech* is the component of language which is articulated.

In order to learn to talk, the child needs normal hearing, intact language pathways in the brain, normal oral structures and, in addition, a certain intellectual ability and the ability to relate to others. Problems in any of these areas cause a delay or difficulties in the development of speech or language.

Words normally first appear at around the first birthday, and are strung together into two-word phrases by the age of 2 years. Language then develops rapidly, although it is not always initially intelligible to strangers. Parents are often the first to express concern about their child's language development.

As a guide, children need to be evaluated if they have fewer than six words at the age of 18 months, no two- or three-word sentences by 2½ years, or still unintelligible speech at 4 years. Earlier indicators of possible difficulties are the absence of double-syllable babble at a year and persistent mouthing and drooling at 18 months. Evaluation of children for speech and language problems is a complex process and beyond toddlerhood often needs the expertise of a speech and language therapist. Nonetheless, doctors should be able to identify language difficulties and know when referral is needed.

A common variant, known as *maturational delay,* is when the child appears to understand well but is late in talking – with a delay of 3–6 months. It is frequently familial, and late talkers are subsequently more likely to have difficulty in learning to read (dyslexia). Children living in socially disadvantaged homes often have language delay, and this is particularly true for neglected and emotionally deprived children. Maturational delay needs to be distinguished from language delay associated with *global intellectual developmental disorders,* when delay in fine motor skills and social skills such as toilet training are also usually present.

Stammering (or stuttering) is very common. It usually occurs at about the age of 3 years, when the child's thought processes outstrip their ability to express themselves. Language development is normal, the stammer is purely a difficulty in articulation. It is referred to as 'normal non-fluency' and is usually outgrown if not too much attention is paid to the problem. If it proves to be persistent, school-age children can be helped by speech therapy.

If a child cannot hear clearly, obviously speech cannot follow. *Conductive hearing loss* resulting from secretory otitis media (glue ear) is the commonest cause of hearing deficit (see p. 146). Once hearing improves, catch-up in language skills occurs. However, if correction does not take place during the critical early years, irreversible difficulties in quality of speech and language may occur. *Neurosensory deafness* is a less common problem, and should be detected by audiological surveillance before language is affected. Hearing screening is now routinely performed after birth in most centres.

The term *language disorder* refers to when language development follows an abnormal pattern rather than being simply delayed. Receptive or expressive language may be affected. These children are at risk for specific developmental learning disorder such as dyslexia, and may even require special education. Speech therapy is important.

It is common for a combination of difficulties to occur. For example, children with a cleft lip are also quite likely to have a conductive hearing loss, and when children with global developmental delay have autistic tendencies their communication difficulties are compounded.

History – must ask!

Even children with normal language skills are shy about talking to strangers, and attempting to assess a child with a language difficulty directly is very likely to be unproductive, so a good history from the parents is essential.

- *Is this a speech or a language problem?* In a speech disorder words are unintelligible, but the child's comprehension of language is normal. If both comprehension and speech are delayed it is likely that there is a language difficulty of some sort.
- *Is there global delay?* Language strongly reflects a child's ability to learn in a more global sense. Children with severe disorders of intellectual development have poor language skills, but are delayed in their fine motor and social skills too.
- *Is there a hearing deficit?* Language cannot develop if a child cannot hear. You must check whether the parents feel the child has difficulty hearing.
- *Are there non-verbal communication difficulties?* In order to acquire language children need to have well-developed communication skills. Autistic children are poor at relating with others from a very young age.

In addition to focusing on language skills, your history should include the following:
- a complete developmental history;
- past medical history including perinatal events;
- a family history of deafness and language delay.

Physical examination – must check!

- Observation. You can glean valuable information by watching the child at play. You may hear him talk, and you can observe the relationship with the parents. Imaginative play with toys such as dolls, cars and tea-sets gives valuable clues about the child's intelligence.

- Developmental examination. When you assess language, you must try to assess both comprehension and expressive language. Asking questions about pictures and directing the child in play are useful techniques. You should also assess motor and social skills.
- Mouth and ears. The focus of your physical examination should be on the ears and mouth. Look for secretory otitis media, and try to evaluate hearing. Anatomical anomalies are usually obvious on inspection of the mouth.

Investigations

It is mandatory to carry out a good hearing evaluation on any child with suspected language difficulties. This should be performed by a trained audiologist.

If you confirm language difficulties on your clinical evaluation, a formal assessment by a speech and language therapist is required.

Key points: Speech and language difficulty

- Assess hearing
- Decide if this is a speech (articulation) or language difficulty
- Decide if the delay is restricted to language or whether there is a global delay
- Look for evidence of a communication disorder (autism)

Clues to the diagnosis of children with language delay and difficulties

	Language development	Other developmental areas	Ability to form interpersonal relationships
Stammer	Comprehension and expressive language is normal, but speech is immature, stuttered or unintelligible	Normal	Normal
Hearing deficit	Comprehension and expressive language delayed	Normal but hearing response reduced	Normal
Maturational delay	Expressive language delayed	Normal	Normal
Disorders of intellectual development	Comprehension and expressive language delayed	Delayed	Often normal
Autism	Comprehension and expressive language delayed	Disordered and delayed	Abnormal
Language disorders	Language delayed but also disordered	Usually delayed	Normal

Delay in learning to walk

Commoner causes of delayed walking*

Delay in motor maturation
Delayed motor maturation (often familial)
Severe disorders of intellectual development

Abnormalities of muscle tone or power
Cerebral palsy
Hypotonia of any cause
Muscular dystrophy
Other neuromuscular disorders

*Obesity and congenital dislocation of the hip are not causes of
delayed walking.

Independent walking is acquired on average at the age of 13 months, although many children walk some months before this. Black babies tend to walk earlier than white. Walking is considered to be delayed if it has not been achieved by the age of 18 months. Delay in walking can result either from delay in maturation of the neuromuscular system or as a result of pathology affecting muscle tone or strength.

You need to determine if the delay is isolated to gross motor skills, or whether there is a more global developmental problem. The quality of motor development to date and a neurological examination should indicate if the problem is simple delay, or if neurological or neuromuscular pathology are present. Look for aetiological factors that might account for the delay.

Environmental factors can delay the onset of walking, but emotional deprivation tends to affect gross motor skills less than other developmental skills. In the past, when institutionalized children were restricted to their cots, delay in gross motor skills was common. A similar process is seen in children who have been ill, casted in plaster, and confined to bed for an extended period. Provided they are given the opportunity to be active, catch-up is seen.

Delayed motor maturation is simply a descriptive term for the child who starts to walk late, but is normal in other respects. There is often a family history of late walking, and on examination motor skills are delayed but normal in terms of quality. Mild hypotonia may be present. The diagnosis is made on clinical grounds, and by exclusion of pathology. Parents should be reassured that the child will eventually walk, and the prognosis is good, although clumsiness may become apparent and later skills such as running and cycling may be delayed. If there is delay in other developmental areas, a more general disorder of intellectual development should be suspected.

Delayed walking may be the presenting feature of milder forms of *cerebral palsy*: hemiplegia and spastic diplegia. In more severe cerebral palsy, concerns about developmental progress are likely to have been aroused long before the child is expected to walk. The prognosis depends on the degree of spasticity, but most children with hemiplegia or diplegia eventually learn to walk, although the gait is not normal.

History – must ask!

Your history should follow the pattern outlined for the presentation of any developmental problem (see p. 252). Make a clear assessment of all four developmental areas. A careful history of motor skills should include the baby's ability to sit supported or unsupported, roll over from both front and back, get to the sitting position independently, crawl, pull to stand and cruise.

A family history of late walking is important as this provides support for the benign diagnosis of maturational delay. It is also important to identify environmental factors such as deprivation or lack of opportunity to exercise gross motor skills.

Physical examination – must check!

Your physical examination should confirm the developmental history, and identify any abnormal neuromuscular signs. Attempt to assess the child's developmental skills well to clarify whether the delay is generalised or isolated to gross motor skills. A great deal of information can be obtained by placing the child on the floor with some toys in easy reach, while you take the history. You can then observe the child in natural activity, before doing a more formal evaluation.

Your neurological examination should be thorough. Look for abnormalities in tone, deep tendon reflexes, strength, asymmetry of movements and the presence of primitive reflexes.

Investigations

If the delay in walking is isolated and the child in other respects has normal development, the only investigation required is a creatinine phosphokinase level (CPK or CK) as late walking may be the earliest manifestation of muscular dystrophy (see later).

If you find signs of cerebral palsy or hypotonia, investigations may be required.

🔑 **Key points: Delayed walking**

- Determine whether the delay is isolated to gross motor skills or whether there is a more global developmental problem
- Identify any abnormal neurological findings
- Identify any responsible aetiological factors

Clues to the diagnosis of the child with delayed walking

	History	Other developmental milestones	General physical examination	Neurological signs
Delayed motor maturation	Family history of delayed walking	Normal	Normal	Normal (or mildly decreased tone)
Severe disorder of intellectual development		Delayed, usually to a greater degree than gross motor	Dysmorphic features, microcephaly etc. may be found	Normal (or decreased tone)
Environmental factors	Lack of opportunity	May be delayed	Normal	Normal
Hypertonia–cerebral palsy		Often delayed		Increased tone and tendon reflexes in affected limb
Muscular dystrophy	Other family members affected	Normal	Later on, maybe large but weak calf muscles	Later on, weakness of the hip girdle muscles, Gower sign

Global developmental delay

Causes of global developmental delay

Cause	Example
Chromosomal abnormalities	Down syndrome Fragile X
Dysmorphic syndromes	Williams; Beckwith-Wiedemann
Injury	
Prenatal	Fetal alcohol syndrome
Perinatal	TORCH, Zika virus infection (see p. 435)
Postnatal	Hypoxic–ischaemic insult
	Meningitis
	Non-accidental injury
	Neglect
Central nervous malformations	Neural tube defects
	Hydrocephalus
Endocrine and metabolic defects	Hypothyroidism
Neurodegenerative disorders	Tay-Sachs
Neurocutaneous syndromes	Tuberous sclerosis
Idiopathic	

The term *global developmental delay* refers to a delay in acquiring all developmental milestones, but particularly language, fine motor, and social skills. It is extremely worrying when this occurs as it usually indicates severe disorder of intellectual development. Gross motor skills may also be delayed, though they do not reflect intellectual capacity in the same way as the other skills, and are sometimes spared.

The purpose of the clinical evaluation is first of all to ascertain whether the child truly has global developmental delay, and to what extent each area is affected. The next stage is to seek an underlying cause and consider whether investigations are likely to be helpful.

In about one-third of children with global developmental delay, no specific cause is identified, although advances in genetics mean this is changing. *Down syndrome* (not usually a diagnostic challenge), Fragile X syndrome, and *fetal alcohol syndrome* are important causes. Some *inborn errors of metabolism* present with developmental delay, as can *neurodegenerative conditions* – the latter characterised by relentless neurological deterioration. Congenital *hypothyroidism,* once a serious cause, is no longer seen since the introduction of neonatal screening. *Intrauterine infections* such as rubella, cytomegalovirus (CMV), and toxoplasmosis infection cause severe fetal damage and can present with global developmental delay.

Emotional abuse and neglect can have serious consequences for children's developmental progress, which is often accompanied by failure to thrive (see pp. 283, 291). The child may be apathetic, with evidence of physical neglect or injury.

History – must ask!

- *What are the child's current skills?* Obtain a detailed history of the child's current abilities in all four areas. Ask the parents if they have any concerns about the child's hearing or vision.
- *When did the child achieve earlier milestones?* It is important to identify whether development was initially appropriate or whether there were concerns early on. Developmental difficulties may have followed trauma or an illness.
- *Has there been regression in skills?* Children with disorders of intellectual development tend to have a slow but steady acquisition of skills. Regression of skills suggests a neurodegenerative disorder.
- *Past medical history.* A detailed perinatal history is particularly important. Ask about alcohol consumption, medications, prematurity, pregnancy health, foreign travel (Zika) and neonatal complications. The links between developmental difficulties and postnatal events such as meningitis or head trauma are usually obvious.
- *Family history.* A family history of disorders of intellectual development or consanguinity is important as it suggests a possible genetic cause for the problem.

Physical examination – must check!

A detailed developmental evaluation, followed by a complete physical examination focusing on neurological findings is needed. Assess all four developmental areas (see pp. 100–5). In addition, focus on the following:

- *Growth.* Many children with developmental problems are short. If actual fall-off in growth has occurred, you should consider hypothyroidism and non-organic failure to thrive.
- *Microcephaly.* Microcephaly is a common, often non-specific finding, but if present at birth it suggests intrauterine infections, fetal alcohol syndrome or a genetic disorder. If it develops in the first year of life in association with developmental delay, a neurodegenerative disorder or perinatal cause should be suspected.
- *Dysmorphic signs.* Not uncommonly global developmental delay is associated with congenital anomalies and dysmorphic features. If present they suggestive a genetic defect, chromosomal anomaly or teratogenic effect.
- *General appearance.* Signs of neglect such as an undernourished appearance, skin and hair in poor condition, uncleanliness, and irritative rashes in the skinfolds may indicate psychosocial factors responsible for the delay.

- *Skin.* Examine the skin for signs such as café-au-lait spots, depigmented patches, and port-wine stains, which are indicative of neurocutaneous syndromes.
- *Hepatosplenomegaly.* The finding of an enlarged liver or spleen suggests a metabolic disorder.

Neurological examination

Features of particular importance are the following:
- *Hypotonia.* This is often a non-specific finding. It occurs in Down syndrome.
- *Signs of cerebral palsy* (see p. 262). Cerebral palsy affects motor skills but disorder in intellectual development also commonly occurs.
- *Hearing and vision.*
- *Ocular abnormalities.* The finding of eye abnormalities such as cataracts suggests a metabolic disorder.

Investigations

Chromosomal analysis and thyroid function tests should be performed in every child with global developmental delay. More sophisticated investigation of biochemical and metabolic function, infection; DNA testing or brain imaging may be indicated in some. NGS (next generation sequencing) including whole exome sequencing, and comparative genome array hybridization (CGA) are new techniques for identifying genetic diseases which were previously undiagnosable.

Management

Every attempt should be made to identify a cause for the delay. Although there is rarely specific treatment, parents are helped by having a diagnosis, and there may be genetic implications for subsequent pregnancies.

The term 'developmental delay' is sometimes used euphemistically as a diagnosis in itself. This is inappropriate. A child should be described as being delayed only up to the point when the diagnosis of a disorder in intellectual development becomes clear (usually well before the age of 3 years). The management of children with global developmental delay is covered in detail in the section on disorders of intellectual development (see p. 267).

Key points: Global developmental delay

- Correct for prematurity if the child is less than 2 years old
- Confirm that the delay is global
- Assess the extent of the delay in each area
- Determine if there is regression of skills
- Attempt to identify a cause for the delay by examination and investigations
- Refer for a child development team assessment

Clues to the diagnosis of a child with global developmental delay

Condition	History	Physical examination	Other features
Down syndrome	Older maternal age is a risk factor	Characteristic facial features, single palmar crease, Brushfield spots, hypotonia	Congenital heart disease, anal/duodenal atresia, growth should be followed on Down charts
Fragile X	Other boys in the family affected	Long face, prominent ears, large jaw, large testes at puberty	Fits, behaviour problems
Fetal alcohol syndrome	Possible history of alcohol in pregnancy, intrauterine growth retardation (IUGR)	Short palpebral fissures, maxillary hypoplasia, thin upper lip, microcephaly	Cardiac defects, minor joint and limb abnormalities
Dysmorphic syndromes	Family history; consanguinity	Dysmorphic features, +/– congenital anomalies	Poor growth common
Abuse and neglect	Family possibly known to social services	Possible signs of neglect or old injuries	Failure to thrive common
Inborn errors of metabolism	Consanguinity, neonatal seizures, hypoglycaemia, vomiting, coma	Sometimes coarse features, hepatosplenomegaly, microcephaly, failure to thrive	Developmental regression may occur
Congenital hypothyroidism	Failure to screen after birth	May have features of cretinism. Plateauing of growth	Constipation, slow reflex relaxation
Neurodegenerative disorders*	Developmental regression	May have coarse features, microcephaly develops	Fits, visual and intellectual deterioration
Idiopathic disorders of intellectual development	May be a familial background	Mild dysmorphic features common	
Intrauterine infections*	Possible history of contact in pregnancy, IUGR, foreign travel	Visual or hearing deficits common, microcephaly	Rash, retinitis, congenital heart disease
Neurocutaneous* syndromes	Often familial	Characteristic skin lesions	Often have specific medical complications

* Features vary according to the type of disorder.

Developmental conditions and disabilities

Autism

Autism is a pervasive developmental disorder characterised by varying degrees of social, language, personality and behavioural dysfunction. The symptoms relate to impairment in social interaction and communication, restricted interests and repetitive behaviour. Other aspects, such as atypical eating, are also common. There is a spectrum of severity, ranging from severe disorder in intellectual development, in which language development is very delayed, to children with normal intelligence and 'social pragmatic communication disorder' (DSM-5) (which overlaps with what was formerly called Asperger syndrome). Some autistic individuals can display extraordinary abilities in highly focused areas such as numerical calculation, and graphical–numerical memory. Such individuals are called 'savants'. Autism has a strong genetic basis, although the genetics of autism are complex.

Clinical features   Characteristically the child fails to develop social relationships. This may be noticed at a very young age when the baby may not make eye-contact or smile as expected, or may not be as 'cuddly' as expected, although in others it appears to develop as toddlers. There is very little communication, both verbal and non-verbal, and eye contact is avoided. Ritualistic, repetitive and obsessional behaviour is also characteristic.

Management   Autism is one of the hardest conditions for a family to cope with. Children at the severe end of the spectrum have very difficult behaviour and can only attend special school. Others who are of normal intelligence cope educationally in mainstream school but have problems making friends and joining in socially. Intensive developmental therapy at a specialised centre is often recommended if available. Input is usually provided by a multidisciplinary team involving a social worker, speech and occupational therapists, and a child psychologist.

Prognosis   Children at the severe end of the spectrum need lifelong support and can never achieve independence. Children with autistic spectrum tendencies have social difficulties and are less likely to marry and be full members of society.

 See NICE guideline: Autism spectrum disorder in under-19s: recognition, referral and diagnosis
https://www.nice.org.uk/guidance/cg128

Attention deficit disorder

Attention deficit disorder (ADD or ADHD) refers to a difficulty in focusing on tasks or activities. Inattention, hyperactivity, and impulsivity are the key behaviours, although the diagnosis is also made if hyperactivity (see p. 388) is not a feature. The condition is far commoner in boys than girls. The diagnosis is made far more frequently than in the past and the reasons for this are not entirely clear.

Clinical features   The child is fidgety, has a difficult time remaining in his or her seat at school, is easily distracted and impulsive, has difficulty following instructions, talks excessively and flits from one activity to another. Daydreaming is more obvious if hyperactivity is not a feature. There is often a history of being colicky, temperamentally difficult babies.

Diagnosis   The diagnosis needs to be made in consultation with teachers. The features of ADD may be similar to those of fatigue, and so it is crucial to ensure that the child is getting enough sleep. Occasionally absence seizures like petit-mal maybe mistaken for ADD. ADD-like features may also be part of a broader behavioural or psychological problem, and such co-morbidities must be carefully excluded. Discipline and social issues in school also need to be carefully addressed. In recent years a variety of computer-based and other types of formal testing have been advocated for more accurate diagnosis and follow-up.

Management   The child benefits from a regular daily routine with simple clear rules, and firm limits enforced fairly and sympathetically. Overstimulation and overfatigue should be avoided. In school a structured programme is required, with good home communication to ensure consistency. Pedagogic planning and close cooperation of the school staff is important to ensure an interesting curriculum pitched at the right intellectual level as well as consistent enforcement of discipline.

Attention deficit problems, particularly if associated with hyperactivity, can be very stressful to the family and counselling may be needed. A variety of central nervous system stimulants such as methylphenidate prescribed during school hours, as well as non-stimulants, have been shown to be helpful in selected cases. Therapies such as megavitamins and fad diets have not been proved to be effective.

Prognosis   Both the hyperactivity and attention difficulties tend to improve through adolescence, but the educational deficit may persist as a handicap later in life.

See NICE guideline: ADHD: diagnosis and management
https://www.nice.org.uk/guidance/cg72

Cerebral palsy

Cerebral palsy is a disorder of movement and posture caused by an early permanent and non-progressive cerebral lesion in the first two years of life. Fifty per cent of children with cerebral palsy also have a combination of epilepsy, hearing and vision problems, intellectual, or feeding difficulties. Cerebral palsy affects two to three per 1000 children and is the commonest cause of physical disability in childhood.

Aetiology/pathology (see Table 14.3)

Although the brain lesion itself in cerebral palsy is non-progressive, the clinical picture changes as the child grows and develops. The underlying brain lesion may result from different insults occurring at various times in the developing brain. The clinical picture resulting from these insults varies depending on the area of the brain involved.

Spastic cerebral palsy is the commonest form and results from damage to the cerebral motor cortex or its connections. *Dystonic (athetoid) cerebral palsy* results from damage to the basal ganglia and is characterised by irregular and involuntary movements which may be continuous or occur on voluntary movement. *Ataxic cerebral palsy* is rare and results from damage to the cerebellum. It is characterised by hypotonia, incoordination, intention tremor, and frequently with disordered intellectual development and speech impairment.

Table 14.3 Causes of cerebral palsy
Prenatal
Cerebral malformations
Congenital infection (p. 258)
Metabolic defects
Perinatal
Complications of prematurity
Intrapartum trauma
Hemorrhagic or hypoxic–ischaemic insult* (p. 430)
Postnatal (if incurred before 24 months of age)
Non-accidental injury
Accidental head trauma
Meningitis/encephalitis
Cardiopulmonary arrest

* In term babies this is an uncommon cause. Cerebral palsy should not be attributed to these insults unless they were severe and followed by neurological problems in the neonatal period. Most babies who have experienced mild to moderate distress in the perinatal period do not develop cerebral palsy, whereas most children with cerebral palsy have a normal birth history.

Clinical features of spastic cerebral palsy

Spastic cerebral palsy is classified according to the limbs affected (Figure 14.1). Clasp-knife hypertonia, brisk deep tendon reflexes, ankle clonus and a Babinski response (extensor plantar) are found in the affected limbs.

Hemiplegia

In hemiplegia (Figures 14.1a, 14.2), only one side of the body is affected, and the arm is often more involved than the leg. During infancy there are decreased spontaneous movements on the affected side. Walking is usually delayed until 18–24 months, and when it develops there is a characteristic gait. The child often walks on tiptoes because of the increased tone, and the affected arm is held in a dystonic posture when running.

Diplegia

Diplegia (Figure 14.1b) is the commonest type of cerebral palsy seen in survivors of severe prematurity. Both legs are involved, and the arms are less affected, if at all. The first indication of a problem often occurs when the baby starts to crawl, and the legs tend to drag behind. There is excessive adduction of the hips and the parents may find difficulty in putting on a nappy.

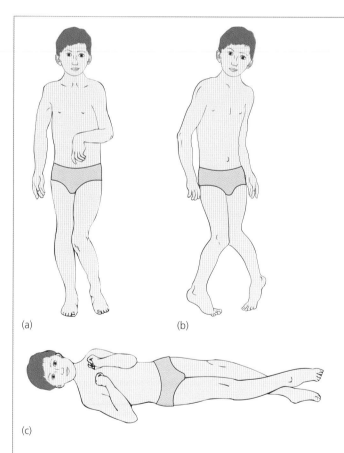

(a)   (b)

(c)

Figure 14.1 Types of cerebral palsy: (a) hemiplegia, (b) diplegia and (c) total body impairment.

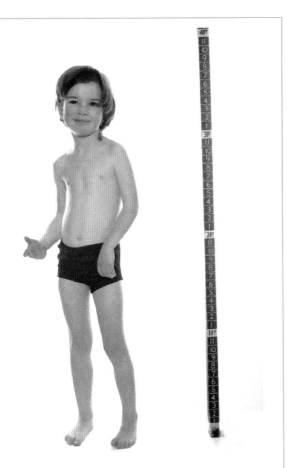

Figure 14.2 A child with left hemiplegia. Note the flexed posture of the arm and circumduction of the leg.

When the baby is suspended under the arms, the legs take up a scissoring posture. Walking is delayed, and the gait is characteristic. The feet are held in the equinovarus position and the child walks on tiptoes.

Total body impairment

Total body impairment (Figure 14.1c) is the most severe form of cerebral palsy because of marked motor impairment of all extremities and the high association with severe disorder of intellectual development and fits. Swallowing difficulties and gastro-oesophageal reflux are also common and often lead to aspiration pneumonia. Microcephaly is common, and flexion contractures of the knees and elbows are often present by late childhood. Associated disabilities, especially speech and visual problems, are particularly prevalent.

Associated problems

Children with cerebral palsy commonly have additional problems, especially if they have the quadriplegic or severe hemiplegic form of the condition. These problems include the following:

- severe disorder of intellectual development;
- epilepsy;
- visual impairment;
- squint;
- hearing loss;
- speech disorders;
- behaviour disorders;
- feeding difficulties;
- undernutrition and poor growth;
- respiratory problems;
- dislocated hips.

How cerebral palsy presents and the diagnosis is made

Follow-up of babies who have suffered a cerebral insult perinatally is the commonest way in which cerebral palsy is diagnosed; others may be detected through child health surveillance. In the neonatal period the diagnosis may be suspected if a baby has difficulty sucking, irritability, convulsions or an abnormal neurological examination. However, many of these infants subsequently develop normally, so it is important that cerebral palsy is not mistakenly diagnosed too early.

The diagnosis is usually made late in the first year of life when the following features emerge:

- *Abnormalities of tone.* Initially the tone may be quite reduced, but eventually spasticity develops.
- *Delays in motor development.* Marked head lag and delays in sitting and rolling over are usually found.
- *Abnormal patterns of development.* Movements are not only delayed but also abnormal in quality.
- *Persistence of primitive reflexes.* Primitive reflexes such as the Moro, grasp and asymmetric tonic neck reflex (see p. 93) persist beyond the age at which they normally disappear.

The diagnosis is made on clinical grounds. As the clinical picture takes time to evolve, repeated examinations are often required to establish the diagnosis. Once made, a multidisciplinary assessment is needed to define the extent of the difficulties.

Investigations

The aetiology of the cerebral palsy is often evident from the history. Rarely, further investigation is required to rule out progressive disorders. Computed tomography (CT) or magnetic resonance imaging (MRI) scans may be useful in demonstrating cerebral malformations, delineating the extent of structural lesions and ruling out very rare progressive or treatable causes such as tumours.

Management of cerebral palsy (see Box 14.1)

The goals of managing cerebral palsy fall into two categories: those specific to cerebral palsy, and those related to any child with a disability. As regards cerebral palsy itself, the effects of spasticity and the development of contractures must be minimized by regular physiotherapy. Providing the child with aids may help them to be

Box 14.1 Managing the child with cerebral palsy

- Aim to minimize the effects of spasticity and development of contractures
- Identify and manage any associated problems
- Ensure the child is provided with appropriate support for their special educational needs
- Ensure the family has adequate support: financial, practical and emotional
- Try to maximize the child's integration into society

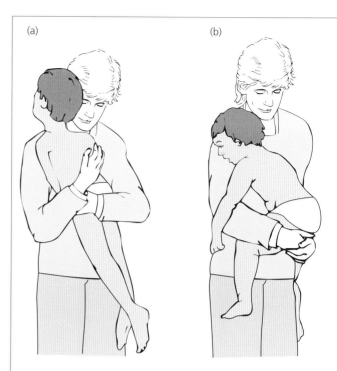

Figure 14.3 Holding a child with cerebral palsy. (a) Incorrect technique. (b) Correct technique.

independently mobile. The associated problems that commonly occur in cerebral palsy must be actively sought and management provided.

As for any child with a disability, appropriate schooling and educational resources must be provided to meet any special educational needs. One must ensure that the family are provided with adequate financial, practical and emotional support, and the child must be helped to integrate as much as possible into society.

Practical aspects of management

Most children with cerebral palsy have multiple difficulties and require multidisciplinary input. This is best provided by a child development team, in order to ensure good liaison between professionals and parents, and to structure a coordinated programme of treatment to meet all the child's needs.

Physiotherapy

The role of the physiotherapist is crucial. It is the physiotherapist who advises on handling and mobilization (Figure 14.3) in daily activities such as feeding, carrying, dressing and bathing in ways that will limit the effects of abnormal muscle tone. Exercises designed to prevent the development of deforming contractures are taught and a variety of aids, such as firm boots, lightweight splints and walking frames can be employed.

Occupational therapy

The occupational therapist's role overlaps with the physiotherapist. The occupational therapist is trained to advise on special equipment such as wheelchairs and seating, and also on play materials and activities that best encourage the child's hand function.

Speech therapy

The speech and language therapist is involved in advising on feeding and language. In the early months, advice may be required for feeding and swallowing difficulties. Later, a thorough assessment of the child's developing speech and language is often required and help given on all aspects of communication, including non-verbal systems when necessary.

Medication

Drugs, other than anticonvulsants for epilepsy, have a limited role in cerebral palsy. The treatment of tone disorders is important and baclofen (for spasticity) and trihexyphenidyl (for dystonia) are first-line management. Botulinum injections for spasticity, intrathecal baclofen for spasticity and dystonia are second-line treatment. Selective dorsal rhizotomy for spasticity and deep brain stimulation for dystonia are newer and more invasive treatments

Orthopaedic surgery

Even with adequate physiotherapy, orthopaedic deformities may develop as a result of long-standing muscle weakness or spasticity. Dislocation of the hips may occur as a result of spasticity in the thigh adductors, and fixed equinus deformity of the ankle as a result of calf muscle spasticity. Both of these may require orthopaedic surgery.

Cerebral palsy at a glance

Definition

Cerebral palsy is a disorder of movement caused by a permanent, non-progressive lesion in the developing brain

Epidemiology

2–3 per 1000 children

Aetiology/pathophysiology

Cerebral palsy is caused by pre-, peri- or postnatal insults to the brain. Types include spastic (commonest), dystonic and ataxic cerebral palsy

Clinical features of spastic cerebral palsy

Hemiplegic, monoplegic diplegic, and quadriplegic forms occur

Neurological signs in affected limbs

- clasp-knife hypertonia (**a**)
- brisk deep tendon reflexes (**b**)
- ankle clonus (**c**)
- Babinski response (extensor plantar) (**d**)

How the diagnosis is made

The diagnosis is clinical, based on findings of abnormalities of tone, delays in motor development, abnormal movement patterns and persistent primitive reflexes. Diagnosis may be suspected in neonates, but can only be made months later

Common associated problems

Gastro-oesophageal reflux

Disorders of intellectual development (mild or severe)

Epilepsy

Visual impairment

Hearing impairment

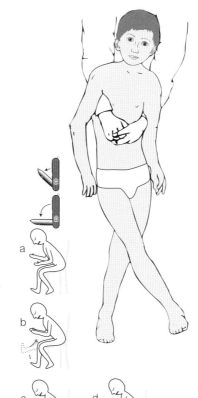

Management

- Multidisciplinary assessment and management
- Phsyiotherapy is essential
- Occupational and speech therapy
- Special equipment needs must be met
- Drugs and surgery have a limited place
- Support for the family involving voluntary agencies and social services
- Special educational needs – in mainstream school, if physical access and resources for learning difficulties are adequate. Otherwise, special school for the physically or learning disabled

Points for routine follow-up

Monitor:

- developmental progress
- medical problems
- development of contractures or dislocation
- behavioural difficulties
- nutritional status

Each child needs a structured programme addressing all needs

Liaison between professionals is important

Prognosis

Depends on degree and type of cerebral palsy, level of learning disability and presence of other associated problems

Degree of independent living achieved relates to:

- type and extent of cerebral palsy
- degree of learning disability
- presence of associated problems, e.g. visual impairment, epilepsy

Nutrition

Undernutrition commonly occurs in children with cerebral palsy, and can reduce the chances of achieving physical and intellectual potential. Food must be given in a form appropriate to the child's ability to chew and swallow. Energy-rich supplements and medical treatment for reflux, if present, may be needed. If the child is unable to eat adequate amounts, a gastrostomy may be needed.

Issues for the family

The family has to cope with all the difficulties facing any family with a child with disabilities (p. 49). However, cerebral palsy, if severe, places particularly heavy demands on the family in terms of time and input. Everyday tasks such as dressing and bathing take time, and feeding, in particular, may take hours each day. The child also needs regular physiotherapy at home, and needs to attend for appointments, both for medical follow-up and therapy. In view of this, the family is in need of support, which often goes beyond what family and friends can supply. It is important that they are aware of the support offered by voluntary and social service agencies in terms of babysitting, respite care and benefits.

Very rarely cerebral palsy has a genetic basis. In most cases parents need reassurance that the chance of recurrence is not substantially greater than that for the general population.

Issues for the school

Children with milder forms of cerebral palsy can cope at mainstream school, provided minor developmental learning disorders and physical access are addressed. Children with more severe cerebral palsy will need special schooling either in a school for children with physical disabilities, or one for children with severe disorders of intellectual development.

Duchenne muscular dystrophy

Duchenne muscular dystrophy is the commonest hereditary neuromuscular disease. It is a progressive disorder resulting in death in the early twenties. It is caused by mutations in the dystrophin gene, which are inherited as an X-linked recessive trait.

Clinical features   Baby boys are normal at birth, but careful examination reveals marked and persistent head-lag in the early

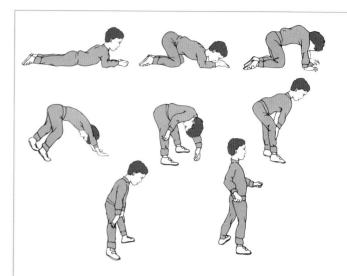

Figure 14.4 Gower sign: from lying down the boy uses his hands to 'climb up' his legs.

months. Walking delay is usually only identified retrospectively. Symptoms appear between the ages of 4 and 6 years and are progressive. They consist of frequent falls, a lordotic waddling gait, and difficulty climbing stairs. On examination the child has enlarged but weak calf muscles. The Gower sign is characteristic (Figure 14.4); on rising from a lying position the boy uses his hands to 'climb up' his legs to get to an upright posture. Plasma creatine kinase level is elevated by at least 10 times the normal level.

Diagnosis   This is via mutation analysis. Muscle biopsy is rarely needed but this may be required to distinguish rarer forms of dystrophy or myopathy.

Management   The child needs physiotherapy, support and help through school. Genetic counselling is extremely important for the family as 50% of boys will be affected. Early detection of an elevated CPK level in late walkers allows planning for future pregnancies, as prenatal diagnosis is possible.

Prognosis   Most of these boys are unable to walk by the age of 8–11 years and become confined to a wheelchair. Chest muscles are also affected. Respiratory insufficiency can be improved by oral steroids or overnight non-invasive breathing support. New stem-cell based and genetic therapies are being actively developed. Life expectancy is improving, but remains poor, with death precipitated by respiratory infections by the mid twenties and early thirties.

Duchenne muscular dystrophy at a glance

Epidemiology
Commonest hereditary
  neuromuscular disease
Boys only affected

Aetiology
X-linked recessive trait
Dystrophin gene defect

History
Frequent falls
Difficulty climbing stairs
Delay in acquired walking*

Physical examination
Lordotic waddling gait
Enlarged, weak calf muscles
Positive Gower sign

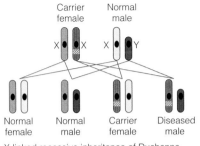

Carrier
female

Normal
male

Normal
female

Normal
male

Carrier
female

Diseased
male

X-linked recessive inheritance of Duchenne
muscular dystrophy (DMD)

Molecular pathophysiology

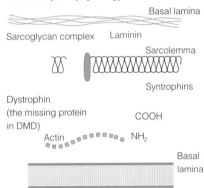

Basal lamina

Sarcoglycan complex   Laminin

Sarcolemma

Syntrophins

Dystrophin
(the missing protein
in DMD)

COOH

Actin   NH₂

Basal
lamina

Skeletal muscle fibre

Confirmatory investigations
Elevated creatinine kinase
EMG shows myopathic changes
Muscle biopsy shows
  characteristic histology

Differential diagnosis
Other muscular dystrophies

Management
Physiotherapy
Genetic counselling (prenatal
  diagnosis available)

Prognosis
Progressive deterioration
Confined to wheelchair by age
  8–11 years
Involvement of chest muscles
  – respiratory infections
Death usually occurs in 20s or
  early 30s although some may
  live until 40s with good care
Experimental treatment with stem
  cells may delay progress

NB *Signs and symptoms are
variable.

Disorders of intellectual development

The term 'disorders of intellectual development' has replaced the terms 'learning disabilities' or 'intellectual disability', 'mental retardation' and 'mental handicap'. Various degrees of disorder occur and are classified into mild, moderate, severe and profound according to intellectual limitations and the degree of independence anticipated or achieved. Individuals with *severe disorders of intellectual development* can learn minimal self care and simple conversation skills, and need much supervision throughout their lives. Those with *profound disorder of intellectual development* require total supervision, few become toilet trained and language development is generally minimal.

The prevalence of severe disorders of intellectual development is about four children per 1000. Children with severe disorder are spread throughout the social classes, and usually have an organic basis for their problem. This contrasts with children with milder disorders of intellectual development, where mostly no organic cause is found and where there is a predominance of children from lower socio-economic classes.

Aetiology/pathophysiology

In about one-quarter of children with significant disorder, no specific cause is identified. However, this picture is changing as a result of advances in the field of genetics such as exome sequencing. Diagnoses are now being made in children who in the past were thought to have idiopathic disorders. Where significant congenital anomalies and dysmorphic features are found, the diagnostic process has been helped by the development of computerized databases.

Chromosome disorders (predominantly Down syndrome and fragile X) are the commonest cause of severe disorders of intellectual development. (see Table 14.4). *Fragile X* is important as a genetic cause in boys. The chromosomal anomaly consists of a 'fragile site' at the end of one of the long arms of the X-chromosome. Diagnosis is by DNA analysis of the number of triple base repeats in the locus. The diagnosis should be sought in any boy who has unexplained moderate or severe intellectual disorder. Some girls carrying the chromosome have mild intellectual disorder.

Fetal alcohol syndrome (Figure 14.5) is another relatively common condition. It is caused by a moderate to high intake

Table 14.4 Causes of severe disorders of intellectual development

Chromosome disorders	30%
Other identifiable syndromes	20%
Cerebral palsy, infantile spasms, post-meningitis	20%
Metabolic or degenerative diseases	<1%
Idiopathic	25%

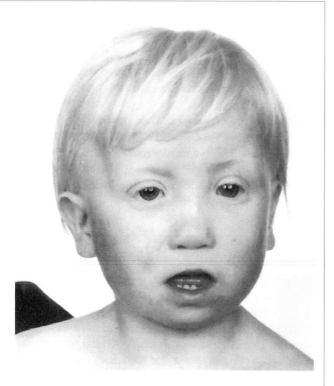

Figure 14.5 A 3-year-old boy with fetal alcohol syndrome. Note the absent philtrum and short thin upper lip, saddle-shaped nose and maxillary hypoplasia.

of alcohol during pregnancy, with the severity of the features related to the quantity of alcohol consumed. The clinical features are characterised by poor growth and microcephaly, a characteristic facial appearance and cardiac defects.

Intrauterine infections such as rubella, cytomegalovirus (CMV) and toxoplasmosis still occur. If infection with these agents occurs for the first time during pregnancy, severe fetal damage can result, leading to multiple disability.

Other causes include the *inborn errors of metabolism,* a group of disorders caused by single gene mutations, usually inherited in an autosomal recessive or maternal inheritance manner. They may present in a variety of ways, of which developmental delay is one. As individual conditions they are very rare. Phenylketonuria is the commonest. Neonatal screening can detect many inborn errors, and this is being ever more widely applied. (p. 32).

Neurodegenerative diseases lead to progressive deterioration of neurological function. The causes are heterogeneous and include biochemical defects, chronic viral infections and toxic substances, although many remain of unknown aetiology. The course for all of these conditions is one of relentless and inevitable neurological deterioration.

Emotional abuse and neglect have serious consequences for a child's developmental progress. Developmental delay is often associated with failure to thrive (see pp. 283, 291), apathy and evidence of physical neglect. Disorder of intellectual development can be a consequence even if the child is removed from the home.

Clinical features

In early childhood, disorder in intellectual development is seen as a delay in reaching developmental milestones, particularly those relating to language and social tasks. The progress achieved by any child is highly variable and depends on the underlying condition, any associated disabilities, as well as, to some extent, the educational and therapeutic input received. Other factors which affect progress are physical health, a healthy parent–child attachment and a cohesive family unit within a supportive social network.

Severe disorders are often accompanied by problems that further limit the child's abilities. These include epilepsy, impairment of vision and hearing, communication deficits and attention deficit hyperactivity disorder. Feeding problems and failure to thrive may also be an issue.

How severe disorders in intellectual development present

Babies with recognizable syndromes, such as Down, are usually diagnosed at birth and the degree of their intellectual disorder predicted with some confidence. However, the overwhelming majority of children with disorders in intellectual development are identified later when they fail to meet their developmental milestones. Children with severe disorder show marked delays in the first year, but children with less severe disorders typically have normal motor development and present with delayed speech and language in the toddler years.

Management of a child with a severe disorder of intellectual development (see Box 14.2)

Perhaps the major goal in the management of children with severe disorders of intellectual development is to support and help the family in coming to terms with the diagnosis and their child's limitations. This is often easier when a specific diagnosis can be made, although that is not always possible. Associated problems need to be identified and the developmental progress of the child followed. Other aspects of management involve providing appropriate educational and therapeutic input throughout the paediatric years.

Once the diagnosis of a severe disorder of intellectual development has been made, the most successful approach involves

> ### Box 14.2 Managing the child with a severe disorder of intellectual development
>
> - Diagnose the underlying condition where possible, and assess and manage associated problems
> - Follow the child's developmental progress
> - Provide good general paediatric care
> - Ensure appropriate input is provided in the preschool years and that appropriate school placement is found
> - Provide a supportive framework for the child and parents

an interdisciplinary effort directed towards education, social activities, behaviour problems and any associated deficits.

Diagnosis of an underlying cause

Diagnosing of an underlying cause is unlikely to affect the child's prognosis, although a growing number of metabolic disorders can now be prevented or treated with appropriate diet and medications. Diagnosis is of great importance to the family, allows for more accurate genetic counseling and alerts one to the possibility of associated problems. The process of diagnosing severe disorders of intellectual development is discussed in the section on the child presenting with global developmental delay (p. 258).

General paediatric care

The child with severe disorders of intellectual development requires the same general paediatric care as any other child. This includes immunisations, following their growth and developmental parameters, maintaining dental hygiene and treating intercurrent illnesses.

Early intervention and educational programmes

It is important to begin an educational programme early to stimulate cognitive, language and motor development. In the preschool years this may take a number of directions. Therapists from the child development team provide advice to the family on play activities and suitable toys, give guidance in the development of simple skills such as feeding, washing and dressing, and instruct parents on the principles of language development, introducing alternative communication systems where appropriate. Planned programmes such as the Portage system, where a trained worker comes to the home on a regular basis, may also be available. Attendance at special nurseries, such as Mencap, can be stimulating for the child while providing contacts with other families in similar circumstances.

School

At the nursery and primary school level many children with severe disorders of intellectual development can cope and benefit from placement in a mainstream school, with appropriate help provided. Other children, particularly if they have additional disabilities, may be better placed in a special educational setting. Children with severe disorders of intellectual development require an Education and Health Care Plan (EHCP) (see p. 51) to ensure that their needs are met.

Behaviour management

Behaviour problems occur with greater frequency in children with developmental disabilities. In milder disorders of intellectual development this may include attention difficulties or hyperactivity (see pp. 261, 388), and in children with severe disorders, stereotypic or self-injurious behaviour. Psychological help in these circumstances is needed, and occasionally medication, too.

Routine review of a child with a severe disorder of intellectual development

The child with severe disorders of intellectual development should have a routine paediatric review, even if perceived to be healthy. Developmental progress should be followed, particularly in the child without a specific diagnosis, as developmental regression suggests an unrecognised degenerative process. Some conditions such as Down syndrome or congenital CMV infection require routine investigations or hearing tests, as these children are at higher risk for certain problems. Behavioural problems may need special attention. Liaison with other professionals is of great importance, and the family is likely to need on going support.

Issues for the family

The diagnosis of a severe disorder of intellectual development is devastating, and families require particularly sensitive support (see p. 51) at diagnosis and beyond. Each stage of the child's development brings its own issues. Adolescence is usually a particularly difficult time when issues related to sexuality, vocational training and community living must be addressed.

Genetic counselling is important, whether there is a clearly inherited disorder or not, as the family will want to know the chances of having another affected child. In children with no identified cause, the risks of another sibling being affected is approximately 1–2%. However, if multiple congenital anomalies are also present the risk falls to 0.5–1%.

Issues for the school

Education for children with severe disorders of intellectual development must be realistic, and should include teaching skills such as personal care, hygiene and safety, development of acceptable social behaviour and maximizing independence. On leaving school, various facilities should be available for the young adult with disorders of intellectual development, including an adult training centre, special hostels, communities and vocational training schemes.

Disorders of intellectual development at a glance

Definition
Learning disabilities are
  considered severe if minimal
  self-care and simple
  conversation at most are
  achievable, and supervision is
  needed in adult life

Prevalence
4 children per 1000

Aetiology/pathophysiology
Chromosome disorders:
  30% (**a**)
Identifiable disorders or
  syndromes: 20% (**b**)
Associated with cerebral palsy,
  microcephaly, infantile
  spasms (**c**)
Postnatal cerebral insults:
  20% (**d**)
Idiopathic: 25%

**Presentation and how the
  diagnosis is made**
Malformations at birth, or later
  when developmental delay is
  evident

Clinical features
• Reduced intellectual
  functioning
• Delay in reaching developmental milestones in early
  childhood, particularly
  language and social skills
• Dysmorphic features may be
  evident*

*Symptoms and signs are variable

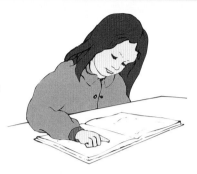
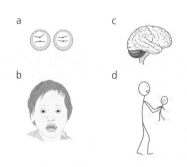

Associated problems
Epilepsy
Vision and hearing deficits
Communication problems
Attention deficit/hyperactivity
Feeding problems and failure to
  thrive
Specific diagnoses may have
  own complications

Management
• Needs to be multidisciplinary
• Diagnosis of underlying cause
  (see Table 14.4)
• General paediatric care must
  not be neglected
• Early intervention and
  educational programmes to
  stimulate cognitive, language
  and motor development
This may be by individual
  therapists, planned home
  programmes or nursery
• School – Education plan
  required and placement in
  mainstream or special school
• Behaviour difficulties must be
  addressed
• Support and benefits
  (see p. 51)

Points for routine follow-up
Developmental progress and
  physical growth need review
Some conditions require
  screening for specific
  associated problems
Liaison with other professionals
  is important
The family needs support

Prognosis
Depends on underlying cause
  and degree of intellectual
  disorder
Degree of independent living
  achieved relates to:
• level of learning disability
• underlying aetiology

Down syndrome

Down syndrome is the commonest congenital anomaly associated with global developmental delay. The underlying
chromosomal abnormality in most cases is trisomy of chromosome 21. The extra chromosome is usually of maternal
origin, and the incidence of Down syndrome increases with
maternal age (2% at age 38 years). Pre-natal screening by
ultrasound for nuchal translucency, biochemical marker testing and more recently fetal DNA in maternal blood can
detect most pregnancies with Down syndrome and some
other chromosomal anomalies. The parents need skilled and
sympathetic counselling in such cases in order to decide
whether to terminate pregnancy.

Clinical features   The features of Down syndrome are easily
recognised – hypotonia, upward sloping palpable fissures,
epicanthic folds, Brushfield spots (speckled iris), a protruding
tongue, flat occiput, single palmar creases, and mild to moderate developmental delay where social skills often exceed the
other milestones (Figure 14.6). One-third of babies with Down
syndrome are born with gastrointestinal problems, most commonly duodenal atresia, and one-third have cardiac anomalies
(most commonly atrioventricular canal defects). Secretory otitis
media, strabismus, hypothyroidism, atlantoaxial instability and
leukaemia occur more commonly than in normal children.

Management   The medical management of Down syndrome demands a routine cardiac evaluation at birth. Routine

audiological and thyroid tests are needed throughout childhood and ophthalmological assessment if there is any evidence of a squint. The child's growth needs to be followed on special Down growth charts. The family requires genetic counselling.

Prognosis   Children with Down syndrome have varying degrees of disordered intellectual development. They can usually be integrated into a mainstream primary school with extra provision made for their educational needs. Individuals with Down syndrome are at risk for early-onset Alzheimer disease.

Neurocutaneous syndromes

The neurocutaneous syndromes are a heterogeneous group of disorders characterised by neurological dysfunction and skin lesions. In some individuals there may be severe disorders of intellectual development and in others intelligence is normal. Examples include neurofibromatosis, tuberous sclerosis, and Sturge-Weber syndrome. The genetic basis of these conditions is now known

---

👁 Down syndrome at a glance

Epidemiology
Commonest congenital anomaly
  associated with learning
  disability
Unscreened incidence
  (1 per 650 births)
  increases with maternal age

Aetiology
Trisomy of chromosome 21
Rarely translocation
  involving chromosome 21

Antenatal diagnosis
Triple test early in pregnancy,
  followed by nuchal skin fold
  thickness, then amniocentesis
  for those at high risk
  Fetal DNA in maternal blood

Clinical features
Mild to moderate developmental
  delay
Upward sloping palpebral
  fissures
Epicanthal folds
Brushfield spots
Protruding tongue
Flat occiput
Single palmar creases
Hypotonia
Small stature
High incidence of
malformations (cardiac, GI)

Confirmatory investigations
Chromosome analysis shows
  trisomy
21 with non-dysjunction,
  translocation or mosaicism

Maternal age	Unscreened incidence
20	1 in 1700 births
40	1 in 100 births
44	1 in 40 births

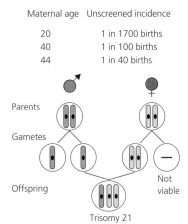

Parents

Gametes

Offspring

Not
viable

Trisomy 21

Genetics: extra chromosome 21
(Translocation between chromosome 14
and 21 is rarer)

Differential diagnosis
Facial features are usually
  clinically evident from birth

Management
Cardiac evaluation at birth
Referral to ophthalmology if
  squint is present
Routine audiological and thyroid
  tests
Genetic counselling for family
Arranging for special
  educational needs

Complications
Cardiac anomalies
Duodenal atresia
Secretory otitis media
Strabismus
Hypothyroidism
Atlantoaxial instability
Leukaemia

Prognosis
Individuals have varying
  degrees of intellectual
  developmental disorder
Children can usually be
  integrated into mainstream
  primary school
At risk from Alzheimer disease
  in adult life

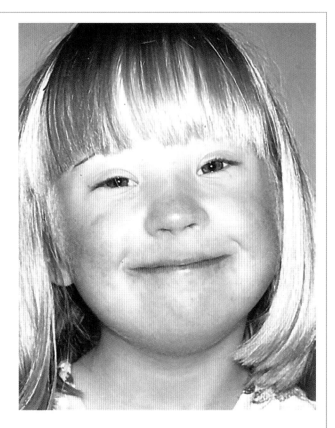

Figure 14.6 A 5-year-old girl with Down syndrome.

Table 14.5 Children at risk for hearing impairment
Severe prematurity
History of meningitis
History of recurrent otitis media
Significantly delayed or unclear speech
Family history of deafness
Parental consanguinity and ethnic predilection
Parental suspicion of deafness
Children with cerebral palsy
Children with cleft palate
Children with absent or deformed ears

Table 14.6 Causes of deafness in school children
Conductive deafness
Glue ear following otitis media and adenoidal hypertrophy
Impacted cerumen
Sensorineural deafness
Damage to the cochlear or auditory nerve
Genetic
Various types (50%)
Intrauterine
Congenital infection, e.g. rubella, cytomegalovirus (CMV)
Perinatal (12%)
Birth asphyxia
Severe hyperbilirubinaemia
Postnatal (30%)
Meningitis
Encephalitis
Head Injury

Hearing impairment

About 4% of school children have a hearing loss. Two per 1000 children have moderate deafness and require a hearing aid, and a further one per 1000 is severely deaf requiring special education. Some children are at a higher risk for hearing impairment, as shown in Table 14.5.

Aetiology/pathophysiology

See Table 14.6. Conductive deafness is an extremely common problem in childhood. It usually results from persistent effusions in the middle ear (a complication of otitis media, see p. 145), and is known as chronic secretory otitis media or glue ear. Impacted cerumen may also impair hearing, and this should always be excluded before a hearing test is done. Sensorineural deafness occurs as a result of damage to the cochlear or auditory nerve. It is rarer, but a cause of more significant disability.

Presentation and diagnosis

Babies with neurosensory deafness are now being identified in many areas through the introduction of newborn hearing screening. Children may also present when parents become concerned that their child is not responding to sound, or if the child's speech and language development is delayed. If the hearing loss is secondary to secretory otitis media, the tympanic membranes look dull and may be bulging or retracted.

The hearing deficit is confirmed by audiological testing (see p. 34). If a child is unable to cooperate, or if an objective test is required, brain stem evoked responses (BSER), an electrophysiological measure, is carried out.

Clinical features

The clinical features vary with the severity of the hearing deficit and the age at which it presents. If it is congenital, the child is delayed in talking. If the onset is later, the child may present with behavioural difficulties which may not be immediately identified as a result of lack of hearing. Deafness is particularly common in certain medical conditions such as cerebral palsy.

Chronic secretory otitis media may be characterised by fluctuating hearing loss, as the middle ear fluid may resolve only to return with each upper respiratory tract infection (URTI).

Hearing deficits frequently occur in association with severe disorders of intellectual development, visual deficits and neurological disorders.

Managing the hearing impaired child

If the hearing deficit is secondary to secretory otitis media, the management is surgical (see below and Box 14.3). Neurosensory loss is only rarely correctable surgically, and the most important aspect of management therefore is to promote the child's ability to communicate from an early age. If the hearing deficit is significant this will usually require sign language, which is used in conjunction with oral speech.

Deafness is an enormous social barrier, and an important part of management must be to encourage the child to participate fully in school and society at large.

Conductive hearing loss

Medical treatment in the form of decongestants and antihistamines are ineffectual in the management of middle ear effusion. If the effusion is causing persistent hearing loss, surgical intervention is required. Tiny plastic tubes (grommets) are inserted into the tympanic membrane to aerate the middle ear and drain the fluid. Adenoidectomy may be performed at the same time. When grommets are in place, the child must take care not to allow water to enter the ear canal at bath time or when swimming. The grommets usually eventually fall out spontaneously. They may not need to be replaced as the condition resolves as the child grows.

Sensorineural deafness

Hearing aids

A hearing aid is a device which amplifies sound. It may be worn behind the ear (Figure 14.7) or in a pocket or harness. Some aids have special features such as amplification of low or high frequencies and circuits to reduce intense peaks of noise. Most aids can be used with the 'loop' wiring system which transmits the teacher's voice, bypassing background noise. Selection of the

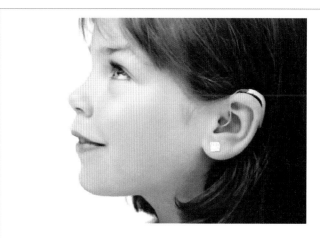

Figure 14.7 A 10-year-old girl with neurosensory deafness wearing bilateral hearing aids.

most suitable aid is made by a paediatric audiologist, who also teaches the family about its management and maintenance.

Communication

In the past there has been some controversy over teaching sign language on the basis that children must learn to live in a hearing world. However, it is now generally accepted that providing an alternative non-verbal means of communication increases a child's ability to relate to others, reduces the isolation and frustration of being unable to hear, and even encourages language development. Sign language is taught in conjunction with oral speech. Lip-reading is also valuable, and electronic analyzers are a new development which can help the child to speak more clearly by converting voice patterns to visual displays.

Education

The peripatetic teacher of the deaf, who is employed by the local education authority, is responsible for the child's early education and management, and later in advising on school placement.

Issues for the family

If the hearing deficit is sensorineural, the parents need to learn how to communicate with their deaf child and promote the child's communication skills. Some causes of deafness are genetic, and in these circumstances genetic counselling is required.

Issues for the school

Many moderately deaf children can attend a normal school. The child is helped by sitting near to the teacher in order to maximize concentration. The 'loop' wiring system is a valuable development. More severely affected children require specialist education either at a school for the deaf or at a partially hearing unit attached to a mainstream school.

Box 14.3 Managing the child with hearing loss

Conductive hearing loss
- Correct by placing grommets

Sensorineural hearing loss
- Ensure the child has a means of communication
- This may involve sign language
- Maximize hearing by use of a hearing aid
- Ensure schooling is appropriate and that support is provided
- Cochlear transplant may be considered

Hearing impairment at a glance

Prevalence

4% of children have hearing deficits mostly acquired after ear disease

3 per 1000 are moderately or severely impaired

2-3 babies per 1000 born with deafness per year

Aetiology/pathophysiology

Most mild to moderate hearing loss is conductive and a result of secretory otitis media

Sensorineural deafness may be genetic, a result of pre- or perinatal problems, or follow a cerebral insult later in life

Clinical features

Lack of response to speech

Delayed speech

Behavioural problems

Associated problems

Learning difficulties

Neurological disorders

Visual deficits

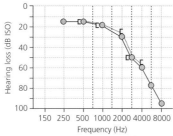

(a) A pure tone audiogram showing high frequency sensorineural deafness

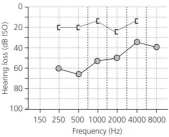

(b) A pure tone audiogram showing conductive deafness. The bone conduction is normal but the air conductive curve is impaired. There is 20–30 dB hearing loss

Presentation and how the diagnosis is made

Child health surveillance

Parental concern

Practical aspects of management

Grommets for conductive hearing loss

Hearing aids

Communication

Education

Issues for the family

Communication with child may involve learning sign language

Genetic counselling

Issues for the school

Moderately deaf children can attend a normal school

The severely deaf require specialist education at a school for the deaf or a partially hearing unit attached to a normal school

The blind or partially sighted child

Blindness and partial sight are best defined functionally rather than by the degree of visual acuity. A child is defined as blind if he or she requires education by methods which cannot involve sight. If the child is of adequate intelligence this will include Braille. A child is defined as partially sighted if he or she requires special education but can use methods which depend on sight, such as large-print books. In practice, most blind children have some vision even if it is only recognition of light and dark. One in 2500 children is registered blind or partially sighted. Fifty per cent have additional handicaps.

Aetiology/pathophysiology

The commonest causes of blindness are optic atrophy, congenital cataracts, and choroidoretinal degeneration. In almost half of cases the cause is genetically determined, and in one third it is related to perinatal problems such as retinopathy of prematurity (see p. 454).

Clinical features

The eyes may be obviously abnormal in appearance, and nystagmus or roving, purposeless eye movements may be present. Babies who have a visual deficit from birth follow an altered pattern of development. Smiling tends to occur at the usual age, but is less consistent and reliable and, as the baby develops, his or her response to sound is unaccompanied by turning towards the source. Motor skills, both gross and fine are likely to be delayed. Hand regard is poor, and reaching for objects and the development of a fine pincer grip is slow. Early language development may be normal, but the acquisition of vocabulary and more complex language may be delayed.

The child with visual deficits frequently develops mannerisms such as eye poking, eye rubbing and rocking. These are known as 'blindisms' and probably occur as they induce pleasurable visual gratification of retinal origin. Neither these mannerisms nor the delayed development should be regarded as evidence in themselves of significant disorder of intellectual development.

Intelligence has an important influence on the child's ability to cope with visual difficulties. However, 50% of children with visual deficits have additional disabilities such as hearing deficits or severe disorder of intellectual development and do less well.

Presentation and diagnosis

Babies may be identified in the neonatal period if, for example, cataracts are found (p. 431), or nystagmus or roving, purposeless eye movements are present. Every newborn must have the 'red reflex' examined. A white pupil is an ominous sign of chorioretinitis, retinal dysplasia or detachment, cataract, corneal opacity and even congenital retinoblastoma. If, however, the eyes appear normal, it is frequently the mother who first suspects a problem when she fails to elicit eye contact. Children may also be identified in the course of child health surveillance (see p. 35). It must be emphasised that a parent who raises concern about poor vision should be taken seriously.

If a visual defect is suspected, examination by an ophthalmologist is indicated. In the young child, visual evoked response (VER) testing is often required. The VER is an electrophysiological method of evaluating the response to light and special visual stimuli.

Managing the child with visual impairment

Management is directed towards providing early intervention in order to promote developmental progress, reduce blindisms and to increase parental confidence. See Box 14.4. The family needs supportive services and the child requires appropriate educational resources.

A peripatetic teacher is provided either by the local authority or the Royal National Institute for the Blind (UK) or similar voluntary organisations to advise parents in the preschool years.

At school level, improvements in equipment have occurred in recent years so that the child with partial sight may now be able to cope in a mainstream school. These improvements include better optical aids, good illumination, and reading material in very large type. Braille remains the essential method of reading for the child with a severe visual deficit, providing disordered intellectual development is not present.

Mobility training is an essential part of education. As the child matures, instruction must be given in travel outside of school, initially under supervision and then independently.

Visual impairment at a glance

Definition
A child is defined as blind if education can only be provided by methods not involving sight, e.g. Braille. A child is partially sighted if educational methods such as large-print books can be used

Epidemiology
1 in 2500 children are registered blind or partially sighted 50% have additional handicaps

Aetiology/pathophysiology
Commonest causes are:
Optic atrophy (**a**)
Congenital cataracts (**b**)
Choroidoretinal degeneration (**c**)
Retrolental fibrodysplasia in premature infants

Clinical features
- The eyes may look abnormal or have unusual movements
- If the deficit is congenital, early smiling is inconsistent and there is no turning towards sound
- Reaching for objects and the pincer grip is delayed
- Early language may be normal, but complex language may be delayed
- ' Blindisms ' (eye poking, eye rubbing and rocking) may occur

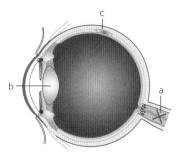

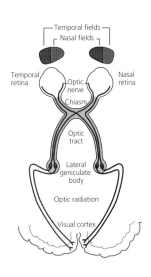

Associated problems
Hearing deficit or severe learning difficulties are common

Presentation and how the diagnosis is made
Malformations at birth, or later when developmental delay is evident

Practical aspects of management
Early intervention to improve developmental progress, reduce blindisms and increase parental confidence
Preschool: a peripatetic teacher from the Royal National Institute for the Blind
Advice on appropriate schooling
Mobility training
Supportive services

Issues for the family
Advice on non-visual stimulation and child-rearing
Adaptation of the home

Issues for the school
Mainstream nursery and nursery school with supportive services are often appropriate
Beyond this, mainstream school, a partially sighted unit, or a school for the blind (depending on learning abilities)

Box 14.4 Managing the visually impaired child

- Provide early intervention in order to improve developmental progress
- Support the family and increase parental confidence
- Provide appropriate educational resources

Issues for the family

Parents of a blind child need help at a very early stage. They must be taught to stimulate their infant using non-visual means, such as touch and speech, and must continue to provide stimulation through the early years with appropriate play materials. The home is likely to require adaptation so that the child can explore this environment safely. Genetic counselling may be needed.

Issues for the school

Mainstream nursery and nursery school are often appropriate for the child with a visual handicap, provided support from the peripatetic teacher is available. Beyond this, factors such as the child's intellect and ability to make use of residual vision, the wishes of the family and the long-term prognosis determine whether placement should be in a mainstream school, partially sighted unit or a school for the blind.

To test your knowledge on this part of the book, please see Chapter 26

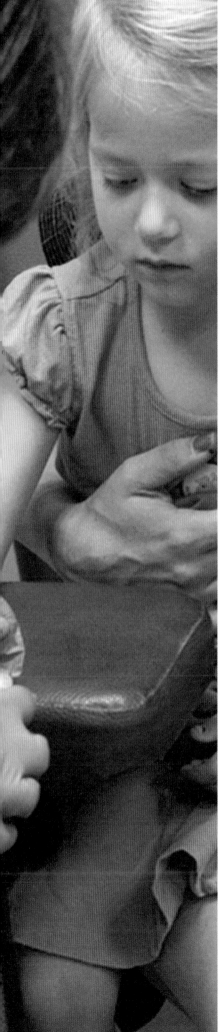

CHAPTER 15

Growth, endocrine and metabolic disorders

I knew a little elfman once
Down where the lilies blow.
I asked him why he was so small,
And why he didn't grow
He slightly frowned, and with his eyes
He looked me through and through:
'I'm quite as big for me,' he said,
'As you are big for you.'
John Kendrick Bangs
(1862–1922)

Symptoms and signs of growth, endocrine and metabolic disorders

Essential Paediatrics and Child Health, Fourth Edition. Mary Rudolf, Anthony Luder and Kerry Jeavons.
© 2020 John Wiley & Sons Ltd. Published 2020 by John Wiley & Sons Ltd.
Companion website: www.wiley.com/go/rudolf/paediatrics

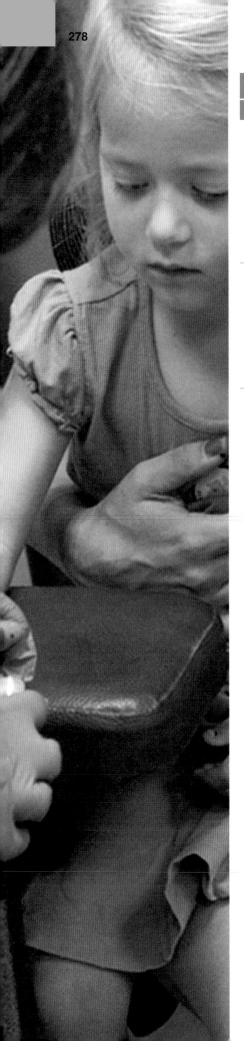

KEY COMPETENCES
YOU MUST ...

Know and understand

- The differential diagnosis of children presenting with short stature, poor growth, obesity and abnormal head size
- How to manage the important and common endocrinological and metabolic disorders of childhood
- How to diagnose the common and important conditions responsible for poor growth and poor weight gain in infants and children
- The principles of managing diabetes mellitus including ketoacidosis

Be able to

- Weigh and measure a baby and child accurately and correct for prematurity
- Calculate BMI
- Plot measures on an appropriate growth chart
- Identify when a child's growth or weight gain is of concern
- Measure blood glucose using a home monitor
- Provide sensitive guidance for a child who is suffering from obesity

Appreciate that

- Short stature is most often a normal or familial trait not requiring intervention
- Weight faltering (FTT), causes significant parental stress and anxiety especially when there are eating difficulties
- Diabetes, as a chronic illness, has a major impact on the child and family
- Good diabetic control is central to minimizing devastating complications

Symptoms and signs of growth, endocrine and metabolic disorders

Finding your way around ...

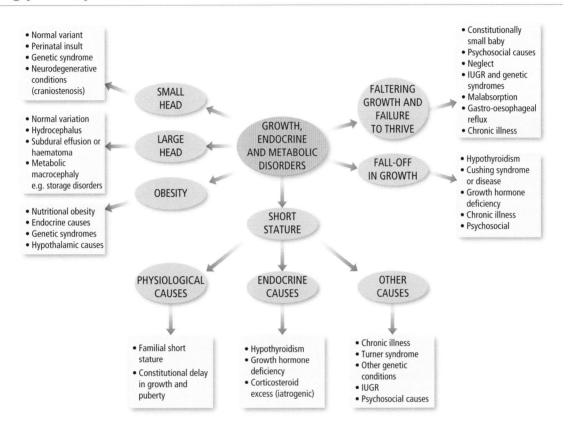

Short stature

Important causes of short stature	Chronic illness
Familial causes	• Inflammatory bowel disease, coeliac disease, chronic renal disease may be occult
Familial short stature (also known as 'constitutional short stature')	Genetic
Constitutional delay of growth and puberty	• Turner syndrome
	• Down syndrome
Pathological causes	• Other genetic and metabolic syndromes
Endocrine	• Skeletal dysplasias
• Hypothyroidism	Intrauterine growth retardation
• Corticosteroid excess (including therapeutic steroids)	Psychosocial
• Growth hormone deficiency	

At birth, a baby's weight and length are influenced mainly by intrauterine factors, and do not correlate well with parental heights. Over the next year or two the baby's growth adjusts, so that by the age of 2 years most children have attained their genetically destined centile. From then until the onset of puberty children usually grow steadily along their centile with little deviation. During puberty it is normal for centiles to be crossed again until final height is achieved, which usually is located close to midway between the parental centiles. Normal growth reflects a child's wellbeing, and any deviation may be indicative of adverse physical or psychosocial factors. Guidelines for concern about a child's growth are shown in the Red Flag box.

Guidelines for concern beyond the age of 2 years

- **The short or tall child.** Height or weight beyond the dotted lines on the growth chart (>99.6th or <0.4th centiles, see Figure 5.6) are outside the normal range and pathology is likely to be found. Although many of these children are healthy, an evaluation needs to be considered.
- **Crossing of centiles**. As a rule of thumb, one should be concerned if two centile lines are crossed.
- **Discrepancy between height and weight.** There is a great deal of variation as regards leanness and obesity. The child who is very thin or overweight may have a problem.
- **Discrepancy with parental heights.** A child should be evaluated if there is a large discrepancy between the child's height centile and the midparental centile (an average of the parents' centiles). The child of tall parents who has a growth problem should not wait until he or she falls below the second centile to be evaluated.
- **Parental or professional concern.** A good clinical evaluation should be carried out in any child where the parents or other professionals are concerned about growth.

Given the social disadvantage of being short, especially for a man, it is not surprising that short stature commonly causes concern. In most short children height is simply a variant of normal, and delay in physical development (constitutional delay) is often a factor. When a short child presents, it is important to exclude organic problems, particularly if a fall-off in growth is observed over time.

Any chronic illness can lead to stunting of growth; however, chronic illnesses rarely present with short stature as the primary complaint since the features of the illness are usually all too evident. The exceptions are inflammatory bowel disease coeliac disease (see p. 207) and chronic renal disease, which can all present with poor growth in advance of other clinical features. Children with genetic syndromes often are short, and Turner syndrome (gonadal dysgenesis) is important to consider in short girls.

Endocrinological causes of short stature include hypothyroidism, growth hormone deficiency, and corticosteroid excess. Hypothyroidism has a profound effect on growth, and the presenting feature is often short stature. Cushing syndrome and disease are extremely rare in childhood, although iatrogenic growth suppression from exogenous steroids is not uncommon.

Adverse psychosocial factors can severely affect a child's growth. In the young child it is referred to as *failure to thrive* (p. 397). The true incidence of psychosocial short stature is unknown, but it is likely that it is quite common. Children often have a growth spurt on being placed in foster care, even if growth has been apparently normal.

The most important aspect of the evaluation of the child with short stature is the history and physical examination, together with careful measurements of height. The purpose of the evaluation should not only be to discover underlying pathological conditions, but also to understand the impact that short stature has on the child.

History – must ask!

The history needs to focus on symptoms suggestive of underlying conditions such as intracranial pathology, hormone deficiency, chronic illness and gastrointestinal symptoms.

- *Medical history.* You need a careful review of medical symptoms, particularly focusing on headache, diarrhoea and abdominal pain, constipation, cough, wheeze and fatigue. Chronic conditions such as asthma, arthritis or diabetes are obviously relevant, as is any chronic medication.
- *Family history.* A child's growth cannot be interpreted without reference to parental and siblings' heights. A child's height normally falls close to the centile between the parents' height centiles, and if there is a marked disparity a cause should be sought. Enquire into parental onset of puberty as constitutional delay is common and often familial. Most mothers can recall their age at menarche, and it is considered late if it occurred after the age of 14 years. Onset of paternal puberty is harder to identify but the age when shaving began can be useful.
- *Birth history.* A child born severely preterm or small for gestational age (SGA) may have reduced growth potential, particularly if height as well as weight is affected.
- *Psychosocial history.* Psychosocial factors can severely stunt a child's growth, and you must be alert to the possibility of emotional neglect and abuse. When assessing any short child you should also find out about any social or emotional difficulties *resulting* from their stature.

Table 15.1 Investigations in a child with short stature

Investigation	Relevance
Blood count and CRP	Inflammatory bowel disease
Urea and electrolytes, blood and urine pH	Chronic renal disease
Coeliac antibodies (anti TTG)	Screening test for coeliac disease
Thyroxine and thyroid-stimulating hormone	Hypothyroidism
Karyotype (in girls)	Turner syndrome
Growth hormone tests, IGF1, IGFBP3	Hypopituitarism, growth hormone deficiency
X-ray of the wrist for bone age* (see Figure 15.1)	Delayed bone age suggests growth and maturational delay, hypothyroidism, growth hormone deficiency or corticosteroid excess. A prediction of adult height can be made from it

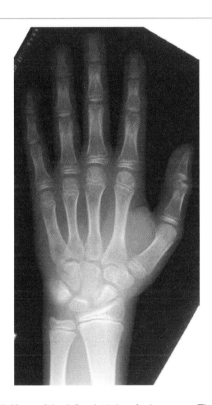

Figure 15.1 X-ray of the left wrist taken for bone age. The development of the various bones is assessed to give an estimate of the child's skeletal maturity.

Physical examination – must check!

A very thorough examination is required, focusing particularly on the following:

- *Pattern of growth.* Review previous growth measurements as they provide important clues to the aetiology of the condition. Fall-off in growth often indicates a medical condition requiring treatment.
- *Anthropometric measures.* Take careful measures of length (to age 24 months) or height and weight and plot them on a growth chart (see p. 284).
- *General examination.* Signs of hypothyroidism (see Table 15.4), body disproportion, signs of Turner syndrome (see below) and dysmorphism are particularly important to identify. Examine each organ system in turn, looking for evidence of occult disease.

Investigations

Your clinical evaluation should guide any investigations. If you find a decrease in growth velocity, investigations are always required (Table 15.1).

Managing the short child

The majority of short children will have a physiological cause for their stature: either 'familial short stature', or constitutional delay. In such cases the family needs reassurance that there is no underlying pathological problem. In addition, it is important to address any psychosocial difficulties the child is having, and occasionally psychological counselling is required. These difficulties are uncommon before adolescence, but become particularly problematic for teenage boys. The use of growth hormone in children with physiological short stature is controversial and probably gives little benefit to final adult height.

Key points: Short stature

- A good history and physical examination will identify most pathological causes of short stature
- The child's height must be related to the parents' heights
- Emotional and social consequences of the short stature should be identified

Clues to the diagnosis of short stature*

	Growth pattern	History	Physical examination	Bone age
Familial (constitutional) short stature	Steady growth below the centile lines	Short parents	Normal	Normal
Constitutional delay of growth and puberty	Usually short with fall-off of growth in early teens	Family history of delayed puberty/menarche	Delay in developing secondary sex characteristics	Delayed
Endocrine disorders (hypothyroidism, Cushing, growth hormone deficiency)	Fall-off of growth	Symptoms of hypothyroidism; on inhaled or oral steroids; symptoms of steroid excess; symptoms of brain tumour;	Proportionate short stature and fine features (GH); signs of hypothyroidism or Cushing. Rarely signs of brain tumour	Very delayed
Chronic illness	Fall-off of growth	Symptoms of inflammatory bowel disease, malabsorption, fatigue	Ill looking. Symptoms of underlying illness, although inflammatory bowel disease and chronic renal failure may be occult	Delayed +/–
Genetic syndromes	Growth below centiles		Signs of Turner or other dysmorphism	Variable
Skeletal dysplasia	Very short, variable growth rate	May be family history or consanguinity	Disproportionate dwarfism; fractures; skeletal deformity	Dysplastic or osteopenic bones
Intrauterine growth retardation	Short from birth	Small for gestational age	Normal but small	Normal
Psychosocial	Variable depending on social circumstances	Adverse circumstances	Unhappy, signs of neglect or abuse	Usually normal

* There are three ages to consider: Chronological age (CA); Bone age (BA); Height age (HA, the age at which the child's height is on the 50th percentile) In normal children, the typical pattern is CA=HA=BA. In children with familial short stature, and genetic syndromes (e.g. Turner) the typical pattern is CA= BA>HA, In children with maturational delay of growth and puberty, the typical pattern is CA>HA=BA. In children with hypothyroidism and GH deficiency, the typical pattern is CA>HA>>BA.

Plateauing in growth

Causes of fall-off in growth

Endocrine
Hypothyroidism (see pp. 295–6)
Corticosteroid excess (see p. 296)
Growth hormone deficiency (see p. 296)

Chronic illness (see p. 46)
Inflammatory bowel and coeliac disease, and chronic renal failure may be occult

Psychosocial causes (see Chapter 22)

A less common problem than short stature is fall-off in growth. This relates to a slow growth rate over time rather than short stature at single points in time. If the child is from a tall family, he or she may not be short in relation to peers. Fall-off in growth is always worrying and merits investigation.

The clinical approach and management are the same as those described in the previous section, but the chance of finding pathology is higher.

Weight and growth faltering

Causes of failure to thrive and growth faltering

Organic
Gastro-oesophageal reflux
Malabsorption
Chronic illness
Endocrine dysfunction

Genetic
Genetic constitution
Intrauterine growth retardation
Genetic syndromes

Environmental/psychosocial (non-organic)
Inadequate access to food (poverty)
Maternal depression/psychiatric disorder
Disturbed maternal–infant attachment
Eating difficulties
Neglect

There is no universal definition of failure to thrive. Failure to thrive implies both a failure to grow and a failure of emotional and developmental progress. Children with failure to thrive may show weight 'faltering' or weight loss as well as decelerated growth rate. The term is usually used in reference to toddlers or babies, although it may also be used in connection with an older child, and may also refer to height. Because infants commonly cross centiles during the first 2 years of life, expertise is required to differentiate the normal infant from the one with worrying weight faltering.

The following can act as guidelines as to when a clinical evaluation is advisable:

- weight below the 2nd centile;
- height below the 2nd centile;
- crossing down two centile channels for height or weight.

Small parents tend to have small children, and the small healthy normal child of short parents should not generally arouse concern. Usually in this case growth is steady along the lower centiles, but the large baby born to small parents may cross down centile lines before settling on the destined line. Growth retardation may occur if a fetus experiences adverse uterine conditions. When this occurs early in gestation, length, and head circumference in addition to weight can be affected (proportional growth failure). In this circumstance the potential for postnatal growth may also be jeopardized. This circumstance leads to a baby being small compared to expected size at any given gestational age (SGA). Note, this is not the same as prematurity, which means being born before 37 weeks gestation. Around 20% of SGA babies experience marked growth failure after birth.

A child may falter in weight for either organic or psychosocial reasons. In the past children were classified as having organic (OFTT) or non-organic failure to thrive (NOFTT). 'Weight faltering' or 'growth faltering' is preferred with FTT reserved for children with psychosocial causes for poor weight gain. Children more often than not do not fall simply into non-organic or organic, and it is important to identify all the factors involved rather than to simplistically seek one cause.

Children and babies with any chronic illness can falter in growth. They rarely present as a diagnostic dilemma as the manifestations of the disease are usually evident. However, organic failure to thrive may be compounded by psychosocial difficulties, and these need to be addressed. Very rarely, chronic disease can be occult and present as weight or growth faltering. Classically this may be seen with renal endocrine or metabolic disease, some cases of coeliac disease, some genetic disorders and malformations.

Vomiting and posseting are common complaints in a baby, and usually do not deleteriously affect growth. However, reflux in association with oesophagitis can cause poor weight gain. Malabsorption is another important cause of poor growth, and symptoms of diarrhoea and colic provide diagnostic clues. The commonest childhood causes of malabsorption include coeliac disease (see p. 207) and cystic fibrosis (see p. 175). In the former, the rate of weight gain characteristically falls off coincident with the introduction of gluten to the diet.

It is very distressing for the family when a young child fails to gain weight well, and your evaluation needs to be carried out sensitively. The purpose of the evaluation is first to differentiate the child demonstrating normal growth patterns from the child with a problem, and then to identify the contributing factors, whether organic or non-organic.

History – must ask!

- Nutritional history. You should include questions about any feeding difficulties, which may have been present from birth but often develop at weaning and in the toddler years. Eating difficulties may be the cause of poor weight gain. However, eating difficulties may also be generated from anxiety that naturally occurs when a baby grows poorly because of other causes. It is helpful to ask the mother to keep a food diary for a few days, recording all that the baby has eaten.
- Review of symptoms. Most organic conditions are identifiable by history. Diarrhoea, colic, vomiting, irritability, fatigue, fevers, rashes and chronic cough are the most important features to elicit.
- Past medical history. The birth history is important. A low birthweight may indicate adverse prenatal conditions which affect growth potential. Recurrent illness of any nature may affect growth.
- Developmental history. This is needed for two reasons. First, failure to thrive can affect a baby's developmental progress and, secondly, the child who has neurodevelopmental problems often has associated eating difficulties which may limit nutritional intake.
- Family history. Relate the child's growth to that of other family members. Growth patterns of the parents and close relatives, as well as current height and weight, are important to elucidate. Medical problems affecting other children in

the family may suggest a diagnosis. A good social history should identify psychosocial problems that may be causing or at least contributing to the problem.

Physical examination – must check!

- General observations. The baby's appearance is important. The healthy small baby will look very different from the neglected or ill child. The child who is malnourished for whatever reason will appear thin, with wasted buttocks, a protuberant abdomen and sparse hair. A neglected child may look unclean and uncared for. Observations must also extend to the mother and how she relates to the baby, which can provide valuable clues to maternal–infant attachment difficulties.

- Growth. Plot growth on a growth chart and compare them with previous measurements. The pattern of growth can be very helpful in the diagnostic process (Figure 15.2).

- You need to carry out a full physical examination to complement the history. Occasionally, clinical signs alone can indicate a cause for the poor growth.

- Look for signs of protein, calorie, vitamin and mineral deficiency.

Figure 15.2 Growth charts of babies showing different forms of weight faltering: (a) intrauterine growth retardation (IUGR); (b) coeliac disease; (c) large baby at birth; (d) psychosocial failure to thrive.

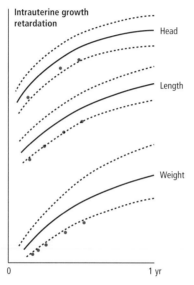

(a) • Low birth-weight baby
   • Many IUGR babies show catch-up but this baby clearly has not, and may have reduced growth potential
   • The IUGR probably started early in pregnancy because OFC and length are also affected

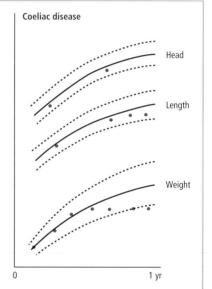

(b) • Note fall-off in weight at time of weaning when wheat was introduced
   • The fall-off in length occurs later

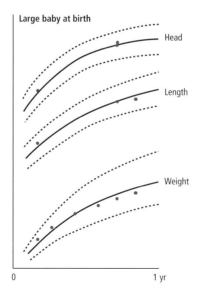

(c) • The growth of a normal baby born large for gestational age, showing crossing down of centiles in the first year in order to reach his destined centile

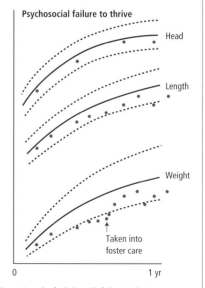

(d) • Growth of a baby with failure to thrive resulting from psychosocial deprivation
   • Catch-up growth occurred when he was taken into foster care

Table 15.2 Investigations to consider in the evaluation of weight faltering

Investigation	What you are looking for
Full blood count, ferritin	Iron deficiency is common in failure to thrive and can cause anorexia
Urea and electrolytes, urine examination	Unsuspected renal disease or failure
Stool for elastase	Low faecal elastase and the presence of fat globules suggest malabsorption
Coeliac antibodies and jejunal biopsy, Sweat test	Coeliac disease and cystic fibrosis are causes of malabsorption
Thyroid hormone and thyroid-stimulating hormone	Congenital hypothyroidism causes poor growth and developmental delay
Karyotype	Chromosomal abnormalities are often associated with short stature and dysmorphism
Hospitalisation	Hospitalisation can be a form of investigation Observation of baby and mother over time can provide clues to the aetiology

Investigations

There is good evidence that 'fishing' for a diagnosis by carrying out multiple investigations is a futile exercise. Investigations should only be carried out if clues to a problem are obtained on history and physical examination. The only exceptions are a blood count, ferritin level and general urine examination including pH. Iron deficiency is extremely common in this group of children, and can affect both development and appetite. Renal disease may be occult and have very few overt clues. Other investigations which may be helpful, if clinically justified, are shown in Table 15.2.

Managing weight faltering

The ability to nurture a baby is perhaps the most basic attribute of parenting. When a child fails to thrive it usually causes extreme distress, anxiety and feelings of inadequacy. It is important therefore that a normal, healthy but small baby is not wrongly labelled as having a problem. On the other hand, it is important that both organic and psychosocial problems are identified and addressed, as failure to thrive has important consequences on the child's developmental progress as well as growth. A thorough clinical evaluation, together with information from the health visitor, can usually sort out the problem. Occasionally it may be helpful to admit the baby to hospital for observation.

Key points: Weight faltering and failure to thrive

- Differentiate the normal baby who is crossing centiles from the baby who is failing to thrive
- Identify any symptoms and signs that suggest an organic condition
- Only perform laboratory investigations if there are clinical leads in the history and physical examination
- Identify psychosocial problems that might be affecting the baby's growth

Clues to the differential diagnosis of weight and growth faltering

	Growth pattern*	History	Physical examination
Constitutional	Steady growth below centiles, or 'catch-down' for larger baby	Short parent(s)	Normal
Psychosocial	Crossing down of centiles at any age	Eating difficulties common Maternal depression may be present	Usually normal Poor or disturbed maternal–infant attachment may be evident, exclude abuse
Coeliac disease	Crossing down of centiles classically occurring at introduction of wheat solids, weight loss	Frequent stools or diarrhoea, but constipation may also occur Irritability	Distended abdomen Wasted buttocks (late sign)

(Continued)

Clues to the differential diagnosis of weight and growth faltering (*Continued*)

	Growth pattern*	History	Physical examination
Cystic fibrosis	Crossing down of centiles	Appetite often fine Chest infections Frequent loose fatty stools	Protuberant abdomen Decreased muscle mass Chest signs possible, clubbing, Poorly child
Gastro-oesophageal reflux	Crossing down centiles early in life	Vomiting, irritability, occasionally apnoea	Normal
Intrauterine growth retardation	Low birthweight with subsequent poor weight gain. Length and head circumference may be reduced	Possible placental insufficiency, difficult pregnancy, smoking, alcohol	Small normal. Look for signs of intrauterine infection (TORCH)
Neglect	Crossing down of centiles, catch up if removed from home	Difficult or troubled family circumstances	Poorly cared for, nappy rash, developmental delay common

* Usually refers to weight in the first instance.

Obesity

Causes of obesity in childhood

Common
Nutritional

Rare
Hypothyroidism
Cushing syndrome or disease
Various genetic syndromes

Obesity is increasing as a problem in childhood. The vast majority of overweight children have nutritional obesity, and this diagnosis can be simply made on the basis of the clinical evaluation. The importance of identifying obesity in childhood is principally in order to provide support and advice and to attempt to prevent the complications of obesity later in life. Although there is a folk belief that obesity is caused by a child's 'glands', this is very rarely the case.

Weight alone is not a measure of obesity in childhood, but must be related to the child's height. Your clinical evaluation should firstly focus on excluding the rare endocrine and genetic causes of obesity. As all of these are accompanied by poor growth, they can be excluded on clinical grounds fairly easily. You then need to assess those aspects of the child's lifestyle that predispose to obesity and any emotional and behavioural difficulties the child is having.

History – must ask!

- *Diet.* Ask what the child and family eat and drink on a normal day, bearing in mind that this may be a sensitive issue. The child may be snacking at school or with friends and neighbours. Nonetheless it can form a basis for advice.
- *Lifestyle.* Ask about physical activity during the day and also about sedentary activities.
- *Sleep problems.* Sleep apnoea is a common complication of obesity so ask about snoring, and lethargy or tiredness during the day.
- *Complications.* Musculoskeletal symptoms are common due to the increased load on the joints. It is rare for diabetes or cardiovascular disease to develop in childhood, although there may be biochemical indicators present.
- *Emotional and behavioural problems.* Social and school problems are very common. Children may be bullied or be bullies, or may suffer from significant depression.
- *Learning difficulties.* Children with a genetic syndrome associated with obesity are likely to have special educational needs or be developmentally delayed.
- *Physical symptoms.* Ask about any physical symptoms that might suggest hypothyrodism (Table 15.4) or Cushing disease (p. 296) as a cause.
- *Family history.* As obesity is a familial condition (genetically and environmentally), a family history is important. It is important to ask about any family members who have developed or died from diabetes or early heart disease.

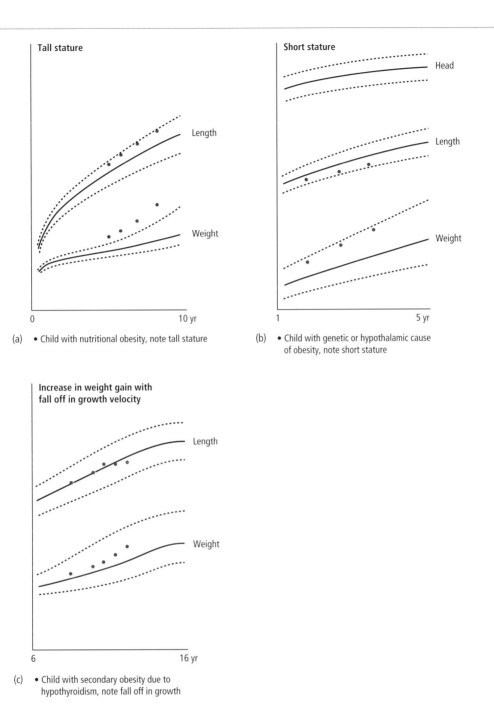

Figure 15.3 Growth patterns in obesity. (a) Child with nutritional obesity: note tall stature. (b) Child with genetic or hypothalamic cause of obesity: note short stature. (c) Child with secondary obesity due to hypothyroidism: note increase in weight gain with fall-off in growth velocity.

Physical examination – must check!

- *Growth.* This is the most important indicator of a non-nutritional cause. In nutritional obesity the child is often relatively tall. With pathological causes, the child is either short or demonstrates a fall-off in height as the weight increases. You should also calculate the body mass index (BMI) and plot this

on a BMI chart (see Figure 5.8). Figure 15.3 illustrates the growth patterns seen with different causes of obesity.

- *Signs of an endocrinological cause.* In the child with poor growth, look for signs of hypothyroidism (goitre – see Figures 15.6 and 15.7 and Table 15.4; developmental delay; slow return of deep tendon reflexes; bradycardia) and steroid excess (moon face, buffalo hump, striae, hypertension, bruising).

Table 15.3 Investigations that may be indicated in the obese child

	Investigation	Relevance
Looking for a cause	T4, TSH	Low T4 and high TSH are found in hypothyroidism
	Urinary free cortisol	High in Cushing disease
	Karyotype and DNA analysis	Genetic syndrome
	MRI of the brain	Hypothalamic cause
Looking for consequences of obesity	Urinary glucose, fasting glucose and insulin or an oral glucose tolerance test	Diabetes
	Fasting lipid screen	Hyperlipidaemia
	Liver function tests	Fatty liver

- *Signs of dysmorphic syndromes.* Certain dysmorphic syndromes are characterised by obesity. These children are invariably short. Look in particular for microcephaly, hypogonadism, hypotonia and congenital anomalies.
- *Signs of complications.* Check the blood pressure and look for acanthosis nigricans (a dark velvety appearance at the neck and axillae) as this is a sign of insulin resistance. Hepatomegaly may indicate fatty liver.

Investigations

Investigations are required if you are concerned that there is a non-nutritional cause for the obesity, particularly if the child is short, dysmorphic, is demonstrating a fall-off in height or has learning difficulties. In this case thyroid function tests, diurnal cortisol levels and genetic studies are indicated. If the child is very obese, investigation for heart disease, diabetes and steatohepatitis may be needed. Possible investigations are shown in Table 15.3.

Managing obesity

Lifestyle management is the mainstay of treating obesity (see p. 292) (see Figure 15.5). At present there are no medications licensed for use in children.

Key points: Obesity

- Exclude rare causes of obesity, remembering that most children with an organic cause will be growing poorly
- Calculate the BMI and plot on BMI growth charts
- Assess the child for early complications resulting from obesity
- Obtain a clear picture of the child's lifestyle, focusing on physical activity and diet
- Find out about emotional and behavioural problems

The large head

Causes of a large or enlarging head

Normal variation (often familial)
Hydrocephalus
Subdural effusion or haematomas
Feature of certain dysmorphic syndromes

The head grows rapidly in the first 2 years of life and then growth slows down, but continues to grow throughout childhood. In the early years the sutures are open, and then fuse around the age of 6 years. Prior to fusion they can separate in response to raised intracranial pressure. The posterior fontanelle usually closes by 8 weeks of age, and the anterior by 12–18 months.

Head size is not directly proportional to body size, but large children are more likely to have large heads, and vice versa. As in body growth, it is not unusual for head circumference measurements to cross centiles in the first year. However, when this occurs clinical assessment is needed to exclude pathological causes.

A large head is usually a normal variant, and often is a familial feature. An unusually large head may indicate hydrocephalus, in which case evidence of raised intracranial pressure may be present. Large heads may also be a feature of certain genetic syndromes.

History – must ask!

- *Is the baby developing normally?* Abnormal developmental progress in a child with a large head is strongly indicative of pathology.
- *Are there symptoms of raised intracranial pressure?* The baby with hydrocephalus or subdural effusion is likely to be irritable and lethargic, have a poor appetite and vomit.

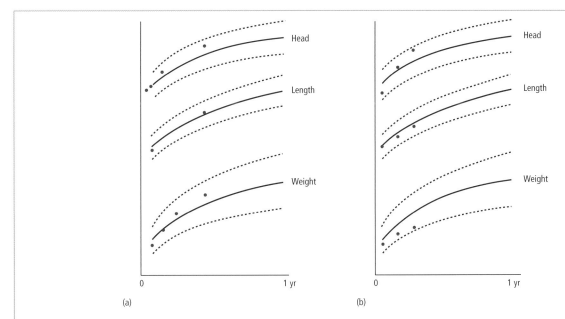

Figure 15.4 (a) Normal increase in head circumference in a rapidly growing baby and (b) the development of hydrocephalus.

Physical examination – must check!

- *Growth measures*. The pattern of head growth is important. Crossing of centile lines is more concerning than steady growth of a large head. Length and weight indicate whether the head is disproportionately large (Figure 15.4).
- *Signs of hydrocephalus*. The child with hydrocephalus has characteristic features (see p. 245).
- *Development*. A developmental examination should accompany the developmental history.
- *Neurological examination*. Raised intracranial pressure may be accompanied by hypertonia of the legs, abnormal tendon and deep reflexes, and nerve palsy. The retina and optic disc should be carefully examined for pallor, papilloedema, cherry red spot and haemorrhge.

Investigations

If raised intracranial pressure is suspected, immediate investigation is required. If the anterior fontanelle is still open, a cranial ultrasound can be performed to detect hydrocephalus, effusions or haemorrhage. A CT provides more anatomical detail, is often available rapidly and is the best immediate choice if the fontanelles are closed. Magnetic resonance imaging (MRI) is particularly useful for posterior fossa disease, genetic malformations and neurodegenerative disease, but is usually not immediately available.

Management

Frequent measurements of head circumference can generate anxiety, and should not be performed if the head size is considered to be a variant of normal. If pathology is suspected, investigations should be carried out and the baby referred for specialised treatment.

> #### 🔑 Key points: The large head
>
> - An enlarging head is more concerning than a steadily growing large head
> - Parental head size is helpful in deciding if this is a normal variant
> - Assess the baby's developmental skills
> - Evidence of raised intracranial pressure indicates hydrocephalus or subdural collection of fluid

The small head (microcephaly)

> #### Causes of microcephaly or poor head growth
>
> *Normal variant (often familial)*
>
> *Limited brain growth*
> Perinatal insult to the brain, e.g. hypoxic–ischaemic insult
> Malformations and genetic syndromes usually associated with delayed development or learning disability
> Neurodegenerative conditions
>
> *Craniosynostosis (very rare)*

A small head can be familial and of no concern, but as the head grows in response to brain growth, a small head often indicates limited brain growth. For this reason microcephaly is a feature of many dysmorphic syndromes, the commonest being Down syndrome. Congenital, perinatal and acquired disorders can be responsible for poor growth of the head:

Congenital

- congenital infections (see p. 435);
- genetic disorder or syndrome;

- antenatal toxins, such as alcohol;
- metabolic disorders (may manifest before or after birth)

Perinatal

- hypoxic–ischaemic encephalopathy (see pp. 429–30);

Acquired

- malnutrition;
- encephalitis and meningitis.

Very rarely, poor head growth occurs as a result of premature fusion of cranial sutures (craniosynostosis). If only some of the sutures are involved, the skull may grow in a distorted manner; if all the sutures are involved, skull growth is restricted, resulting in raised intracranial pressure. Treatment is with early neurosurgery.

History – must ask!

- *Is the baby developing normally?* If a baby is developing normally, it is unlikely that the head size is a cause for concern. If developmental delay is present, the baby needs to be evaluated for the disorders listed above.
- *Past medical history.* The perinatal history may throw light on factors such as infection, alcohol or hypoxic–ischaemic events which may have affected brain growth.

Physical examination – must check!

- *Growth measures.* The length and weight of the baby indicate whether the head size is disproportionately small. The pattern and form of head growth is important. Crossing of centile lines is more concerning than steady growth of a small head.
- *Parental head size.* Microcephaly in normal individuals is often familial.
- *Developmental skills.* Confirm the developmental history by carrying out a good developmental assessment.
- *Dysmorphic features.* Dysmorphic features suggest the diagnosis of a genetic syndrome. The sutures are prominent and fontanelles may be prematurely closed in craniosynostosis.
- *Neurological* Neurodegeneration may be associated with abnormal tone. Optic disc pallor may occur in craniosynostosis.

Investigations

A skull CT shows premature fusion of the sutures if craniosynostosis is present. A karyotype, DNA analysis and neurometabolic screen are indicated if you suspect a neurodegenerative, inherited or dysmorphic syndrome.

Management

If craniosynostosis is demonstrated, the child should be referred for urgent neurosurgical intervention. If you suspect developmental disability, close follow-up is required (see p. 254).

 Key points: The small head

- Determine whether the child is developing normally
- Check parental head size

Growth, metabolic and endocrine disorders

Constitutional short stature

As stature is largely genetically determined, short parents tend to have short children. 'Constitutional' or 'familial' short stature is the term used for children who are short because of their genetic constitution.

Clinical features   The history and physical examination is normal, and the bone age is appropriate for age. Social difficulties are common in the adolescent years, particularly for boys.

Management and prognosis   Reassurance is often all that is required. Occasionally children need psychological support in the adolescent years. There are social disadvantages to being short.

Constitutional delay of growth and puberty

Children with constitutional delay are often called 'late developers' or 'late bloomers'. The delay may be associated with constitutional short stature, in which circumstance the child may have particular difficulty coping with their height. It is not uncommonly a cause of being bullied, especially for boys.

Clinical features   Children are normal at birth but are short during childhood and reach puberty late, their final height depending on their genetic constitution, which may be normal. A family history of delayed puberty and menarche is often obtained. The bone age is delayed.

Management and prognosis   Most families simply require reassurance that final height will not be affected. Occasionally teenage boys find the social pressures to be so great that it is helpful to artificially trigger puberty early, thus causing an early growth spurt. Treatment does not have an effect on final height.

Environmental (previously non-organic) failure to thrive

The commonest causes for weight faltering and failure to thrive are psychosocial. The problems include difficulties in the home, limitations in the parents' ability to parent, disturbed attachment between the mother and child, maternal depression/psychiatric disorder and eating difficulties. Neglect is the underlying factor in only a few children.

Clinical features   Weight gain is usually affected first, but eventually a reduction in linear growth and head circumference follows and the child's developmental progress may be delayed.

Children with failure to thrive or weight faltering range across a spectrum of backgrounds. At one end of the spectrum is the child from a caring home who appears well looked after. The parents are anxious and concerned and interact well with the child. The problems are often eating difficulties, where the child has a minimal appetite or refuses to eat, meals are very stressful and the parents have been drawn into excessive measures (sometimes force feeding) to persuade the child to eat. At the other end of the spectrum is the neglected child who shows physical signs of poor care and emotional attachment. In this case the problem is often denied and compliance with intervention is poor.

Management   Management must fit the problem. Most families can be helped by appropriate intervention, usually consisting of dietary advice and psychological support. Practical support can ease the stress, and nursery placement can be very helpful in this regard as well as helping to resolve eating difficulties. In those cases where neglect is the cause and the family are not amenable to help, social services must be involved (see pp. 40, 395).

Prognosis   With appropriate intervention, the problem usually resolves or at least stabilizes. A few children need to be removed from their homes.

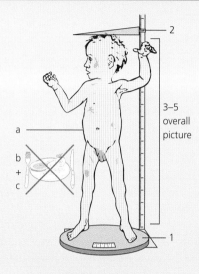

Environmental failure to thrive at a glance

Epidemiology
2% hospital admissions

Definition
Diagnosis is considered when height or weight below 2nd centile or cross down two centiles and organic causes have been excluded

Aetiology/pathophysiology
Psychosocial problems such as
- disturbed maternal–child attachment
- maternal depression/psychiatric disorder
- eating difficulties
- neglect

History
- Poor weight gain (a)
- Eating difficulties* (b)
- Inadequate diet* (c)
- Maternal anxiety/depression*

NB *Signs and symptoms are variable.

Physical examination
- Fall-off in weight velocity (1)
- Fall-off in linear growth and head circumference* (2)
- Developmental delay* (3)
- Signs of malnutrition: thin child, wasted buttocks, thin hair* (4)
- Signs of neglect: dirty, unkempt, nappy rash, unusual reaction to strangers* (5)

Confirmatory investigations
Exclusion of organic causes (see Causes box, p. 283)
Iron status (iron deficiency is common)
Good weight gain in hospital with standard diet

Differential diagnosis
Organic causes of failure to thrive (see Causes box, p. 283)

Management
Dietary advice
Psychological support
Social support (nursery placement particularly effective)
Referral to social services in some cases

Prognosis
With good early intervention, the process is likely to reverse
Without intervention the child is at severe risk for emotional and intellectual deficits and poor growth

Intrauterine growth retardation

Intrauterine growth retardation can result from a variety of causes (see p. 436). The impact on postnatal growth depends on the stage of pregnancy at which growth retardation occurred. If the insult occurred early in gestation, the baby is born not only underweight but also short and often with a small head. Many short newborns have a reduced growth potential and remain short throughout life. If catch-up growth occurs, it does so in the first 2 or 3 years.

Nutritional obesity

The metabolic factors that predispose some individuals to becoming obese have yet to be determined. Certainly, the correlation between nutrient intake and development of obesity is not simple.

Clinical features   The child with nutritional obesity tends to be tall for his or her age, and tends to develop puberty early, so that final height is not excessively tall. Boys' genitalia may appear deceptively small if buried in fat. Knock-knees are common. Striae and acanthosis nigricans may develop in severe cases and should prompt a search for endocrinopathies. Hypertension may occur but be difficult to assess due to adiposity. Children with obesity have a high incidence of emotional and behavioural difficulties.

Management   Rapid decreases in weight should not be attempted, and during the growing years maintenance of weight, while the child increases in height, is a reasonable goal (Figure 15.5). Gimmick and strict diets may be initially effective but often the benefits are short lived and may even be hazardous. The family needs encouragement to take a whole-family approach towards a healthier lifestyle, rather than targeting the child with the weight problem.

Lifestyle management programmes, if available in the community, can be a helpful way to tackle diet and eating behaviour and encourage an increase in physical activity. If the child is reluctant to participate in organized sports, everyday exercise such as walking to school may be more acceptable. Children affected by obesity are often the victims of teasing by peers, and psychological disturbance is common. Even if weight control is not successful,

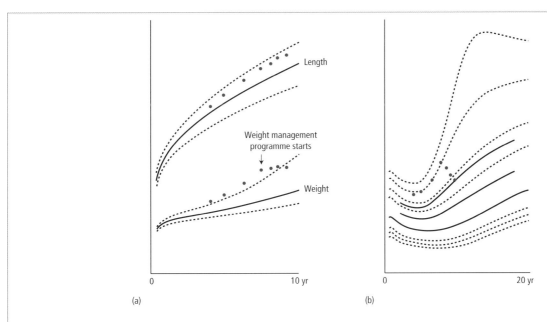

Figure 15.5 (a) Growth chart of a child affected by obesity. The goal of treatment is to reduce the rate of weight gain (but not actual weight loss) so that the child continues to grow. (b) BMI chart of the same child, showing marked reduction in BMI with lifestyle management.

continuous support is necessary to help these children cope with their condition. Adolescents over 14 years with severe intractable obesity may be candidates for bariatric surgery.

Prognosis Despite medical intervention, reduction of obesity once it is well established is difficult. Psychological difficulties may well persist into the adult years. Society deals harshly with the obese, and studies show that obesity is a handicap later in life.

In childhood, overt medical complications are few, although metabolic markers for cardiovascular disease, diabetes and fatty liver are common. Children affected by obesity are more susceptible to musculoskeletal strain and slipped capital femoral epiphyses (see p. 315). Rarely, insulin-resistant diabetes mellitus develops in childhood. If these children become obese as adults, the morbidity is significant, with diabetes and hypertension common, leading to early mortality from ischaemic heart disease, renal failure and strokes. Gallstones and certain cancers are also more prevalent.

Prevention As in most conditions, prevention is better than cure. There is some evidence that breast-feeding in infancy is protective, and promotion of good nutrition in the early years, when food habits are developing, is important. Physical activity needs to be encouraged in all children, not simply the obese. There is a need for these health issues to be addressed in school, particularly during adolescence, when a high intake of high-fat foods and decrease in exercise is common. If intervention is provided early in the course of obesity, weight control is likely to be more successful.

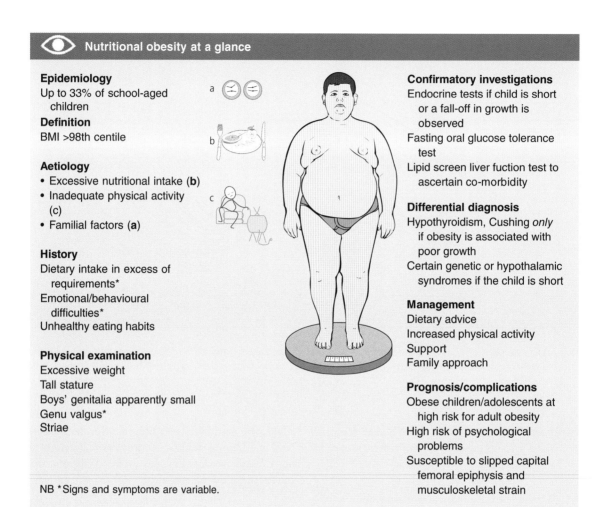

Nutritional obesity at a glance

Epidemiology
Up to 33% of school-aged
children

Definition
BMI >98th centile

Aetiology
• Excessive nutritional intake (**b**)
• Inadequate physical activity
(**c**)
• Familial factors (**a**)

History
Dietary intake in excess of
requirements*
Emotional/behavioural
difficulties*
Unhealthy eating habits

Physical examination
Excessive weight
Tall stature
Boys' genitalia apparently small
Genu valgus*
Striae

Confirmatory investigations
Endocrine tests if child is short
or a fall-off in growth is
observed
Fasting oral glucose tolerance
test
Lipid screen liver fuction test to
ascertain co-morbidity

Differential diagnosis
Hypothyroidism, Cushing *only*
if obesity is associated with
poor growth
Certain genetic or hypothalamic
syndromes if the child is short

Management
Dietary advice
Increased physical activity
Support
Family approach

Prognosis/complications
Obese children/adolescents at
high risk for adult obesity
High risk of psychological
problems
Susceptible to slipped capital
femoral epiphysis and
musculoskeletal strain

NB *Signs and symptoms are variable.

Congenital hypothyroidism

Lack of thyroid hormone in the first years of life has a devastating effect on both growth and development. However, since neonatal screening began nearly 50 years ago (see p. 32), congenital hypothyroidism is now very rare. The underlying pathological defect is either abnormal development of the thyroid gland or inborn errors of thyroxine metabolism.

Babies usually appear normal at birth, and rarely have the characteristic features of cretinism, which include coarse facies, hypotonia, a large tongue, an umbilical hernia, constipation, prolonged jaundice and a hoarse cry (Figure 15.6). In the older baby or child, delayed development, lethargy and short stature are found. Thyroid function tests reveal low T4 and high thyroid-stimulating hormone levels. Thyroid replacement is required throughout life and must be monitored carefully as the child grows. If therapy is started in the first few weeks of life, and compliance good, the prognosis is excellent.

Thyroiditis

Thyroiditis is more common in girls than boys.

Clinical features In Hashimoto (auto-immune) thyroiditis, the gland is diffusely enlarged, smooth and non-tender, although nodules may occur. The onset is usually insidious, with the goitre noticed as an incidental finding or observation (see Figures 15.7 and 15.8). The child may be clinically euthyroid or hypothyroid (see Table 15.4), although thyroid overactivity (tremor, palpitations, diarrhoea, sweating) is sometimes seen at the onset (Graves disease). Hypothyroidism is manifested by deceleration of growth with a marked delay in bone age, lethargy, constipation, dry skin and sluggish deep tendon reflexes. School work may not appear to suffer, although following treatment the child is often transformed into a more spirited child.

Occasionally thyroiditis may be infectious in origin and self-limited. A goitre especially if assymetric or nodular should prompt exclusion of cystic or malignant disease. Mild physiologic thyroid enlargement may be seen in puberty and pregnancy.

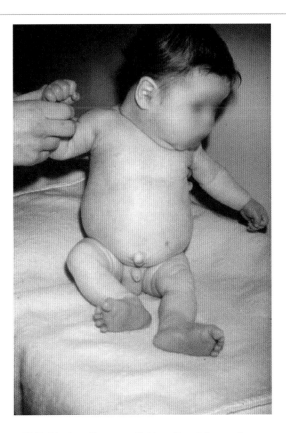

Figure 15.6 A baby with congenital hypothyroidism: note coarse facies and the umbilical hernia.

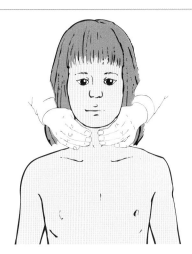

Figure 15.8 Palpation of the thyroid gland. Stand behind the child and ask the child to swallow.

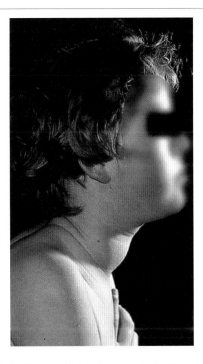

Figure 15.7 A 12-year-old girl who presented with a swelling in the neck, which proved to be due to thyroiditis.

Table 15.4 Signs of hypo- and hyperthyroidism
Hypothyroidism
Sluggishness
Constipation
Dry skin
Poor growth
Developmental delay
Underachievement at school
Bradycardia, hypotension
Delayed tendon reflex relaxation
Hyperthyroidism
Nervousness
Hyperactivity
Increased appetite with weight loss
Tremor
Increased sweating
Tachycardia and hypertension
Lid lag and retraction

Investigations Laboratory investigations show either normal thyroid function tests, or evidence of primary hypothyroidism with a normal or low T4 and elevated thyroid-stimulating hormone (TSH). Antithyroid antibodies (antimicrosomal and antithyroglobulin) may be present.

Management If there is evidence of hypothyroidism, replacement treatment with thyroxine is indicated. The goitre usually shows some decrease in size. Even if untreated, all children require follow-up of their thyroid status. If nodules persist despite treatment, biopsy should be performed as thyroid cancer can develop.

Acquired hypothyroidism at a glance

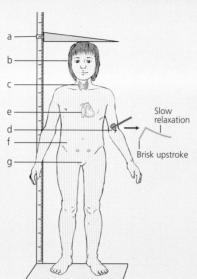

Epidemiology
More common in girls than
boys

Aetiology/pathophysiology
Auto-immune (Hashimoto)
thyroiditis (TSH deficiency
very rare)

History
Constipation*
Fall-off in school performance*
Cold intolerance*

Physical examination
• Fall-off in growth or short
stature (**a**)
• Dry skin and thin dry hair (**b**)
• Goitre (**c**)
• Slow relaxing reflexes (**d**)
• Bradycardia (**e**)
• Obesity* (**f**)
• Delayed puberty* (**g**)

NB *Signs and symptoms are variable.

Slow
relaxation

Brisk upstroke

Confirmatory investigations
Low T4
High TSH
Antithyroid antibodies

Differential diagnosis
Other causes of short stature
(see Table 15.1)
Other causes of fall-off in
growth (see Causes box,
p. 283)
Other causes of goitre

Management
Thyroxine replacement for life
Monitor growth and
development
Monitor thyroid function tests
regularly

Prognosis
Good prognosis, provided there
is compliance with treatment

Growth hormone deficiency

Growth hormone deficiency is a rare cause of short stature and
insensitivity to GH even rarer. GHD may occur secondary to
lesions of the pituitary such as tumours or cranial irradiation,
and it can be isolated or accompanied by deficiency of other
pituitary hormones.

Clinical features   Growth hormone deficiency causes slow
linear growth, with a delay in bone age. Insulin-like growth
factor 1 (IGF1) and Insulin-like growth factor binding protein
3 (IGFBP3) are useful screening tests. GH deficiency is confirmed by provocative growth hormone testing. Brain imaging
is needed to identify any underlying hypothalamic or pituitary
pathology.

Management   Growth hormone deficiency is treated with
daily subcutaneous injections of synthetic growth hormone
until the child stops growing. Underlying lesions, if any, need

to be treated. GH may also be administered in a variety of
genetic and other causes of short stature.

Prognosis   As regards growth, the prognosis is dependent
on the age at which growth hormone therapy was initiated; the
younger the child, the greater the chances that final height will
be in the normal range. In secondary growth hormone deficiency, the prognosis is related to the underlying lesion.

Cushing syndrome and corticosteroid excess

Cushing syndrome and disease, resulting in excessive levels of
cortisol in the blood, are extremely rare in childhood, growth
suppression from exogenous steroids being much more common. In children requiring long-term high-dose steroid therapy, the deleterious effects on growth can often be minimized
by giving the steroids on alternate days.

Turner syndrome

Turner syndrome (gonadal dysgenesis) is an important cause of short stature and delayed puberty in girls. It is a genetic disorder caused by the absence of one X-chromosome. The resulting phenotype is female, with gonads which are merely streaks of fibrous tissue. Mosaicism is common. Intelligence is usually normal but learning difficulties are described commonly.

Clinical features   See Figure 15.9. As neonates, babies with Turner syndrome often have marked webbing of the neck and lymphoedematous hands and feet. In childhood, short stature is marked and the classic features of webbing of the neck, shield-shaped chest, wide-spaced nipples and a wide carrying angle, may or may not be evident. Aortic valve disease and coarctation of the aorta are characteristic. Renal and eye anomalies may be present. Some girls are only diagnosed in adolescence when puberty fails to occur.

Management   During childhood, growth can be promoted by small doses of growth hormone and oestrogen. Puberty must be initiated and maintained by oestrogen therapy.

Prognosis   Women with Turner syndrome, despite treatment, are generally short. Recent advances in infertility treatment have resulted in a few women becoming pregnant through in vitro fertilization with donated ova.

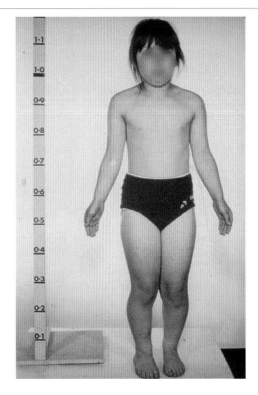

Figure 15.9 A 10-year-old girl with Turner syndrome. Note the short stature, webbing of the neck, shield shaped chest and wide carrying angle.

👁 Turner syndrome at a glance

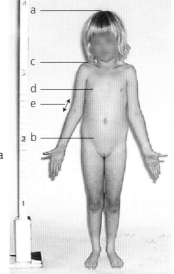

Epidemiology
One in 2500 female births

Aetiology/pathophysiology
45 XO karyotype leads to streak gonads (gonadal dysgenesis) and failure of oestrogen production
Mosaicism is common

Clinical features

- In neonates limb and neck oedema
- Short stature (**a**)
- Absent, incomplete or delayed puberty (**b**)
- Webbing of the neck (**c**)
- Shield-shaped chest, widely spaced nipples (**d**)
- Wide carrying angle (**e**)
- Systolic murmur (left outflow obstruction)
- Classic features are often absent*

Confirmatory investigations
Chromosome analysis
May be diagnosed at amniocentesis

NB *Signs and symptoms are variable.

Differential diagnosis
Other causes of short stature (see Table 15.1)
Other causes of delayed puberty (see Table 25.6)

Management
Promotion of growth in childhood by low-dose growth hormone and oestrogen therapy
Induction of puberty and maintenance with oestrogen replacement therapy

Associated problems
Bicuspid aortic valve
Coarctation of the aorta
Renal malformations

Prognosis
Generally remain short despite treatment
New advances provide some chance of fertility

Diabetes mellitus

Diabetes is an important condition as it has such a major impact on the child and family in terms of daily life, the possibility of unpredictable emergencies and the severity of the medical problems that occur later in life. In recent years the incidence of the disease has been increasing steadily in many parts of the world.

Aetiology and pathophysiology of diabetes

Type I or juvenile diabetes mellitus results from insulin deficiency. In childhood this almost always is a consequence of failure of the beta cells in the islets of Langerhans secondary to auto-immune destruction. The aetiology contrasts with so-called adult-onset diabetes (type 2), which usually results from peripheral resistance to the action of insulin and high rather than low insulin levels occur.

The underlying reason for beta cell destruction has yet to be fully elucidated. It is likely that the process is initiated by environmental factors, possibly viral, which affect genetically susceptible individuals. An auto-immune process has been implicated.

The lack of insulin results in an inability to utilize glucose, causing hyperglycaemia and breakdown of fat with ketosis. High levels of blood sugar cause a hyperosmolar state. The resultant osmotic diuresis causes polyuria and dehydration, precipitating thirst and polydipsia. Despite the high glucose levels, the calories cannot be utilized and their loss in the urine causes weight loss. As insulin levels are low, fat is broken down to ketones and ketoacidosis ensues.

Diabetic complications

Four long-term complications occur in diabetes and account for its major morbidity:

- retinopathy (the commonest cause of blindness in developed countries);
- nephropathy (affects 25–40% of diabetic individuals);
- neuropathy;
- heart disease.

Complications tend to occur some years after onset and so are uncommon in the childhood years. They are related to the degree of long-term glycaemic control, and therefore every effort must be made to maintain the child in as close to a euglycaemic state as possible. In addition to these complications, hypothyroidism, other auto-immune diseases and coeliac disease occur more commonly in children with diabetes.

Initial presentation of diabetes

Symptoms are usually present for only a number of weeks before the diagnosis is made. This contrasts with type 2 diabetes, where symptoms may occur for months or even years before diagnosis. Most children are diagnosed following recognition of the symptoms of polyuria (which may cause nocturnal enuresis), polydipsia, thirst and weight loss. Accompanying symptoms may include lethargy, anorexia, and constipation, and if prolonged also vomiting, abdominal pain and the features of diabetic ketoacidosis (DKA) (see Figure 15.11).

Physical examination is often not helpful but may confirm weight loss, and there may be signs of dehydration and the smell of acetone on the breath. The diagnosis is confirmed by the finding of hyperglycaemia, either on random blood sampling or by urine testing. A blood sugar of over 11.1 mmol/L (200 mg/dL) in the presence of a typical clinical picture is diagnostic and no further tests, such as fasting blood sugar or glucose tolerance tests, are needed.

Referral to a paediatric specialist team is always required. The child is usually admitted to hospital for a few days even if not in ketoacidosis, as intensive education is essential for both the child and the family. Normoglycaemia is usually easily achieved by subcutaneous insulin injections and oral rehydration. If marked dehydration and ketoacidosis are present, these demand treatment as described in Table 15.6. Care must be taken not to precipitate hypoglycaemia.

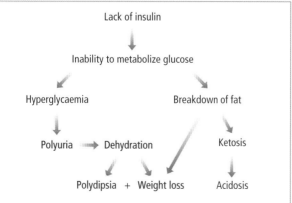

Figure 15.10 Glucose metabolism and the clinical features of diabetes (shown in yellow).

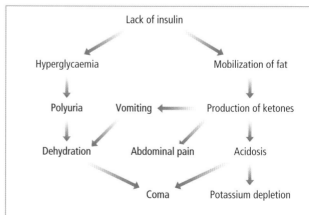

Figure 15.11 Metabolic cycle leading to the features of diabetic ketoacidosis (shown in yellow).

The diabetic team

The team of professionals required to manage diabetes successfully in childhood usually consists of:

- a paediatrician with a special interest in diabetes;
- a diabetes nurse specialist;
- a dietitian;
- a social worker.

In some teams a psychologist or psychiatrist, chiropodist and dentist are also involved.

Education of the child and parents

The diagnosis of diabetes involves a change in lifestyle, probably more than any other chronic medical condition. Education following diagnosis is crucial for establishing and maintaining these changes. The family needs to acquire the following skills:

- insulin administration;
- blood glucose monitoring;
- testing urine for ketones;
- nutritional understanding and a dietary plan;
- an understanding of the relationship between food, insulin, exercise and infection;
- ability to identify and manage hypoglycaemic attacks;
- grasping the importance of good control;
- knowing how to obtain advice at any time.

The school too should be visited to ensure that staff likewise understand and are trained to cope.

Management of diabetes

Management requires replacement of insulin, with the aim of mimicking the physiological state exactly. This includes the use of short and long acting insulins, and pumps and continuous glucose monitoring devices with computer control when necessary. The goal is to avoid the immediate symptoms and dangers of hyperglycaemia and hypoglycaemia, and also the long-term complications of diabetes.

The aim, as for any chronic condition of childhood, is to encourage the child to live as normal a life as possible while accepting the limitations that good management demands (Box 15.1; see also pp. 47–8). As a lifelong condition the child needs to learn to take responsibility for all aspects of the condition (see Box 15.2).

Medication

Insulin preparations have varying durations of action (see Table 15.5). The goal is to approximate insulin levels to physiological insulin secretion. This is achieved by mixing short- and long-acting insulins. The commonest insulin regimen is called 'basal–bolus', and consists of once-a-day long-acting insulin to give a basal background of insulin, with boluses of fast-acting insulin with each meal. The bolus doses are often determined by the parent assessing the approximate carbohydrate content of each meal, a process termed 'carbohydrate counting'.

Box 15.1 Goals in managing diabetes

- Good metabolic control – maintaining blood glucose levels as normal as possible, without episodes of DKA and a minimum of hypoglycaemic events
- A good understanding of the condition by the family such that they can competently manage the child's diabetes and adjust insulin requirements to diet, exercise, stress and infection
- Minimize complications
- Normal growth and development with full participation in school and social activities
- Work towards the child taking maximal responsibility for his or her diabetes as appropriate for age and intelligence

---

Box 15.2 Medical management of diabetes

Insulin
- Insulin is given subcutaneously by syringe or pre-mixed insulin 'pen', or continuously by pump.
- A mixture of short- and medium-acting insulin is given to approximate to the fluxes in insulin that occur physiologically
- At least two injections a day are needed to ensure good control
- The insulin dose should be adjusted on the basis of blood glucose monitoring and HbA1c levels

Hypoglycaemia
- Treat with carbohydrate snack or dextrose tablets if the child is able to eat
- Apply glucose gel to buccal mucosa if level of consciousness does not permit oral intake
- If unconscious, give glucagon intramuscularly if available
- Intravenous glucose can be given in hospital (10–25% only)

Diabetic ketoacidosis
- Rehydrate with normal saline and replace electrolytes, especially potassium
- Give continuous low-dose intravenous insulin until glucose levels fall to 12 mmol/L and then continue with the addition of dextrose to clear ketones and correct acidosis
- When clear and able to drink fluids, change to short-acting insulin using a sliding scale, or child's regular regimen
- Treat any precipitating infection

Children usually require 0.5–1.0 units of insulin/kg per day, giving approximately half of the dose as fast-acting boluses and half as a once-a-day basal dose. These proportions need to be adjusted on a regular basis according to blood glucose

Table 15.5 Types of insulin preparation and their action

Type of insulin	Onset	Peak	Duration
Rapid-acting	5–10 minutes	45–75 minutes	2–4 hours
Short-acting	30 minutes	2–4 hours	Up to 8 hours
Medium- to long-acting	1–2 hours	4–12 hours*	16–35 hours*

* Some long-acting insulins provide a steady 24 hour action without peaks. Newer ultra-long acting insulins act up to 42 hours.

measurements, which should be monitored regularly. Insulin is usually given before meals to match the rise in insulin with the rise in postprandial glucose. Figure 15.12 shows the relationship of blood glucose and insulin levels to meals and insulin injections.

Insulin is given subcutaneously by syringe or by using preloaded insulin 'pens' (Figure 15.13). The site of injection is unimportant but children are encouraged to rotate the site between upper arms, thighs, abdomen and buttocks in order to avoid lipoatrophy and lipohypertrophy, which are unsightly

and can affect absorption. Older children and adults are now increasingly fitted with insulin pumps which provide continuous infusion combined with maximum bolus flexibility as well as monitoring (Figure 15.14).

Dietary management

The other mainstay of treatment is diet. Families often see this as a major restriction, but in fact the requirements are simply a normal 'healthy' diet, high in fibre, in amounts sufficient to promote normal growth. High-sugar foods are kept to a minimum as they cause excessive swings in glucose levels. In children, unlike adults, it is important not to adjust food intake to counteract rises in blood sugar, as this may jeopardize growth. Unless obesity is an issue, the child's requirements should be guided by appetite and hunger, and the dietary recommendations and insulin dose adjusted accordingly. Families require the guidance of a dietitian, particularly in the early stages.

Blood glucose monitoring

Adjustments in insulin dose are guided by regular blood glucose monitoring (Figure 15.15 and 15.16) using a monitor. Most children adjust to the demands of testing, and it is usually recommended to test at least three to four times per day, 2 days per week, and whenever the child has hypo- or hyperglycaemic symptoms. Results are recorded in a diary (Figure 15.17) and allow for sensible adjustments in insulin dose, the goal being to keep glucose levels close to the normal range of 4–6 mmol/L. Most devices also measure ketones.

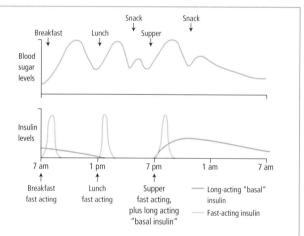

Figure 15.12 Relationship of blood glucose and insulin levels to meals and insulin injections.

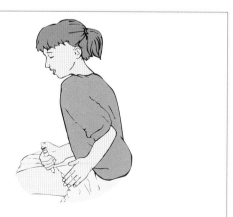

Figure 15.13 A girl with diabetes injecting insulin with a pen.

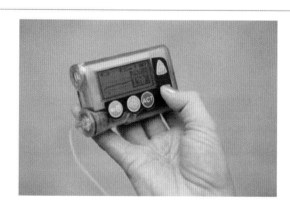

Figure 15.14 An insulin infusion pump.

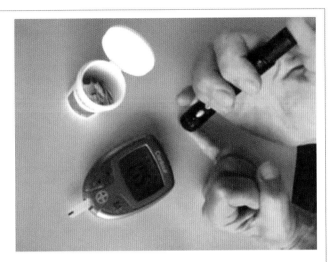

Figure 15.15 Blood glucose monitoring. A drop of blood is obtained and dropped on to a blood monitoring strip which is inserted into a meter for reading.

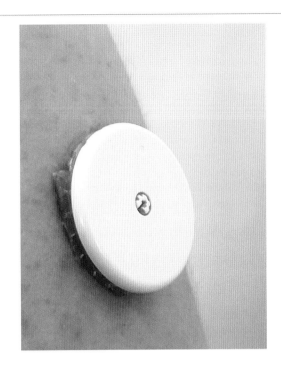

Figure 15.16 A continuous blood glucose monitor.

In the last few years, continuous glucose monitoring linked to computer and digital devices have become increasingly popular and affordable, and these are now becoming the standard of care in industrialized countries. They provide for automatic monitoring, trend alarms and can even be linked to pumps to provide an 'artificial pancreas'. Future technological improvements and new insulin preparations are revolutionizing management as well as safety and accuracy. Patients still need to know when and how to test for ketosis by measuring ketone levels in urine or blood using reagent strips.

Date	Insulin injection							Blood								Urine				Comments
Time	Insulin glargine (Lantus)	15 minutes before Breakfast / Insulin aspart	15 minutes before morning snack	15 minutes before Lunch / Insulin aspart	15 minutes before afternoon tea	15 minutes before Supper / Insulin aspart	15 minutes before evening snack	Before breakfast	2 hours after breakfast	Before midday meal	2 hours after midday meal	Before evening meal	2 hours after evening meal	Before bed	During night	Before breakfast	Before midday meal	Before evening meal	Before bed	
1st	28u	18u		18u		18u		5.1	8.4			5.8		7.1						
4th								5.2		6.3		5.5	6.4		4.5					
7th								6.0	8.5			4.7		6.5						
9th								5.1	8.3			5.2		7.6						
11th										5.1	7.3			8.2						

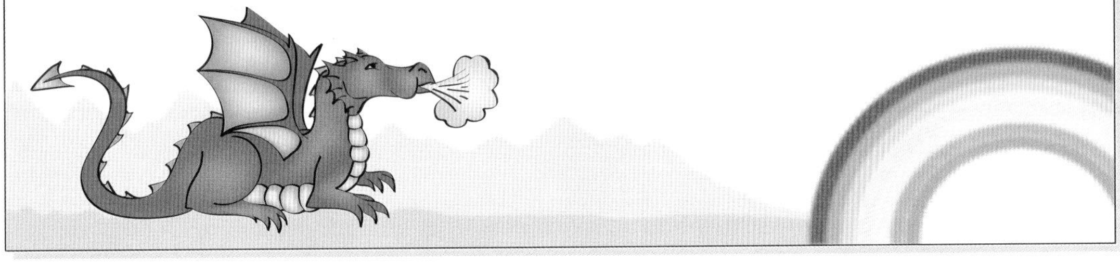

Figure 15.17 Diabetic diary showing good control.

Glycosylated haemoglobin (HbA1c)

Blood glucose monitoring is very dependent on compliance. Glycosylated haemoglobin (HbA1c) levels have the advantage of providing an objective measure of control, are the benchmark for changes in management and give motivation to both the family and the physician. HbA1c integrates the prevailing blood glucose levels over the previous couple of months. In simplistic terms the HbA1c fraction of haemoglobin becomes irreversibly 'sticky' (or glycosylated) in proportion to the degree of hyperglycaemia. In normal individuals 4–6% of the HbA1c fraction is glycosylated. For diabetic individuals in good control, HbA1c levels are almost normal, and levels above 7% require close monitoring.

Management of acute problems

Diabetic ketoacidosis (DKA)

Diabetic ketoacidosis is a medical emergency and must be treated immediately. It is precipitated when insulin levels fall below the child's requirements. This may occur as a result of non-compliance or because of increased requirements, as occurs with infection. Some individuals, particularly adolescents, have brittle diabetes and develop ketoacidosis very easily. The cycle of events is shown in Figure 15.10 (see also p. 113).

Treatment should be carried out where possible in intensive-care surroundings to permit close monitoring and frequent adjustments to therapy, carefully following protocols. Skill and experience are required, the particular dangers being hypokalaemia or cerebral oedema, which may cause death. Management consists of careful rehydration, provision of insulin, replacement of electrolytes and treatment of any precipitating infection (Table 15.6).

Hypoglycaemia

Virtually all diabetic children experience some hypoglycaemic attacks at some time. They are an almost inevitable accompaniment to management that emphasises good control. The symptoms and signs include pallor, hunger, sweating, trembling and tachycardia, and may proceed to drowsiness, mental confusion, seizures and coma. Hypoglycaemia is easily differentiated from ketoacidosis as it occurs over a span of minutes as opposed to hours or days.

Common causes include errors in insulin dose, inadequate caloric intake and physical activity in the absence of food intake. It is treated, if the child is conscious, by giving dextrose tablets or a carbohydrate-containing snack or drink. If the child is unable to drink or eat, glucose gel can be squeezed on to the buccal mucosa. The family should also be taught how to inject glucagon (which releases hepatic glucose stores) intramuscularly if the child is unconscious. Intravenous 10% glucose solution is administered if medical personnel are available.

It is important that the family understands precipitating factors of the attack, and that adjustments in snacks or insulin dose

Table 15.6 Management of diabetic ketoacidosis (recommended intensive care environment)
General resuscitation if in shock (see p. 408)
Clinical assessment including weight and signs of infection
Aim to normalise metabolic status gradually over 24-48 hours
Cardiac monitor
Intravenous line and investigations (glucose, blood gases, electrolytes, full blood count, cultures)
Rehydration (see p. 418)
Normal saline should be used initially
Care must be taken, as overzealous fluid replacement can precipitate lethal cerebral oedema
Bicarbonate is used sparingly to avoid paradoxical CNS acidosis and oedema
Insulin
Low-dose intravenous insulin is given continuously by pump
Blood glucose monitoring must be carried out frequently to enable titration of the insulin dose. Once the blood glucose level has fallen, dextrose is added to the solution and insulin continued as it is still required to clear the ketones and normalise pH
Electrolytes
Acidosis drives the potassium out of the cells and depletion occurs as a result of diuresis. Potassium must be replaced and is added to the intravenous solution once the child has passed urine (so ensuring functional kidneys)
Identification of infection
Clinical and laboratory search for infection is required
When the diabetic ketoacidosis is under control, subcutaneous insulin can be introduced, initially using regular doses of short-acting insulin on a sliding scale, followed by the child's normal dose. Oral fluids followed by a regular diet can be introduced

are considered. Nocturnal hypoglycaemia is particularly hazardous as it may be overlooked when the child and family are asleep.

Routine follow-up of the child with diabetes (see Checklist)

In most areas special diabetes clinics are established, which often incorporate education sessions and opportunities for families to meet as well as routinely reviewing the child's diabetic condition. There are particular periods when families are likely to need extra advice and input:

- *At diagnosis.* Initially glucose control is usually smooth as the child often has some reserves of insulin which buffer glucose swings. This is called the honeymoon period and may last for several months.

- *In toddlerhood.* These years are characterised by typically unreasonable behavior. Particular difficulties include picky eating and food refusal. A particular problem is differentiating hypoglycaemia from normal temper tantrums. Blood glucose tests differentiate the two.
- *In the adolescent years.* The stresses of adolescence, hormonal changes, often erratic lifestyle and compliance all contribute to disrupting diabetic control.
- *During illness.* Illness places an extra stress on the child and demands extra insulin. It is often the trigger for diabetic ketoacidosis. The first sign of an infection can be a rise in glucose levels.
- *During stress.* Stress, whether physical such as in accidents, or psychological, increases insulin demands.

✓ Checklist for review of a child with diabetes

If the child is new to you or the clinic, check:
- ☐ Family's understanding of diabetes and their ability to make adjustments in insulin dose and use devices competently
- ☐ Who gives the insulin and whether by pen, syringe or pump. How often are pump tubes and needles checked.
- ☐ Blood glucose monitoring is being performed
- ☐ School is well informed
- ☐ Family is aware of the British Diabetes Association

At routine follow-up, review:
History
Review diary and ask about:
- ☐ Blood glucose levels
- ☐ Symptoms of hypo- and hyperglycaemia
- ☐ Dietary difficulties
- ☐ Problems at school, related or unrelated to diabetes
- ☐ If in poor control, assess compliance with injections and diet, and any new stresses

Physical examination
- ☐ Height and weight
- ☐ Injection sites for lipoatrophy or hypertrophy
- ☐ Fundi and blood pressure

Investigations
- ☐ HbA1c
- ☐ Thyroid function tests if thyromegaly or fall-off in growth
- ☐ Ophthalmological exam yearly from 8 years after onset

Action
- ☐ Advise on adjustments in insulin and diet
- ☐ Encourage child to take more responsibility as he or she grows
- ☐ Counsel about particular issues such as:
  - food refusal in toddlers
  - compliance, smoking, alcohol and contraception in adolescence

Discussion of treatment and monitoring options

A full physical examination is not required at every review. Growth monitoring is important, both as a measure of control and also as an indication of hypothyroidism or coeliac disease. Injection sites, fundi and blood pressure should be measured. Glycosylated haemoglobin is most helpful if a recent level is available. Assessment of thyroid function and coeliac disease is required if a fall-off in growth is observed.

A well-kept diary is vital if continuous monitoring is not done. If the child is in poor control, any new stresses should be

sought and compliance with injections and diet should be gently ascertained.

The visit should not only focus on advice about adjustments in insulin and diet. Over the years, children need to be encouraged to take on more responsibility. The transition to adult care needs to be smooth so that adult life can be faced with good support.

👁 The child with type 1 diabetes at a glance

Epidemiology
More than 20 000 children in the UK
Incidence rising in recent years

Aetiology/pathophysiology
Destruction of the beta cells in
the islets of Langerhans,
resulting in insulin deficiency

How the diagnosis is made
Children usually present with
ketoacidosis, polyuria,
polydipsia and weight loss.
Diagnosis is confirmed by
finding raised blood sugar
levels. A glucose tolerance
test is not required in children

Clinical features
Poor control (hyperglycaemia)
History
- Polydipsia
- Polyuria and enuresis
- Hypoglycaemic episodes*

Physical examination
- Poor growth
- Lipoatrophy/dystrophy

Investigations
- High blood sugar
- High HbA1c

Ketoacidosis
History
- Thirst and polyuria
- Vomiting
- Abdominal pain

Physical examination
- Acetone smell on breath
- Dehydration
- Kussmaul breathing
- Hypovolaemic shock*
- Drowsiness/coma*

Investigations
- Very high blood sugar,
  ketonuria
- Blood gases – metabolic
  acidosis
- Urea and electrolytes
  deranged

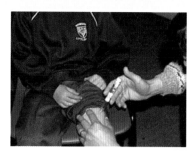
Injecting insulin using a pen

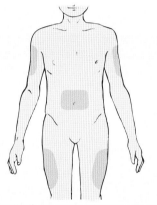
Sites for injections

Clinical features (cont.)
Hypoglycaemia
History
- Hunger
- Shakiness

Physical examination
- Pallor
- Sweating
- Tachycardia
- Tremor
- Drowsiness
- Seizures
- Coma

Investigations
- Low blood sugar often
  followed by rebound high
  blood sugar

General management
A specialist team should be
involved

Initial management: correction
of metabolic state and
education of the family
Medication:
Insulin (see Table 15.5 and Box
15.2)
Nutritional control
Monitoring:
Blood glucose by finger prick at
home
Continous computerised glucose
monitoring becoming
widespread
HbAlc levels
Education:
Self-management of diabetic
control
Injection technique
Insulin pumps and continous
patient controlled sc. infusion
becoming widespread
Diet
Coping with hypo/
hyperglycaemia
Liaison with school

Management of acute problems
Hypoglycaemia (see Box 15.2)
Diabetic ketoacidosis (see Table
15.6 and Box 15.2)

Points for routine follow-up
Monitor
- diary of symptoms of hypo-
  and hyperglycaemia
- digital displays of glucose
  levels, trends and events
- dietary difficulties
- intercurrent illness and stress
- growth
- injection sites
- blood pressure
- fundi

Investigations
HbA1c, thyroid function tests,
ophthalmological exam

Prognosis
Lifelong condition.
Complications of retinopathy,
nephropathy, neuropathy and
atherosclerosis are not
usually seen until beyond
childhood and are related to
the degree of diabetic control
attained

Prognosis and long-term issues

The prognosis no longer depends on overcoming the potentially life-threatening problems of hypoglycaemia and ketoacidosis, but on the long-term complications which develop years if not decades after onset. Education given at the onset of diabetes is critical and ongoing support is needed. On the medical front, arguably the most important person is the diabetic nurse specialist. Diabetes UK gives families the opportunity to be mutually supportive, and children often find it helpful to attend their camps.

Although diabetes is not a genetic disease, there is an increased risk of about one in 20 for first-degree relatives. Special care is required during pregnancy, as there are risks for the fetus if control is not exemplary. Teenage girls therefore need advice about contraception and planning pregnancies.

The school has to be aware of children with diabetes and understand the implications. The diabetes nurse specialist should make a point of going to the school at the outset to prepare staff for the newly diabetic child's return, and re-education is needed over time and when there is a change of school. The school must be able to recognise and manage hypoglycaemia, and cope with the dietary requirements of snacks at odd times. Staff can also be very helpful in reporting untoward symptoms and non-compliance.

 See NICE guideline: Diabetes (type 1 and type 2) in children and young people: diagnosis and management
https://www.nice.org.uk/guidance/ng18

Type 2 (adult or maturity-onset) diabetes mellitus.

With the increase in obesity in children and adolescents, the incidence of type 2 diabetes has begun to increase in the paediatric age group. Rarely type 2 diabetes may be monogenic, as for example with the Maturity Onset Diabetes in the Young (MODY) which is an autosomal dominant condition.

Although insulin secretion is insufficient for needs, the dominant issue in this condition is resistance to insulin action and sometimes dyshormonogenesis involving glucagon and other hormones. The major cause is severe obesity combined with lack of physical activity. Genetic factors are more important in type 2 as opposed to type 1 diabetes, and it is common to find other family members with the disorder. The symptoms of the disorder are similar to type 1 but typically present in a slower and more indolent fashion, and DKA is unusual.

Clinical features

Most children with type 2 diabetes mellitus are obese or extremely obese at diagnosis. Polyuria and polydipsia, if present is mild, and there is little or no weight loss. Children are usually diagnosed around the age of 10 years and are in middle to late puberty. Rarely ketoacidosis may be evident at presentation. There is frequently a family history of type 2 diabetes mellitus.

Acanthosis, a cutaneous finding characterised by velvety hyperpigmented patches most prominent in intertrigenous areas is common. Polycystic ovarian syndrome (PCOS), characterised by hyperandrogenism and chronic anovulation may be present in girls. Lipid disorders and hypertension also occur more frequently in children with type 2 diabetes mellitus.

Management

A full clinical evaluation with emphasis on the skin, orthopaedic, cardiac, vascular, neurological, hepatic and renal systems is important to detect and document complications and provide baseline information for future follow-up. Biochemical and metabolic evaluation is similar to type 1 with the added importance of stressing lipid and cholesterol status, together with exclusion of steatohepatitis.

The bedrock of management is patient and family education. Obese children are at risk for social and school problems and the addition of diabetes adds to the problem. The major task is weight control and reduction and this requires a long-term family-orientated approach. The combined efforts of physician, dietitian, nurse, teacher and often psychologist may be required. Physical activity should be strongly encouraged without insisting on humiliating competitive sports.

Oral hypoglycaemic agents are effective and routinely used in type 2 diabetes. Nevertheless, with the improvements in insulin technology and delivery, insulin may be added successfully to the management plan. Some drugs are not registered for the paediatric age group. Bariatric surgery has been successfully used in older adolescents with intractable obesity and diabetes.

Since the long-term consequences of diabetes are compounded by obesity, it is vital to educate the child into healthy routines and attitudes while still young.

Prognosis

The struggle with obesity is likely to be life-long. It is however possible to be optimistic if the child and family realize that to a large extent the future health of the patient is in their hands.

To test your knowledge on this part of the book, please see Chapter 26

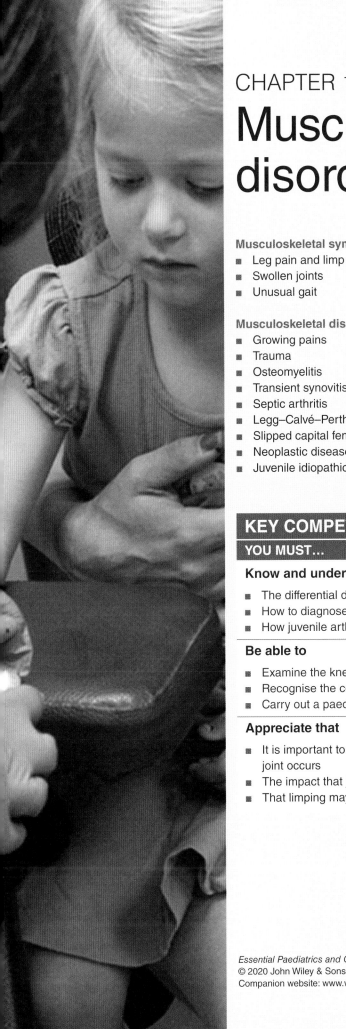

CHAPTER 16

Musculoskeletal disorders

A general pain of all the joints … The disease lies concealed for a long time, when the pain and the disease are kindled up by any slight cause … It is incredible how far the mischief spreads.

Aretaeus, 1st century AD

KEY COMPETENCES

YOU MUST...

Know and understand

- The differential diagnosis of children presenting with leg pain, limp or swollen joints
- How to diagnose and manage important and common musculoskeletal disorders
- How juvenile arthritis presents

Be able to

- Examine the knee and hip joints competently
- Recognise the common conditions that can alter gait
- Carry out a paediatric rheumatological screening assessment, such as pGALS

Appreciate that

- It is important to diagnose and treat rapidly septic arthritis before destruction of the joint occurs
- The impact that juvenile idiopathic arthritis has on the child and family
- That limping may be a trivial phenomenon or a sign of systemic disease

Essential Paediatrics and Child Health, Fourth Edition. Mary Rudolf, Anthony Luder and Kerry Jeavons.
© 2020 John Wiley & Sons Ltd. Published 2020 by John Wiley & Sons Ltd.
Companion website: www.wiley.com/go/rudolf/paediatrics

Musculoskeletal symptoms and signs

Finding your way around ...

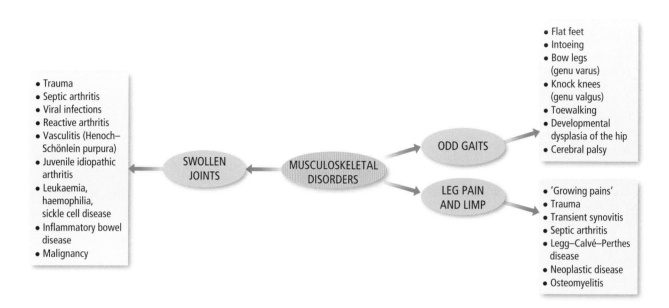

Online Interactive Q11

Leg pain and limp

Causes of leg pain and/or limp

Inflammatory
Transient synovitis
Septic arthritis
Osteomyelitis and diskitis

Orthopaedic
Trauma
Legg–Calvé–Perthes disease
Slipped capital femoral epiphysis
Developmental dysplasia of the hip (DDH)

Neurological
Neuropathy
Chronic Regional Pain Syndrome (CRPS, 'sympathetic dystrophy')
Spinal cord malformation or disease

Genetic
Bone dysplasias

Neoplastic and haematological
Sickle cell anaemia
Leukaemia
Tumours
Gaucher disease

Functional
Growing pains
Hypermobility of the joints

The complaint of leg pain alone, unaccompanied by physical signs, is usually non-organic in nature. Limp, however, is likely to have an underlying organic explanation. *Transient synovitis* is the commonest cause of limp and must be distinguished from *septic arthritis*, can lead to destruction of the joint.

Trauma when acute is an obvious cause of pain; however, chronic pain can result from stress fractures or prolonged healing of muscle haematoma. The pain of *osteomyelitis* is usually very localized and accompanied by swelling, erythema, and tenderness, but it may present subclinically. Haematological disease is an important if less common cause of limb pain. It includes *sickle cell anaemia, haemophilia* and Gaucher disease (p. 310, which is frequently overlooked). *Juvenile idiopathic arthritis* and the *collagen vascular diseases* tend to present with swelling of the joints rather than arthralgia. Both *Legg–Calvé–Perthe disease* (avascular necrosis of the femoral head) and *slipped capital femoral epiphyses* are paediatric causes of leg pain. *Neoplastic disease*, such as leukaemia or osteosarcoma, is the most potentially serious cause. *Growing pains* are a common complaint in healthy children and are characterised by nocturnal pain usually in the lower leg and usually bilateral. Hypermobility of the joints and chronic regional pain syndromes are other 'non-organic' causes of limb pain in children.

In a child presenting with acute or recurrent leg pain, a good history and physical examination should differentiate non-organic from organic causes. Investigations may be required to identify the aetiology where organic disease is suspected.

History – must ask!

Focus on the characteristics of the pain and any systemic symptoms that the child might have.

- *Is there pain?* Pain from organic causes tends to be persistent, occurring day and night, and interrupts play as well as schooling. Particularly significant is a limp or refusal to walk. Organic pain is often unilateral or located to a joint. By contrast, non-organic pain usually occurs at night and primarily on school days. It does not interfere with normal activities, and the parents report a normal gait. It is often bilateral and located between joints.
- *Are there systemic symptoms?* Systemic symptoms such as weight loss, fever, night sweats, rash and diarrhoea point to organic causes.

Physical examination – must check!

Examine the child lying down and then walking. Remember that pain in the hip may be referred to the knee, so that a child presenting with knee pain requires a full examination of the leg and groin.

- *The limb.* Look for signs of point tenderness, redness, swelling and muscle weakness or atrophy. Examine the joints for limitation of movement. In non-organic pain the examination is normal, although you may see minor changes such as coolness or mottling of the leg.
- Neurological examination. Limp may be a sign of weakness so test for power, and examine reflexes.
- *General examination.* Look for evidence of fever, rash, pallor, lymphadenopathy or organomegaly, which suggest infectious or systemic causes.

Investigations

If the leg pain is thought to be pathological, the investigations listed in Table 16.1 may be indicated.

Managing leg pain

In the child where no organic cause is suspected, the approach described in Box 11.1, p. 195, may be helpful.

Table 16.1 Laboratory tests helpful in diagnosing leg pain

Investigation	What you are looking for
Blood count	Leukaemia
	Infections
	Haematological diseases
	Collagen vascular disease
Inflammatory markers: plasma viscosity, ferritin, C-reactive protein, erythrocyte sedimentation rate	Infections
	Collagen vascular disease
	Inflammatory bowel disease
	Tumours
Blood culture	Osteomyelitis
	Septic arthritis
Muscle enzymes	Myositis and trauma
Serum fibrinogen	Familial Mediterranean Fever
Ultrasound	Transient synovitis
	Arthritic effusion
	Osteomyelitis
X-ray	Bone tumours
	Trauma
	Avascular necrosis
	Slipped capital femoral epiphysis
Bone scan	Osteomyelitis
	Stress and spiral fractures
	Malignant tumours
	Avascular necrosis
MRI	Tumours
	Soft tissue infection
	Trauma
Bone marrow	Sickle cell anaemia
	Leukaemia
	Gaucher disease

 Key points: Leg pain or a limp

- Organic and non-organic causes can be differentiated on clinical grounds
- Important features suggesting organic disease are limp or refusal to walk, and any physical signs
- Pain in the hip is referred to the knee, so children with knee pain require a full examination of the leg and groin

Clues to the differential diagnosis of leg pain

	Organic	Functional
Characteristics	Day and night	Only at night ('growing pains')
	Interrupts play	Primarily school days
	Often unilateral	No interference with normal activities
	Usually located in joint	Often located between joints
	Limp or refusal to walk	Unilateral or bilateral
		Normal gait
History	Weight loss	Otherwise healthy child
	Fever	
	Night sweats	
	Rash	
	Diarrhoea	
Physical examination	Point tenderness	Normal examination or minor changes such as
	Redness	coolness or mottling of leg
	Swelling	
	Limitation of movement	
	Muscle weakness or atrophy	
	Fever, rash, pallor, lymphadenopathy, organomegaly	

Swollen joints

Causes of swollen joints

Trauma	Intra-articular bleeding or effusion
Infection	Septic arthritis, viral
Reactive and post-infective arthritis	Post-streptococcal or gastrointestinal infections, rheumatic fever
Auto-immune disease	Henoch–Schönlein purpura, juvenile idiopathic arthritis, systemic lupus erythematosus
Haematological disease	Haemophilia, sickle cell disease, Gaucher
Seronegative arthritis	Ulcerative colitis, Crohn disease, psoriasis
Malignancy	Leukaemia
Genetic	Familial Mediterranean Fever

Swollen joints from causes other than trauma are not very common in childhood. They include viral or reactive causes, but more serious pathology must be excluded, the most critical being *septic arthritis*, which demands urgent diagnosis and treatment. Rheumatic fever varies in frequency over time but should not be forgotten.

A number of conditions can lead to persistent or recurrent joint swelling. *Juvenile chronic arthritis* (JCA), a chronic condition of childhood, is the most important and has three different patterns of presentation. Children with *psoriasis, ulcerative colitis,* or *Crohn disease* can also experience arthritis, the latter of which which tend to coincide with periods of active bowel disease. *Leukaemia* and other malignancies occasionally present with swelling of one or more joints and pain, which is often severe.

Haemarthrosis affecting elbows, knees and ankles is a hallmark of *haemophilia*. The bleeding often seems to be spontaneous, but does not form a diagnostic problem as children present earlier in life with obvious bleeding. Children with *sickle cell disease* may develop symmetrical, painful swelling of the hands and feet as a result of vaso-occlusive crises. *Henoch–Schönlein purpura,* a diffuse allergic vasculitis characterised by a distinctive rash (see Figure 19.14), is often accompanied by pain in the joints with or without swelling. *Gaucher disease* mimics other diseases and its diagnosis is frequently delayed its hallmarks.

Viral infections, notably rubella, can resemble chronic rheumatic disease. *Reactive arthritis* is a sterile arthritis affecting one or more joints which may follow any streptococcal infection or bacterial gastroenteritis. The arthritis is generally transient and the outcome good.

As ever, a thorough clinical evaluation is essential, as the history and distribution of the joints involved provide clues to the underlying problem. The paediatric Gait, Arms, Legs and Spine assessment (pGALS) is a useful validated screening examination rheumatological or musculoskeletal disorders are suspected in school-age children (see p. 93).

History – must ask!

- *Joint symptoms.* Stiffness is an important complaint which may be localized or generalised. In most inflammatory arthropathies, the stiffness that occurs in the morning or after periods of inactivity is alleviated by activity, whereas mechanical problems are exacerbated by activity. A history of pain or swelling of other joints is obviously relevant.
- *Systemic symptoms.* Once you have discounted trauma, you must establish whether the child's symptoms are specific to the joint(s) or whether there are clues present, such as fever, anorexia, weight loss, rash, weakness and fatigue, that suggest a systemic cause.
- *Past medical and family history.* Important information in the past medical and family history includes inflammatory bowel disease, auto-immune conditions, blood dyscrasias and psoriasis: these are all associated with arthritis.

Physical examination – must check!

- *Musculoskeletal system.* Your examination should include all four limbs, temporomandibular joints and the spine using the pGALS approach. Carefully examine the affected joints by inspection and palpation, looking for skin colour changes, heat, tenderness, range of motion and asymmetry. Look for fluid and measure the circumference of any swollen joint. In the young child it is very helpful to observe normal active motion, especially gait, to pinpoint the joints involved.
- *General examination.* Unless there is a clear history of localized trauma to the joint, the child needs a full physical examination looking for signs such as fever, anaemia, hepatosplenomegaly, cardiac murmurs and rash, which might be associated with systemic disease.

Table 16.2 Useful investigations in the child with swollen joints and their relevance

Investigation	Relevance
Full blood count	Elevated white count and shift to the left with bacterial infection
	Anaemia in collagen vascular diseases, inflammatory bowel disease, malignancy
	Characteristic features of the haemoglobinopathies
CRP, ferritin, fibrinogen, ESR	Elevated in bacterial infection, very high in collagen vascular disease and inflammatory bowel disease
Blood culture	Positive in septic arthritis
ASO titre	Indicative of recent streptococcal infection – reactive arthritis or, rarely, rheumatic fever
Viral titres	Viral arthritis
Rheumatoid factor and antinuclear antibodies	Negative in most forms of juvenile chronic arthritis
X-ray of the joint	Characteristic depending on the underlying aetiology
Joint aspiration	Microscopy and culture to exclude/confirm septic arthritis. May be helpful in other conditions

ESR, erythrocyte sedimentation rate.

Investigations

Most children presenting with arthritis or joint swelling require investigations. These are described in Table 16.2.

 Key points: Swollen joints

- Trauma is the commonest cause of an isolated swollen joint
- If the joint is acutely swollen, rule out septic arthritis as the cause
- Elicit any systemic symptoms
- Clues to the underlying diagnosis are provided by the history and distribution of the joints involved
- An isolated swollen joint that does not settle within a few days should be X-rayed to rule out a bone tumour

Unusual gait

Causes of abnormal gait

Common
Flat feet
Intoeing
Bow legs and knock-knees
Toe walking

Less common but important
Congenital dislocation of the hip
Cerebral palsy

Parents not uncommonly have concerns about the shape of their child's legs or their gait. They are rarely of significance, and reassurance is usually all that is required. The child should be observed walking independently and without a nappy, trousers, socks, or shoes, and then on standing still, from in front and from behind. All the joints should be examined lying down (see p. 93).

Flat feet   Most babies have flat feet, the arch gradually developing through childhood. Flat feet in childhood are painless and need no therapy.

Intoeing   Intoeing (see Figure 16.1) may occur as a result of rotation of the leg at the hip (femoral anteversion), at the tibia (medial tibial torsion) or in the foot (metatarsus adductus). The diagnosis is made clinically. The only condition which requires orthopaedic intervention is metatarsus adductus, as buying shoes is problematic if the feet are curved. Otherwise intoeing usually resolves by 4 or 5 years of age.

Bow legs and knock-knees   During the first 2 years the legs are naturally bowed in shape. During the third and fourth year a physiological knock-knee pattern emerges, which straightens by

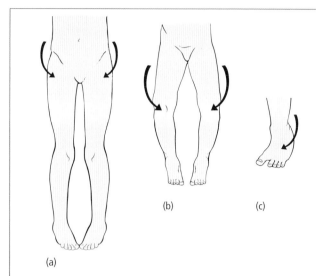

Figure 16.1 Types of intoeing: (a) femoral anteversion, (b) tibial torsion, and (c) metatarsus adductus.

the age of 10 years, although may persist in the obese. Bow legs are rarely indicative of rickets or other pathology.

Toewalking   Some children start to walk on their toes. This is usually a normal variant, but is occasionally a sign of cerebral palsy, which can be determined by neurological examination of the legs.

Congenital dislocation of the hip   This is usually detected through screening before the child starts to walk, but should be considered if there is a limp (see p. 454).

Cerebral palsy   Occasionally mild forms of cerebral palsy present with an abnormal hemiplegic or diplegic gait (see pp. 87, 262). The diagnosis is made clinically by the finding of spasticity, increased deep tendon reflexes, and an extensor plantar response in affected legs.

Musculoskeletal disorders

Growing pains

'Growing pains' is a term used for the common complaint of leg pain in children where organic disease has been excluded. The complaint tends to occur in the 3- to 6-year-old age group. The term is a misnomer as the pain does not appear to be related to growth, but may be caused by oedema in the fascial sheaths.

Clinical features   Limp is not a feature. The pain classically occurs at night, most often in the lower leg and is symmetrical, often after a day of vigorous activity. These children also not infrequently experience headaches and abdominal pain. It has been suggested that there may be a link with migraine.

Management   Symptoms usually respond to heat and massage and may need simple analgesia. As in all cases of functional pain, psychosomatic factors should be considered. The approach described in Box 11.1, p. 195, may be helpful.

Trauma

Trauma is a common cause of joint pain and swelling in childhood, and in this case the cause of the swelling is obvious. Two paediatric forms of joint trauma are worthy of particular mention.

Pulled elbow or '*nursemaid's*' *elbow* is a common mishap which occurs in the toddler age group. The child may not complain of pain but refuses to use the arm and holds it in a flexed position. The precipitating cause is sudden forceful traction on the arm, causing radial dislocation at the elbow. This usually happens when a reluctant child is dragged by the arm, or trips while being held by the hand (Figure 16.2). The condition is treated by simply supinating the arm while flexed at 90° causing the head of the ulnar to click back into place. No post-reduction fixation is necessary. The parents need to be alerted to the cause in order to avoid recurrence.

The other traumatic joint problem peculiar to childhood is *fracture of the growth plate* or *Salter-Harris* type fracture. When a child traumatizes a joint, the most vulnerable structure is the growth plate, rather than the ligaments. Children presenting with swelling of a joint following trauma may well have a fracture through the growth plate rather than a ligamentous sprain. The fracture is not easily seen on X-ray. Treatment consists of immobilizing the joint for some weeks.

Osteomyelitis

Osteomyelitis most often affects the metaphyses of long bones and is usually haematogenous in origin. The commonest

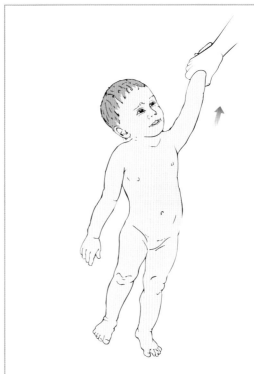

Figure 16.2 Nursemaid's elbow. Sudden forceful traction dislocates the elbow joint.

organisms are *Staphylococcus aureus*, *Kingella kingae* and *Streptococcus pyogenes*. *Haemophilus influenza* is now rare in immunised children.

Clinical features   Children may present with fever and pain or PUO, and the infected limb is obviously tender and held immobile. Swelling and redness eventually appear. The adjacent joint may contain a sterile 'sympathetic' effusion. Inflammatory markers are elevated and there is leucocytosis with a left shift.

Management   Repeated blood culture determines the causative organism in 25–50% of cases. X-rays are not of any diagnostic help in the first 10 days as it takes time for the radiological changes of the subperiosteum to develop. Technetium-pyrophosphate bone scans, however, are useful early in the course of the disease. High-dose intravenous antibiotics are required initially. Once blood inflammatory markers and temperatures settle, the child can be changed to high-dose oral antibiotics, which should be continued for a total of at least 3–6 weeks. If there is no immediate response, surgical exploration and drainage is required. If the infection is inadequately treated, irreversible bone necrosis, draining sinuses and limb deformity can occur.

Osteomyelitis at a glance

Aetiology
Infection of the metaphysis (usually blood-borne)
Organisms: *Staphylococcus aureus Kingella kingae Haemophilus influenzae Streptococcus pyogenes*

History
Fever
Painful limb
In infants disease may be systemic. In older children it may be very indolent

Physical examination
Swelling and redness at site
Sympathetic effusion of adjacent joint*

Confirmatory investigations
High white cell count and erythrocyte sedimentation rate
Blood culture (repeat samples needed)

NB *Signs and symptoms are variable.

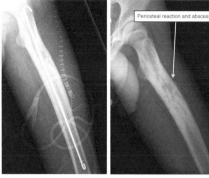

Chronic osteomyelitis of left femur. Note bone destruction and regeneration and sub-periosteal abscess. In the left picture a stabilising antibiotic releasing pin has been inserted.

Bone scan to detect early changes
Subperiosteal changes on X-ray seen only after 10 days

Differential diagnosis
Soft tissue infection
Trauma
Malignancy
Septic arthritis

Management
High-dose antibiotics for 4–6 weeks
Surgical exploration and drainage

Prognosis/complications
If inadequately treated may lead to bone necrosis, draining sinuses, limb deformity

Transient synovitis

Transient synovitis is the commonest cause of limp in young children, usually affecting boys aged 2–8 years. It is a benign condition, the major significance being the possibility of overlooking septic arthritis of the hip.

Clinical features   There is a sudden onset of limp with hip and/or knee pain. A mild URTI may precede the symptoms.

On examination there is limited abduction, extension and internal rotation of the hip. Transient synovitis can be differentiated from septic arthritis by the lack of systemic symptoms and signs, a normal white cell count, normal or only mildly elevated CRP. Diagnosis is confirmed by hip ultrasound examination (see Figure 16.3).

The right hip shows a bulging hip joint, effusion and thickening of the joint capsule compared with the normal left joint.

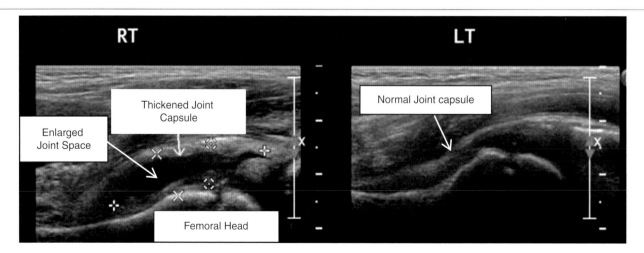

Figure 16.3 Ultrasound of hips in transient synovitis showing thickened joint capsule and enlarged joint space.

Management and prognosis Transient synovitis lasts for a few days or weeks and treatment consists of rest and simple analgesia.

Septic arthritis

Septic arthritis is a serious cause of joint swelling which, if untreated, rapidly leads to destruction of the joint. Infection usually affects the larger weight-bearing joints such as hip, knee and ankle. The commonest organism is a staphylococcus, but *Kingella kingae, St. pneumonia or gram negative organisms* may also be responsible. These organisms are blood-borne.

Clinical features Children present with fever and a hot, tender, swollen joint. Occasionally more than one joint may be involved. Movement of the joint is limited and extremely painful. When the hip is involved, the leg is held in a flexed and abducted posture and may not appear swollen or hot to the touch due to the thick muscle and soft-tissue covering. In neonatal septic arthritis, the baby usually looks very ill and holds the limb immobile ('pseudo-paralysis').

Investigations Supportive evidence of bacterial infection may be found in the white cell count and elevated inflammatory markers and C-reactive protein. Ultrasound or X-ray of the joint may show widening of the joint space caused by fluid accumulation, debris in the joint space and in some cases signs of an adjacent osteomyelitis. Aspiration of the joint should be carried out urgently for microscopy and culture. The joint fluid is purulent with organisms found on Gram's stain.

Management Treatment involves intravenous antibiotics and surgical decompression. Intravenous cefuroxime is the treatment of choice. The joint needs to be splinted in the acute stage. Once temperatures and inflammatory markers settle, antibiotics are switched to the oral route and 2–4 weeks of therapy are necessary. As soon as pain has subsided, a full range of joint mobility needs to be encouraged, with physiotherapy to prevent joint flexion deformities.

Prognosis With early and effective treatment, the prognosis is very good. If the diagnosis is delayed, destruction of the joint may occur. This is most likely in the neonate.

Legg–Calvé–Perthe disease

Legg–Calvé–Perthe disease (avascular necrosis of the femoral head) is a relatively common condition affecting children, principally boys, between the ages of 4 and 10 years. It may follow on from an episode of transient synovitis. The aetiology of the avascular necrosis is unknown.

Clinical features The condition often presents with painless limp which may be intermittent, but once a crush fracture develops, pain in the hip or knee are major features.

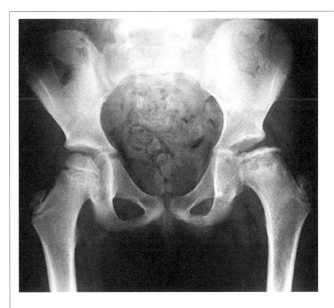

Figure 16.4 X-ray of the hips of a 5-year-old child with Legg–Calvé–Perthe disease. Note the increased density, flattening and fragmentation of the left capital femoral epiphysis.

Diagnosis is made by X-ray (Figure 16.4) or technetium-pyrophosphate bone scan, which typically shows 'cold' hypovascularity.

Management and prognosis Treatment involves bracing or traction and recovery may take 2–3 years.

Slipped capital femoral epiphysis

Slipped capital femoral epiphysis is a condition classically occurring in overweight sedentary teenage boys.

Clinical features Pain is experienced in the groin or medial side of the knee, often gradual in onset. On examination the hip is held in abduction and external rotation with limitation of internal rotation. X-ray confirms the diagnosis (Figure 16.5).

Management Treatment is surgical.

Neoplastic disease

Neoplastic disease is the most potentially serious of all causes of limb pain, and should always be considered if limb pain or limp persists for more than a few days. Malignant tumours usually initially present with pain, and in some cases are palpable as a tender mass, which is seen as a destructive bony lesion on X-ray. Benign tumours also occur and may also present as a mass or pain. Leukaemic bone disease is harder to diagnose. The pain is described as deep and throbbing and often wakes the child at night. Diagnosis is often made on the blood count, but X-rays are only sometimes helpful.

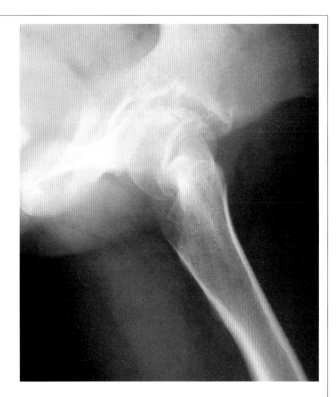

Figure 16.5 X-ray of an obese boy with slipped capital femoral epiphysis.

Juvenile idiopathic arthritis

Juvenile idiopathic arthritis (JIA) is the commonest rheumatic disease of childhood and is a major cause of chronic disability. It is characterised by synovitis of the peripheral joints, with soft tissue swelling and effusion. There are three main patterns of presentation – systemic, poly- and pauci-articular arthritis. Each form has distinctive clinical features and the prognoses differ. The various features are summarized in Table 16.3.

Systemic juvenile idiopathic arthritis (Still disease)

The systemic form is the rarest type of JIA. It often presents as a diagnostic puzzle as the child may not have any joint symptoms at the outset. He or she looks ill with a remitting fever, variable rash, hepatosplenomegaly, weight loss or abdominal pain. When the fever drops the child may look remarkably well. Joint symptoms may be overlooked in view of the other systemic features. Sepsis and malignancy are often considered in the diagnosis. Laboratory findings such as normocytic anaemia, neutrophilia, thrombocytosis and raised inflammatory markers (particularly ferritin) are characteristic although non-specific. Rheumatoid factor is negative, making the diagnosis at times difficult to confirm.

Polyarticular juvenile idiopathic arthritis

Children with polyarticular JIA present with painful swelling and restricted movement of five or more large and small joints within 6 months. This is commonly symmetrically distributed. Systemic features are not prominent, although poor weight gain and mild anaemia may occur. Morning stiffness is common and young children may be quite irritable. Rheumatoid factor is usually negative, although antinuclear antibodies may be positive. The prognosis for this type of JIA is generally good.

Pauciarticular juvenile idiopathic arthritis

Pauciarticular JIA commonly affects girls under the age of 4 years. By definition it involves few (fewer than five) joints, commonly knees, ankles and elbows. Systemic symptoms are minimal and the appearance of the joints is identical to those in the polyarticular form. Rheumatoid factor is negative, although antinuclear antibodies may be positive.

The important distinction between the two latter forms, apart from the number of joints involved, is the risk of chronic iridocyclitis. In pauciarticular arthritis, inflammation of the inner structures of the eye may lead to loss of vision and even permanent blindness. The changes are only detectable by slit lamp examination, and for this reason regular ophthalmological examinations are necessary. See Figure 16.6.

Table 16.3 Features of juvenile idiopathic arthritis					
Type	Characteristics	Sex ratio	Rheumatoid factor/ ANA*	Iridocyclitis	Severe arthritis
Systemic	Large and small joints affected	M>F	Negative	No	25%
Polyarticular	Large and small joints affected	F>M	RhF negative, ANA may be positive	No	12%
Pauciarticular	<5 joints, usually large	F>M	RhF negative, ANA may be positive	High risk	Not usually

* ANA, antinuclear antibody.

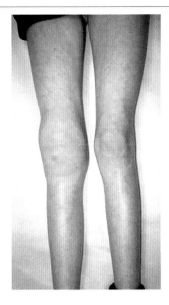

Figure 16.6 A 10-year-old girl with pauciarticular juvenile idiopathic arthritis affecting the right knee.

 Juvenile idiopathic arthritis at a glance

Epidemiology
Three patterns occur: systemic (Still disease) and pauciarticular in young children; polyarticular in older children

Aetiology
Immune disorder

Clinical features
A. Systemic JIA:

History
- fever and shaking chills
- malaise
- weight loss
- arthralgia*

Physical examination
- ill child
- high, spiking fever
- hepatosplenomegaly

Lymphadenopathy
- salmon pink rash*
- arthritis at onset*

B. Pauciarticular JIA:
History
- painful swollen joints

Physical examination
- <5 swollen joints (knees, ankles or elbows)

C. Polyarticular JIA:
History
- painful swollen joints
- poor weight gain

Physical examination
- swollen, tender large and small joints

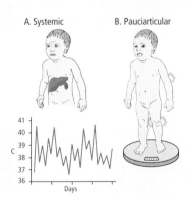

A. Systemic   B. Pauciarticular

C. Polyarticular

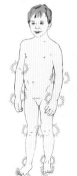

NB Rule out sepsis

Confirmatory investigations
High inflammatory rate markers e.g. CRP, Ferritin, ESR

Anaemia with high white cell count

Rheumatoid factor – negative ANA (antinuclear antibody) may be positive in pauci - and polyarticular types

X-ray: soft tissue swelling, periostitis, early loss of cartilage, bone destruction and fusion

Differential diagnosis
Sepsis and malignancy in systemic type

Other causes of swollen joints in pauci- and polyarticular types (see Causes box, p. 286)

Management
Reduction of inflammation using non-steroidal anti-inflammatory drugs

Early use of disease modifying drugs including biological drugs and cytotoxics (methotrexate)

Steroids for acute severe disease
Intra-articular steroids for pauciarticular disease
Physio- and occupational therapy
Psychosocial support

Prognosis/complications
- Generally good, with eventual resolution of arthritis in most
- 25% of systemic type develop chronic disabling arthritis
- Pauciarticular form at high risk for acute chronic iridocyclitis

NB* Signs and symptoms are variable.

Management of the child with juvenile idiopathic arthritis

The aims of management are twofold:
- to preserve joint function;
- to help the child to achieve optimal psychosocial adjustment.

The goals of medical treatment are to reduce joint inflammation, maintain function and prevent deformity. Non-steroidal anti-inflammatory drugs are used to suppress the inflammation. Corticosteroids are indicated for severe systemic disease unresponsive to other therapies. Steroid injection into selected joints may be helpful, but should not be used repeatedly. Disease modifying drugs such as hydroxychloroquine, penicillamine, gold injections, methotrexate and immune regulatory drugs are used in severe disease and increasingly as first line agents. New biological agents such as TNF inhibitors are promising alternatives.

Physical and occupational therapy are important to improve movement and physical strength in affected joints and to maintain the function of the child as a whole. Treatment consists of daily exercises, hydrotherapy, and day and night splints.

The family needs support, and children should be encouraged to lead as normal and self-sufficient lives as possible. Unpredictable exacerbations are disheartening, and families need encouragement to work at maintaining joint mobility. The prognosis in the various subgroups differs, but overall most children have a good prognosis with no or only minor disability in adulthood. Children with residual handicaps need help in vocational planning.

To test your knowledge on this part of the book, please see Chapter 26

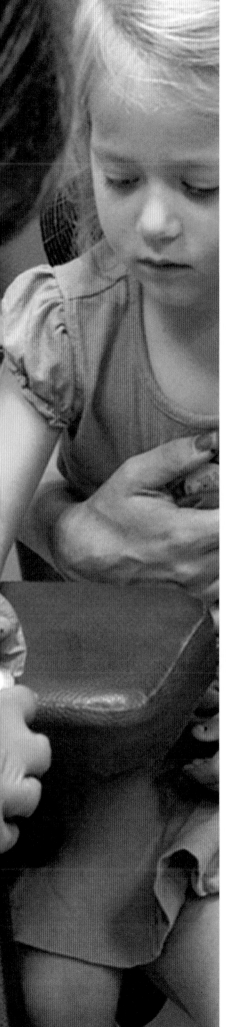

CHAPTER 17

Renal and urinary tract disorders

And this little piggy went Wee, Wee, Wee all the way home.
English nursery rhyme

Renal and urinary symptoms and signs

Renal and urinary conditions

KEY COMPETENCES

YOU MUST...

Know and understand

The differential diagnosis of children presenting with dysuria, wetting, polyuria and haematuria

- How to diagnose and manage the important and common conditions of the urinary tract
- The criteria for diagnosing UTI on urine culture
- How wetting is managed

Be able to

- Dipstick a urine specimen
- Interpret urinalysis findings
- Advise parents of a child with dysuria due to perineal irritation

Appreciate that

- The problem of enuresis is common in children and teenagers
- Chronic renal disease places a considerable burden on children and their families

Essential Paediatrics and Child Health, Fourth Edition. Mary Rudolf, Anthony Luder and Kerry Jeavons.
© 2020 John Wiley & Sons Ltd. Published 2020 by John Wiley & Sons Ltd.
Companion website: www.wiley.com/go/rudolf/paediatrics

Renal and urinary symptoms and signs

Finding your way around …

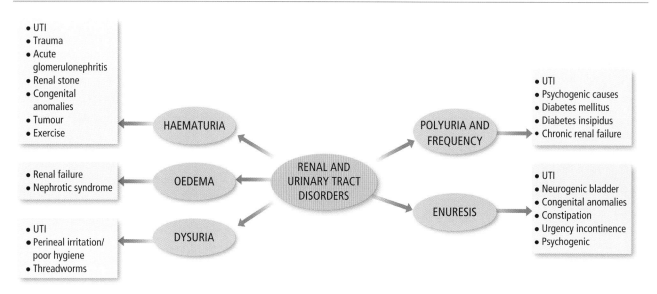

Dysuria

Causes of dysuria	
Urinary tract infections (see p. 326)	Irritation secondary to threadworm infestation (p. 215)
Irritation secondary to poor hygiene	
Sensitivity to bubble baths or washing powder	

Dysuria, or pain on micturition, is commonly experienced by little girls secondary to vulval irritation and inflammation. Poor hygiene, bubble bath sensitivity and threadworms all irritate the delicate skin and mucous membranes and cause soreness. Poor hygiene may be a particular problem in young girls who have just achieved independent toileting but may not wipe themselves well or wash carefully. Paradoxically, bubble baths and soaps also cause dysuria by irritating the sensitive skin in this area.

Other causes include vaginal foreign bodies (e.g. tissue paper) and urinary tract infection (UTI), which is less frequently a cause but needs to be considered, particularly if fever is also present. Itching and soreness can be a problem for girls infested with threadworms, when the worms emerge from the anus and enter the perineal area. Candida infection is often overdiagnosed as a cause of dysuria in children who are out of nappies. Sexual abuse may present with ano-urinary symptoms.

History – must ask!

A history of UTIs or symptoms such as frequency, fever (particularly with rigors) and abdominal or loin pain suggest urine infection. Anal itching indicates irritation from threadworms.

Physical examination – must check

The perineal area should be inspected for signs of inflammation, bruising and poor hygiene, and evidence of a discharge may be found in underwear.

Investigations (see also p. 114)

Urine dipstick and urinalysis may be helpful, although it may well show protein, red and white cells from irritation even if there is no urine infection. If it tests positive for nitrites, infection is more likely. A urine culture is needed to assess if a

Box 17.1 Advice for girls with dysuria

- Take daily baths or wash with simple, non-perfumed soap or, if not too dirty, water alone
- Avoid bubble baths and talcum powder
- Only wear pure cotton knickers and preferably wear skirts. Constricting clothing such as nylon tights or tight trousers trap moisture and exacerbate irritation
- A barrier cream or nappy cream may help
- An empirical trial of mebendazole against threadworms can be given

UTI is present. If itching is a problem, the child needs to be investigated for threadworms (see Figure 11.9) or empirically treated with mebendazole.

Management

The management, if there is no urinary infection, lies in improving hygiene and reducing factors which lead to inflammation of the area (see Box 17.1). Treatment of urine infections is covered on p. 326.

Wetting

Wetting while asleep is called *enuresis*; however, it is often called *nocturnal enuresis* (NE) for clarity. Wetting by day is called daytime wetting or daytime urinary incontinence. Nocturnal enuresis may exist alone, but not uncommonly it coexists with day wetting. Treatment of nocturnal enuresis differs in those with nocturnal enuresis alone from those who also have day wetting.

Daytime urinary incontinence – day wetting

Causes of day wetting

Physiological
Overactive bladder (*urge incontinence*) – usually with nocturnal enuresis

Organic
Urinary tract infection
Neurogenic bladder
Congenital anomalies
Constipation (or, rarely, other pelvic masses)

Psychogenic

Day wetting can be defined as a lack of bladder control during the day in a child old enough to maintain bladder continence. Most children with day wetting also have nocturnal enuresis – the combination often having a genetic or inherited basis. In our

culture, daytime bladder control usually occurs by the age of 2½ years, but it can be delayed beyond this without being abnormal.

The commonest cause of daytime wetting is an *overactive bladder* causing urgency, and frequency of micturition. The bladder contracts dramatically, unpredictably, and often frequently, usually when relatively empty, without any warning, causing a sudden urge to void. The child may wet a few drops of urine. To minimize wetting, the child will tighten pelvic floor muscles and display 'avoidance' manoeuvres (sometimes called 'Vincent's curtsey') often misunderstood by bystanders as the child delaying or avoiding going to the toilet. Running the gauntlet to the toilet can paradoxically increase the risk of wetting because running is incompatible with tightening of pelvic floor muscles. Children in this predicament, when asked if they need to go to the toilet, might dissemble and maintain that 'they don't need to go', thus infuriating their already frustrated parents.

Children may be too shy or embarrassed to ask permission to go to the toilet, especially if they have repeatedly been falsely accused of 'waiting until the last moment'. Day wetting may be part of a wider behavioural problem or externalizing disorder, such as ADHD. Psychosocial triggers and stress have traditionally been over-emphasised as a cause.

Day wetting, often with nocturnal enuresis, may be associated with encopresis, although the causal link is unclear. Dealing with the bowel problem is a prerequisite to solving the urinary problems. Day wetting with NE usually has a genetic basis (see below); however, there is genotype/phenotype mismatch, that is different family members with presumably the same gene may have different combinations of night-time and daytime wetting. While daytime wetting usually indicates an overactive bladder, one should exclude an unlikely organic cause (often on clinical grounds). The potential organic causes include UTI (usually presenting with symptoms of dysuria, frequency, abdominal pain and/or fever, rather than enuresis alone); diabetes mellitus; or neurological dysfunction or neurogenic bladder (more likely in the presence of concurrent neurological problems such as cerebral palsy or spina bifida, and gait disturbance or inadequate bowel control).

A *neurogenic bladder* can range from a spastic small bladder which empties suddenly without warning, to a large hypotonic bladder which fills to capacity and overflows. The cause can be either an upper or lower motor neuron lesion. Urgency of micturition makes neurogenic bladder most unlikely. Clinical features of neurogenic bladder are a distended bladder, abnormal perianal sensation and anal tone, and abnormal neurological findings in the legs. The finding of hairy patches or lipoma overlying the lower spine suggests a spinal anomaly responsible for the problem. In addition to incontinence, neurogenic bladder dysfunction can cause chronic kidney disease.

Urinary incontinence can be caused by congenital urinary tract anomalies (see p. 334 for details).

Pelvic masses, the commonest being faecal impaction, may lead to day wetting, mainly due to bladder over-activity. Children, and adults, may experience frequency and sometimes urgency when excited or frightened. Rarely, urinary frequency can be an indicator of more serious emotional problems and stress.

History – must ask!

- *Is there nocturnal enuresis, and if so is it primary or secondary?* Enuresis is primary if bladder control has not yet been attained for a continuous period of 6 months, and secondary if a relapse has occurred after achieving primary continence.
- *Is the child ever dry?* Most day wetting is intermittent through the day, but if there is continuous dampness or leakage of urine, you must suspect an organic problem such as an ectopic ureter.
- *Is there daytime frequency, urgency or 'delaying manoeuvres' (Vincent's Curtsey)?* Such a triad suggests an overactive bladder, usually (but not always) found with nocturnal enuresis. The volume of the daytime wetting is usually small. The parents and teachers often mistakenly think that the child 'waits until the last minute' and is by implication lazy or too busy to stop what they are doing in order to go to the toilet on time. Explaining the phenomenon, not only to parents but to wider family, carers and teachers relieves the child of an undue burden. Day wetting without urgency makes an overactive bladder much less likely.
- *Are there other symptoms?* Acute onset dysuria, frequency and haematuria or a prior UTI suggest a UTI. 'Emptying' problems such as straining, weak or intermittent stream, a feeling of incomplete emptying, post-micturition dribble, infrequent voiding, and genital or lower urinary tract pain are specialist continence or urological issues. Suspect a neurogenic bladder if the child has coexisting bowel and/or gait difficulties.

Physical examination – must check!

Examine the genitalia, abdomen, anus and legs, and if possible observe the urinary stream (in girls it is easier to listen than observe).

- *The abdomen.* Bladder outlet obstruction will cause a distended bladder. This can be caused by abdominal masses, usually hard faeces. A neurogenic bladder will often be palpable and expressable (i.e. voiding can be induced by manual pressure).
- *The genitalia.* If the history suggests continuous wetting, inspect the vulval area for seepage of urine. In a boy, phimosis, hypospadias, and a dribbling, deviated or stuttering stream may all suggest partial obstruction to flow.

> ### Box 17.2 Expected bladder capacity (EBC) in children under 12 years:
>
> (Age in years + 1) x 30 mL/void.
> Repeated voided volumes under EBC suggest an overactive bladder

- *The back and legs.* Examine the back for a midline lipoma, hairy patch, or spinal deformity, and the legs for neurological signs which would suggest spina bifida occulta (see p. 452) causing neurogenic bladder.
- *The anus.* Abnormal perianal sensation and anal tone suggest a neurogenic bladder, and a pelvic mass obstructing the urinary outlet may be felt. It may be best to postpone this threatening examination until the child is more familiar with the examiner.

Laboratory and clinical investigations

The only baseline test required is urinalysis (including for glycosuria) and urine culture. If organic causes are suspected, urinary tract ultrasound, with pre- and post-voiding bladder volume is the first line of investigation. The normal residual volume is less than 15 mL.

The diagnosis of overactive bladder is suggested by a history of urgent voiding, frequency, and small volume wetting. Relative confirmation is obtained with a 48-hour diary of voided volumes, to verify that the child often voids amounts below the expected bladder capacity (see Box 17.2).

> ### 🔑 Key points: Wetting
>
> - Establish if the nocturnal enuresis is primary or secondary.
> - Check if there is a history of frequency, urgency or day wetting to suggest overactive bladder.
> - Ask about a parental history of bed wetting when they were children – nocturnal enuresis is usually familial.
> - Constipation can cause or aggravate the tendency to NE or day wetting.
> - Continuous leakage of urine indicates an anatomic cause
> - Features of a neurogenic bladder include a distended bladder, abnormal perianal sensation and anal tone, and abnormal neurological findings in the legs

Q Clues to the diagnosis of wetting

Condition	Type of incontinence	Other features
Urinary tract infection (UTI)	Secondary	Frequency, dysuria
Neurogenic bladder	Primary or secondary, depending on problem	Distended bladder, abnormal perianal sensation and anal tone, abnormal neurological findings in the legs, spinal deformity, lipoma or sacral hairy patch
Congenital anomalies	Primary (or secondary if triggered by UTI)	Continuous leakage of urine Distended bladder Urinary tract infection in the preschool years
Constipation	Secondary	Infrequent stools. Faecal mass palpable in abdomen and per rectum
Physiological	Primary or secondary	Family history of bed wetting
Psychogenic	Primary or secondary	Over emphasised. Stress such as sibling birth or starting school. Behavioural problems

Polyuria

Causes of frequent and excessive urination

Psychogenic (polydipsia)
Diabetes mellitus
Diabetes insipidus and tubular dysfunction
(Chronic renal failure)

Polyuria and frequency may be difficult to differentiate on clinical grounds, hence a 48-hour diary of voiding volumes compared to Expected Bladder Capacity (EBC) may be of use (see 'Laboratory and clinical investigations' above). Repeated voided volumes above EBC suggest polyuria.

The commonest cause of *polyuria* is polydipsia. Obviously, a child who drinks excessively will pass very large quantities of dilute urine. Usually the problem is simply one of habit, particularly in the toddler who is attached to a bottle.

Very rarely, polydipsia can be a sign of significant pathology. Children with diabetes mellitus commonly present with symptoms of acute polyuria, polydipsia, and weight loss and are usually diagnosed within a few weeks of the onset, often before diabetic acidosis has developed.

Diabetes insipidus is a rare condition in which there is an inability to concentrate urine. Rare tubular disorders of tubular concentration like Fanconi syndrome and renal tubular acidosis usually present in infancy, and may have other abnormalities associated with the disease. Polyuria also occurs in chronic renal failure, but is unlikely to be the presenting symptom.

History – must ask!

- *Pattern of urination.* You may be able to differentiate frequency and polyuria by taking a good history. In any child who has only recently attained bladder control, any condition causing polyuria or frequency is likely to cause enuresis. If symptoms are absent through the night, a psychogenic cause is more likely. UTIs may be associated with frequency and urgency as well as dysuria, abdominal pain and fever, although they may also be asymptomatic.
- *Thirst and pattern of drinking.* True polyuria with an organic cause will cause thirst, even at night, secondary to dehydration. Such children will often drink any fluid available to them. Conversely the child with habitual drinking will not usually wake at night to drink and is usually more selective in what they drink.
- *Behaviour.* Ask about behavioural and emotional issues.
- *Past medical history.* A history of poor growth and weight loss are significant in identifying the child with a chronic illness.

Physical examination – must check!

The physical examination rarely contributes to the diagnosis of urinary symptoms. Height and weight measurements are important if only to provide a baseline for the future. Any signs of dehydration and weight loss are clearly concerning. It is good practice to examine the abdomen for bladder distension, kidney size and abdominal masses. A thorough examination of the genitalia and perineum is cardinal.

Investigations

Bedside urinalysis – Glycosuria suggests diabetes mellitus or renal glycosuria. Urinary nitrites and/or white cells point to a UTI. Low specific gravity is seen in diabetes insipidus and psychogenic polydipsia.

Psychogenic polydipsia can usually be differentiated from diabetes insipidus by a trial of fluid restriction. In psychogenic polydipsia, fluid restriction usually decreases urine output with an increase in urine concentration (specific gravity). In long-standing cases, however, the kidneys may become 'washed out' and may take time to recover normal concentrating capacity. In diabetes insipidus a trial of fluid withdrawal will usually still result in dilute urine, which can rapidly cause severe dehydration, hence the trial must be carried out in hospital.

Haematuria

Online Interactive Q6

Causes of haematuria
Familial
Urinary tract infection
Trauma
Acute glomerulonephritis
Stones and hypercalciuria
Congenital anomalies
Tumour
Bleeding disorder
Exercise
Drugs

Macroscopic haematuria is gross and evident to the eye, and may be tea or cola coloured or bright red with clots. Microscopic haematuria is identified on dipstick or microscopy of the urinary sediment. It may occur as an isolated symptom or accompanied by signs of a systemic disorder. The commonest cause of asymptomatic microscopic haematuria (although it may also be macroscopic) is benign familial haematuria, now better referred to as Thin Basement Membrane Disease (TBMD). UTI is also frequently implicated. An important, but less common cause is acute glomerulonephritis, in which glomerular damage is inflicted by the formation of immune complexes (mostly IgG, complement or IgA). The most common aetiology of this is following a streptococcal infection. Gross or microscopic haematuria may also follow vigorous exercise. The source of bleeding is probably in the lower urinary tract. It resolves within 48 hours of cessation of exercise.

Blunt or penetrating injury to the abdomen may injure the kidney and cause haematuria, and if there is a urinary tract malformation, even minor trauma to the flank can result in bleeding. Renal stones are rarer and can result from chronic infection or excessive secretion of calcium and other metabolites or disorders of urine pH. The commonest renal tumour in childhood is Wilms tumour (Figure 17.1), which may present with haematuria, but more commonly presents with a loin mass.

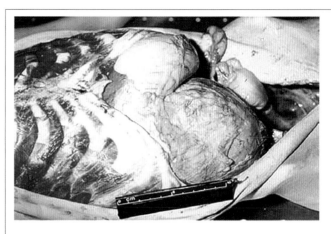

Figure 17.1 Post-mortem photograph of an infant with Wilms tumour.

History – must ask!

- *What colour is the urine?* The colour of the urine indicates the site of damage. Haematuria originating from the kidney is brown or cola-coloured, and that originating from the bladder or urethra has a red to pink colour and may contain clots. Renal haematuria tends to have a consistent colour throughout micturition, whereas bleeding from the lower tract may clear during micturition. Not all red urine is caused by blood – urine may turn red due to drugs (e.g. rifampicin) or on eating certain foods, notably beetroot and blackberries.
- *Are there other urinary symptoms?* Frequency, urgency, fever and dysuria suggest a UTI.
- *Is there pain?* Abdominal pain or renal colic suggest a clot, calculus, or obstructive malformation.
- *Was there a precipitating factor?* Trauma to the loin or abdomen can cause kidney damage. Upper respiratory tract or skin infections often precede acute glomerulonephritis. Intense exercise may precipitate haematuria.
- *Family history.* A family history of haematuria, a bleeding disorder, hypertension or kidney disease may be relevant.

Physical examination – must check!

- *Blood pressure.* It is mandatory to measure blood pressure in any child presenting with haematuria. Hypertension suggests renal disease.
- *Oedema.* Look for oedema periorbitally, at the ankles, scrotum, and sacrum, and search for ascites or pleural effusion. It can be a feature of glomerulonephritis or nephrosis.
- *Renal mass.* Palpate the abdomen carefully for tenderness, and for renal masses. If you find a mass, the most likely diagnoses are hydronephrosis, polycystic kidneys or tumour.

Investigations

See Table 17.1. A dipstick urine test is not precise. If haematuria is suspected or identified, urinalysis is required on the

Table 17.1 Investigations and their relevance in haematuria

Investigation	Relevance
Urinalysis	Red cell casts and proteinuria indicate a glomerular lesion. Pyuria and bacteriuria point to infection
Urine culture	Urinary tract infection
Full blood count	Anaemia
ASO titre and throat culture	Recent streptococcal infection often precedes acute glomerulonephritis
Serum creatinine, urea and electrolytes	Elevated creatinine and urea indicate impaired renal function
24-hour urine for creatinine, protein and calcium	Creatinine clearance quantifies the degree of renal impairment
Serum C3 and C4 level	Low C3 with normal C4 is specific for post-streptococcal glomerulonephritis
ANF/autoantibodies	Positive in systemic lupus erythematosus
Abdominal/pelvic ultrasound or MRI/CT	Structural abnormalities of the kidney
Renal biopsy	Required if haematuria is persistent with proteinuria, hypertension or impaired renal function

sediment of a centrifuged sample of urine. The presence of red cell casts and proteinuria indicate the glomeruli to be the source of the bleeding.

Urinalysis and culture are required in any child with haematuria, but beyond this step, further investigations are guided by clinical evaluation. If acute glomerulonephritis is suspected, confirmation of streptococcal infection is required by throat culture, antistreptolysin (ASO) titre and complement (C3, C4) levels, and serum creatinine concentration to assess renal function. Further investigations are only required in this condition if renal failure ensues or the course is atypical for post-streptococcal disease. Investigations of stones, tumours and malformations require imaging by MRI, CT or isotope scanning.

 Key points: Haematuria

- Identify the site of the urinary tract damage by the colour of the urine and microscopy of the sediment
- Measure blood pressure
- Palpate carefully for renal masses

Oedema

Generalised oedema in childhood is an uncommon problem. Acute oedema may result from a severe allergic reaction but when persistent it invariably results from hypoproteinaemia due to any cause especially nephrotic syndrome, or from some other form of renal disorder. It is important to remember that peripheral oedema is not a feature of congestive heart failure in childhood, which is manifested by respiratory distress and hepatomegaly rather than oedema.

Clues to the diagnosis of haematuria

Condition	Urine	Symptoms	Possible signs
Urinary tract infection	Bloody	Dysuria, frequency, urgency	
Glomerulonephritis	Smoky, tea/cola-coloured, granular, and red cell casts	Malaise, oliguria	Hypertension, oedema
Renal stone	Bloody	Renal colic	
Tumour	Bloody	Abdominal pain	Renal mass
Congenital anomalies	Bloody	Painless	Renal mass

Renal and urinary conditions

Urinary tract infection

Acute urinary tract infection is the commonest bacterial infection in childhood and occurs in 3% of girls and 1% of boys. *Escherichia coli* is the causative organism in 90% of cases. A clear diagnosis of UTI is important as it may be the first sign of a congenital anomaly of the urinary tract or vesicoureteric reflux (VUR) which, if untreated, may lead to renal scarring or failure.

Clinical features   Symptoms are often non-specific and include fever, irritability, vomiting and diarrhoea. In the neonate, prolonged jaundice, apnoea, weight loss and collapse may be the presenting signs. Older children are more likely to present with more specific symptoms including dysuria, frequency, bed-wetting and loin pain. Dysuria and frequency as isolated symptoms are very common and are often not caused by UTI, but this must always be excluded. Clinically, it may be impossible to differentiate between cystitis and pyelonephritis in young children as both may present with fever, although rigors and systemic symptoms are suggestive of pyelonephritis.

Diagnosis   UTI can only be reliably diagnosed by identifying a pure growth of bacteria in a urine specimen. Unfortunately, the collection of uncontaminated urine may be difficult. In older, cooperative, and continent children a mid-stream urine sample is the most reliable method. An alternative in younger children is a 'clean catch' specimen. Stimulation by tickling or gently pressing on the suprapubic region may encourage the passage of urine. Sterile urine collection pads placed in the nappy, or a bag specimen of urine is often taken in babies, but even with careful cleansing of the genital region, bacterial contamination often occurs. If there is a doubt as to whether organisms in the urine are the result of contamination, a catheter or suprapubic aspirate is necessary. The growth of >10^5 colony-forming units together with >50 white cell count in a fresh urine specimen indicates UTI. Any organisms present in a suprapubic specimen indicate UTI (see also p. 114).

Management   See Box 17.3. The principles of management can be summarized as antibiotics, copious fluid intake, and analgesia appropriate to the degree of pain. In all cases a urine sample should be obtained for culture prior to commencing antibiotics. Local microbiological guidelines should

---

Box 17.3 Managing the child with a urinary tract infection

- Always obtain a urine sample for culture before starting antibiotics
- Prescribe the appropriate antibiotic for the organism found on culture
- In an infant <3 months of age, or in older children with signs of systemic illness, give intravenous antibiotics
- Investigate children with atypical or recurrent UTIs
- Consider prophylactic antibiotics at low dose in children with recurrent UTIs
- Treat any constipation and give advice on hygiene, maintaining a good fluid intake and not delaying voiding

---

be followed to cover for regional bacterial resistance patterns. It is also important to note microbiological sensitivities for any recent infections that the child may have had. In an infant below 3 months of age, or an older child who is acutely ill (including when upper tract infection is suspected), intravenous antibiotics are necessary. Advice should be given to the parents to reduce the risk of further UTIs. If symptoms resolve, there is no need for a follow-up urine culture after completion of the course of antibiotics. Antibiotic prophylaxis is now only recommended following recurrent UTIs. Advice should be given to the parents to reduce the risk of further UTIs. This includes drinking adequate fluid volumes, avoiding constipation, discussing environmental difficulties in using the toilets (e.g. too scared to ask in school or bullying in toilets), and ensuring wiping front to back.

Investigations   See Table 17.2. Infants less than 6 months of age with a single confirmed UTI require an ultrasound of their urinary tract, even if they respond rapidly to antibiotics. Children with atypical or recurrent UTIs need further investigation. The first-line investigation is an ultrasound scan, which can identify renal tract anomalies such as megaureters and bladder abnormalities. DMSA radioisotope scans, performed 4–6 months after acute infection, are used to detect renal scarring. A micturating cystourethrogram (MCUG) (Figure 17.2) is indicated in infants less than 6 months of age, or older

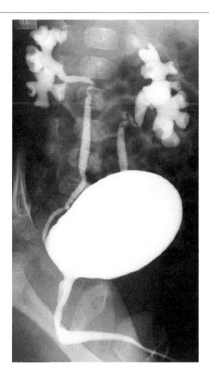

Figure 17.2 Micturating cystourethrogram (MCUG) in a child with recurrent urinary tract infection. Gross bilateral vesicoureteric reflux (VUR) is seen as the child micturates.

children when there are specific concerns, to look for bladder neck outflow and vesicoureteric reflux. MCUG is an unpleasant procedure as it requires catheterisation, and should be covered with a short course of oral antibiotics. It must not be performed immediately after a UTI as the acute infection can cause transient ureteric reflux.

Persistent proteinuria in the presence of sterile urine suggests renal compromise, possibly as the result of the UTI. If present, biochemical assessment of renal function (creatinine clearance) should be monitored.

Prognosis   Recurrence of UTI occurs in 50% of girls within 5 years. If it becomes a recurring problem, and vesicoureteric reflux has been excluded, long-term prophylactic antibiotics may be required. Permanent renal damage as a result of UTI is rare in children, but in infants, infection, particularly in the presence of vesicoureteric reflux, may cause permanent renal scarring with loss of function. Renal scarring is associated with hypertension in adult life and, rarely, chronic renal failure. Chronic pyelonephritis is usually a result of untreated reflux.

 Urinary tract infection at a glance

Epidemiology
3% of girls, 1% boys

Aetiology
Escherichia coli causative
organism in 90%

History
Non-specific symptoms in
infants
Fever*
Dysuria
Frequency
Enuresis
Abdominal/loin pain

Physical examination
Often normal

NB *Signs and symptoms are
variable

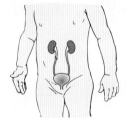

Confirmatory investigations
• Clean urine for culture (in babies
catheter or suprapubic aspirate
may be needed)

• >10^5 colony-forming units on
culture (any number if
suprapubic specimen)
and >50 white cell count
• Dipstick may show haematuria and proteinuria

Differential diagnosis
Any febrile illness in babies
Poor perineal hygiene in older
girls

Management
Rapid sterilization of urine with
antibiotics (IV in neonate or ill
child)
Encourage fluid intake
Investigation of renal structure
and vesicoureteric reflux (see
Table 17.2)

Prognosis/complications
10–20% develop hypertension if
scarring of the kidney occurs
Chronic renal failure very rare

Table 17.2 Investigations required according to urinary tract infection characteristics

UTI type	UTI in infant under 6 months	Atypical UTI	Recurrent UTI
Features	• Single confirmed UTI • Respond rapidly to treatment	• Seriously ill • Septicaemia • Poor urine flow • Abdominal or bladder mass • Raised serum creatinine • Failure to respond to antibiotics within 48 hours • Non *E. coli* organisms	• 3 or more episodes of cystitis/lower urinary tract infection • 2 or more episodes of urinary tract infection if any episode involved upper urinary tract
Investigations required	• Ultrasound urinary tract	• Ultrasound urinary tract during acute episode • DMSA scan 4–6 months later if age <3 years • MCUG if age <6 months	• Ultrasound urinary tract • DMSA scan 4–6 months later • MCUG if age <6 months

See NICE guideline: Urinary tract infections in under 16s: diagnosis and management
https://www.nice.org.uk/guidance/cg54

Vesicoureteric reflux

Vesicoureteric reflux (VUR) refers to reflux of urine from the bladder up the ureter on micturition. It can be found in children who present with atypical or recurrent UTI, and its importance lies in the risk of renal scarring (reflux nephropathy).

Clinical features and diagnosis   There are no specific clinical features of VUR. It is identified by investigation following atypical or recurrent UTI, or may be suspected in a fetus found to have dilated renal pelvices or scarring on antenatal ultrasound screening. It is diagnosed by a MCUG (Figure 17.2) and graded as shown in Figure 17.3.

Management   The majority of children with VUR tend to improve as they get older. Long-term prophylactic antibiotics are the recommended treatment, with careful surveillance for normal renal growth. Mild degrees of VUR tend to resolve, but children with grade 3 reflux require very close surveillance and may require surgical reimplantation of the ureter into the bladder, particularly if repeated UTI occurs on prophylactic treatment.

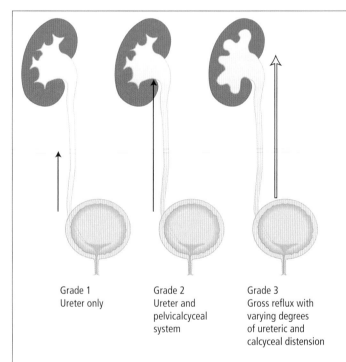

Grade 1
Ureter only

Grade 2
Ureter and pelvicalyceal system

Grade 3
Gross reflux with varying degrees of ureteric and calcyceal distension

Figure 17.3 Grading severity of VUR detected by MCUG. For clarity only one side is shown.

Prognosis   More than half of children with severe VUR have renal scars. Renal scarring carries a 10–20% risk of hypertension in adult life, and, less commonly, chronic renal failure.

Vesicoureteric reflux at a glance

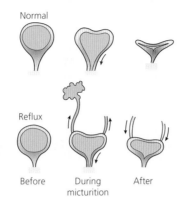

Epidemiology
30% children presenting with UTI

Aetiology
Incompetence of the valvular mechanism at the vesicoureteric junction, allowing reflux of infected urine to the kidneys

History
None

Physical examination
None

Normal

Reflux

Before   During micturition   After

Confirmatory investigations
Identified on micturating cystourethrogram following UTI

Management
Long-term antibiotic prophylaxis with surveillance of renal growth
Surgery may be needed for severe reflux

Prognosis/complications
>50% of children with VUR have renal scars
Renal scarring carries 10–20% risk of hypertension when adult

Nocturnal enuresis

Nocturnal enuresis (NE) or bedwetting can be defined as being a problem when it occurs more than one night a month, arguably, after age 5 years. NE may be primary (dryness not achieved continuously for at least 6 months) or secondary (a relapse after achieving primary bladder control for 6 months). It is very common, occurring in 15% of children at 4–5 years old, 7% at 7 years old, 2% at 12 years old and 1% at 18 years old.

The underpinning cause is usually familial. If one parent remembers wetting the bed after age 5, each of their children has about a 40% of also wetting. If both parents remember, then the incidence increases to about 75% for each child. Gene linkage analysis of large families has implicated several genetic loci in causing NE.

The pathophysiology is a combination of:
1. Nocturnal polyuria – often due to a relative deficiency of nocturnal ADH release
2. Heavy sleep – poor arousal to the stimulus of a full bladder
3. Poor bladder filling (overactive bladder) – see above

Secondary NE is occasionally associated with organic or psychological causes such as urine infection, sexual abuse, diabetes mellitus/insipidus, obstructive sleep hypoventilation, neurogenic bladder, or externalizing disorders such as attention-deficit/hyperactivity disorder (ADHD) or conduct disorder. Large family studies, however, have shown that secondary NE is usually no different aetiologically from primary, with undue emphasis on the difference being unwarranted.

Nocturnal enuresis persisting into adolescence is more commonly seen in those with past or present overactive bladder or those with secondary enuresis.

Clinical features   Boys are affected more than girls (3:2). Parents who were affected as children may sometimes conceal this information from their children and even blame the child needlessly as they themselves were blamed. This denies the child sympathy, and obscures a simple explanation for an otherwise enigmatic problem. There are no signs on physical examination. Children who also have symptoms of overactive bladder by day are often mistakenly thought to be lazy, unfocused, or defiant.

Investigations   Urinalysis and culture are negative.

Management   Treatment of the child with nocturnal enuresis alone, differs from that who also has daytime wetting, urgency or frequency. Those with daytime symptoms usually have an overactive bladder (see 'wetting' above).

For NE alone, intervention is usually delayed until a child approaches age 7 years. Prior to that, the emphasis should be on demystifying the problem, removing all blame from the child, and defusing tension within the family and embarrassment for the child. Parental exasperation usually evaporates with an explanation of the inherited and physiological nature of NE and that it is not within the child's voluntary control. An age-appropriate explanation to the child of the problem and its prevalence will ease a heavy daily burden that they may carry.

Preliminary tactics   Prior to consulting doctors, parents have usually tried tactics such as fluid restriction in the evening and lifting a child from bed to urinate at night. These manoeuvres may decrease the number of wash loads per week, but there is evidence that they do not alter the underlying tendency to wetting.

Behavioural management   *Star charts* (see p. 384) and rewards for dry nights, have traditionally been used to motivate children to dryness but the results of large studies into their effectiveness have mostly been disappointing. Rewards risk reinforcing the incorrect message that the child has voluntary control, subject to the right motivation.

Figure 17.4 An enuresis alarm.

An *enuresis alarm* is the most effective treatment for children with NE alone (with no daytime symptoms of urgency, or wetting). A sensor is placed in the child's undergarments (the personal alarm) or under the bedsheet (the pad and bell alarm). Urine triggers the sensor and a loud alarm rings next to the bed, hopefully waking the child. (Figure 17.4). Parents must initially help the child wake. The child completes voiding in the toilet (even if the bladder is empty) after which bedding is changed and the alarm reapplied. The alarm is usually used for a period of 8–12 weeks. For children with NE alone, success rates are of the order of 80% and relapse rates are below 20%. The mode of action is unclear. The alarm was once thought to work by classical conditioning – if so, the child should attain dryness by waking at night prior to wetting. However, in practice most children become dry by sleeping through the night and waking dry the next morning.

Medication

Nocturnal enuresis with no day symptoms of overactive bladder

Vasopressin: Available as an oral tablet or a sublingual 'melt' (absorbed by sublingual blood vessels). It is most likely to succeed in those with NE alone. In this group remission rate is about 80% but the relapse rate is very high – hence it is mostly considered palliative rather than curative. It can also be used as a short-term stopgap for occasions, such as at cub camp or staying with a friend.

Tricyclics: Tricyclics are no longer used outside of specialist clinics because of low remission rate, high relapse rate and the potential for fatal cardiotoxicity in accidental overdose.

Nocturnal enuresis with daytime symptoms of overactive bladder

Anticholinergics: Oxybutynin is an anti-muscarinic agent useful in children with NE and daytime urgency and frequency +/- wetting. It is used for about 6 months, usually resulting in improvement of day symptoms and sometimes the NE as well. Should the NE persist after treatment, an alarm or vasopressin may be added.

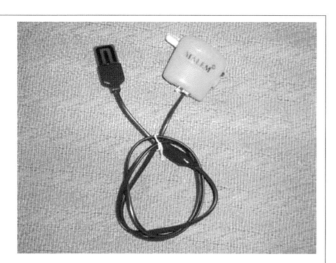

Nocturnal enuresis at a glance

Epidemiology
7% at 7 years old decreasing to 2% at 12 years old
More common in boys

Aetiology
Various physiological mechanisms suggested
Genetic factors prominent

History
May be primary or secondary enuresis
Enuresis more often cause of stress than caused by stress
Family history of enuresis*

Physical examination
Normal

NB *Signs and symptoms are variable

Confirmatory investigations
Rule out UTI

Differential diagnosis
Rarely can be UTI

Management
Intervention usually only indicated for children aged 7 + years
Behavioural incentives
Enuresis alarm
Vasopressin

Complications
Good with appropriate management, although 1% still enuretic at 18 years

 See NICE guideline: Bedwetting in under 19s
https://www.nice.org.uk/guidance/cg111

Acute glomerulonephritis

Acute glomerulonephritis results from immunological damage to the glomerulus. The commonest form in childhood occurs as a result of the formation of immune complexes following infection by a nephritogenic form of group A *Streptococcus*. Haematuria characteristically occurs 1–2 weeks after a throat or skin infection. Other forms of glomerulonephritis are much rarer and need only be considered if the course of the illness is atypical.

Clinical features   The presenting complaint is the appearance of smoky or cola-coloured urine. The child may otherwise be asymptomatic, although malaise, headache, and vague loin discomfort may occur. Oedema may be seen around the eyes, and the backs of the hands and feet. Urine microscopy shows gross haematuria with granular and red cell casts. Proteinuria is also evident. In most children mild oliguria only occurs, but the course may be complicated by renal failure, hypertension, seizures and heart failure.

Management   Evidence that the condition is the post-streptococcal form is sought by taking a throat swab and ASO titre. Low complement (C3) levels in the presence of normal C4 is pathognomonic. There is no specific therapy for glomerulonephritis, and the management is similar to that of acute renal failure. Creatinine clearance and fluid balance need to be monitored, and if oliguria develops, salt and water restriction is imposed. Diuretics and hypotensive drugs are needed if there is hypertension, and rarely peritoneal dialysis is required.

Eradication of streptococcal infection with penicillin is recommended to limit the spread of nephritogenic organisms, but there is no evidence that it affects the course of the disease. Members of the family may also be cultured and, if necessary, treated with penicillin.

Prognosis   The long-term prognosis for post-streptococcal glomerulonephritis is excellent. IgA nephropathy may cause prolonged microscopic haematuria and occasionally renal failure. Other forms have a poorer prognosis. The illness usually resolves in 10–14 days, but if renal impairment persists, a renal biopsy is justified to define the nature of the glomerular pathology.

 Acute glomerulonephritis at a glance

Prevalence
Age 3+ years

Aetiology
Immunological damage to the glomerulus, usually caused by immune complexes resulting from streptococcal infection

History
Smoky/cola-coloured urine (**a**)
Malaise/headache* (**b**)
Loin discomfort * (**c**)
Throat or skin infection 1 –2 weeks previously * (**d**)

Physical examination
Oedema* : periorbital and backs of hands/feet (**1**)
Hypertension* (**2**)

Confirmatory investigations
Gross haematuria
Urinalysis: haematuria, proteinuria
Urine microscopy: granular and red cell casts
Throat swab/ASO titre for streptococcal infection
Low C3 (as opposed to normal in nephrotic syndrome)

NB * Signs and symptoms are variable

Differential diagnosis
UTI
Other causes of haematuria (see Causes box, p. 324)

Management
Monitor fluid balance and creatinine clearance

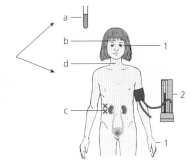

Salt and water restriction if oliguric
Diuretics and hypotensive agents for hypertension
Rarely dialysis
Penicillin to eradicate Streptococcus in child and family
Renal biopsy if course is atypical

Prognosis/complications
Good prognosis for post-streptococcal glomerulonephritis
Usually resolved by 10 –14 days
Complications include:
• renal failure
• hypertension
• seizures
• heart failure

Pathophysiology

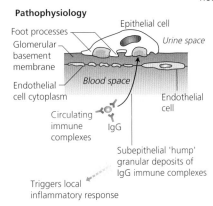

Nephrotic syndrome

The nephrotic syndrome is characterised by proteinuria, hypoproteinaemia, oedema and hyperlipidaemia. The underlying pathology is an increase in glomerular capillary wall permeability, which leads to urinary protein loss, and as a result of hypoalbuminaemia oedema develops. Three histological patterns are seen in nephrotic syndrome, the commonest being 'minimal change', which is seen in 85% of cases.

Clinical features   Figure 17.5. Nephrotic episodes may follow a viral URTI. Periorbital or pitting oedema of the legs is usually noticed first. With time it becomes more generalised and is associated with weight gain, ascites, pleural effusion and declining urinary output. Symptoms of anorexia, abdominal pain and diarrhoea are common, but hypertension is rare. An increased susceptibility to infection occurs.

Investigations   Typical results of investigations are shown in Table 17.3. Renal biopsy is only necessary if the clinical picture does not appear to be typical of minimal change nephrotic syndrome, or if the child does not respond to steroids within a month.

Management   It is usual to hospitalize the child for diagnostic, therapeutic and educational purposes. Excessive fluid intake is discouraged, and sodium intake is limited to 'no added salt'. Steroid treatment (prednisolone) is given to induce remission, which may take 2 weeks to occur. Recovery is monitored by daily weights and proteinuria. Low-dose steroids are continued for 4–6 weeks. During steroid treatment children are at risk if exposed to chicken pox or live vaccines. Prophylactic penicillin is given because of the risk of infection when hypoproteinaemic (antibodies are lost in the urine).

Approximately 75% of children who initially respond to steroids experience a subsequent relapse with proteinuria. Children who frequently relapse or who show signs of steroid toxicity should be treated with cyclophosphamide. A renal biopsy is not necessary unless the child is resistant to steroid treatment.

Prognosis   Most children experience relapses over the subsequent 10 years or so, which must be treated in the same way as the initial episode. The long-term prognosis for minimal change nephrotic syndrome is good and residual renal impairment is rare. The prognosis for other forms of nephrotic syndrome is more guarded.

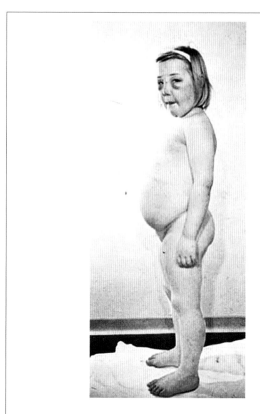

Figure 17.5 A girl with severe nephrotic syndrome.

Table 17.3 Typical investigations in nephrotic syndrome	
Urinalysis	3+ or 4+ or protein/ microscopic haematuria
Serum albumin	Low
Serum cholesterol and triglycerides	High
C3 levels	Normal

Nephrotic syndrome at a glance

Epidemiology
'Minimal change' form most
common

Aetiology
Idiopathic
Increase in glomerular
permeability leads to
proteinuria,
hypoalbuminaemia and
oedema

History
Puffiness (**a**)
Anorexia (**b**)
Abdominal pain* (**c**)
Diarrhoea* (**d**)
Preceding URTI*

Physical examination
Pitting oedema of the legs (**e**)
Periorbital oedema (**f**)
Weight gain
Ascites and pleural effusion*
Reduced urine output

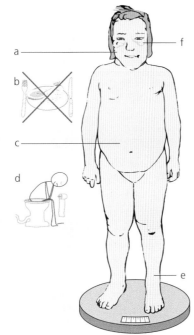

NB *Signs and symptoms are variable.

Confirmatory investigations
Proteinuria +/− haematuria
Low serum albumin
High cholesterol
High triglycerides
Normal C3
Renal biopsy if presentation
atypical or poor response to
steroids

Differential diagnosis
Other causes of oedema are
extremely rare

Management
Hospitalize, monitor weight and
urinary protein loss
Moderate fluid and salt intake
Steroids to induce remission
Low-dose steroids for 3–6
months (NB child at risk for
severe chicken pox)
Prophylactic penicillin
Cyclophosphamide if steroids
ineffective

Prognosis/complications
Relapses are common
Long-term prognosis good for
minimal change
Other forms can lead to renal
impairment

Haemolytic uraemic syndrome (HUS)

HUS is the most frequent cause of acute kidney injury (AKI) in children. It is a rare disorder almost exclusively encountered in young children, characterised by microangiopathic haemolytic anaemia, nephropathy and thrombocytopenia. It is usually associated with infectious diarrhoea from a shiga toxin producing strain of bacteria, classically *E. coli* 0157:H7 (Shiga-Toxin *E. coli* 'STEC-HUS'). Atypical HUS occurs in the absence of STEC, associated with congenital abnormalities of the complement cascade. HUS can also occasionally occur as a rare complication of a pneumococcal infection.

The pathophysiology of the syndrome is triggered by endothelial damage, which leads to microvascular thrombosis, especially in the glomeruli, and hence a reduction in remaining circulating platelets (similar to that in disseminated intravascular coagulation, DIC). These intraluminal clots also physically damage the red blood cells, which leads to anaemia (as the red cell numbers diminish), jaundice and uraemia due to the byproducts of haemolysis.

Clinical features   Children usually present with abdominal pain and diarrhoea (frequently bloody). This then progresses over around 4–7 days to pallor, jaundice, anuria and oedema as the kidney injury becomes apparent. There may be local outbreaks of STEC-HUS, often associated with petting zoos, farms or food establishments. Microthrombi can also occur in the brain, causing neurological symptoms and complications, such as encephalopathy or coma; in the pancreas, causing an increased risk of pancreatitis and diabetes mellitus; or in the heart, causing cardiac ischaemia.

Investigations   Any child presenting with bloody diarrhoea should have full blood count, clotting and renal function tests performed. Stool should also be sent urgently for culture and toxin assessment, and public health departments should be notified as contact tracing may be required.

In confirmed HUS careful renal function monitoring is crucial, including electrolyte and renal function tests; blood pressure monitoring; fluid balance and daily weights. It is important to assess accurate body surface area through height measurements.

Management At least half of all affected children will require renal replacement therapy (e.g. haemo- or peritoneal dialysis); however, treatment for STEC-HUS is supportive. The acute kidney injury usually takes around 1–3 weeks to improve and extremely tight fluid balance is required to reduce the risk of secondary complications. Red cell transfusions and antihypertensives are often required, and dietetic input is needed in order to avoid starvation states. Antidiarrhoeal medications and antibiotics should be avoided. Monoclonal antibody therapy is occasionally used for atypical HUS.

Prognosis STEC-HUS has a mortality rate of around 5% acutely, and around a quarter of all children affected will have a long-term complication. This is usually renal, such as persistent proteinuria or hypertension, although diabetes mellitus and neurological complications can occur. Some children have intestinal complications, such as intussusception, as a result of the initial colitis phase. The prognosis in atypical HUS is worse, with acute mortality rates at 25% and with half of the children requiring long-term renal replacement therapy. Care must be taken to avoid ongoing transmission as STEC can be shed in the faeces for up to a month after acute infection.

Congenital anomalies of the kidney and urinary tract (CAKUT)

Congenital renal anomalies occur in around 1 in 500 infants. There is a wide spectrum, with the more severe abnormalities often being detected on antenatal scans. Common anomalies include a horse-shoe kidney, where the two kidneys are fused at the lower pole across the midline; renal agenesis; or renal hypoplasia. CAKUT is more common if a first-degree relative is affected.

Clinical features Many anomalies are discovered during assessment for recurrent urinary tract infections; however, they may be asymptomatic and discovered only when hypertension develops.

The commonest congenital urinary tract anomalies causing urinary incontinence are ectopic ureters in girls and posterior urethral valves in boys. The ectopic ureter commonly ends in the vagina, causing continuous dampness and dribbling without urgency of micturition. Posterior urethral valves cause lower urinary tract obstruction and bladder distension with overflow incontinence without urgency. Both conditions are treated surgically.

Some infants, however, are severely affected and may present in utero with oligohydramnios, because the amniotic fluid is primarily produced from fetal 'urine'. The lack of amniotic fluid, which the fetus 'breathes' in utero, causes pulmonary hypoplasia which is usually fatal shortly after birth. The sequence of bilateral renal agenesis leading to pulmonary hypoplasia is known as 'Potter syndrome/sequence'.

Investigations Investigations to detect, or exclude, congenital renal and ureteric abnormalities include ultrasound scan, micturating cytourethrogram (MCUG) and DMSA scans.

The ultrasound can detect echogenic kidneys, suggesting inflammation, congenital anomalies, and will occasionally detect signs of vesicoureteric reflux (VUR). The MCUG needs to be carried out with antibiotic cover as it involves inserting a urinary catheter and injecting a radio-opaque dye into the bladder. This test will indicate VUR, and in a boy it can be used to assess for urethral strictures, when the catheter is removed and the child micturates. The DMSA scan requires an IV cannula into which a radiolabeled isotope is injected. The kidneys then filter this out and the resultant image will show any areas of the kidney which are scarred and therefore not functioning. As the evolution of scars takes some time it should not be checked until at least 4–6 weeks after the latest urinary tract infection. DMSA scans are read from behind (e.g. image on the left is the left kidney), in contrast to X-ray images.

Management Many renal anomalies may not require any further management; however, some will require surgical correction or lifestyle advice to protect the kidneys. Hypoplastic, poorly functioning kidneys may be surgical removed, as they can lead to hypertension.

Prognosis Given that there is a spectrum of abnormalities the spectrum varies depending on the severity of the anomaly.

Acute kidney impairment (AKI) and chronic kidney disease (CKD)

Acute kidney injury (AKI) can be caused by pre-renal causes (hypotension causing reduced renal blood flow, e.g. from severe gastroenteritis, sepsis or blood loss); intrinsic renal causes (such as nephrotoxic drugs, glomerulonephritis or scarring) or post-renal causes (where urinary backflow pressure damages the kidneys, e.g. posterior urethral valves or urethral damage). It is common in children who require intensive care, with up to 30% of all PICU admissions having some degree of AKI. AKI is defined as the acute impairment of renal function with reduced glomerular filtration rate (GFR), and hence impaired electrolyte, acid-base and fluid balance control.

CKD has five stages, with a glomerular filtration rate of less than 15 mL/min/1.73m^2 as grade 5. A renal function of GFR less than 60 mL/min/1.73m^2 (stage 3) for 3 months or more is classified as CKD. Around half of all CKD in children is caused by CAKUT, especially in younger children. In teenagers, chronic glomerulonephritis is a more common cause.

Clinical features Symptoms of AKI include reduced urine output (less than 0.5mL/kg/hr in an older child or less than 1mL/kg/hr in a neonate); however, all too often AKI is under-recognised. Further tests often reveal raised creatinine and urea, metabolic acidosis, proteinuria and hypertension, although this depends on the cause.

It is important to consider the risk factors for AKI and then to be vigilant for its development. In the neonatal unit this includes hypoxic ischaemic encephalopathy (HIE), renal artery/vein thrombosis (often as a result of umbilical lines), and nephrotoxic drugs (e.g. gentamicin). In the older child, AKI may result from NSAID use associated with dehydration/hypovolaemia, HUS, acute glomerulonephritis or acute tubular necrosis.

CKD can be difficult to detect in children unless considered, with the insidious symptoms such as failure to thrive, vomiting or polyuria. It may present with hypertension, often when blood pressure is checked incidentally, or following hypertensive symptoms such as seizure or headache.

Investigations   Investigations for AKI and CKD will initially need to establish the cause of the deficit, and then to ensure that the remaining functions of the kidneys are optimized.

Tests to help elucidate the cause of AKI include urine dip/microscopy, blood film, stool samples (if diarrhoea), complement levels, ANCA, ANA, anti-glomerular basement membrane titres, creatinine kinase, and occasionally renal biopsies. AKI monitoring and management involves daily weights, blood pressure monitoring, strict fluid balance (catheterisation or weighing nappies), urine dipstick testing, urea, electrolytes and creatinine (often several times a day in the acute phase), calcium, phosphate, bicarbonate, pH, chloride, albumin, glucose and full blood count.

Children with CKD require frequent assessment of blood pressure, full blood count, vitamin D and bone profile, height, and renal function as above in order to optimize management.

Management   Many children with AKI will recover through careful fluid balance and management of electrolytes and blood pressure.

Children with CKD require dietetic advice to ensure that their diet is low in salt, and has an adequate balance of energy from fats, carbohydrates and protein. Excessive protein will lead to an increase in urea, which can be harmful. Vitamins, specifically Vitamin D, need to be supplemented and medications used to control calcium, phosphate and PTH levels. As the kidney also produces erythropoietin (EPO) to stimulate red cell development, children with CKD may also need iron or EPO supplementation to prevent anaemia. Short stature can also be a complication of CKD and nutritional management +/- growth hormone may be required. Hypertension is common and frequently requires the use of antihypertensives.

Children who would be suitable to have a renal transplant may be offered renal replacement therapy once the kidneys are unable to maintain homeostasis. Renal replacement therapy (RRT) is either in the form of peritoneal dialysis or haemodialysis. In peritoneal dialysis, a tube is surgically inserted into the peritoneal cavity and specific sterile fluid is flushed into the peritoneum which then allows diffusion of waste products from the blood into the fluid, which is then removed. The fluid may be circulated by a pump cycle, usually at home. Haemodialysis involves central line insertion in younger children or the joining of two blood vessels in the forearm to make a fistula. Blood is then pumped through the haemodialysis machine which functions as an artificial kidney. Haemodialysis requires attendance at hospital several times a week for several hours at a time. Renal transplant is required once the kidneys fail to function and this may be from a friend or relative (living donor) or from a deceased donor. After transplantation anti-rejection drugs are required for life.

Prognosis   Many children with AKI will recover; however, if they have had a significant renal insult, they will need lifelong monitoring to assess for signs of hypertension and proteinuria, and should have periodic renal function tests to ensure that scarring has not developed.

To test your knowledge on this part of the book, please see Chapter 26

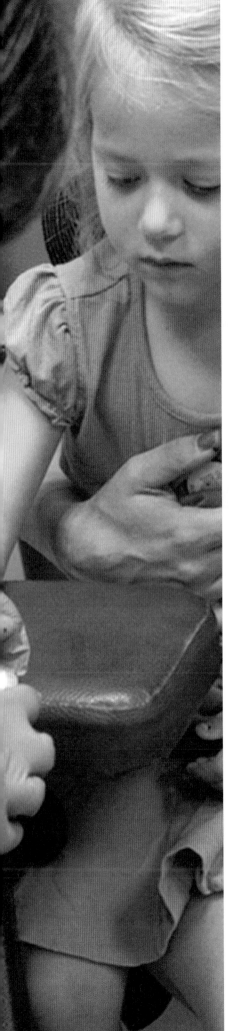

CHAPTER 18
Genitalia

There was a young infant named Paul
Who seemed to have only one ball
But kind doctor Hynd
Was able to find
That there really were two after all.

Anon.

KEY COMPETENCES
YOU MUST...

Know and understand

- The differential diagnosis of children presenting with ambiguous genitalia, testicular pain, scrotal swellings, swellings in the groin and impalpable testes
- How to diagnose and manage important and common disorders affecting the genitalia

Be able to

- Competently examine for retractile or undescended testes
- Distinguish a hydrocoele from an inguinal hernia

Appreciate that

- Sensitivity is required when examining the genitalia beyond infancy
- Testicular torsion is a medical emergency
- Ambiguous genitalia may be a medical emergency, can cause significant confusion and distress in families, and require multi-professional teams for successful management

Essential Paediatrics and Child Health, Fourth Edition. Mary Rudolf, Anthony Luder and Kerry Jeavons.
© 2020 John Wiley & Sons Ltd. Published 2020 by John Wiley & Sons Ltd.
Companion website: www.wiley.com/go/rudolf/paediatrics

Symptoms and signs relating to the genitalia

Finding your way around …

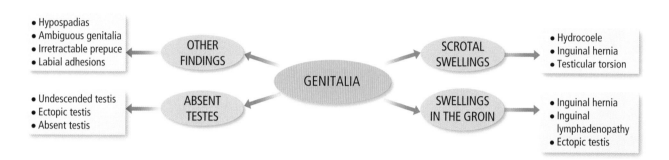

Scrotal swellings

Causes of scrotal swellings
Hydrocoele
Inguinal hernia
Testicular torsion
Epididymo-orchitis
Scrotal oedema and cellulitis
Testicular tumour

A swelling in the scrotum may present for attention because of parental concern, or may be an incidental finding identified during child health surveillance.

History – must ask!

- *Characteristics.* An inguinal hernia characteristically causes intermittent swelling, particularly when intra-abdominal pressure is increased, as in crying or straining. Hernias (unless incarcerated) and hydrocoeles are painless, although parents may think a hernial swelling is painful as it tends to occur when the baby cries. Testicular torsion, in contrast, is acutely painful. Hydrocoeles are often present at birth, tend to shrink but may show little variation in size over time. Epididymo-orchitis and cellulitis cause painful, hot swellings often with overlying oedema and erythema.

Physical examination – must check!

- *Observation.* The boy with testicular torsion and epididymo-orchitis or cellulitis is obviously in acute pain. The swelling caused by an inguinal hernia extends up into the groin, whereas the hydrocoele usually does not.
- *Palpation.* On palpation the inguinal hernia can be felt to reach up to the inguinal region, and reduction of an inguinal or inguinoscrotal mass, whether spontaneously or by manipulation, is diagnostic of a hernia. The testis is palpable separate from the hernial swelling. A hydrocoele, in contrast, does not usually extend up into the groin and the testis cannot be palpated through the fluid. Neither is usually tender, although the hernia becomes so if incarcerated. An inflamed testis or scrotum is tender, warm and red. A testicular torsion is so tender that palpation is not possible. The cremasteric reflex is absent and the testis rides 'high' and horizontal in the scrotum. Testicular torsion **is an emergency** since the testis may infarct in a matter of hours unless surgically resolved.
- *Transillumination.* When a torch is held to the scrotum, a hydrocoele transilluminates, whereas a hernia does not.

Investigations

The differentiation between these conditions is clinical. No investigations are indicated, although occasionally ultrasound is used if there is diagnostic uncertainty.

Clues to diagnosing scrotal swellings

	Hernia	Hydrocoele	Torsion	Epididymo-orchitis/cellulitis	Testicular tumour
Usual age	Infants, particularly premature	Babies	Any age, commonest 14–16 years	Adolescence	Rare; Adolescence
Pain	No (unless incarcerated)	No	Intense	Yes	No
Extends to groin	Yes	Usually not	No	No	No
Transilluminates	No	Yes	No	No	No

Swellings in the groin

Causes of swelling in the groin

Inguinal hernia
Inguinal lymphadenopathy
Ectopic testis
Bleeding or aneurysm

Like scrotal swellings, lumps in the groin are distinguishable clinically. The features of *inguinal hernias* are described in the previous section. In contrast, the *inguinal lymph node* has a firm consistency with clear borders. It may be tender, and a responsible infected lesion may be found on the legs, or buttocks or anus. If an enlarged lymph gland is found, the child must be fully examined for more generalised lymphadenopathy and hepatosplenomegaly, which if found may be suggestive of a serious cause such as lymphoma.

Rarely, the lump may be an *ectopic testis*, and the scrotum should be examined for the presence of both testes. Small 'shotty' inguinal nodes are very common in young children, and are related to the degree of minor trauma that the legs incur at this age. They are of no significance. Trauma can cause an inguinal haematoma, which may grow to a surprising size, is tender and blue. Aneurysms are rare and pulsatile.

Impalpable testes

Causes of impalpable testes

Undescended or ectopic testes
Retractile testes
True testicular absence

The commonest reason for a testis or testes to be impalpable is an exaggerated cremasteric reflex which retracts the testes high into the scrotum. Retractile testes can be brought down by careful palpation when the child is relaxed in a warm room, and scrotal examination is made easier if the child is in a squatting or cross-legged position. Often more than one examination is required to establish whether the testis is truly absent from the scrotum. A poorly developed hemi-scrotum suggests that the testis is undescended and not retracted.

Cryptorchidism (undescended testes) is an important condition to identify in babies and is screened for during child health surveillance, as there is a risk of infertility and malignancy if it is left uncorrected. Undescended testes may descend into the scrotum spontaneously before the age of 1 year. Beyond that age, if the testes cannot be palpated and brought down into the scrotum, orchidopexy is required. Surgery should be carried out before the age of 1 year to minimize the risk of complications.

Approximately 20% of non-palpable testes are absent. In most cases this is presumed to be a result of a vascular accident. If absent bilaterally, Disorders of Sex Development (DSD) must be considered and the chromosomal sex confirmed.

 Key points: Impalpable testes

- Examine the child in a warm room with warm hands
- Scrotal examination is facilitated if the child is in a squatting or cross-legged position

👁 Cryptorchidism (undescended/ectopic testes) at a glance

Epidemiology
1–2% boys

Aetiology
Incomplete or maldescent
of the testis during
gestation
Hypopituitarism may cause
bilateral cryptorchidism

History
Asymptomatic

Physical examination
Examine with child relaxed
in a warm room
Testis impalpable, or high in
inguinal region or scrotum
Inguinal hernia*

NB *Signs and symptoms
are variable.

Embryology of testicular descent

(a) **In utero**

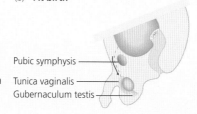

Testis (under peritoneum)
Gubernaculum testis
Pubic symphysis
Processus vaginalis
Scrotal swelling
Rectum

(b) **At birth**

Pubic symphysis
Tunica vaginalis
Gubernaculum testis

Confirmatory investigations
Usually a clinical diagnosis
Ultrasound may help in locating
the testis
Hormonal testing if testes
impalpable bilaterally

Differential diagnosis
Retractile testes

Management
Orchidopexy before 2 years old

Prognosis/complications
There is a risk of malignancy in
the undescended testis, and
infertility in adulthood if left
uncorrected

Conditions affecting the genitalia

Hydrocoele

A hydrocoele is an accumulation of fluid in the tunica vaginalis. Hydrocoeles do not fluctuate in size, unless they communicate with the peritoneal cavity. Most hydrocoeles resolve by the age of 1 year, but occasionally large ones persist and require surgical treatment. Rarely, the development of a hydrocoele in an older boy is indicative of malignancy.

Inguinal hernia

Inguinal hernias in childhood are indirect. They are far more common in boys and result from persistent patency of the processus vaginalis, which normally closes at birth (Figure 18.1). They are particularly common in premature infants.

Clinical features   A swelling is evident in the groin which may extend down into the scrotum (Figure 18.2).

It tends to be most obvious when intra-abdominal pressure is raised as a result of crying, straining or coughing, and often disappears when the baby or child is relaxed and lying down. A hernia is usually not painful unless incarcerated, in which case signs of intestinal obstruction may occur. The observation of an inguinal or inguinoscrotal mass that reduces spontaneously or on manipulation is diagnostic of a hernia. Bilateral inguinal hernias in a phenotypic female should raise the possibility of a DSD (androgen insensitivity).

Management   Management of a hernia is surgical. Rarely, if a hernia is incarcerated and irreducible, this must be carried out as an emergency. More commonly the hernia can be gently reduced by the doctor or parent (relaxing the child in a warm bath or with a drink can help). Surgery can then be carried out as an elective procedure.

 Inguinal hernia at a glance

Epidemiology
Boys more than girls,
   particularly premature infants

Aetiology
Herniation of bowel through a
   defect caused by a
   persistently patent processus
   vaginalis

History
Swelling in groin particularly
   prominent on crying/straining
Painful only if incarcerated

Physical examination
Swelling in groin extending to
   scrotum
No transillumination
Reducible by manipulation
   unless incarcerated

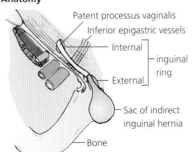

Anatomy

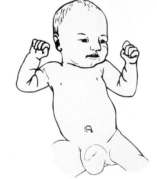

Patent processus vaginalis
Inferior epigastric vessels
Internal ⎤
   ⎥ inguinal
   ⎥ ring
External ⎦
Sac of indirect
   inguinal hernia
Bone

Confirmatory investigations
The diagnosis is clinical

Differential diagnosis
Hydrocoele

Management
Reduce by manipulation, and
   plan elective surgery
Instruct parents about signs of
   incarceration
Urgent surgery if hernia
   becomes strangulated

Prognosis/complications
Risk of strangulation of bowel
   and testis is low
Excellent prognosis following
   surgery

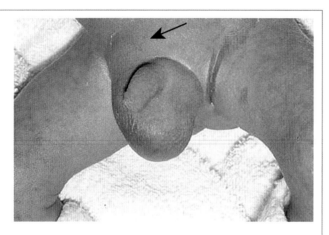

Figure 18.1 Anatomical development of an inguinal hernia and hydrocoele.

Normal:
processus vaginalis
closed

Hydrocoele:
processus vaginalis
closed. Collection of
fluid in the tunica
vaginalis

Hernia:
processus vaginalis
open, allowing bowel
to pass through into
the scrotum

Figure 18.2 Right inguinal hernia.

Undescended and ectopic testes

Undescended and ectopic testes can only be differentiated from each other at operation, and both conditions are referred to as cryptorchidism. Testes usually descend from their fetal intra-abdominal position through the processus vaginalis and into the scrotum during the seventh month of gestation (see Figure 18.1). The undescended testicle is found along the normal path of descent and the processus vaginalis is usually patent. If bilateral, the diagnosis of hypopituitarism should be considered. The ectopic testis is one that has completed its descent through the inguinal canal, but lands up at the wrong destination, usually in the groin.

Clinical features.   The distinction between retractile testes and cryptorchidism is discussed above. One or both testes may be affected. Undescended testes are more common in premature babies than in term babies, and are often accompanied by an inguinal hernia.

Management and prognosis.   Surgery should be performed before the age of 1 year, as by this age the number of germ cells in undescended testes is already reduced and the risk of infertility is increased whether the cryptorchidism is unilateral or bilateral. There is also an increased risk of testicular tumour occurring in the third and fourth decade if surgery is delayed.

Testicular torsion

Testicular torsion occurs at any age, but with a peak in early adolescence. The testes are unusually mobile and torsion results when the testis rotates on the spermatic cord. Prompt diagnosis and treatment is required for the testis to survive.

Clinical features.   The boy presents with acute pain and swelling of the scrotum. On examination the scrotum looks tender and swollen, the testis is cold but rides high and horizontal in the scrotum, and the cremasteric reflex is absent. Examination may be resisted.

Management and prognosis.   Testicular torsion is an emergency. Prompt surgical exploration is required to untwist and fix the testis to the scrotum. If this takes place within 6 hours, the majority of gonads survive. The contralateral testis must also be fixed as it is also prone to torsion.

Hypospadias

Hypospadias is a condition in which the urethra is abnormally sited. See Figures 18.3 and 18.4. It occurs in approximately one in 500 boys. The meatus may be sited anywhere from the ventral aspect of the glans penis (the commonest type) to the penoscrotal junction or even the perineum. With increasing degrees of severity, the penis is curved ventrally (chordee).

Severe cases require repair to allow the boy to void standing, to allow future sexual function and to avoid the psychological consequences of malformed genitalia. Management is

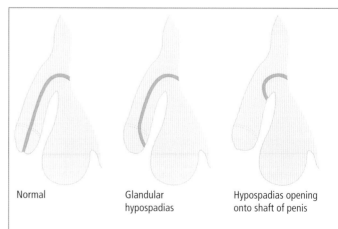

Normal

Glandular
hypospadias

Hypospadias opening
onto shaft of penis

Figure 18.3 Hypospadias showing sites of opening of the meatus.

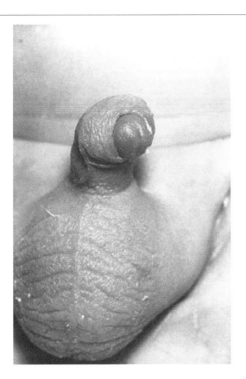

Figure 18.4 Hypospadias. The meatus is at the junction of the glans and shaft.

surgical reconstruction before the age of 2 years. Severe cases require reconstruction using the foreskin and the parents must be advised not to have the child circumcised.

Ambiguous genitalia

Rarely, babies are born with ambiguous genitalia and indeterminate sex (disorders of sexual development; DSD) This should be considered to be a medical emergency as it may be associated with major electrolyte imbalance (congenital adrenal hyperplasia). The indeterminate nature of the child's gender should be discussed with the parents and a decision regarding gender only made when investigations are complete. This depends as much on the surgical possibility of producing a functional penis as the genetic sex. Delay in naming the child is advised until gender determination is made. DSD are caused by endocrine, chromosomal and Mendelian disorders. The diagnostic approach is complex and is beyond the scope of this book. It should be stressed that future sexual identity, sexual role, sexual proclivity, chromosomal sex and phenotypic sex are all separate but interlinked characteristics, and one does not necessarily predict another. It may be very difficult to explain these issues to a family, especially during the stressful time after birth.

Irretractable prepuce

In the majority of boys the prepuce becomes retractable by the age of 3 years. Inability to retract before this age is not pathological. True phimosis (the inability to retract the prepuce) can be congenital or a sequel of inflammation, and requires surgery.

Female genital disorders

Ovarian cysts and torsion

Ovarian cysts are very common in adolescents and most are due to hormonal action (follicular and corpus luteum cysts). They may be asymptomatic or cause pain or irregular vaginal bleeding. Polycystic ovaries often present with obesity, hirsuitism, hypertension, and glucose intolerance. Endometriosis causes chronic pelvic pain. Tumours are rare and include dermoid cysts and benign cystadenomas, which may grow very large. Ovarian cancer is very rare in the paediatric age group. Occasionally an ovary may present with torsion and the picture is then one of an acute abdomen.

Labial adhesions

The labia majora are sometimes found to be adherent in young girls who are still in nappies. The adhesions probably develop as a result of irritation secondary to nappy rash and low oestrogen levels in this age group. The adhesions usually self-resolve, but occasionally an emollient or oestrogen cream is used.

To test your knowledge on this part of the book, please see Chapter 26

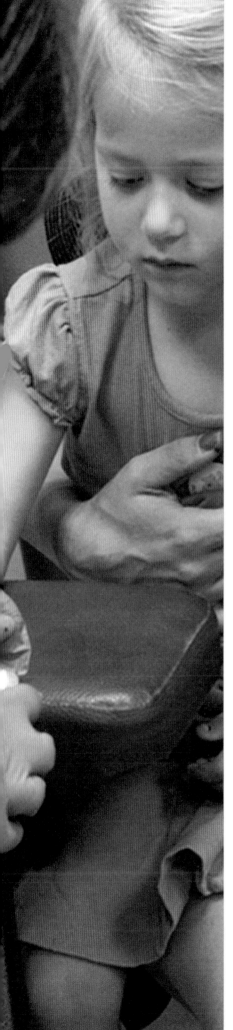

CHAPTER 19

Dermatology and rashes

If there is a white spot on the skin, ... then the priest shall quarantine the affected person for 7 days
Leviticus 13:4

If the skin is covered with dull white spots, it is a simple rash ......
Leviticus 13:39

KEY COMPETENCES

YOU MUST...

Know and understand

- The differential diagnosis of children presenting with acute and chronic rashes, nappy rash, itching and infectious skin lesions
- The common congenital birthmarks and skin lesions
- How to diagnose and manage common dermatological disorders, especially dermatitis

Be able to

- Differentiate and describe lesions of the skin
- Identify the common childhood exanthems clinically
- Recognise common birth marks
- Advise a parent about caring for a baby's nappy rash

Appreciate that

- There are social consequences of having a chronic skin condition
- Excessive use of topical steroid creams has important unwanted effects
- Purpuric and petechial rashes may be indicative of life-threatening conditions

Essential Paediatrics and Child Health, Fourth Edition. Mary Rudolf, Anthony Luder and Kerry Jeavons.
© 2020 John Wiley & Sons Ltd. Published 2020 by John Wiley & Sons Ltd.
Companion website: www.wiley.com/go/rudolf/paediatrics

Dermatological symptoms and signs

Finding your way around ...

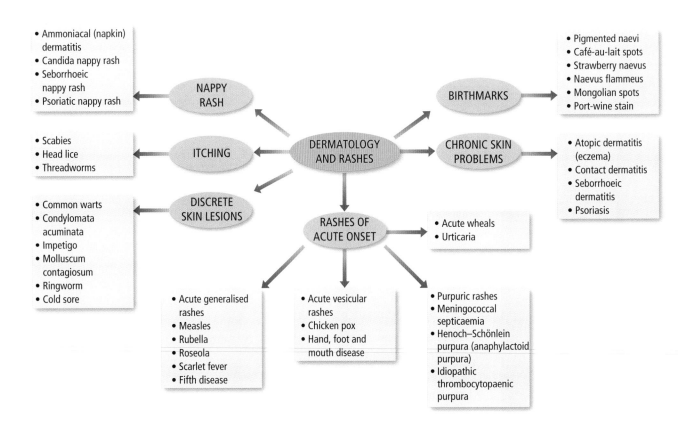

Parents commonly bring their child to the doctor for diagnosis of rashes and skin lesions. In most situations a diagnosis can be made clinically, and treatment, if required, can be given without further investigation. Experience is required to identify these skin manifestations, and the process of identification is rather like identifying wildflowers or bird-spotting – if you have encountered it before, you are likely to recognise it again. It is important, however, to learn to describe the features, just as in bird-spotting; this increases one's powers of observation and enhances the learning process.

The various types of skin lesion are described and illustrated in Table 19.1.

Unlike with almost any other condition in medicine, it is reasonable to examine the child presenting with a rash or skin lesion *before* embarking on a detailed history.

Description of the rash or lesion

If you are unsure of the correct dermatological term for lesions, you should carefully describe them. The following features are important to include:

- raised or flat;
- crusty or scaly;
- colour;
- blanching on pressure;
- size of the lesions;
- distribution (discrete, generalised or limited to certain sites in the body).

Other features

The child's age, changes in the rash over time, current health and any accompanying features contribute to the diagnosis.

Table 19.1 Types of skin lesion

Type of lesion	Description	Example
Macules	Discrete flat lesions of up to 1 cm in diameter that are different in colour from the surrounding skin; they may be pigmented, depigmented pink or red in colour. Characteristically acute macules fade on pressure	Rubella Roseola
Patches	Discrete flat lesions above 1 cm in diameter. They may be of any colour.	Salmon patch birthmark Chagrin patch in tuberous sclerosis
Papules	Solid palpable projections above the surface of the skin Maculopapular: A mixture of macules and papules which tend to be confluent	Insect bite Measles Drug rash
Nodules	Raised palpable lesions larger than papules and deeper	Pyogenic granuloma Lipoma Sebaceous cyst
Plaques	Raised lesions bigger than 1 cm in diameter	Psoriasis
Purpura and petechiae	Purple lesions caused by small haemorrhages in the superficial layers of the skin. In general, they indicate a serious condition. Characteristically they *do not fade on pressure*. Petechiae are less than 0.5 cm in diameter and purpura are over 0.5 cm.	Meningococcal septicaemia Idiopathic thrombocytopenic purpura Henoch – Schönlein purpura Leukaemia
Ecchymosis	Larger subcutaneous bleeds often a number of centimetres in diameter	Bleeding diathesis Trauma
Telangiectasis	An abnormal overgrowth of cutaneous blood vessels. If they emerge from a central feeding arteriole, they are referred to as 'spider naevi'	Liver disease Ataxia telangiectasia
Vesicles	Raised fluid filled lesions <1.0 cm in diameter	Chicken pox

(continued)

Table 19.1 Types of skin lesion (*continued*)

Type of lesion	Description	Example
Bullae	Fluid filled lesion greater than 1 cm in diameter	Impetigo
Pustules	Round raised lesion filled with pus	Infected bite
Crusts	A dry lesion in which pus, exudate or serum has dried up	Haemorrhagic scab
Wheals	Raised lesions with a flat top and pale centre of variable size	Urticaria
Desquamation or scales	A loss of epidermal cells producing a 'scaly' eruption	Post-scarlet fever Post-Kawasaki fever
Erosion	A shallow lesion marked by denuding of the epithelium	Trauma
Ulcer	A deeper and more persistent loss of epithelial and deeper tissue layers	Pressure ulcer
Fissure	A narrow deep crack in the skin	Icthyosis
Excoriation	A scrape or abrasion of the skin	Rubbing trauma

On the basis of this brief evaluation, the problem can be classified according to the following criteria:

- acute onset of rash;
- chronic rashes;
- nappy rash;
- individual skin lesions;
- birthmarks;
- itchy conditions.

Each of these is discussed in the following sections.

Acute rashes

Type of rash	Examples
Macular and maculopapular	Exanthems of childhood infections (see below) Allergy
Vesicular	Chicken pox Hand, foot and mouth disease
Purpuric	Meningococcal septicaemia Henoch–Schönlein purpura (see p. 364) Idiopathic thrombocytopenic purpura (see p. 378)
Wheals	Urticaria

Most children presenting with acute onset of a rash have one of the common infectious diseases of childhood and are unwell with a temperature. These conditions are covered in Chapter 9.

Purpuric conditions always need attention as they may be a sign of a life-threatening condition and must be identified promptly. See Figures 19.1 and 19.2.

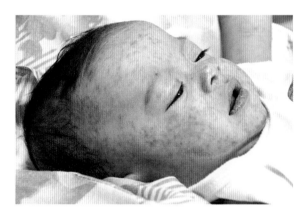

Measles – maculopapular rash.

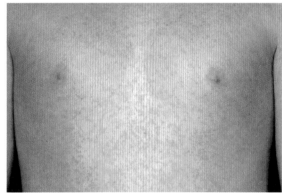

Rubella – small macular lesions.

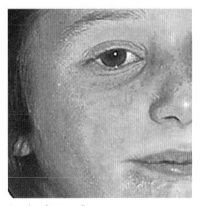

Scarlet fever – fine punctate maculopapular rash.

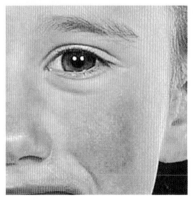

Fifth disease – 'slapped cheek' rash.

Figure 19.1 Acute macular and maculopapular rashes.

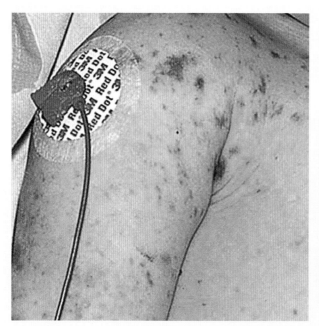

Meningococcaemia. Note the typical purpuric rash.

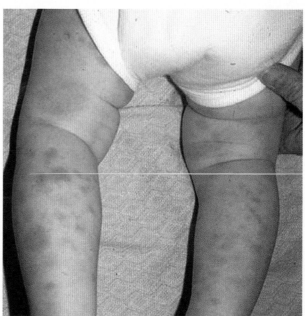

Henoch–Schönlein purpura. Note the typical distribution.

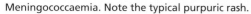

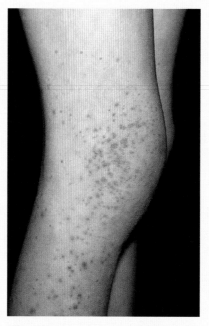

Idiopathic thrombocytopenic purpura.
Note the petechial rash.

Figure 19.2 Acute purpuric and petechial rashes.

History – must ask!

- *Is the child ill or febrile?* Most of the exanthematous diseases are accompanied by fever and malaise (see Chapter 9). In Henoch–Schönlein purpura (HSP) and idiopathic thrombocytopenic purpura (ITP) fever is usually absent.
- *Is the rash itchy?* Itchiness suggests an allergic response, or chicken pox if the rash is vesicular. If you suspect allergy, ask about possible allergens such as food, washing powder, soaps and lotions. However, it is rare to identify the allergen.
- *Are there associated symptoms?* These are particularly important in the purpuric conditions. In ITP there may be bruising, and bleeding from the gums and nose. In HSP, arthritis and abdominal pain, melaena and haematuria commonly occur. In hives, wheezing or stridor may rarely be present.
- *Past medical history.* A history of a previous attack of an infectious disease makes a further attack unlikely, but there is a high incidence of inaccurate diagnoses, particularly with maculopapular rashes. It is obviously relevant to ask about the child's immunisation history. An atypical rash commonly follows some 10 days after measles, mumps and rubella (MMR) vaccination.
- *Contact with anyone ill.* Enquire whether anyone else in the family, or at school or nursery has been diagnosed as having an infectious disease.

Physical examination – must check!

You need to describe the rash carefully, focusing on the following:
- *Characteristics.* Is the rash macular, papular, maculopapular, purpuric or petechial, vesicular or wheals? An important part of the examination is to test the rash for blanching, as purpuric and petechial rashes do not blanch on pressure whereas maculopapular rashes do.
- *Distribution.* Measles and rubella both start on the face and work their way down the body. Roseola and chicken pox are mostly on the trunk. Both HSP and fifth disease have characteristic distributions. A rash that begins on the periphery and works its way to the centre is called centripetal; the opposite is centrifugal. An example of centripetal rash is rickettsia, and example of centrifugal is measles.
- *The presence of an enanthem.* Look in the mouth for an enanthem (see p. 137), for example Koplik spots in measles.

Investigations

In general, the viral exanthems do not need a serological confirmation of the diagnosis, unless for public health reasons. An exception is if rubella is suspected in a pregnant girl. If meningococcal septicaemia is suspected, blood cultures, meningococcal PCR, clotting screen, full blood count and calcium profile are performed urgently. If the rash is petechial, a platelet count is required to make the diagnosis of thrombocytopenia.

Management

Prior to the advent of immunisation, there was little difficulty in recognizing the childhood exanthems as they were so common. It is important to recognise them so that appropriate advice about incubation periods and isolation can be made (Table 9.2). Maculopapular rashes are often overdiagnosed clinically as being caused by measles or rubella. As these diagnoses are difficult to make unless in the midst of an epidemic, it is preferable to make the diagnosis of viral exanthem rather than a wrong diagnosis. If accurate diagnosis is required, confirmation by serological testing is necessary.

If meningococcal septicaemia is suspected (see p. 154), the child should immediately be given intramuscular penicillin as rapid deterioration can occur, and urgent admission to hospital arranged. The child with suspected ITP also requires urgent hospital evaluation and admission if the platelet count is dangerously low.

 Key points: Acute rashes

- Decide if the rash is macular, maculopapular, vesicular, purpuric or wheals
- Determine if the child is febrile or ill
- If the rash is petechial or purpuric and the child is unwell, treat with penicillin IM and admit for investigation
- Beware of making a specific diagnosis of measles or rubella clinically. Without serological confirmation, 'viral exanthem' should be diagnosed

Clues to diagnosing acute generalised rashes in childhood

	Type of rash	Characteristics of the rash	Other features
Measles	Maculopapular	Begins on the face and spreads downwards, centrifugal	Koplik spots, coryza, cough and conjunctivitis, ill child
Rubella	Macular	Tiny pink macules on the face and trunk, works downwards, centrifugal	Well child, lymphadenopathy sometimes
Roseola	Macular	Faint pink rash on the trunk, centrifugal	Rash occurs after fever defervesces
Scarlet fever	Maculopapular	Fine punctate red rash with sandpapery feel, followed by peeling	Strawberry tongue, perioral pallor, tonsillitis
Fifth disease	Maculopapular	'Slapped cheek' appearance. Lace-like rash on the arms, trunk and thighs, centripetal	Well child, lasts up to weeks
Allergic reaction	Papular	Itchy rash, often generalised	The allergen is usually not identified
Chicken pox	Vesicular	Occurs in crops on face and trunk. Papules, vesicles and crusts are present, centrifugal	Shallow ulcers of the mucous membranes
Meningococcal septicaemia	Purpuric	Morbilliform, petechial or purpuric, often centripetal	May progress rapidly to shock and coma
Henoch–Schönlein purpura	Purpuric	Typical rash characteristically distributed over the buttocks, thighs and legs, centripetal	Abdominal pain, arthralgia, melaena, haematuria. Child usually appears well
Idiopathic thrombocytopenic purpura	Petechial	Petechial rash over body, with bruising	Bleeding from other sites, e.g. venepuncture, gums, nose. Child usually appears well
Urticaria	Wheals	Well circumscribed, itchy wheals of different sizes	Rarely accompanied by wheezing or anaphylactic shock

Chronic skin rashes

Common chronic skin rashes

Eczema (atopic dermatitis)
Contact dermatitis
Seborrhoeic dermatitis
Psoriasis

Most chronic skin conditions in childhood are eczematous. See Figure 19.3. Acute eczema (the generic term used to designate a particular type of skin reaction) is characterised by erythema, weeping and microvesicle formation within the epidermis. Chronic eczema is characterised by thickened, dry, scaly, coarse skin (lichenification). The commonest type of eczema in children is atopic dermatitis, although contact dermatitis and seborrhoeic dermatitis are also relatively common.

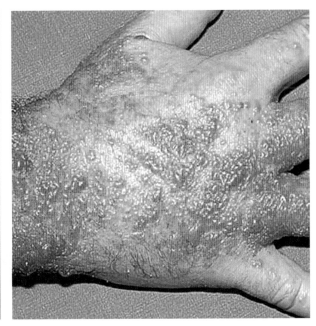

Atopic dermatitis – note flexural involvement.

Contact dermatitis.

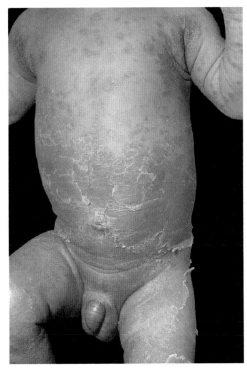

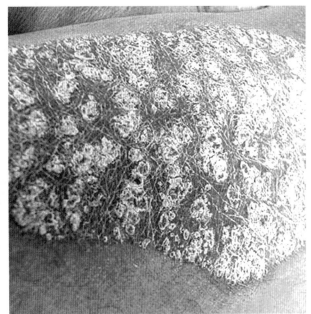

Seborrhoeic dermatitis.

Psoriasis – characteristic silvery/white plaques.

Figure 19.3 Common chronic skin conditions.

Most children presenting with a chronic skin rash have atopic dermatitis, but it is important to learn to distinguish other rashes.

History – must ask!

- *Is the rash itchy?* Itchiness is characteristic of atopic and contact dermatitis. It may also be present in seborrhoeic dermatitis.
- *Are there precipitating factors?* Certain foods such as cow's milk, wheat and eggs may precipitate or exacerbate atopic dermatitis. Saliva, citrus juices, bubble bath, detergents, occlusive synthetic shoes and topical medication are common irritants that cause contact dermatitis.
- *Is there a family history?* Children with eczema often have a family history of atopy. The presence of psoriasis in a parent may support a diagnosis of psoriatic rash in a child. A recent history of scabies in the family or at school would suggest a diagnosis of scabies rather than atopic dermatitis.

Physical examination – must check!

- *Characteristics of the rash.* Examine the child completely so that you can assess the rash and its distribution adequately.

Note that the pattern of involvement of atopic dermatitis changes during childhood.
- *Other helpful features.* The presence of cradle cap or a rash behind the ears and skin folds suggests seborrhoeic dermatitis. Nail pitting or joint involvement point towards psoriasis.

Management of chronic skin complaints

The skin is visible, so skin disease poses an additional problem not usually found in diseases of other systems. This means that the child and family are subject to the stares and curiosity of others, and possibly stigmatization. It is important to remember that management should involve not only the skin condition but the whole child too.

Topical corticosteroids form an important part of the management of a variety of chronic skin conditions. They must be used with care as long-term use, particularly of the fluorinated variety, leads to atrophy of the skin and an increase in hair growth in some patients. Small amounts of cream applied frequently is more effective than large amounts applied infrequently. The more potent topical steroids should not be applied to the face. If they are applied over the body using occlusive dressings, systemic absorption with adrenal suppression can occur.

🔍 Clues to diagnosing chronic skin conditions

	Atopic dermatitis	Contact dermatitis	Seborrhoeic dermatitis	Psoriasis
Lesions	Erythema, weepiness and crusting leading to dry, thickened scaling skin	Erythema and weeping	Dry scaly and erythematous; red plaques may be present	Plaques of thick silvery or white scales with sharp borders
Distribution	See 'At A Glance' Box p. 359	At sites of contact with the irritant	Face, scalp, neck, axillae and nappy area	Scalp, knees, elbows and genitalia
Itchiness	+++	+++	+/−	−
Other features	Starts in infancy; family history of atopy		Cradle cap	Nail pitting, arthritis

---

Nappy rash

Causes of nappy rash

Ammoniacal dermatitis	Seborrhoeic dermatitis
Candidiasis	Psoriasis

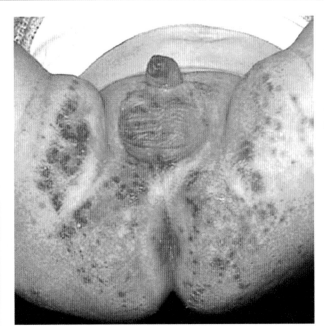

Ammoniacal nappy rash.

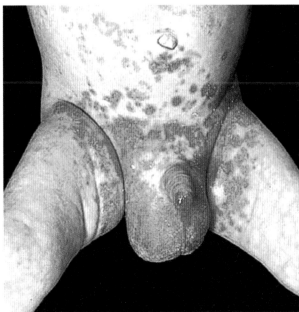

Candida nappy rash – note rash involving the inguinal folds with satellite lesions.

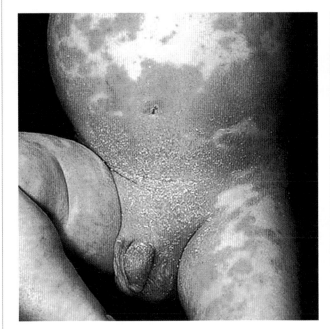

Seborrhoeic dermatitis – note pink and greasy looking lesions.

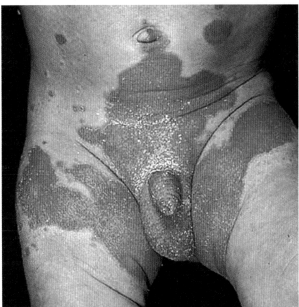

Psoriatic nappy rash.

Figure 19.4 Nappy rashes.

See Figure 19.4. The nappy area is very prone to rash as it is an area that is warm and moist, usually tightly enclosed in an occlusive waterproof covering, and is in contact with urine, which is an irritant. Mostly the rash is a simple irritative rash, commonly with candidiasis superimposed, but in a prolonged, resistant rash, conditions such as seborrhoeic dermatitis and psoriasis should be considered. The baby needs to be examined, paying particular attention to the intertriginous areas, scalp and mouth.

🔍 Clues to distinguishing nappy rashes

Ammoniacal dermatitis	Erythematous +/− papulovesicular or bullous lesions, fissures and erosions
	Patchy or confluent
	Skin folds characteristically spared
Candida	Bright red, with sharply demarcated edge and satellite lesions
	Inguinal folds involved
	Oral thrush may be found
Seborrhoeic dermatitis	Pink, greasy lesions with yellow scale
	Often in the skin folds
	Cradle cap may be found
Psoriatic nappy rash	Like seborrhoeic dermatitis
	Positive family history for psoriasis

Itching

Conditions causing itching

Atopic dermatitis
Contact dermatitis
Urticaria
Scabies
Chicken pox (seborrhoeic dermatitis)
Head lice
Threadworms

Itching is an unpleasant symptom which, if generalised, is usually associated with a rash. Certain measures can help reduce the discomfort of itching, whatever the cause. Cool baths are soothing, and tight synthetic or woollen clothing should be avoided. Topical antihistamine gels or cooling agents like calamine may be helpful. It is important to discourage scratching, and fingernails should be kept short and clean to minimize secondary infection. Systemic sedative antihistamines prescribed at night can increase the chances of a more restful night.

Infectious skin lesions

Common infectious skin lesions

Warts
Impetigo
Molluscum contagiosum
Tinea
Herpes simplex (cold sores)
Birthmarks

Diagnosis of these common lesions requires visual recognition (Figure 19.5). You should learn to distinguish them by studying the photographs, and looking for characteristic distinguishing features.

🔍 Clues to diagnosing infectious skin lesions

Common warts	Roughened keratotic lesions with an irregular surface
Impetigo	Sticky, heaped-up, honey-coloured crusts
Molluscum contagiosum	Pearly, dome-shaped papules, with central umbilicus
Tinea corporis	Dry, scaly papule which spreads centrifugally with central clearing
Cold sore	Single or grouped vesicles/pustules sited periorally

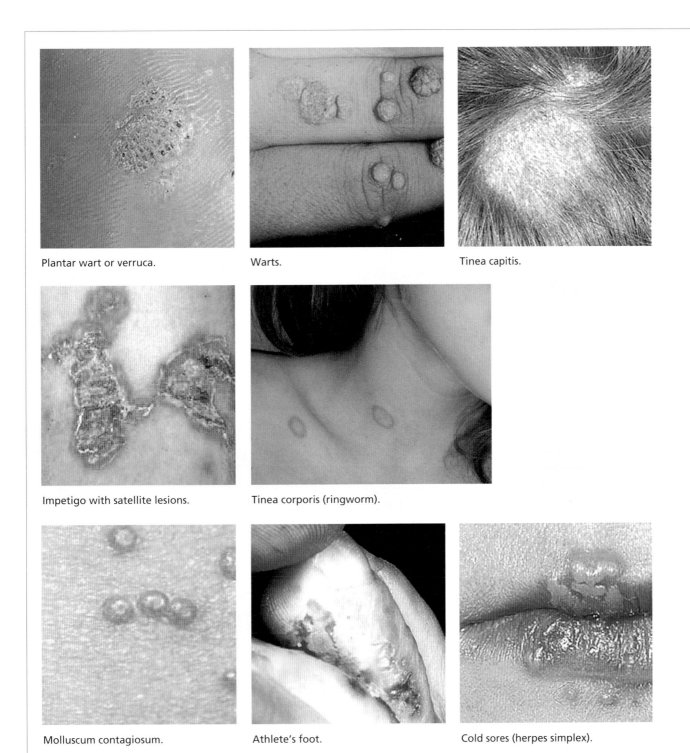

Plantar wart or verruca.

Warts.

Tinea capitis.

Impetigo with satellite lesions.

Tinea corporis (ringworm).

Molluscum contagiosum.

Athlete's foot.

Cold sores (herpes simplex).

Figure 19.5 Infectious skin lesions.

Dermatological conditions and other rashes

Atopic dermatitis (eczema)

Atopic dermatitis (see Figure 19.6) is an inflammatory skin condition characterised by erythema, oedema, intense itching, exudation, crusting, and scaling. There appears to be a genetically determined predisposition, and infants with atopic dermatitis tend to subsequently develop allergic rhinitis and asthma. It most often begins in the first 2–3 months of life, and the onset frequently coincides with the introduction of certain foods such as cow's milk, wheat, and eggs into the diet. There is some evidence that genetically susceptible infants have a reduced risk of developing eczema if they are exclusively breast-fed. There is often a family history of atopy.

Clinical features   The clinical features vary according to the stage of childhood. In infancy the lesions are erythematous, weepy patches on the cheeks which subsequently extend to the rest of the face, neck, wrists, hands and extensor surfaces of the extremities. Pruritus is marked, and the infant makes efforts to scratch by face-rubbing on the sheets. This leads to weeping and crusting, and commonly secondary infection.

By preschool age (3–5 years) there is a tendency towards remission, although some children have persistent mild to moderate dermatitis in the popliteal and antecubital fossae, on the wrists, behind the ears, and on the face and neck.

During school years recurrence tends to occur, with antecubital and popliteal involvement and extension to the neck, forehead, eyelids, wrists, and dorsa of the hands and feet. The skin becomes dry and thickened and the face can take on a whitish hue. Hyperpigmentation, scaling and lichenification become prominent.

Investigations   The diagnosis is a clinical one. Serum IgE levels are often raised and eosinophilia may be present. Although skin testing is frequently positive, it is rarely helpful clinically.

Management   See Box 19.1. Scratching has a major role in the production of skin lesions, and treatment is directed at trying to interrupt the itch–scratch–itch cycle. Dietary restriction is controversial and generally of limited value. Arbitrary exclusion of a number of foods can lead to malnutrition.

During an acute flare-up wet dressings are helpful as they have an anti-inflammatory and antipruritic effect. Topical steroids are then applied between dressing changes. Antihistamines can be useful for their sedative and antipruritic effect. Scratching often causes infection even if this is not obviously apparent, and so topical or oral antibiotics are often required.

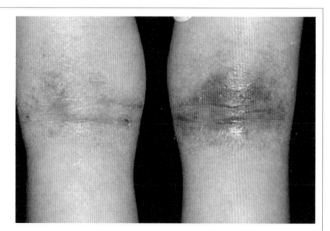

Figure 19.6 Atopic dermatitis. The legs of a child with atopic dermatitis, showing flexural involvement.

> **Box 19.1 Advice for children with atopic eczema**
>
> - Avoid food and environmental factors known to trigger itching (but arbitrary exclusion of numerous foods from infants' diets is irrational and can lead to malnutrition)
> - Avoid extremes of temperature and humidity
> - Keep fingernails short to help control scratching
> - Clothes should be of smooth cotton and avoid wearing wool
> - Avoid medicated soap, though a superfatted, simple soap is acceptable
> - Bath oils and creams are intended to seal moisture into the skin. Apply them after the child has soaked in the bath for 15 minutes or so
> - Bleach baths have been shown to be effective in preventing secondary infection and ameliorating eczema
> - A pet-free household is advisable, given the common development of asthma in atopic children
> - Breast-feeding with avoidance of cow's milk protein for the first several months is advisable in subsequent siblings

After the acute phase, while the dermatitis is still active, topical steroids are applied in the form of creams or ointments. The more potent steroid creams must be kept to a minimum to control the disease and should not be applied to the face. Systemic corticosteroids are only rarely used.

Lubricants are used after application of steroid creams and continued on a prophylactic basis to keep the skin moist. Bath oils can be added to the bath water after the child has soaked well, so that moisture is sealed into the well-hydrated skin. Bleach baths have been shown to be effective in treating eczema and preventing secondary infection. Another important drug class are the topical calcineurin inhibitors (TCIs) such as tacrolimus. These are effective in mild to moderate eczema and avoid the side effects of steroids.

Prognosis   The course of atopic dermatitis is fluctuating; fortunately the condition resolves entirely in some 50% of infants by the age of 2 years. A few cases continue to be problematic beyond childhood. Reasonable control of this chronic condition can usually be achieved in most children.

See NICE guideline: Atopic eczema in under 12s: diagnosis and management
https://www.nice.org.uk/guidance/cg57

Atopic dermatitis at a glance

Epidemiology
Often starts in infancy but clinical picture changes with age

Aetiology
Atopic condition

History
Itchy rash
Often begins at age 2 –3 months
Family history of atopy *
Associated allergic rhinitis, asthma*

Physical examination
Infant
Erythematous, weeping, crusting lesions
Sites: patches on cheeks → rest of face, neck, wrists, hands, extensor surfaces of arms and legs

Preschool
Mild to moderate dermatitis
Sites: popliteal and antecubital fossae, wrists, behind ears, face and neck

School age
More severe, with hyperpigmentation, lichenification, scaling
Sites: popliteal and antecubital fossae, forehead, eyelids, wrists, dorsa of hands and feet

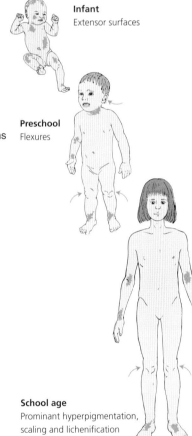

Infant
Extensor surfaces

Preschool
Flexures

School age
Prominant hyperpigmentation, scaling and lichenification

Confirmatory investigations
None
High serum IgE, eosinophilia, elevated specific IgE to specific allergens may be found

Differential diagnosis
Scabies
Contact dermatitis
Seborrhoea
Psoriasis

Management
Acute flare-up:
• prevent scratching
• wet dressings
• topical steroids (as least potent as possible)
• topical calcineurin inhibitors (TCI) eg tacrolimus effective in mild to moderate eczema
• antihistamines
• antibiotics for secondary infection (often needed)
Prophylaxis:
• lubricants
• bath oil
• bleach baths effective as prophylactic

Course/prognosis
Fluctuates
Control achieved in most children
Resolves in 50% infants by age 2 years
A few cases continue to be problematic beyond childhood

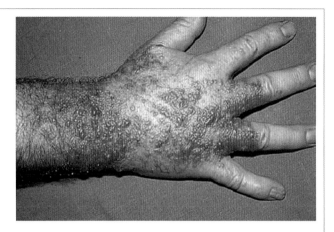

Figure 19.7 Contact dermatitis. A severe rash that erupted on contact with holly.

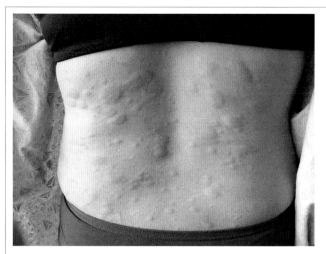

Figure 19.8 Urticaria (hives). Note the characteristic, well-circumscribed wheals. Source: Lovelyday Vandy/Shutterstock.com.

Contact dermatitis

Clinically, contact dermatitis may be indistinguishable from atopic dermatitis, although a detailed history, the sites involved, and the age of the child often provide clues. See Figure 19.7. It can either be caused by irritants or, in susceptible individuals, by allergens. It results from prolonged or repetitive contact with a variety of substances that include saliva, citrus juices, bubble bath, detergents and occlusive synthetic shoes. Topical medications, jewellery and chemicals used in the manufacture of clothing are all potential allergens.

Clinical features Saliva may cause dermatitis on the face and neckfolds of a drooling child. It also occurs in older children who habitually lick their lips. 'Trainer' or 'sneaker' dermatitis can result from the leaching out of chemicals in the shoe rubber by excessive sweating. Bubble baths can be a cause of severe pruritus.

Management In general, contact dermatitis clears on removal of the irritant or allergen and temporary treatment with a topical corticosteroid preparation.

Urticaria (hives)

Urticaria is an allergic reaction characterised by well-circumscribed but sometimes coalescent wheals of various sizes (Figure 19.8). It is usually difficult to identify the allergen. Certain individuals may develop urticaria when exposed to insect bites (papular urticaria), cold, exercise, hot showers and anxiety.

Clinical features The lesions may be intensely pruritic. Each wheal resolves within 2 days, but new ones continue to occur and urticaria may become chronic, persisting for many weeks. In angioneurotic oedema deeper tissues are also involved, including the upper respiratory and gastrointestinal tract. Urticaria may also be seen in the child presenting in anaphylactic shock.

Management In most instances urticaria is a self-limited condition requiring no treatment, other than that aimed at reducing itching. Antihistamines are the drug of first choice. The allergen is usually not identified, although it is worth taking a good food and drug history.

Seborrhoeic dermatitis

Seborrhoeic dermatitis is a chronic inflammatory condition which is commonest during infancy and adolescence. See Figure 19.9. It is often most troublesome in the first year of life.

Clinical features Cradle cap is the commonest manifestation and is seen as diffuse or focal scaling and yellow crusting of the scalp. A dry scaly erythematous dermatitis may also involve the face, neck, axillae and nappy area and behind the ears. If the scaling is prominent it may look like psoriasis, and red scaly plaques may appear. Itching may or may not be present. Seborrhoeic nappy rash is characterised by pink, greasy lesions with a yellow scale. It is most commonly seen in the intertriginous areas.

Management Scalp lesions are usually controlled with topical salicylate ointment, which is very effective at removing scales, and antiseborrhoeic shampoo. Inflamed lesions respond to topical corticosteroid therapy. Secondary bacterial infections and superimposed candidiasis are not uncommon. Seborrhoeic nappy rash usually responds to mild topical corticosteroid cream.

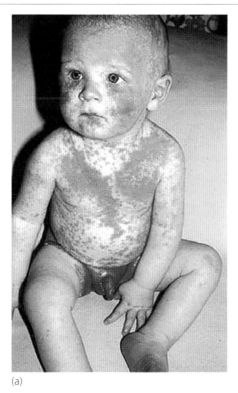
(a)

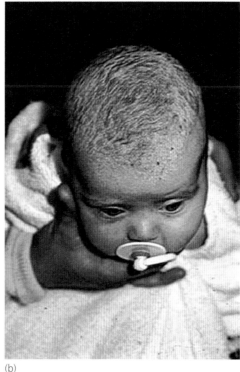
(b)

Figure 19.9 Seborrhoeic dermatitis. (a) Note the baby's erythematous rash involving the face, neck, chest and nappy area. (b) Severe cradle cap in a baby, with widespread scaling and crusting of the scalp.

Psoriasis

Psoriasis is a common chronic skin disorder among adults, one third of whom become affected during childhood. See Figures 19.10 and 19.11. Girls are more affected than boys and there is usually a family history.

Clinical features   The lesions consist of erythematous papules which coalesce to form plaques of thick silvery or white scales and sharply demarcated borders. They tend to occur on the scalp, knees, elbows, umbilicus and genitalia. Nail involvement, a valuable diagnostic sign, is characterised by pitting of the nail plate. Guttate psoriasis is a variant affecting children where multiple small oval or round lesions appear over the body, often following a recent streptococcal infection. Psoriasis in the infant can present as a persistent nappy rash, similar to that of seborrhoeic dermatitis.

Management   Therapy is mainly palliative and should be kept to a minimum. The application of coal tar preparations such as dithranol is a mainstay of treatment. Phototherapy with or without psoralens is very helpful. Topical corticosteroids are effective but must be used with caution. Methotrexate is important for sufferers with systemic complications such as arthritis. A variety of more specific drugs including biological agents have come into use in recent years.

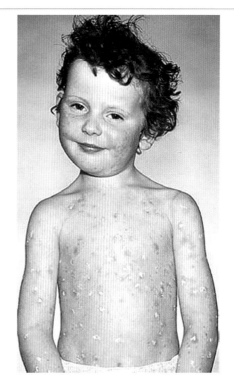

Figure 19.10 Psoriasis. Note the characteristic silvery/white plaques over the upper body.

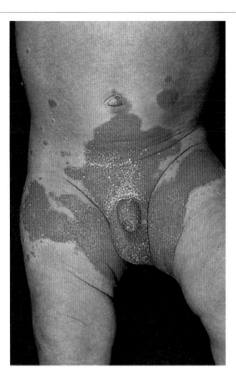

Figure 19.11 Psoriatic nappy rash.

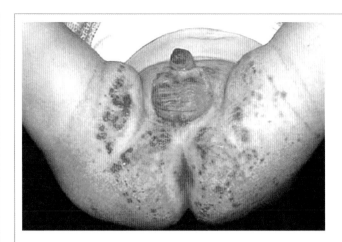

Figure 19.12 Ammoniacal nappy rash.

Ammoniacal (napkin) dermatitis

Nappy rash can be considered the prototype of irritant contact dermatitis. See Figure 19.12. The rash results as a reaction to overhydration of the skin, friction, maceration, and prolonged contact with urine, faeces, nappy detergents and chemicals. Since the widespread use of disposable nappies, nappy rash has been less prevalent.

Clinical features   The rash is erythematous, often with papulovesicular or bullous lesions, fissures, and erosions. The eruption can be patchy or confluent, but the skin folds are characteristically spared as they are in less contact with urine than the exposed areas are. Secondary infection with bacteria and yeasts is common.

Management   The rash often responds to simple measures, including regular changing and washing of the genitalia with warm water and mild soap, exposure of the area to air as much as possible, and the application of protective creams such as zinc and castor oil ointment. When these measures do not suffice, limited application of mild hydrocortisone cream can be used. As superimposed candida infection is so common, use of anticandidal agents is also justified.

 Nappy rash at a glance

Epidemiology
Universal

Aetiology
Prolonged contact with urine, faeces, detergents, chemicals
Candidal superinfection common

Physical examination
Erythema
Patchy or confluent
Sparing of skin folds (unless candida present too)
Papules, vesicles, bullae, fissures, erosions*
Oral thrush*

NB *Signs and symptoms are variable.

Confirmatory investigations
None

Differential diagnosis
Candida
Seborrhoeic nappy rash
Psoriatic nappy rash

Management
Regular changing and washing area
Exposure to air
Protective creams
Consider use of mild hydrocortisone cream, anticandida creams

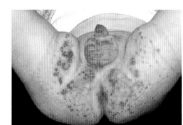

Candida nappy rash (Figure 19.13a)

Candida superinfection of other rashes is common. See Figure 19.13. It also commonly follows a course of oral antibi-otics as the gut flora is changed, so allowing the candida to flourish opportunistically.

Clinical features   Candidal dermatitis classically appears as a bright red rash with a sharply demarcated edge and satellite lesions beyond the border. Unlike in ammoniacal dermatitis, the inguinal folds are usually involved as the warm moist area promotes growth of the yeast.

Thrush (oral candidiasis) may be found on inspection of the mouth. It appears as white 'curds' coating the tongue, gums and buccal mucosa (Figure 19.13b).

Management   The diagnosis is usually made on clinical grounds, but confirmation can be made on potassium hydroxide (KOH) preparation. Treatment consists of application of an anticandidal agent such as miconazole, at each nappy change, until the rash has resolved.

If oral thrush is present oral miconazole gel should be prescribed.

Henoch–Schönlein purpura (anaphylactoid purpura)

Henoch–Schönlein purpura is a form of systemic vasculitis which is presumed to be caused by immune-complex-mediated disease.

Clinical features   The child presents with a purpuric rash in a typical distribution over the buttocks, thighs and legs (Figure 19.14). The lesions are purple, raised and a few millimetres in diameter. Peri-arthritis or arthralgia and abdominal pain are commonly experienced often with oedema and warm erythema, and occasionally melaena occurs. Seventy per cent of the children develop haematuria and/or proteinuria, but the glomerulonephritis is usually asymptomatic and non-progressive.

Management   The diagnosis is usually made by the clinical constellation of the typical rash, and abdominal and joint complaints, with a normal platelet count. Treatment is simply supportive. The rash resolves over a week or two, although microscopic haematuria can persist for over a year. Children with renal manifestations should continue to have urinary examinations and blood pressure measurements at periodic intervals to detect late development of hypertension and renal impairment.

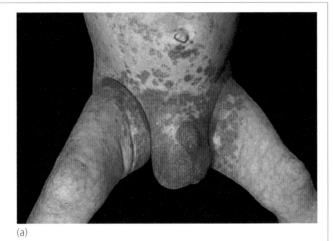
(a)

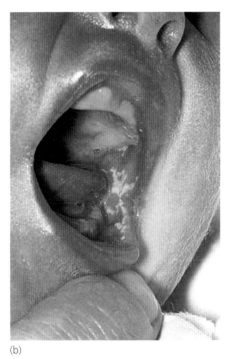
(b)

Figure 19.13 Candidal nappy rash. (a) Note the bright red rash involving the inguinal folds and the satellite lesions. (b) Oral thrush appearing like white curds on the buccal mucosa.

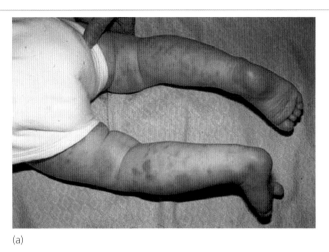
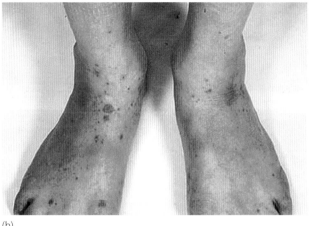

(a)   (b)

Figure 19.14 Henoch–Schönlein purpura. (a) Note the distribution; (b) close-up of the rash over the feet.

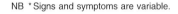

Henoch–Schönlein purpura at a glance

Epidemiology
Any age

Aetiology
Systemic vasculitis presumed to
  be mediated by IgA immune
  complexes

History
Arthralgia*
Abdominal pain *
Melaena*

Physical examination
Purple raised lesions
Typical distribution over
  buttocks, thighs and legs *
Arthritis*

NB * Signs and symptoms are variable.

Confirmatory investigations
Clinical diagnosis
Haematuria/proteinuria in 70%
Normal platelet count

Differential diagnosis
Usually unequivocal
(Septicaemia)
(Bleeding diathesis)

Management
Supportive
Urinalysis and blood pressure
  periodically if renal
  manifestations are present
Steroids useful in abdominal pain
and (rare) CNS involvement

Prognosis/complications
Intussusception may occur in
young children
Rash lasts 1–2 weeks
 Haematuria may persist for
  many months
Hypertension and renal
  impairment may occur

Impetigo

Impetigo (see Figure 19.15) is a skin infection occurring most commonly in children, particularly in the hot humid summer months. The organisms responsible are group A haemolytic streptococci or staphylococci (which commonly also causes a bullous lesion). Infection may be spread to other parts of the body by the fingers, clothing, and towels. Insect bites, dermatitis and scabies serve as portals of entry for the organism, which does not penetrate intact skin.

Clinical features   The skin lesions pass rapidly through a vesiculopustular phase, and following rupture sticky, heaped-up, honey-coloured crusts are formed. The sites involved are usually exposed areas.

Management   Impetigo can be contagious, and in all cases simple rules of hygiene must be followed to prevent spread. Antibiotic cream is prescribed if the number of lesions is small (fewer than five), and is applied after the crusts have been soaked off with warm water and soap. In more extensive impetigo, oral

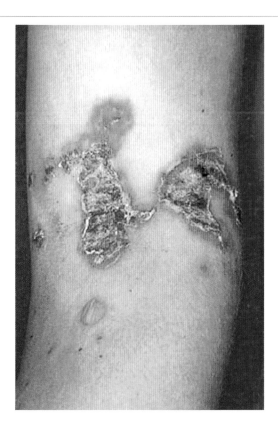

Figure 19.15 Impetigo. Note the honey-crusted lesions. Spread has occurred with satellite lesions.

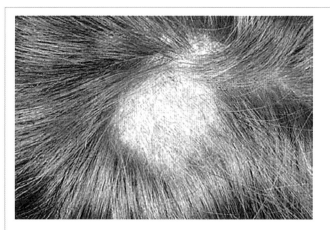

Figure 19.16 Tinea capitis. Note the circumscribed patch of hair loss with patchy scaling of the scalp.

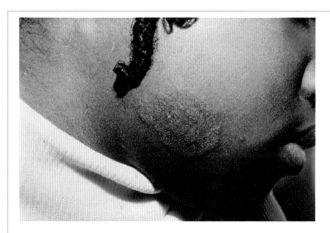

Figure 19.17 Tinea corporis (ring worm) contracted from a pet dog. Note the typical ring-like patches with central clearing.

antibiotics are required, cefalomazin being the drug of choice as it covers both streptococcal and staphylococcal infections

Ringworm (tinea)

Children can be affected by ringworm, which is either anthropophilic (exclusive to humans) or zoophilic (primarily parasites of other animals). Differing organisms cause lesions at different sites.

Tinea capitis

In tinea capitis the child presents with a circumscribed patch of hair loss and patchy scaling of the scalp (Figure 19.16). Close examination shows the hair to be broken off close to the follicle, giving a 'black dot' appearance. It may present as a kerion – a boggy inflammatory mass with local lymphadenopathy. The common form of tinea capitis infection fluoresces brilliant green on Wood's light examination, and can be seen microscopically in a wet-mount KOH preparation. Topical therapy alone is ineffective: griseofulvin needs to be taken orally for at least 4 weeks.

Tinea corporis

Tinea corporis can be acquired from infected persons or pets or simply by contact with shed scales or hairs. The typical lesion (Figure 19.17) begins as a dry scaly papule which spreads centrifugally, clearing centrally as it does so. The diagnosis can be confirmed by microscopical examination of the scrapings in a KOH wet mount. Lesions usually respond to topical antifungal agents applied for 2–4 weeks, but griseofulvin may be required in extensive cases.

Tinea pedis

Tinea pedis (or athlete's foot) (Figure 19.18) is uncommon and is overdiagnosed in young children, where contact dermatitis is a more likely diagnosis. It does occur with some

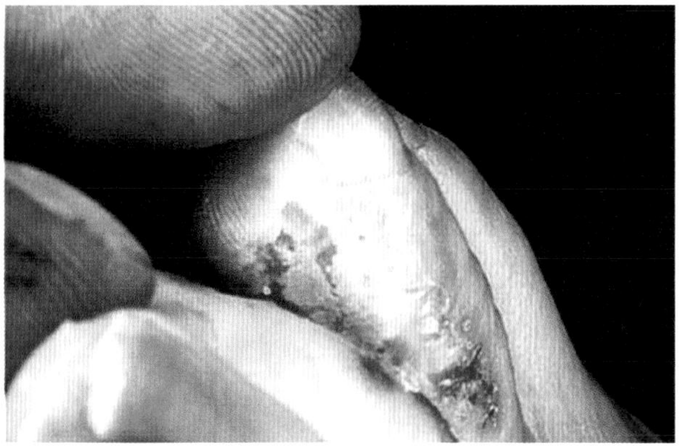

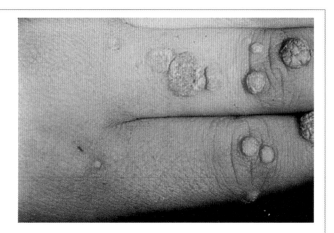

Figure 19.18 Athlete's foot in a teenage boy. Maceration and peeling are seen in the interdigital space.

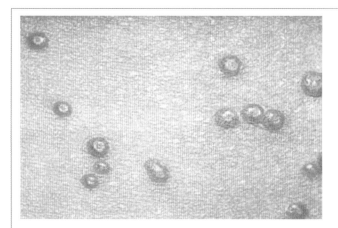

Figure 19.20 Lesions of molluscum contagiosum. Note the characteristic pearly dome-shaped papules.

Figure 19.19 Warts. Note the roughened, irregular, keratotic appearance.

frequency during adolescence. The interdigital spaces between the toes become macerated, with peeling of the surrounding skin. An odour and severe itching are characteristic. Simple measures such as avoidance of occlusive footwear, drying between the toes and the use of antifungal powder usually suffices for most infections.

Common warts

Common warts are harmless and self-limiting. See Figure 19.19. They are transferred by direct contact, but once acquired are spread by autoinoculation.

Clinical features Warts occur most frequently on the hands, face, knees and elbows, and are well-circumscribed papules with a roughened keratotic, irregular surface. If they are situated on the soles of the feet, they are called verrucas or plantar warts, and are usually flush with the surface of the sole because of the pressure of weight bearing. Plantar warts may be painful.

Management Warts tend to disappear spontaneously within two years. No special precautions are indicated for school activities other than swimming, when plantar warts should be covered by a latex sock. If painful, warts can be treated either by the application of a salicylic-acid-based wart paint, or frozen using liquid nitrogen.

Condylomata acuminata

Condylomata acuminata (venereal warts) are moist, fleshy, papillomatous lesions that occur on the perianal mucosa and genitalia. When untreated they proliferate, forming large cauliflower-like masses. They can be transmitted with or without sexual contact, and in prepubertal children they suggest sexual abuse. Cervical infections may become latent and are associated with cervical cancer. Condylomata are treated by repeated application of podophyllin in tincture of iodine.

Molluscum contagiosum

Molluscum contagiosum (Figure 19.20) is a common skin infection caused by a DNA virus. The disease is acquired by direct contact and spread by autoinoculation.

Clinical features The lesions are discrete, pearly, dome-shaped papules which typically have a central umbilication from which a plug of cheesy material can be expressed. The papules may occur anywhere on the body, but particularly on the face, axillae, neck and thighs.

Management Molluscum contagiosum is a self-limited disease, but can persist for months if not years. Treatment, for example with phenol or liquid nitrogen, is generally not required, although should be considered in children who have troublesome local lesions or who also have atopic dermatitis as the infection may spread rapidly.

Cold sore

Recurrent herpes simplex infections are common as cold sores around the mouth (Figure 19.21). The virus persists in a latent form after primary infection and appears as single or grouped vesicles periorally. They tend to recur during respiratory tract infections, menstruation, and stress. There is minimal therapeutic benefit from the use of topical aciclovir. Children do not need to be excluded from day care or school.

Scabies

Scabies infection (Figure 19.22) is caused by a mite which is transmitted by direct contact.

Clinical features The eruption is intensely pruritic, particularly at night, and consists of wheals, papules, vesicles, and a superimposed eczematous dermatitis. A characteristic lesion occurs which, if seen, is pathognomonic for scabies – the mite burrow appears as a thread-like line, commonly seen in the interdigital spaces, but this is often obliterated by scratching. In older children and adults, the head, neck, palms and soles are usually spared, but these areas are often affected in babies.

Management The diagnosis is made by microscopic examination of the mites obtained from scrapings. Treatment requires application of scabicides (malathion or permethrin), but these must be used with extreme caution in babies because of their toxic effects. The eczematous reaction and pruritus may persist for some time because of ongoing hypersensitivity to dead mites. All the household should be treated, and bedding and clothes laundered in hot water.

Head lice (pediculosis capitis)

Head lice (Figure 19.23) are the only common lice infestation in children. They cause intense itching of the scalp. The lice can be transmitted on infested clothing, combs, brushes or direct human contact. The lice themselves are not always visible, but their eggs (or nits) can be readily identified as white specks adherent to the hair shaft, close to the scalp (Figure 19.23a). The adult louse can be extracted by combing the hair with a fine-tooth comb, particularly if this is carried out after washing with conditioner. Combing in this way provides a good preventive measure. Treatment involves the use

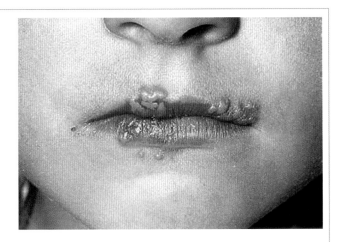

Figure 19.21 Cold sores caused by herpes simplex infection. The lesions are at the pustular stage prior to crusting.

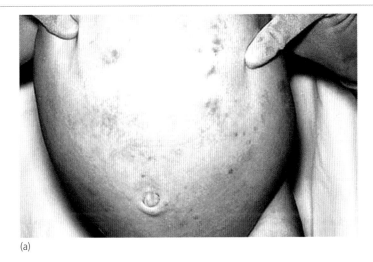
(a)

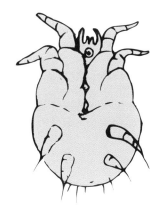
(b)

Figure 19.22 (a) Scabies in an infant; (b) the scabies mite.

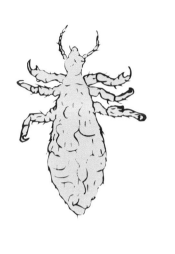

(a)

(b)

Figure 19.23 (a) Nits; (b) a head louse.

of a variety of anti-pediculosis shampoos (e.g. carbaryl). After treatment, removal of nits is not necessary to prevent spread.

Threadworms (enterobiasis)

Threadworm infection causes intense itching of the anus and occasionally the vulval area. It is a common infestation, particularly affecting preschool children. The threadworms reside in the gut, and the gravid females migrate by night to the perianal region to deposit their eggs. Scratching transmits the eggs to the fingers and the eggs become disseminated and ingested.

Clinical features   The infestation may be asymptomatic or may be recognised if a child is seen to be scratching or complains of itching or anal pain.

Management   The diagnosis can sometimes be made by examining the anal area during itching, when a tiny (5mm) white worm may be seen. Alternately, the sticky-tape test can be applied (see Figure 11.9). Sticky tape is applied around the end of a tongue depressor, with the sticky side outermost. This is placed against the child's anus on rising in the morning, and then applied to a glass slide. The threadworm eggs can then be visualized microscopically. Examination of stool specimens does not identify threadworms. Treatment consists of a single dose of mebendazole repeated once after 10 days. The whole family may need to be treated. Reinfection is very common.

Birthmarks

See Figure 19.24.

Pigmented naevi

These naevi are rarely present at birth and start to appear at the age of 2 years. In childhood they are usually flat or only slightly elevated. The risk of malignancy is extremely rare unless they are large congenital naevi.

Café-au-lait spots

Café-au-lait spots are uniformly pigmented, sharply demarcated, macular lesions, which can vary greatly in size. They may be present at birth or develop during childhood. Extensive café au lait spots are a feature of neurofibromatosis (see Figure 19.24).

Strawberry naevus (superficial haemangioma)

These are bright red, protuberant, compressible, sharply demarcated lesions. Almost all of these lesions, even if large, resolve spontaneously. They may increase in size in the first year of life before fading. Oral propranolol is a highly effective and safe modality of treatment for these lesions.

Naevus flammeus (salmon patch)

These are small pink flat lesions that occur most commonly on the eyelids, neck, and forehead. The lesions on the face usually fade and disappear entirely. They are popularly called stork marks – signs left by the beak of the stork at delivery!

Mongolian spots

These are blue or slate-grey lesions which occur most commonly in the sacral area. More than 80% of black and Asian babies are born with them. They usually fade during the first few years of life.

Port-wine stain

Port-wine stains are present at birth. They consist of mature, dilated, dermal capillaries. The lesions are macular, sharply circumscribed, pink to purple in colour and vary in size. If localized to the trigeminal area of the face, the diagnosis of Sturge–Weber syndrome must be considered. In this syndrome there is an underlying meningeal haemangioma and intracranial calcification which can be associated with fits.

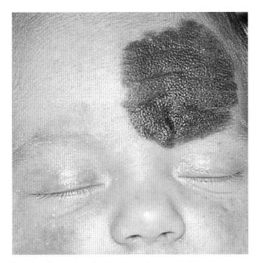
Large pigmented naevus.

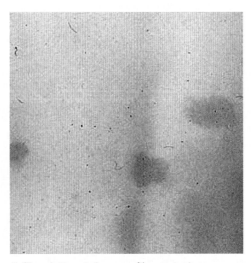
Café au lait spots in neurofibromatosis.

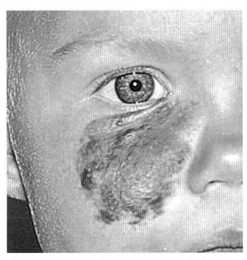
Strawberry naevus (beginning to resolve).

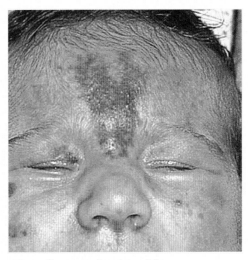
Naevus flammeus ('stork mark').

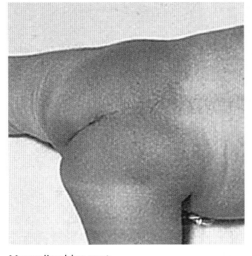
Mongolian blue spot.

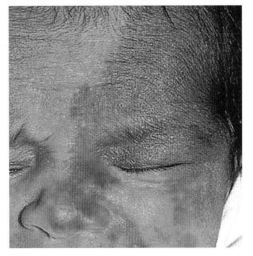
Port-wine stain.

Figure 19.24 Common birthmarks.

To test your knowledge on this part of the book, please see Chapter 26

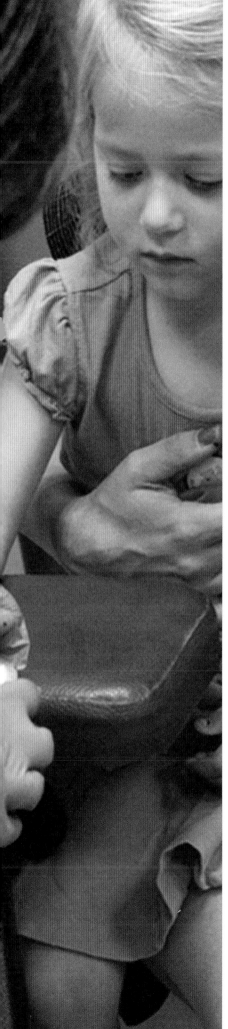

CHAPTER 20

Haematological disorders

And as pale sickness
does invade
Your frailer part, the
breaches made
In that fair lodging, still
more clear
Make the bright guest,
your soul, appear.
Edmund Waller
(1606–1687)

KEY COMPETENCES

YOU MUST...

Know and understand

- The differential diagnosis of children presenting with anaemia, pallor and clotting disorders
- That iron deficiency is very common in young children, its prevention and treatment
- How to manage the important and common haematological conditions in childhood
- When to suspect leukaemia, the principles of its management and outcomes

Be able to

- Investigate and manage a child with microcytic, normocytic and macrocytic anaemia
- Assess a child with easy bruising or excessive bleeding

Appreciate that

- Chronic haematological conditions have an impact on the child and family
- Doctors have an important role in supporting the family of a child with a chronic haematological condition

Essential Paediatrics and Child Health, Fourth Edition. Mary Rudolf, Anthony Luder and Kerry Jeavons.
© 2020 John Wiley & Sons Ltd. Published 2020 by John Wiley & Sons Ltd.
Companion website: www.wiley.com/go/rudolf/paediatrics

Haematological symptoms and signs

Finding your way around...

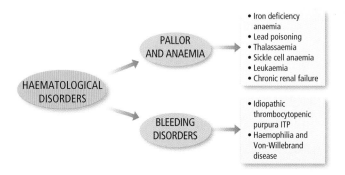

Anaemia and pallor

Causes of anaemia/pallor in childhood

Common causes (hypochromic microcytic)
Iron deficiency anaemia
Thalassaemia trait

Less common causes
Lead poisoning
Haemolysis, e.g. thalassaemia major, sickle cell anaemia
Chronic infection
Chronic renal failure
Malignancy, e.g. leukaemia

Anaemia is usually detected when a blood count is performed routinely or on investigating another problem. It may also be suspected if a child is noted to look pale, lacking in energy, or having a poor appetite. Anaemia may be due to a failure of production, increased destruction (haemolysis) or excessive loss (haemorrhage).

Iron deficiency anaemia is very common in childhood, as it is difficult to maintain sufficient iron stores for growth, when eating inadequate amounts of iron-rich foods, as is common in toddlers. Iron-rich foods include red meats, lentils (beans). Vitamin C aids the absorption of iron.

If a child is ill, other causes of anaemia must be considered. Chronic infection and chronic renal failure give a normochromic normocytic picture. The haemoglobinopathies have characteristic clinical features. Thalassemia causes hypochromic microcytic red blood cell parameters, and in sickle cell anaemia, sickle cells may be evident on the blood film.

The commonest childhood malignancy is leukaemia, which can often be suspected on clinical grounds, and the presence of blast cells in the peripheral blood film.

Haemoglobin levels vary during childhood (Table 7.1, p. 108) and blood counts need to be interpreted accordingly. The neonate starts life with a polycythaemic picture, and a physiological fall occurs in early infancy.

In adulthood, anaemia is always investigated before treatment is started. In childhood, nutritional iron deficiency is so common that it is usual to give a therapeutic trial of iron first, and to investigate only if the response is inadequate, or there are worrying clinical features (see Table 20.1).

If a child fails to respond to iron, and the picture is microcytic and hypochromic, thalassaemia trait or lead toxicity should be considered, and haemoglobin electrophoresis and testing for lead should be carried out (Figure 20.1).

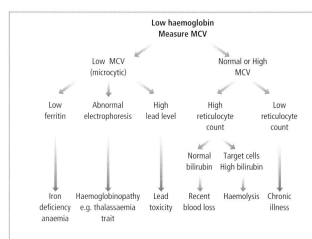

Figure 20.1 Flow diagram to show the investigation of anaemia.

Table 20.1 Possible investigations in the child with anaemia who is ill or unresponsive to iron treatment

Investigation	Relevance
Full blood count	Degree of anaemia
	Type of anaemia (microcytic, hypochromic, etc.)
Blood film	Presence of bizarre cells
	Presence of blast cells (suggest leukaemia)
Ferritin	Low in iron deficiency
Lead level	High in lead toxicity
Haemoglobin electrophoresis	Abnormal in haemoglobinopathies (e.g. thalassaemia, sickle cell anaemia)
Urea and electrolytes	Abnormal in renal failure
Blood and urine culture	Chronic infection
Bone marrow aspiration	Presence of leukaemic cells

Haematological disorders

Iron deficiency anaemia

In the early childhood years, the demand for iron is high to keep up with the rapid growth that occurs at this time. Babies and children commonly have a poor intake of iron-rich foods, and the combination of these two factors results in a high prevalence of iron deficiency. Blood loss may exacerbate the problem if babies are given whole cow's milk too early, as it can induce chronic microscopic bleeding. The incidence of iron deficiency anaemia can be as high as 50% in some populations, depending on dietary and social habits.

Clinical features   Pallor is the most important clue to iron deficiency anaemia. If the haemoglobin level falls significantly, irritability, and anorexia occur. Iron deficiency may also have a detrimental effect on neurological and intellectual functioning. A number of reports suggest that iron deficiency, even in the absence of anaemia, affects attention span, alertness and learning. Severe iron deficiency is associated with pica.

Investigations   The initial finding in iron deficiency is a low ferritin level or a reduced serum iron and raised total iron binding capacity reflecting inadequate iron stores. As the deficiency progresses, the red blood cells become smaller and the haemoglobin content decreases. With increasing severity, the red blood cells become deformed and misshapen and present characteristic microcytosis, hypochromia and poikilocytosis (see Figure 7.2, p. 109).

Management   The treatment is iron salts given orally over 2–3 months so that iron stores are adequately built up. Parents should be advised to limit the consumption of milk and to encourage the consumption of more iron-rich foods. The haemoglobin level starts to increase within 1 week of starting treatment. If it does not, this suggests non-compliance or an incorrect diagnosis.

Prevention   Breast milk provides some protection against the development of iron deficiency. Although it has a relatively low iron content, the iron is absorbed more efficiently because of the iron-binding protein lactoferrin. Since unmodified cow's milk can cause subtle chronic intestinal blood loss, it should not be given during the first year of life. Tea is also inadvisable as it reduces the absorption of iron. In many countries, screening for anaemia is carried out routinely in the first year of life.

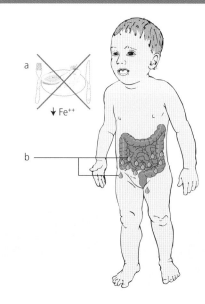

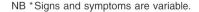

Lead poisoning

Lead affects many enzyme systems, but particularly those involved in haem synthesis. The main sources of lead poisoning used to be lead paint and water from lead pipes. More recently, there has been concern regarding inhalation of atmospheric lead from car exhaust fumes.

Clinical features   Symptoms are usually subtle and non-specific, consisting of irritability, anorexia and decreased play activity. Colic may be present and pica (the chronic ingestion of non-nutrient substances) is a feature of lead poisoning. Acute encephalopathy with vomiting, ataxia and seizures is now rare.

Investigations   The blood picture is one of hypochromic microcytic anaemia. High lead levels confirm the diagnosis. X-ray of the abdomen may demonstrate radiopaque flecks if foreign matter containing lead was recently ingested. X-ray of the long bones may show bands of increased density at the growing ends of the bone (leadlines).

Management   Treatment is directed at removing lead from the body. This is achieved by using lead chelating agents which increase lead excretion. The source of lead must be identified and removed.

Prognosis   Chronic lead exposure has a detrimental effect on intellectual development. Severe lead poisoning carries a high mortality and survivors are often neurologically handicapped.

Thalassaemia

The thalassaemias are a heterogeneous group of inherited anaemias of varying degrees of severity. The underlying genetic defect results in an imbalance of production of the alpha and beta globin chains resulting in ineffective erythropoiesis and haemolysis. Beta thalassaemia is the commonest form, and affects individuals from Asian and Mediterranean backgrounds.

Clinical features   Heterozygous beta thalassaemia (beta thalassaemia trait) produces a mild anaemia and hypochromic microcytic red cell indices. Homozygous thalassaemia (beta thalassaemia major) results in a severe haemolytic anaemia, where compensatory bone marrow hyperplasia produces a characteristic overgrowth of the facial and skull bones (see Figure 20.2). Haemosiderosis with cardiomyopathy, diabetes and skin pigmentation occur as a result of increased iron levels through repeated blood transfusions, although these complications have become reduced since the introduction of desferrioxamine, and more recently, oral chelators.

Investigations   A hypochromic, microcytic anaemia is found in thalassaemia trait, which may be confused with iron deficiency, although both conditions often occur together. In the homozygous state there is severe anaemia, with hypochromia, microcytosis, bizarre fragmented poikilocytes, and target cells. Diagnosis of the type of thalassaemia can be made by haemoglobin electrophoresis; in beta thalassaemia major HbA$_1$ is absent and HbA$_2$ and HbF

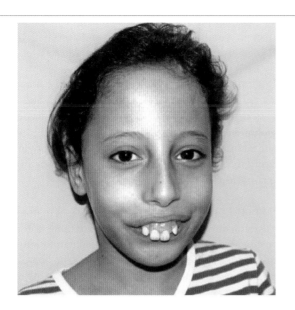

Figure 20.2 A child with thalassaemia. Note the characteristic facial features with frontal bossing and maxillary overgrowth, and skin pigmentation due to haemosiderosis.

greatly increased. In thalassaemia trait there may be a mild anaemia with hypochromic and microcytic red cells. Haemoglobin electrophoresis shows a raised HbA2. Currently, molecular biology and gene sequencing offers a more definitive diagnosis.

Management Thalassaemia trait requires no treatment. Its main importance is the genetic implication and distinguishing it from iron deficiency and lead poisoning. In thalassaemia major, blood transfusions are given on a regular basis to maintain haemoglobin levels and reduce endogenous hematopoiesis. Haemosiderosis (overload with iron) is an inevitable consequence, but can be minimized by the use of subcutaneous or intravenous infusions of the chelating agent desferrioxamine. Oral iron chelating agents have been developed and are also used.

Thalassaemia major at a glance

Epidemiology
Beta thalassaemia is the
   commonest form
In the UK, it is seen
   predominantly in children of
   Greek Cypriot or
   Bangladeshi origin

Aetiology/pathophysiology
A genetic defect of globin chain
   synthesis causing ineffective
   erythropoiesis in the bone
   marrow and premature
   destruction of circulating red
   blood cells by the spleen
Clinical features are related to
   haemosiderosis caused by
   treatment

History
Anaemia and jaundice from
   babyhood
Family history of thalassaemia

Physical examination
• Anaemia (**a**)
• Maxillary overgrowth, frontal
   bossing (**b**)
• Hepatosplenomegaly (**c**)
• Skin pigmentation due to
   haemosiderosis (**d**)
• Short stature and delayed
   puberty (**e**)

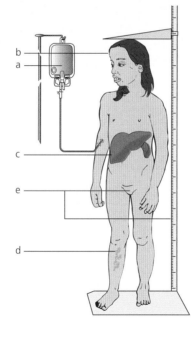

Confirmatory investigations
Hypochromic microcytic
   anaemia
High HbF and HbA$_2$ on
   haemoglobin electrophoresis
Antenatal diagnosis is available

Differential diagnosis
Thalassaemia major: other
   causes of severe haemolytic
   anaemia
Thalassaemia minor: iron
   deficiency, lead toxicity

Management
Regular blood transfusions to
   maintain haemoglobin levels
Subcutaneous intravenous or
   oral iron chelate to excrete
   iron overload
Genetic counselling for family

Prognosis/complications
Without treatment, life
   expectancy is only a few
   years
Haemosiderosis caused by
   frequent blood transfusions
   leads to cardiomyopathy,
   cirrhosis, diabetes and
   endocrinopathies
Thalassaemia minor (the
   heterozygous carrier state) is
   asymptomatic, and detected

Sickle cell anaemia

Sickle cell anaemia is the commonest of the haemoglobinopathies, and principally occurs in black populations. The homozygous condition is referred to as sickle cell anaemia and the heterozygous condition as sickle cell trait. The underlying genetic defect is a substitution of glutamic acid by valine as the 6th amino-acid in the beta globin chain, causing an unstable haemoglobin (HbS). This change is due to a single nucleotide polymorphism of adenosine to thymine. When HbS is deoxygenated, it forms highly structured polymers which cause brittle, spiny red cells. The clinical manifestations of the disease are caused by ischaemic changes, which result from occlusion of blood vessels by masses of sickled cells. There is also increased susceptibility to infectious disease – pneumococcal and *Salmonella typhi*.

Clinical features   Sickle cell anaemia is a serious disease characterised by a chronic haemolytic anaemia. Children experience recurrent, acute, painful crises which can be precipitated by dehydration, hypoxia or acidosis. Painful swelling of the hands and feet is a common early presentation. Repeated splenic infarctions tend to occur in the early years, eventually leaving the child asplenic and susceptible to serious infections. Renal damage leads to a reduced ability to concentrate urine, making dehydration a severe problem. Acute chest syndrome is caused by sickling in the lungs, often associated with infection, and the resulting hypoxia results in a worsening circle of sickling and occlusion of the pulmonary vasculature, require exchange trans-fusion to halt this process. Sickle cell trait is asymptomatic other than in conditions of low oxygen tensions such as occur at high altitude or under general anaesthesia.

Investigations   The peripheral blood smear in the homozygote state typically contains target cells, poikilocytes, and irreversibly sickled cells (Figure 20.3). Diagnosis is made by haemoglobin electrophoresis, and the 'sickle test' (an in vitro test where addition of a reducing agent causes turbidity in the presence of HbSS). This may also be used for screening in susceptible populations.

Management   Treatment of crises is largely symptomatic with analgesics, antibiotics, warmth, adequate fluids and oxygen if required to maintain normal oxygen saturations. In severe cases with a high proportion of HbS (>40%) 'top-up' or exchange transfusion is considered. It is important to maintain immunisation status, and daily lifelong prophylactic penicillin must be given to reduce the risk of pneumococcal disease. Prophylactic treatment with hydroxyurea increases the concentration of HbF at the expense of HbS and has been shown to reduce dramatically the incidence of painful crises and admissions to hospital.

Prognosis   Antenatal screening with specialist counselling of prospective parents is important. Neonatal screening programmes can ensure early identification of affected children and reduce morbidity and mortality by enabling early recognition, treatment of crises and early commencement of pneumococcal prophylaxis.

Sickle cell anaemia at a glance

Epidemiology
Commonest
 haemoglobinopathy
Predominantly seen in black
Americans, Africans,
 Afro-Caribbeans
Autosomal recessive inheritance

Pathogenesis
Genetic mutation of the Hb
 chain results in unstable
 haemoglobin (HbS)
When deoxygenated, HbS
 causes sickling of red cells
 which occlude the
 microcirculation
Crises are precipitated by
 dehydration, hypoxia, acidosis

History
Recurrent acute painful crises
 affecting any organ

Physical examination
Chronic anaemia
Flow murmur
• Jaundice* (**a**)
• Chronic leg ulcers* (**b**)
• Dactylitis (**c**)
• Splenomegaly in young child
 only (**d**)
• Haematuria* (**e**)

Confirmatory investigations
Low haemoglobin, sickle cells
 on smear
HbS and absent HbA on
 haemoglobin electrophoresis
Abnormal liver function tests

NB *Signs and symptoms are variable.

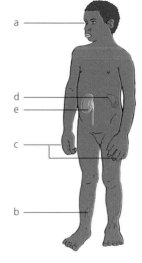

Differential diagnosis
Leukaemia
Arthritis

Complications
Chronic haemolysis
Recurrent painful crises due to
 ischaemic occlusions
Aplastic crises
Sequestration crises causing
 circulatory collapse
Pneumococcal infection due to
 asplenism and *Salmonella*
Osteomyelitis
Renal damage with reduced
 ability to concentrate urine
Gallstones
Heart failure from chronic
 anaemia

Management
Analgesics, antibiotics, warmth,
 fluids during crises

Long-term treatment with
 hydroxyurea increases
 concentration of HbF at the
 expense of HbS. Fewer crises
 and admissions

Blood transfusion if Hb falls
 markedly during an aplastic,
 sequestration or haemolytic
 crisis
Maintenance of immunisations
Penicillin prophylaxis to prevent
 pneumococcal infection
Genetic counselling for family

Prognosis
High mortality from sepsis
 under age 3 years 85%
 survive to age 20 years
Heterozygous state is
 asymptomatic although
 microscopic haematuria
 may be observed. (unless
 in very low oxygen tensions
 as with GA or high altitude)

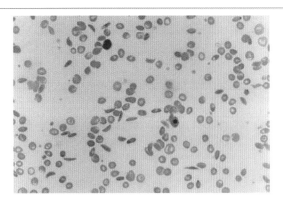

Figure 20.3 Sickle cell anaemia. Peripheral blood smear with target cells, poikilocytes and irreversibly sickled cells.

Splenectomy and hyposplenism

Children who lack an effective spleen are at increased risk of sepsis. Hyposplenism may occur as a result of sickle cell disease (due to autoinfarction), splenectomy for trauma and some metabolic and haematological conditions.

Clinical features   The major risk of hyposplenism is infection, especially due to encapsulated *Streptococcus pneumoniae* or *Haemophilus influenzae*, resulting in overwhelming sepsis or meningitis. This risk is especially high in children under 5 years old. As the spleen is responsible for filtering the blood and early antibody responses, sepsis can progress rapidly, leading to death within 24 hours.

Treatment and prevention   Regular penicillin prophylaxis reduces the risk of infection in hyposplenic children. Pneumococcal vaccination, now part of routine childhood immunisation, should be given pre-splenectomy to those children who missed out previously.

Idiopathic thrombocytopenic purpura (ITP)

ITP presents with petechiae and superficial bruising (Figure 20.4), but mucosal bleeding from the gums and nose may also occur. Although as the name suggests it has no known cause, it nevertheless often follows 1 or 2 weeks after a viral infection, which is thought to trigger an immunological basis underlying the destruction of circulating platelets.

Clinical features   The onset is frequently acute, and apart from the signs of bleeding the child appears clinically well. The most serious complication is intracranial haemorrhage, which is very rare and occurs in less than 1% of cases. One of the features of ITP is that even when the platelet count is in single figures, there is often no clinical bleeding – the platelets remain fully functional and effective.

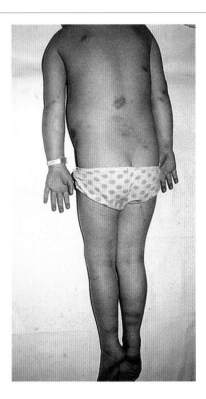

Figure 20.4 Idiopathic thrombocytopenic purpura.

Investigations   Diagnosis is made on the finding of a platelet count which is reduced to below 40×10^9/L and may be below 5×10^9/L. The white cell count is normal and there is generally no anaemia. The blood film may show atypical or reactive (viral) lymphocytes. As the differential diagnosis includes an aplastic or neoplastic process of the bone marrow, bone marrow aspiration should be considered, especially if treatment (see below) is being considered, which may mask a neoplastic process. In ITP a normal or increased number of megakaryocytes is seen, reflecting the increased turnover which occurs as a result of the destruction of platelets peripherally.

Management   In those who have only mild symptoms no treatment is necessary, but where there is a risk of severe bleeding a short course of steroids or immunoglobulin infusion may produce a rise in the platelet count. Platelet transfusion is of little benefit as the transfused platelets survive only briefly. They should be administered, however, if life-threatening haemorrhage occurs.

Prognosis   Idiopathic thrombocytopenic purpura has an excellent prognosis, with 85% having a self-limited course. Severe spontaneous haemorrhage and intracranial bleeding are usually confined to the initial phase of the disease. The majority of children recover spontaneously within 6 months, although ITP becomes chronic for a few children (10-20%). Splenectomy and immunosuppressive therapy may be required in these cases. Recent advances in biological agents provide hope for chronic resistant cases.

👁 Idiopathic thrombocytopenic purpura at a glance

Aetiology
Destruction of circulating platelets by immune mechanism

History
Generally well
Bleeding from nose and gums*
Non-blanching red or purple spots, bruises unrelated to trauma
Preceding viral infection 1–2 weeks before*

Physical examination
Petechial rash (**a**)
Superficial bruising (**b**)

Confirmatory investigations
Low platelet count (<20 × 10^9/L)
Normal white cell count, normal haemoglobin
Bone marrow aspirate shows normal or increased number of megakaryocytes (bone marrow rarely done in typical cases)

NB *Signs and symptoms are variable.

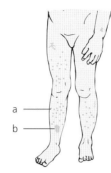

Pathogenesis
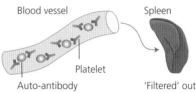
Blood vessel
Spleen
Platelet
Auto-antibody
'Filtered' out in the spleen

Differential diagnosis
Leukaemia
Aplastic anaemia

Management
Monitor platelet count
Short course of steroids or IV gamma globulin for frank bleeding
Platelet transfusion for life-threatening haemorrhage

Prognosis/complications
85% of patients have simple limited course
Spontaneous haemorrhage or intracranial bleeding are the worrying complications
A few patients develop chronic ITP and need splenectomy and immunosuppressive therapy
New biological agents offer hope for resistant cases

Leukaemia

Leukaemia is the most common childhood cancer, accounting for approximately 30% of cases. It characterised by a malignant proliferation of white cell precursors which occupy the bone marrow. These blast cells may also circulate in the blood and deposit in various tissues. The commonest leukaemia in childhood is acute lymphoblastic leukaemia (ALL), in which the blast cells resemble primitive precursors of lymphoid origin: 70% being B-cell precursors and the remainder T-cell. It can occur at any age, but the peak incidence is 2 to 5 years.

Clinical features   The onset is usually insidious with anorexia, irritability and lethargy. As the bone marrow fails, pallor, bleeding and fever occur. Bone pain may be an important presenting complaint. Rarely, signs of increasing intracranial pressure such as headache and vomiting indicate meningeal involvement, or a lump in the testes indicating testicular involvement. On examination, petechiae or mucous membrane bleeding may be present, and lymphadenopathy and splenomegaly may be found.

Investigations   Most patients have a markedly elevated white cell count, anaemia and thrombocytopenia on the peripheral blood smear. Blast cells may be seen (Figure 20.5).

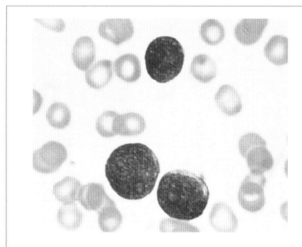

Figure 20.5 Acute lymphoblastic leukaemia (ALL). Peripheral blood smear. Note blast cells.

The definitive diagnosis is made on examination of the bone marrow, which is replaced by leukaemic lymphoblasts.

Management   The basic components of treatment include induction chemotherapy, which is given until the child no longer shows leukaemic cells, prophylactic treatment to the central nervous system, and a continuation of systemic treatment (maintenance therapy) for 2–3 years. The child needs to be followed closely for relapse and, if this occurs, intensive retreatment is required. With increasing intensification of treatment in high risk groups, febrile neutropenia and sepsis is a not uncommon complication, requiring broad-spectrum antibiotics and haematopoeitic growth factors. As in all immunosuppressed patients, whether resulting from the underlying disease or its treatment, vigilance is required especially for school-aged children. Contact with cases of measles and chicken pox is particularly concerning, and treatment with hyper or specific gammaglobulin required.

Prognosis   The prognosis varies with the type of ALL, but the aim is for cure. The current cure rate is greater than 80% even in high risk groups. The prognosis is less favourable if the child is less than 2 or more than 10 years of age; boys have a slightly worse prognosis due to testicular infiltration.

👁 Leukaemia at a glance

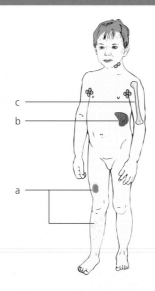

Epidemiology
Commonest childhood
  malignancy
80% of childhood leukaemias
  are acute lymphoblastic
  leukaemia (ALL)

Aetiology
Malignant proliferation of white
  cell precursors

History
Insidious onset
Anorexia, irritability, lethargy
Fever
Bone pain*
Mucous membrane bleeding *

Physical examination
Pallor
• Petechiae, bruising* (a)
• Lymphadenopathy, spleno-
  megaly* (b)
• Bone tenderness* (c)

Confirmatory investigations
Peripheral blood: high white cell
  count, anaemia,
  thrombocytopenia, blast cells
Bone marrow: replaced by
  leukaemic lymphoblasts

Differential diagnosis
Chronic infection
Bleeding diatheses
Other causes of
  lymphadenopathy
Other tumours infiltrating the
  bone marrow

Management
Chemotherapy to induce
  remission
Ongoing less intense
  chemotherapy for 2 years
Prophylaxis (chemotherapy/
  radiation) to the CNS
Close monitoring and treatment
  of relapses
Psychosocial support

Prognosis
Depends on the leukaemia. In
  favourable presentations of
  ALL, 75% are cured. There is
  a less favourable outcome of
  <2 years or >10 years

Haemophilia and Von-Willebrand disease

Haemophilia A (factor VIII deficiency) is a common inherited coagulation disorder, occurring in 1:5000 of newborn males, and inherited as an X-linked recessive condition. Presenting symptoms and signs include prolonged bleeding which may occur after tonsillectomy or circumcision, spontaneous soft tissue and joint haemarthrosis, and muco-cutaneous bleeding, such as epistaxis. Prolongation of the 'intrinsic pathway' is detected by the activated partial thromboplastin test (APTT).

Treatment is mainly with recombinant factor VIII products. Von-Willebrand disease is made up of a common group of autosomal dominant conditions characterised by a deficiency of Von-Willebrand factor (VWF). Bleeding is often mild to moderate with nose bleeds, menorrhagia and bleeding after tooth extraction being typical. Treatment is with vasopressin (DDAVP) or VWF concentrates in severe cases.

To test your knowledge on this part of the book, please see Chapter 26

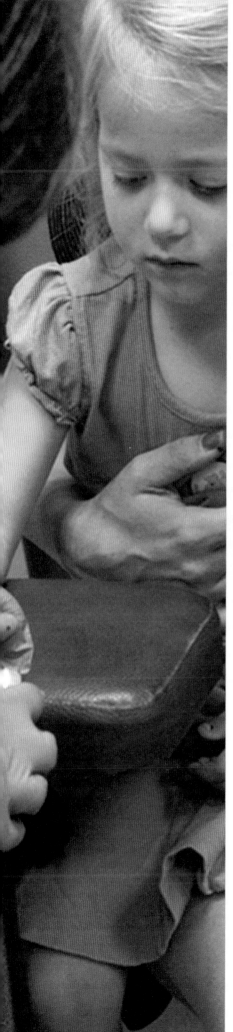

CHAPTER 21

Emotional, behavioural and educational problems

She was not really bad at heart,
But only rather rude and wild;
She was an aggravating child.
'Rebecca, Who Slammed Doors
for Fun', Hilaire Belloc

Emotional, behavioural and educational difficulties

Common behavioural, emotional and educational problems

KEY COMPETENCES

YOU MUST...

Know and understand

- The range of emotional and behavioural problems that commonly occur in childhood
- Effective approaches to managing emotional and behavioural problems in childhood
- Family and school stresses that contribute to the development of behavioural problems
- Circumstances that protect against emotional and behavioural difficulties
- Types of behaviour indicative of serious disturbance

Be able to

- Obtain a good picture of a child's behavioural and emotional difficulties
- Make a good assessment of family circumstances relevant to behavioural and emotional problems

Appreciate that

- Behavioural problems are common, if not universal
- These problems can be extremely stressful for all in the family
- Parenting is a difficult task
- A good evaluation does not focus on the child alone
- Being consistent about limits is an important part of rearing children but praise is more powerful than punishment

Essential Paediatrics and Child Health, Fourth Edition. Mary Rudolf, Anthony Luder and Kerry Jeavons.
© 2020 John Wiley & Sons Ltd. Published 2020 by John Wiley & Sons Ltd.
Companion website: www.wiley.com/go/rudolf/paediatrics

Emotional, behavioural and educational difficulties

Finding your way around...

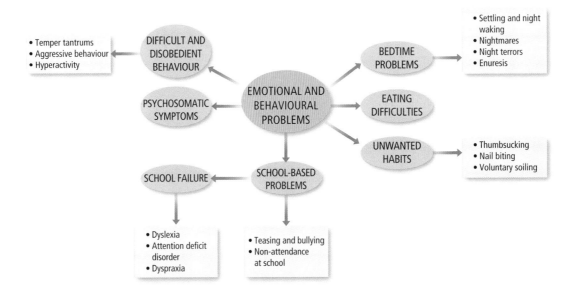

Common emotional, behavioural and educational problems in childhood

Sleeping difficulties
Eating problems
Unwanted habits
Difficult and disobedient behaviour
School-based problems
Psychosomatic symptoms
Enuresis

In recent years parents have been turning increasingly more to their doctors for guidance about a variety of emotional, social and educational problems, so much so that these have been called the 'new morbidities of childhood'. It is important therefore that physicians feel comfortable and competent in addressing them.

Emotional and behavioural problems occur to a degree in all children, but they can become exaggerated for a variety of reasons, either related to the child, or as a result of the way they are handled. Other difficulties arise as a result of stresses in the family, such as death or divorce, or are caused by problems at school.

The problems become pathological when they disturb the child's or family's wellbeing and functioning.

Some childhood behaviours, notably deliberate violent or destructive conduct and self-harm, running away, encopresis and age-inappropriate sexual behaviour are indicative of serious disturbance (see Red Flag box).

Behaviour indicative of serious disturbance

Behaviour	Disturbance
Deliberately destructive	Low self-esteem, hostile relationships
Deliberate self-harm	Severe distress, low self-esteem
Running away	Lack of affection, severe distress
Voluntary encopresis (deliberate soiling in inappropriate places)	Lack of self-worth, inadequate care
Age-inappropriate sexual behaviour	Sexual abuse

Table 21.1 Factors contributing to emotional and behavioural problems

In the child

Difficult temperament

Developmental delay

Poor self-image

School failure

Abuse

In the family

Marital problems

Death of a relative, friend or pet

Poor discipline

Poverty

In school

Change of school

Bullying and social media shaming

Poor peer relationships

Table 21.2 Factors that protect against emotional/behavioural problems

Consistent loving relationships

Adequate income

Stable family relationships

Support outside the family

Factors that contribute to emotional and behavioural problems, and those that protect against their development, are shown in Tables 21.1 and 21.2.

When addressing emotional and behavioural problems, it is essential that the focus does not rest on the child alone. An understanding of the concerns must be seen in the context of the family and the child's environment. Even if these factors are not directly responsible for the problem (and they often are), it is impossible to address the issue without a good understanding of the broader picture. It is also important to remember that handling these problems well takes both time and empathy.

History – must ask!

- *The problem.* Obtain a full picture of the problem or difficulty, with the parents' perceptions of the cause, and how the situation is handled. It is worthwhile to include the child in this process if he or she is old enough.
- *The child.* Gain an understanding of the child's temperament and personality, how the child is viewed by the parents, and how he or she relates to friends and family.
- *Recent events.* Childhood disturbances often occur as a reaction to events in the family. Common triggers include the birth of a sibling, the death of a grandparent or a move to a new house or school.
- *The family.* An understanding of family circumstances is essential. Marital friction is a common source of childhood emotional and behavioural problems, and single parents are likely to have more difficulties in disciplining and coping with their children single-handed. Isolation compounds any problem, and it is important to assess the level of support from relatives and friends.
- *School or nursery.* School life brings its own problems and also affects how the child adjusts to difficulties at home. Peer and teacher relationships are as important to assess as the level of academic achievement.

Management of the child with emotional and behavioural problems

While emotional and behavioural problems differ from one another and from family to family, there is a commonality to approaching their management. Perhaps the most important aspect is to listen well, hearing a full account of the problem. This in itself can be therapeutic, and can lead the family to find solutions themselves. The process of listening cannot be rushed: adequate time must be given.

Many parental concerns relate to normal behaviour, for example, food fads in toddlers or night waking in infants, and it may be adequate simply to provide reassurance. Other concerns relate to difficult behaviour, and guidance regarding effective discipline is required.

The general principles of effective discipline include providing structure and routine in everyday life, setting clear limits of acceptable behaviour, rewarding good behaviour, and being consistent with punishments. Punitive anger is often ineffective and does not encourage the child to learn to control his or her actions and emotions. It is helpful to remind parents that positive results can be obtained by simply 'catching their child being good', rather than always looking to punish negative behaviour (see Box 21.1).

Box 21.1 Parental guidelines for preventing and managing difficult behaviour

- Provide structure and routine in everyday life
- Set clear limits of acceptable behaviour
- Be consistent
- 'Catch your child being good' and reward positive rather than punish negative behaviour
- Enforce the above with love and affection
- Star charts and time out are useful strategies

	1st Week	2nd Week	3rd Week	4th Week	
Monday		★		★	
Tuesday			★	★	
Wednesday	★		★	★	
Thursday		★	★	★	
Friday				★	
Saturday		★	★	★	
Sunday	★			★	

Figure 21.1 A star chart kept by a 4-year-old boy to encourage good behaviour.

Star charts

A useful strategy in overcoming difficult behaviour is using a star chart (Figure 21.1), which can be adapted to improve and motivate a variety of behaviours, such as temper tantrums and disruptive behaviour at school. A calendar is drawn up, and each day the child has behaved as required, a star or smiley face is awarded. When a certain number of stars have been earned, the child is rewarded with a prize. This method can be very effective in reinforcing desirable behaviour, while alleviating focus on the negative.

Time out

Time out is a strategy used during an episode of difficult behaviour. The child is required to stay in a quiet spot for a fixed short period of time. One minute per year of age is a good guide, and a kitchen timer a useful way of enforcing the time. This method allows the child (and the parent) time to cool off, and also gives the parent a clear but limited non-violent means of discipline.

An important aspect of good management is to arrange a follow-up appointment for the parents. Other professionals may also provide support and help. The health visitor is a particular asset for preschool children, and teachers for school-aged children. More intransigent problems may require referral to a child psychologist or psychiatrist.

Key points: Emotional and behavioural problems

- Allow adequate time to make a full assessment
- Ensure that you obtain a full picture of the problem, the child, the family and the environment. If the child is old enough, obtain his or her account too
- Family and school issues must be addressed as well as the child's problems. Where relevant, confer with others involved such as grandparents, teachers, childminders, etc.
- Parents need to be provided with guidelines for effective discipline, to be enforced with love and affection
- Do not wait for a child to grow out of a problem. Even if the problem resolves, the child may remain psychologically disturbed
- Medication has a very limited role and should only be prescribed by specialists

Common behavioural, emotional and educational problems

Difficulties in settling to sleep and waking through the night

Babies and children differ in their requirements for sleep, and parents vary in their ability to tolerate their child waking in the night. A substantial number of children have struggles around bedtime, and reports indicate that as many as one-third of preschool children have disturbed sleep.

In most babies sleeping 'difficulties' are simply habit. Waking during the night is a normal phenomenon; failure to return to sleep independently is not. It usually results from a lack of early establishment of routine, and this develops so that toddlers readily realize that by playing up at bedtime they can receive attention. Feeding and attending to infants who wake at night reinforces this behaviour and makes it intractable. Sleep difficulties can also occur as a result of conflict in the family, or anxieties, such as starting school or fear of dying.

Clinical features   Sleeping problems include a refusal to settle at night and crying through the night. Difficulties in settling commonly develop if babies are only put to bed once they are already asleep, and may also persist when a child wakes at night as a result of being unwell. A common mistake is when parents take their child into their bed or sleep with the child for comfort. Once this pattern is established, it is difficult to break.

Management   Parents may be resigned to sleepless nights and may not be aware that they are capable of controlling the situation. The problem can only be overcome if they are determined to tackle it. This is most easily achieved at an age when the child cannot climb out of bed. Night sedation is not advisable and should only be used as a last resort.

Successful management involves the principles outlined in Box 21.2. A regular routine should be firmly established with parents adopting a calm, understanding but determined attitude, while avoiding angry threats and punishments. Bedtime should be set at a regular time, with time for a quiet, restful pre-bedtime routine, which might include a warm bath, light snack and reading a story. At the set time the child should resolutely be put to bed. If the child cries then, or later through the night, the crying should be ignored, or if that proves to be too stressful for the parent, the child may be checked but no positive attention given. On no account should the child be taken to the parental bed. If the parents are resolute, the sleeping problem resolves within a short period. However, it is usually a stressful undertaking and plenty of support, reassurance and encouragement are required.

Nightmares and night terrors

In a *nightmare* the child wakes as a result of a bad dream, becomes lucid quickly, and usually remembers the dream's content. The child can often simply be reassured and returned to sleep. Nightmares may occur as a result of stresses, and if persistent may need psychological help.

Night terrors (see p. 247) are a sleep problem of the preschool years. By contrast with a nightmare, the child wakes confused, disorientated, and frightened, and fails to recognise the parent. Minutes pass before orientation occurs, and the dream cannot usually be recalled. Night terrors should not be confused with epilepsy. They are short-lived and reassurance alone is required.

Eating difficulties

Most children at some stage or another develop food fads. Difficulties frequently result if there is excessive parental insistence on eating, and anxiety when the child refuses to do so. In fact, most of the worry about children's eating is unnecessary, and the majority of children come through this phase thriving and unscathed. Mismanagement by parents can result in a great deal of conflict and stress at mealtimes, which is particularly distressing as it challenges the parents' basic need to nurture. The problems are compounded if the eating problems are associated with failure to thrive (see p. 283).

Occasionally, severe eating problems are caused by emotional stress and can be associated with problems in the parent–child relationship. Eating disorders in adolescence are discussed in Chapter 25.

Clinical features   Eating difficulties may present early in infancy, or more commonly develop during weaning. They may follow a minor illness, where appetite is naturally

---

Box 21.2 Parental guidelines for preventing and managing sleeping problems

- Set a bedtime
- Have a relaxing bedtime routine
- Say goodnight
- If the child cries, ignore or at least give no positive attention
- Do not feed or give drinks at night
- If the child gets out of bed, return him or her promptly and firmly
- Give positive reinforcement following good nights

reduced, and negative reactions to food are set up as a result of parental insistence to eat. The child then develops adversative behaviour such as refusing to eat, spitting out or throwing food, or even vomiting (Figure 21.2). Parents too often respond by force-feeding, playing games, preparing alternative meals, or persisting with lengthy mealtimes in order to get just another mouthful in.

Management Eating difficulties can be hard to tackle. It is important to reduce parents' anxiety, and it is often helpful to demonstrate that the child is growing normally according to a growth chart. Battles over food are always best avoided, and relaxed, social family meals should be encouraged (see Box 21.3). A high chair is invaluable for the toddler at mealtimes, both for comfort and restraint. The child's appetite should be respected, and no attempts made to make the child eat by bribery, games, or force. With reduction in anxiety and pressure the problem usually resolves. Although the diet often lacks variety, it is usually nutritionally adequate, and prescription of vitamins is not necessary.

Unwanted habits

Children not infrequently indulge in habits that concern their parents. These include thumb-sucking, head-banging, body-rocking, nail-biting, hair-pulling, teeth-grinding and tics. The child may not be able to control these habits, which may be further reinforced by parents attempting to stop the child exhibiting them. As the child grows older, he or she often learns to inhibit the habit, particularly in social situations.

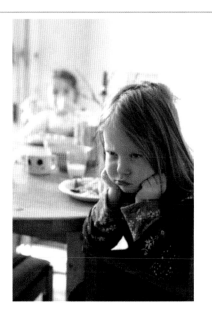

Figure 21.2 Eating difficulties are very common in young children.

> ### Box 21.3 Parental guidelines for preventing and managing eating difficulties
>
> - Be guided by the child's appetite
> - Mealtimes should be relaxed social events
> - Do not resort to bribery, games or force
> - End the meal at the first sign of adverse behaviour
> - Do not provide alternatives if a meal is refused

Thumb-sucking

Thumb-sucking is normal in early infancy. However, beyond a certain age it makes the older child appear immature and may interfere with normal alignment of the teeth. It is a difficult habit to influence, and it is best to ignore it as it resolves over time. The child who actively tries to restrain thumb-sucking should be given praise and encouragement.

Nail-biting

Nail-biting is a difficult habit to break, and it is only possible to influence if the child is resolved to do so. Application of bitter tasting nail varnish can be helpful. In some children nail-biting is a sign of tension.

Masturbation

Masturbation is a normal and pleasurable self-stimulation, but this sometimes presents as a problem, particularly if it occurs publicly. It is more likely to appear when the child is bored, anxious, or tired, and the child can often be distracted at these times. Dressing the child in clothes that make access more difficult may help. The habit should be ignored in younger children. The older child should not be reprimanded, but needs to understand that it is not acceptable to be carried out publicly.

Enuresis – night-time wetting

Failure to achieve nocturnal dryness or regression to wetting may be a sign of stress. For example, birth of a sibling, death in the family, marital conflict, and sexual abuse have all traditionally been implicated as a cause. Wetting is however increasingly understood to mostly have a physical basis – usually an inherited condition, with nocturnal partial deficiency of antidiuretic hormone and difficulty in waking to the stimulus of a full bladder. Most behavioral and self-esteem problems disappear upon successful resolution of the wetting. The prevalence is nonetheless slightly higher in those with externalizing disorders such as ADHD. Undue emphasis on a psycho-behavioral cause is unwarranted. Enuresis is fully discussed in Chapter 17 (p. 321).

Encopresis

Encopresis is due to functional retention of faeces, and subsequent leakage of stool. In the past it was seen as a behavioral disorder often attributed to some stressful trigger. This causal explanation no longer applies in the majority of cases, although stress and behavioral problems are undoubtedly a consequence of having encopresis. Most encopretic children have little voluntary control of their bowel motions and have decreased awareness of the retained faeces (rectal hyposensitivity). Nonetheless there is sometimes an association with externalizing disorders such as ADHD, oppositional defiant disorders, and some behavioural problems, especially in children who do not have retained faeces. Encopresis and soiling are covered in Chapter 11 (p. 198).

Psychosomatic symptoms

Some children manifest emotional problems in the form of somatization or functional symptoms. The commonest of these are abdominal pain in the younger child and headaches in the older child, although both these may indicate simple functional disturbances and not underlying emotional pathology. Organic causes for these complaints should be excluded (see Chapters 11 and 13), as well as seeking for positive indications of an underlying emotional cause.

Difficult and disobedient behaviour

Temper tantrums

Temper tantrums (Figure 21.3) are a normal part of children's development and peak around 18 months to 3 years.

Clinical features   Frustration, anger and tantrums are typical for toddlers, and may involve hitting, biting and other aggressive behaviour. Some babies and toddlers resort to

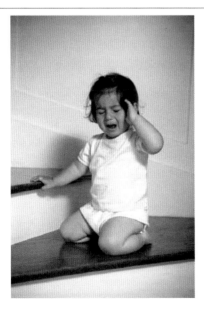

Figure 21.3 A toddler having a temper tantrum. These are best handled firmly and can often by diverted by giving the child a choice of acceptable activity. Time out is a helpful strategy.

breath-holding (see p. 247) as part of the tantrum, and this is often a frightening event to witness.

Management   Parents' response to tantrums is very important. Caregivers who respond to toddler defiance with punitive anger run the risk of reinforcing defiance, and teach the child that out-of-control emotions are a reasonable response to frustration. Temper tantrums need firm handling, without anger and aggression (see Box 21.4). Avoiding high-risk situations like hunger and tiredness, and providing distraction or giving the child a simple choices of activities can often avert them. Once the tantrum is in full cry, it is best to ignore it until the child has calmed down. Time out is an excellent strategy for managing the tantrum after the event.

Aggressive behaviour

Young children often have aggressive outbursts, ranging from temper tantrums to hurting others or destroying toys or furniture. This behaviour usually results from frustration and the child's inability to deal with it. Most children learn to control their aggression, but some fail to do so, and it escalates as a problem, leading to bullying in primary school, and delinquency beyond. If the behaviour is extreme, the psychiatric term 'conduct disorder' is applied.

Clinical features   Several factors contribute to aggression. Boys more than girls, large, active children, and children from larger families tend to show more aggressive behaviour. Marital discord and aggression within the home contribute to its expression, and exposure to aggression on television may also have an effect. There is a relationship between aggression and emotional disturbance, school failure, brain damage and overactivity.

Management   Parents need to be consistent in their management of the child exhibiting aggressive behaviour, and, difficult though it may be, must resist from counteracting aggression with more aggression. Both time out and star charts are positive methods for managing the child. It is important for the doctor to explore whether frustration, disturbance and tensions in the home can be reduced.

> **Box 21.4 Parental guidelines for preventing and managing temper tantrums**
>
> - Prevent tantrums by avoiding high-risk situations such as hunger and tiredness
> - Attempt to divert the tantrum if possible
> - Teach control by example
> - Reward good behaviour
> - Ignore the behaviour and leave the child until calm
> - Use time out as a strategy

For the school-age child, staff at school must be involved in order to address any academic or social problems, and to gain cooperation in instituting behaviour modification. If aggression and bullying (see below) are general problems at school, instituting a school-based intervention can be effective.

Hyperactivity (see also attention deficit disorder, p. 389)

Attention deficit disorder may or may not be associated with hyperactivity. The two together are characterised by poor ability to attend to a task, motor over-activity and impulsivity. In the preschool years, children are naturally active and tend to have a short attention span for activities. How this is viewed often depends on parental perceptions, and a child with high spirits in one family may be perceived as hyperactive in another. Many so-called hyperactive children are able to concentrate well enough if an activity interests them (such as playing a video game) and the overlap with simple lack of discipline may be difficult to distinguish.

Boys tend to manifest hyperactivity more than girls, and there is often a family history. Babies who have been temperamentally difficult are more likely to develop into hyperactive children, and it is more common in children with delay of developmental milestones. Hyperactivity is also seen in children who have never been given limits or taught to develop self-control, and it occurs as a reaction to tensions and problems in the home.

Clinical features   It is important to be aware that hyperactive children may not demonstrate the extent of their hyperactivity in the visit to the doctor, and the history is therefore more important than observation in the clinical setting. Hyperactive children are restless, impulsive and excitable, and fail to focus on any activity for long. They tend to have little sense of danger, and require great vigilance. As such children are unable to concentrate for long on any quiet activity, they often have difficulties on starting school.

Management   Hyperactive children benefit from routine and regularity in everyday life. They need to have firm boundaries set for their behaviour and consistency in discipline. On starting school, the support of the teacher is essential in helping with adjustment. Medical management is discussed on p. 261.

School-based problems

Teasing and bullying

Bullying is a major problem for many children. Overall, about 10% of children report being bullied at least once per week, and 7% of children are identified as bullies. It is important to remember that victims may be bullies themselves and that most bullying goes undetected by parents and teachers. Bullying tends to be more common in primary schools, and varies from school to school according to the ethos.

Clinical features   Children may or may not admit to being a victim of bullying, and it should therefore be considered as a possible cause of distress whenever a schoolchild is disturbed. They may react to bullying by becoming withdrawn or aggressive or developing psychosomatic symptoms. Bullying is a common cause for school refusal.

Management   In schools where bullying is a problem, a whole-school approach is most effective so that the ethos of bullying becomes unacceptable, and both the victims and the bullies are helped. The individual child needs help in handling the situation and increasing self-esteem. Any school refusal must be addressed instantly.

In recent years the abuse of social media to shame and target individuals or disseminate insulting or even explicit material has become a serious issue. Schools and parents need to coordinate closely and educate themselves about these issues. Occasionally social workers and even the police may become involved.

Non-attendance at school

Attendance at school is compulsory and prolonged or unexplained absence may be unlawful. Most absences from school (Table 21.3) occur as a result of illnesses, which are usually minor. These absences may be prolonged through parental anxiety, particularly if the child has a chronic illness (see p. 46). In some circumstances, parents may keep their child at home to help care for younger siblings or elderly relatives, or even to help out at work. The two situations where the doctor may become involved are school refusal and truancy.

Clinical features   The main distinction between school refusal and truancy is that in the former everyone knows where the child is, but in the latter the child's whereabouts are unknown during school hours.

School refusal may result from either separation anxiety or school phobia. Anxiety on separating from parents is common on first starting school, and also may be precipitated by a traumatic event, such as a family death. *School phobia* is usually triggered by distressing events at school, such as problems with

Table 21.3 Reasons for school absence

Illness
Kept at home by parent
School refusal
Truancy

peers or teachers. In both types of school refusal, the child is usually well behaved with no academic problems, although there may be associated neurotic behaviour.

Truancy is commonest in secondary school, particularly in the last years, and is probably universal to a degree. Persistent truancy is associated with generally antisocial behaviour, poor academic achievement and unsettled family background.

Management Management of school absenteeism must involve close collaboration between parents and teachers. In most cases of school refusal, the child should be returned to school as quickly as possible, while addressing underlying problems. Delaying the return only exacerbates the problem. Truancy is harder to tackle and requires a total treatment package. The needs of the child must be met, including any developmental learning disorders such as dyslexia. The education welfare officer should become involved if the truancy is persistent.

School failure

Failure at school has profound effects not only for achievement in adult life and chances of employment, but also for quality of life in the school years. School failure is associated with low self-esteem, behavioural difficulties and psychosomatic disorders. Children may fail at school for a number of reasons, educational, social and medical, that may compound each other (Table 21.4). From the educational point of view it is particularly important to address causes such as dyslexia, attention deficits, and visual or hearing impairments that reduce the

Table 21.4 Causes for failing at school

Educational

Limited intellect

Attention deficit disorder

Hearing or visual deficit

Dyslexia

Dyspraxia

Social

Problems at home

Peer problems

Absence from school

Organic

Hypothyroidism

Lead poisoning

Chronic disease

child's potential to learn, and can lead to frustration and other negative psychological reactions.

Dyslexia

Dyslexia is the commonest type of developmental learning disorder (the term now replacing specific learning difficulty). Dyslexic children are unable to process effectively the information required in order to read. The result is a reading ability below that expected for the child's general level of intelligence. Dyslexia must be differentiated from slow reading as a result of limited intellect or inadequate teaching. It is much more common in boys and there is often a family history.

Clinical features The child often has a history of delay in learning to talk. There may be difficulties other than reading, and spelling is affected more than reading. If the difficulty is not recognised, the child is likely to fail at school and commonly responds by withdrawing or exhibiting disruptive behaviour.

Management If suspected, the diagnosis must be confirmed on testing by an educational psychologist. The child needs individual help in overcoming the difficulty, and may need 'statementing' (see p. 46).

Attention deficit disorder

'Attention deficit disorder' refers to a general difficulty in focusing on tasks or activities. It may or may not occur with hyperactivity (see pp. 261, 388) and is far commoner in boys than girls. These children often have a history of being colicky, temperamentally difficult babies.

Clinical features The child is fidgety, has a difficult time remaining in his or her seat at school, is easily distracted and impulsive, has difficulty following instructions, talks excessively and flits from one activity to another. Daydreaming is more obvious if hyperactivity is not a feature.

Management The child benefits from a regular daily routine with simple clear rules, and firm limits enforced fairly and sympathetically. Overstimulation and overfatigue should be avoided. In school, a structured programme is required with good home communication to ensure consistency. Pedagogic planning is vital as children who are faced with educational material which is too easy become bored and if too difficult become despondent. In both cases attention will drift. Adequate discipline is vital in home and school. Central nervous system stimulants such as methylphenidate, prescribed during school hours, are helpful in selected cases but should only be prescribed within the context of a structured academic programme.

Attention deficit problems, particularly if associated with hyperactivity, can be very stressful to the family and counselling may be needed. Therapies such as megavitamins and low-sugar diets have not been proved to be effective. Diets with no artificial colourings or flavourings remain controversial, but in general do not help the majority of these children.

Prognosis   Both hyperactivity and attention difficulties tend to improve through adolescence, but the educational deficit may persist as a handicap later in life.

Dyspraxia

Clumsiness, or dyspraxia, can cause problems at home and at school. Fine motor incoordination leads to untidy writing, and gross motor incoordination leads to difficulty with sports. The academic and social difficulties that ensue can cause the child considerable unhappiness and lead to behavioural problems if they are not recognised and dealt with helpfully. An occupational therapist can assist the school in devising a programme which will help overcome the difficulties and build self-confidence.

To test your knowledge on this part of the book, please see Chapter 26

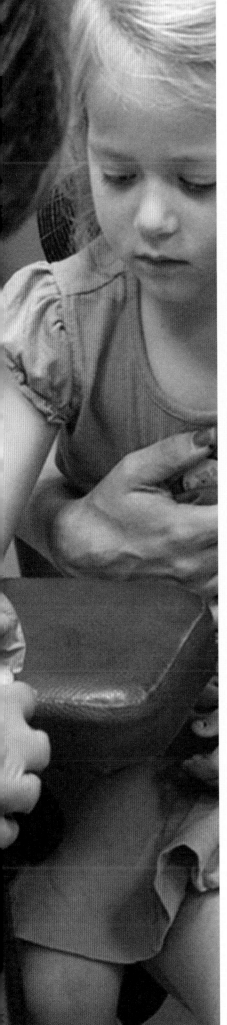

CHAPTER 22

Social paediatrics

There was an old woman who lived in a shoe,
She had so many children she didn't know what to do!
So she gave them some broth without any bread,
And she whipped them all soundly and sent them to bed!

English nursery rhyme

Symptoms and signs of child abuse

Forms of abuse and neglect

KEY COMPETENCES

YOU MUST...

Know and understand

- The various manifestations of child abuse and neglect
- Features that are characteristic of non-accidental injury
- Procedures for raising concerns about abuse or neglect

Be able to

- Describe the symptoms, signs and red flag features for child abuse
- Identify the procedures for raising concerns about child maltreatment

Appreciate that

- All health professionals have a duty of care to report concerns about child maltreatment
- Wrongly diagnosing or overdiagnosis of abuse can also be extremely damaging to families, so assessment should only be carried out by a skilled paediatrician in an appropriate setting
- Abuse and neglect have a devastating impact on children
- Management requires multi-professional expertise

Essential Paediatrics and Child Health, Fourth Edition. Mary Rudolf, Anthony Luder and Kerry Jeavons.
© 2020 John Wiley & Sons Ltd. Published 2020 by John Wiley & Sons Ltd.
Companion website: www.wiley.com/go/rudolf/paediatrics

Symptoms and signs of child abuse

Finding your way around ...

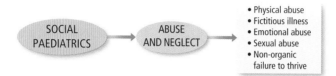

Child abuse is a tragic condition that crosses all social, ethnic and economic boundaries. It can be highly challenging to detect tell-tale clues in 'normative' families. Families may adopt a variety of strategies in order to avoid suspicion and detection.

During the course of child health surveillance children may be identified as being the victims of neglect or abuse. This may emerge on finding characteristic physical signs at a routine examination or a medical appointment or witnessing abnormal behaviour on the part of the child. Older children may take the opportunity of a routine contact with a doctor or nurse to disclose abuse.

The clinical evaluation of children who are suspected victims of abuse or neglect requires skill. Enough time must be allowed so the evaluation is not rushed, and the setting must be private to ensure confidentiality. The doctor's attitude is important as it is vital to gain both the child's and, where possible, the family's trust. There is no place for the doctor to be accusatory in any way. Objective, accurate and detailed records are vital, supplemented when required by photographic and other data.

It is important to emphasise that although medical staff have a crucial role in detecting child abuse, any person, neighbour or concerned citizen who suspects child abuse is required to report this to competent authorities.

Types of child abuse

Physical neglect
Emotional abuse
Non-accidental injury
Sexual abuse
Non-organic failure to thrive (see p. 397)

The evaluation must be thorough, including a full history and physical examination, or important clues may be missed. If injuries are present, it is important to decide whether they were incurred accidentally or could have been inflicted. It is also essential to contact other professionals such as social workers, the GP and the school, who may throw light on the child's home circumstances.

History – must ask!

- *How did the injury occur?* The most important part of the history is the explanation given for any injuries, as this helps you decide whether lesions are likely to be non-accidental (see Red Flag box). Characteristically, in non-accidental injury the explanation given does not match the appearance of the injury and often sounds unconvincing. Injuries occurring in young, non-mobile infants should arouse particular suspicion. There is often a delay before medical advice is sought, and the child may communicate details which conflict with the parental explanation. The history may be taken on repeated occasions by the same or different team members; inconsistencies and changing stories or details should raise suspicions.
- *Past medical history.* A history of previous injuries is obviously relevant. Frequent visits for apparently trivial complaints may cover up abuse.
- *Developmental history and behaviour.* A child's psychosocial development can be severely affected by neglect and abuse, and an assessment can also be useful to serve as a baseline for the future.
- *Social history and family history.* In order to gain a complete picture, you need a full social history. It is important to know who is in the home, and if anyone other than the parents are responsible for caring for the child. Risk factors for child abuse and neglect include unstable homes where there are changes of partner, broken marriages, economic hardship and single-parent or very large families. Other professionals such as health visitors and nursery nurses can often provide important details about the family.

Characteristics of non-accidental injury

- Injuries in very young children
- Explanations which do not match the appearance of the injury and sound unconvincing
- Inconsistent histories
- Multiple types and age of injury
- Injuries which are 'classic' in site or character, or are severe and/or unusual
- Delay in presentation
- Things the child may communicate during the evaluation

Physical examination – must check!

You must always carry out a thorough physical examination with the child undressed.

- *General appearance.* Note how the child looks. He or she may show signs of neglect, such as an unkempt dirty appearance, sores and untreated nappy rash. The child's reaction to you is important. A child who has experienced prolonged abuse may have a 'frozen watchful' appearance: appear motionless, with an expressionless face and wary eyes. The neglected child may be abnormally affectionate to strangers, as if seeking any human contact.
- *Growth.* Abused and neglected children commonly fail to thrive. Height, length, weight, and head circumference need to be measured, plotted and compared with previous measurements.
- *Injuries* (see Box 22.1). Examine the child for signs of injury. Many non-accidental injuries have a characteristic appearance, and multiple injuries at different sites and of different ages are particularly suspect.
  - *Bruises.* Multiple bruises are commonly found on the legs of any toddler, but bruises at other sites may be suspicious. A bruise cannot be aged accurately from a clinical assessment or from a photograph. The pattern of the bruise may indicate how it was acquired (Figure 22.1 a–d). Linear, or patterned bruises are very concerning for abuse and bruises with petechiae are also highly suggestive.
  - *Burns and scalds.* When a toddler accidentally scalds him- or herself the scald is usually irregular and asymmetrical in shape with additional splash marks. Inflicted scalds are classically symmetrical and may cause a doughnut-shaped lesion on the buttocks, which are centrally spared where the base of the bath protects the skin from contact with the hot water (Figure 22.1f). Inflicted cigarette burns cause deep circular ulcers (Figure 22.1e) as compared with the superficial lesions seen with accidental burns. Electric burns may cause significant deep tissue damage with minimal superficial signs.
  - *Bites.* Bites have the shape of a dental impression. These can be used forensically to identify the perpetrator (Figure 22.1g).
  - *Hidden head injuries.* Examine the fundi for retinal haemorrhages (Figure 22.2), as they may occur when a baby is shaken, or suffers direct impact the the head, and can be associated with the presence of subdural haematomas (see p. 246).
  - *Bone injuries* (Figure 22.3). You may find evidence of fractures.
- *Signs of sexual abuse.* This examination should only be carried out by an experienced paediatrician in a setting where the child's privacy can be respected. If the child discloses sexual abuse or is suspected of being a victim, the genitalia and anus must be carefully examined. Signs of sexual abuse may be overt, such as bruising and tears, or may be more

Box 22.1 Clinical features of physical abuse

- Physical neglect
- Failure to thrive
- Bruises
- Fractures
- Burns and scalds
- Bites
- Ligature marks

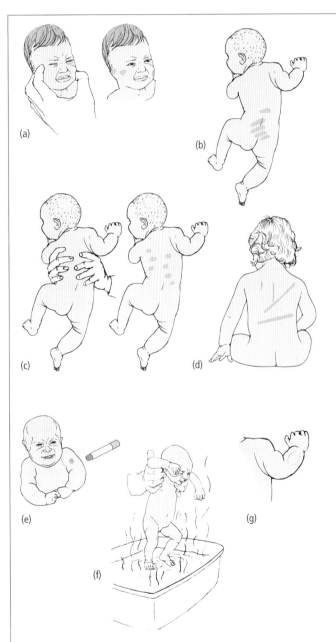

Figure 22.1 Skin lesions indicative of non-accidental injury: (a) facial squeeze, (b) slap marks, (c) grip marks, (d) stick marks, (e) cigarette burns, (f) scalding, and (g) bite marks.

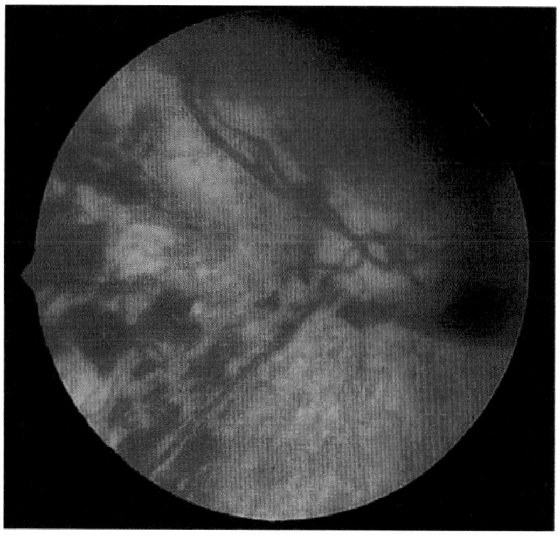

Figure 22.2 Retinal haemorrhages seen in an infant who was admitted with seizures and lethargy following inflicted abusive head trauma.

Table 22.1 Investigations in suspected child abuse	
Investigation	**Relevance**
Photographs	Useful for further consultation and evidence in court
Full blood count, prothrombin time (PT), activated partial thromboplastin time (APTT), thrombin time (TT), fibrinogen, assays of factor VIIIc and Von-Willebrand factor	To rule out thrombocytopenia or other haematological disorder as a cause for excessive bruising
Skeletal survey (X-rays)	Characteristic fractures and fractures at various stages of healing may be found in non-accidental injury
Head CT scan	Particularly important in infants presenting with probable abuse, to detect subdural haemorrhages which may otherwise be easily missed
Pregnancy test and cultures for sexually transmitted disease	In children suspected of sexual abuse, the finding of sexually transmitted disease is strong corroborative evidence (and needs treating)

subtle, but it is important to remember that the absence of physical signs does not in any way mean that a child has not been sexually abused.

Investigations

Table 22.1 shows the investigations which may be helpful in children suspected of being victims of abuse. If suspicious injuries are found, photographs should be taken so that they are available for future consultation and evidence in court.

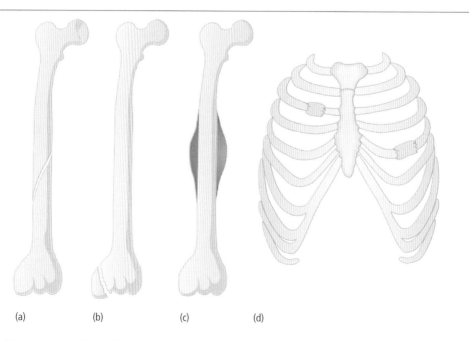

(a) (b) (c) (d)

Figure 22.3 Types of fractures associated with non-accidental injury: (a) spiral fractures, (b) metaphyseal chips, (c) periosteal bleeds, and (d) callus around ribs.

As the implications of non-accidental injury are so serious, rare medical causes of excessive bruising or fragile bones must be ruled out. A full blood count and clotting screen will exclude a haematological cause for bruising. In the case of fractures, osteogenesis imperfecta (brittle bone disease) may be considered and can usually be ruled out on clinical evaluation.

In any child <2 years old suspected of being a victim of abuse or neglect, a skeletal survey (X-ray of the entire body) should be requested to determine whether there have been previous unreported injuries. Fractures that have been inflicted often have a characteristic appearance and tend to occur through the growth plate, as this is the most vulnerable part of growing bones. Spiral fractures are particularly likely to result from violent inflicted trauma. When multiple fractures are found, they are often seen to be at different stages of healing. Repeat imaging taken at a later date may also reveal healing fractures not seen at the acute assessment.

- The child who has disclosed sexual abuse needs to be investigated for sexually transmitted diseases, and forensic samples taken. A pregnancy test is needed in the postpubertal girl who has been raped.

Management of the child suspected of being a victim of abuse (see also Chapter 2)

Where there is any suspicion that a child has suffered abuse or neglect, the child should be referred immediately for the specialist opinion of a paediatrician experienced in child protection work. If the paediatrician concludes that the child has been abused or is at risk of abuse, the social services department is immediately informed. Social workers may be authorized to obtain records from other hospitals and settings to which the child may have presented. In extreme cases Child Protection Officers or the police may be need to be contacted at an early stage.

If the child is deemed to be in danger, or further assessment is required, he or she needs to be admitted to a place of safety, usually a hospital ward or a social services institution, until a fuller inquiry can be made. An emergency care order can be obtained from court if the family resists admission or investigation.

The social work team usually takes the lead in planning the strategy for management. Initial policy is worked out at a case conference, attended by all professionals involved and the parents. Many children are allowed home, initially under supervision and with appropriate support. Occasionally it is necessary to take the child away from the parents. This is generally a difficult decision and requires a court order. The child may be placed with another member of the family, in foster care or, in the case of an older child, a group home.

For the child returned to his or her home, support and supervision must be provided. This may be in the form of placement in a social services day nursery, or voluntary and self-help groups may be available to help the parents overcome their difficulties. Social Care keep a record of children who have been abused or neglected so that professionals can readily determine if a child or others in the family are known to be at risk.

 See NICE guideline: Child maltreatment: when to suspect maltreatment in under 18s
https://www.nice.org.uk/guidance/cg89

 Key points: When abuse is suspected

- Safeguarding children is every health care professional's duty and must appropriately escalate concerns identified
- Evaluations should be conducted in privacy and the child's trust gained
- Helpful information can be obtained from other health professionals and social services
- If injuries are present, indications that they have been inflicted must be sought in the history and physical appearance
- A thorough examination, including growth and general appearance, must be made to identify other injuries, failure to thrive and signs of neglect
- Comprehensive clear notes must be made and where necessary photographs taken as they may be required for evidence

Forms of abuse and neglect

Physical abuse (non-accidental injury)

Parents who abuse their children come from all ethnic and socioeconomic groups. In most cases the abuser is a relative or lives within the home. Most perpetrators have neither psychotic nor criminal personalities, but tend to be unhappy, lonely, angry adults under stress, who have often themselves experienced physical abuse as children. The event often coincides with the loss of a job or a home, marital strife or physical exhaustion.

Clinical features Injuries may range in severity from minor bruises to fatal subdural haematomas. Characteristic injuries are shown in Figures 22.1 and 22.3. Spinous process and scapular fractures also have high specificity for child abuse. Vertebral body, digital and complex skull injuries have moderate specificity.

Management The injuries, if severe, require medical attention. The general management of abused children is discussed above.

👁 Physical abuse at a glance

Epidemiology
Occurs in all ethnic and
  socioeconomic groups

Aetiology
Most perpetrators are close
  contacts of the child, often
  abused themselves as
  children

History
Delay in seeking medical
  advice*
Explanation does not match
  appearance of injury*
Inconsistent history*
Past injuries*

Physical examination
Injuries typical of abuse
Multiple injuries of different
  ages*
Failure to thrive*
Signs of neglect*

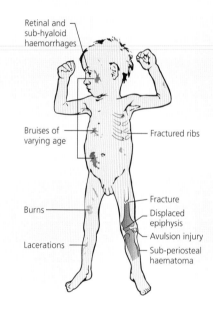

Retinal and sub-hyaloid haemorrhages
Bruises of varying age
Fractured ribs
Burns
Fracture
Displaced epiphysis
Avulsion injury
Lacerations
Sub-periosteal haematoma

Confirmatory investigations
It is essentially a clinical
  diagnosis
Blood dyscrasias need to be
  ruled out by an FBC and
  clotting screen
Skeletal survey is needed to
  assess presence of fractures
Consider head CT

Differential diagnosis
Accidental injury
Blood dyscrasias
Osteogenesis imperfecta very
  rare

Management
Medical care for injury
Involve social services
Admit to place of safety if child
  in ongoing danger
Case conference
Child Protection Register
Removal from home if child
  remains at risk

Prognosis/complications
Without intervention 5% of
  abused children are killed,
  25% are seriously injured
Neurological damage is
  common from repeated CNS
  insults
Emotional/behavioural
  disturbance
Commonly become perpetrators
  of abuse as adults

NB *Signs and symptoms are variable.

Prognosis   About 5% of abused children who are returned to their parents without intervention are killed and 25% seriously injured. Children with severe or repeated injury to the central nervous system may develop brain damage with learning disabilities or epilepsy. Abused children are commonly fearful, aggressive and hyperactive, and many go on to become delinquent, violent and the next generation of abusers.

Emotional abuse and neglect

Emotional abuse can be defined as the frequent rejection, scapegoating, isolation or terrorizing of a child by caretakers. It is usually very difficult to prove and has long-term emotional and developmental consequences for the child.

Clinical features   Emotional abuse is commonly associated with developmental impairment and failure to thrive (see pp. 258, 291). On presentation the child may be apathetic and show evidence of physical neglect such as dirty clothing, unkempt hair and nappy rash. There may be signs of non-accidental injury, and if there is any suggestion of regression of developmental skills, the diagnosis of chronic subdural haematomas (which can occur as a result of abusive head trauma) should be considered.

Management   Intensive input and support is required. Day nursery placement can provide good stimulation, nutrition and care.

Prognosis   The prognosis depends on the degree of the damage incurred and how early the intervention is provided. Children who require removal from the home often have irreversible learning and emotional difficulties.

Sexual abuse

Sexual abuse may take the form of inappropriate touching, forced exposure to sexual acts, vaginal, oral or rectal intercourse, and sexual assault. Secrecy is often enforced by the offender, who is usually male and a family member or acquaintance of the family, but rarely a stranger.

Clinical features   Sexual abuse may come to light if disclosure is made as a result of genital infections or trauma, or if a child exhibits inappropriate sexual behaviour. Signs of trauma may be evident in the mouth, anus or genitalia, but absence of signs is common and less than half of the victims have any substantiating physical evidence.

Management   Particularly sensitive and skilled management is required and should only be undertaken by those experienced in the work. All victims require psychological support, and the offender too may be amenable to help.

Prognosis   With intervention most incest victims can lead normal adult lives. Without intervention they are likely to become seriously disturbed and grow up unable to form close relationships. Victims commonly enter abusive relationships with men later in life and often need psychiatric help.

Non-organic failure to thrive

A proportion of young children whose weight falters or who fail to thrive (see p. 283) do so as a result of neglect, the principal factor being inadequate nutrition. The parent may have mental health problems.

Clinical features   The child looks malnourished and uncared for, and immunisations are often not up to date. Delays in development are common, and signs of physical abuse may be seen. When admitted to hospital these babies often show rapid weight gain.

Management   If the problem is clearly one of neglect, child protection procedures must be initiated.

Prognosis   Without detection and intervention, a small proportion of these children die from starvation. With intervention, catch-up growth may occur, but brain growth may be jeopardized, and emotional and educational problems are common.

Fabricated or induced illness (FII)

In this bizarre form of abuse, which used to be called Munchhausen by proxy, the carer fabricates the child's symptoms or signs. The child is likely to become subject to extensive hospitalization and investigations, and may be in actual physical danger (as when apnoea is fabricated by suffocation or drugs administered without prescription). The diagnosis is difficult to make, but must be suspected if the presentation is unusual and incongruous, and if symptoms and signs emerge in the parent's presence alone. Detection of multiple admissions to various hospitals is an important clue.

Medical neglect

Medical neglect is a difficult area. It includes failure to bring a child for medical treatment or diagnosis, failure to comply with medical advice and treatment, failure or refusal to immunise, and administration of harmful 'remedies'. Children may be severely damaged as a result or even die.

   The underlying causes of medical neglect are manifold. Neglect is a serious medical problem when it results in the child being exposed to serious risk, causes significant deterioration of the child's health, or results in frequent or prolonged periods of hospitalization. Factors that can contribute include poverty or economic hardship, lack of access to care, family chaos and disorganization, and a lack of awareness, knowledge, or skills. Lack of faith in scientific medicine or trust in health care professionals resulting from caregivers' belief systems may also contribute.

Sensitivity is needed to explore the reasons for neglect. Community resources may be drawn in to aid in caring for the child, and where necessary child protective services should be involved. Intervention is a serious step that is usually reserved only for very serious cases of medical neglect, such as when medical treatment is needed for an emergency situation or the child has a life-threatening acute or chronic illness.

To test your knowledge on this part of the book, please see Chapter 26

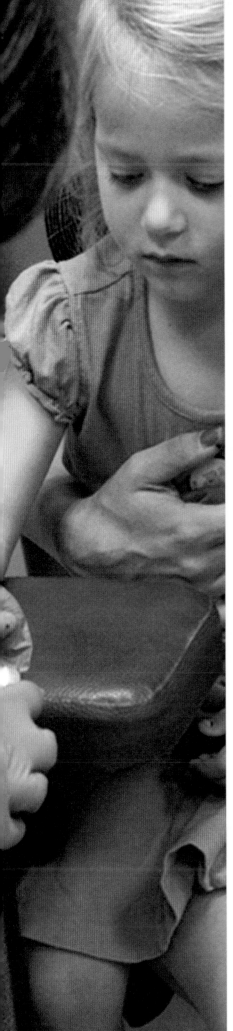

CHAPTER 23

Emergency paediatrics

Elisha came into the house and behold! – the boy was dead, laid out on his bed. He entered and shut the door behind them both. Then he went up...and placed his mouth upon his mouth...and he warmed the flesh of the boy...the boy sneezed seven times, and the boy opened his eyes.

2 Kings 4: 32–34

KEY COMPETENCES

YOU MUST...

Know and understand

- How severely ill children may present using the 'traffic light' system
- How to assess rapidly a child presenting as an emergency using the ABCDDEFG approach
- How to recognise the early signs of sepsis and shock
- The signs of cardio-respiratory failure and the basics of cardiopulmonary resuscitation
- How key emergency paediatric conditions are diagnosed and managed including trauma, poisoning and status epilepticus
- How to estimate clinically the severity of dehydration and principles of treating it

Be able to

- Carry out basic airway management (airway positioning, suction, administration of oxygen, placement of an oral airway and bag-valve mask ventilation)
- Deliver age-appropriate cardio-pulmonary resuscitation
- Calculate the Pediatric Early Warning Score and identify unwell or deteriorating children
- Manage the choking child
- Place the comatose child in the recovery position
- Advise a parent about first aid management of seizures
- Instruct a family in the use of an adrenaline self-injector
- Recognise the need for help and how to obtain it

Appreciate that

- In emergencies management precedes history and full physical examination
- Time is critical in emergencies – the 'golden hour'

Essential Paediatrics and Child Health, Fourth Edition. Mary Rudolf, Anthony Luder and Kerry Jeavons.
© 2020 John Wiley & Sons Ltd. Published 2020 by John Wiley & Sons Ltd.
Companion website: www.wiley.com/go/rudolf/paediatrics

Emergency paediatric presentations

Finding your way around ...

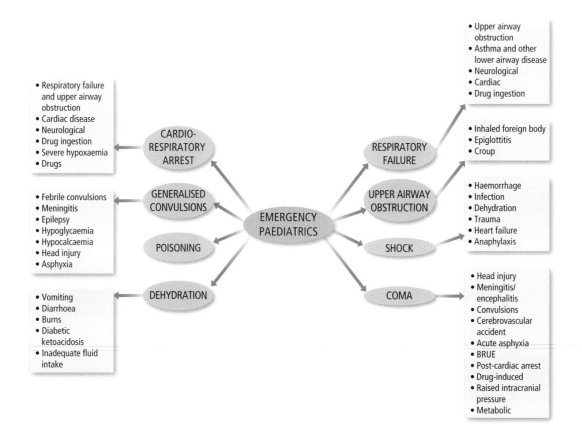

This part of the book discusses the presentation and treatment of children with acute life-threatening disorders and emergency problems. Children may become critically ill very rapidly, and survival depends on rapid recognition of the ill child, appropriate first aid, rapid transfer to hospital and appropriate use of therapies.

The commonest cause of severe illness in children is infection. The immune response may be impaired by prematurity, malnourishment, drugs (steroids in particular), malignant disease and its management and, rarely, an inherited or acquired abnormality in immune function (Table 23.1). AIDS and congenital immune deficiency are very rare cause of immune deficiency in childhood. Newborn babies are particularly prone to infection. This is usually bacterial and acquired perinatally from the mother or nosocomially from carers.

How do acutely ill children present?

Presentation to some extent depends on the age of the child. Babies and young children obviously cannot verbalize their distress. The older child is likely to have more specific symptoms and an ability to describe the site of any pain. Physical signs may also vary with age: for example, signs such as Kernig or neck stiffness are specific in older children, but in very young children they may not occur at all, or only very late in the illness. For these reasons, assessing whether a baby of 6 months of age or less is significantly ill may be difficult. Infants under 6 months old may present with illness or infection with a low temperature, rather than fever; poor feeding; or an irritable cry.

The NICE clinical guideline 'Feverish illness in children under 5 years' (CG160) gives advice on the assessment and management of children with fever (see Table 23.2 below).

Table 23.1 Factors predisposing to the development of severe and acute illness in children

Factor	Risk group
Age	Neonates
	Infants <1 year
Impaired immune function	Premature infants
	Steroid treatment
	Malignancy
	Immune deficiency (AIDS)
	Splenectomy
	Children with Down syndrome
Malnutrition	E.g. malabsorption
Chronic disease	E.g. cystic fibrosis
	Cerebral palsy
Immunisation status	Incomplete vaccination schedule
Exposure to infectious agents	Children in hospital

Table 23.2 Signs of acute and severe illness in older children

Symptom	Features
Toxicity	This includes a high fever with marked facial flushing and confusion
	Hallucinations may occur with high fever
Severe pain	Associated with pallor, tachycardia, immobility or writhing
Change in consciousness level and reduced consciousness (e.g. Glasgow Coma Scale 13/15 or less)	This is always significant of severe illness
Shortness of breath	Causing difficulty in speaking
Dehydration	See p. 416
'Going off their feet'	Any acute difficulty in walking or unsteadiness of gait

It uses a traffic light system for healthcare professionals to use for remote, as well as direct, assessment. It is used to guide management (see Sepsis section below). Older children with severe illness are easier to assess. Signs of acute and potentially severe illness in older children are shown in Table 23.2.

Critically ill children must be rushed to hospital for resuscitation and supportive care without delay as they can deteriorate very rapidly. Clearly, children with the following conditions need urgent hospitalization:

- shock (see p. 408 for definition)
- coma
- acute cyanosis or severe respiratory distress
- severe unexplained pain
- profound apnoea
- major trauma
- progressive non-blanching (petechial or purpuric) rash (see p. 351)
- status epilepticus
- severe poisoning.

Assessment and management in an emergency

See Figure 23.1. Although life-threatening disorders often start insidiously, it is important to remember that progression from minor symptoms to moribund state may occur very rapidly. This is particularly likely if the child has an underlying predisposition to severe illness (Table 23.1).

Infants are particularly susceptible to sepsis, which is usually obtained from passage through the birth canal or through environmental contact with bacteria. Group B Streptococcus (GBS) is a normal vaginal commensal which can cause severe sepsis in infants up to 3 months old (see p. 421).

Children often present with febrile illness, however infants under 6 months may need to be treated more aggressively to assess and manage infection as they have a higher risk of sepsis. In infants of this age other infections, particularly *E. coli* urine infections, frequently spread to meningitis.

The homeostatic physiological balance is relatively fragile in children, and particularly so in infancy. The child has an ability to preserve intravascular volume against abnormal fluid losses as occur in diarrhoea or excessive vomiting, but once these physiological mechanisms have been fully deployed, collapse with shock can rapidly occur.

Unlike in any other aspect of paediatrics, management of the emergency must precede history and examination. After very rapid assessment, the critically ill child must be resuscitated, the airway secured, and the child's condition stabilized. The initial management of the critically ill child is discussed below, but the difference between life and death may depend on the management in the first hour after the collapse.

Once the initial resuscitation has taken place, the child must be carefully assessed for evidence of disease in other

NICE National Institute for Health and Care Excellence

Traffic light system for identifying risk of serious illness

	Green – low risk	Amber – intermediate risk	Red – high risk
Colour (of skin, lips or tongue)	• Normal colour	• Pallor reported by parent/carer	• Pale/mottled/ashen/blue
Activity	• Responds normally to social cues • Content/smiles • Stays awake or awakens quickly • Strong normal cry/not crying	• Not responding normally to social cues • No smile • Wakes only with prolonged stimulation • Decreased activity	• No response to social cues • Appears ill to a healthcare professional • Does not wake or if roused does not stay awake • Weak, high-pitched or continuous cry
Respiratory		• Nasal flaring • Tachypnoea: – RR >50 breaths/minute, age 6–12 months – RR >40 breaths/minute, age >12 months • Oxygen saturation ≤95% in air • Crackles in the chest	• Grunting • Tachypnoea: RR >60 breaths/minute • Moderate or severe chest indrawing
Circulation and hydration	• Normal skin and eyes • Moist mucous membranes	• Tachycardia: – >160 beats/minute, age <12 months – >150 beats/minute, age 12–24 months – >140 beats/minute, age 2–5 years • CRT ≥3 seconds • Dry mucous membranes • Poor feeding in infants • Reduced urine output	• Reduced skin turgor
Other	• None of the amber or red symptoms or signs	• Age 3–6 months, temperature ≥39°C • Fever for ≥5 days • Rigors • Swelling of a limb or joint • Non-weight bearing limb/not using an extremity	• Age <3 months, temperature ≥38°C* • Non-blanching rash • Bulging fontanelle • Neck stiffness • Status epilepticus • Focal neurological signs • Focal seizures

CRT, capillary refill time; RR, respiratory rate
*Some vaccinations have been found to induce fever in children aged under 3 months
This traffic light table should be used in conjunction with the recommendations in theNICE guideline on Feverish illness in children. See http://guidance.nice.org.uk/CG160

Figure 23.1 Traffic Light assessment of children under 5 years of age (NICE clinical guideline on 'Feverish illness in children under 5 years' (CG160)).

systems that may have caused the initial collapse, although the underlying disease may be obvious, as in trauma or asthma.

History – must ask!

Once the child has been stabilized, or whilst colleagues are stabilising, it is important to find out more history in order to consider all the potential causes of the illness.

- *Description of the events leading up to the collapse.* A detailed history from a witness of the collapse may be very helpful. This may be a teacher or a playmate if the child collapsed away from home. Establish whether the child was well immediately before the collapse or whether there was a rapidly progressive illness.
- *Previous medical history.* It is very important to establish whether the child has an underlying illness such as diabetes, allergy or asthma predisposing to collapse. Find out if the child has been on prescription drugs or could have been indulging in substance abuse. In infants, a recent minor illness may be significant, and the severity of diarrhoea and vomiting may have been underestimated by the parents.
- *Specific risk factors for sepsis in infants under 3 months old.* Risk factors for sepsis in infants include prolonged rupture of membranes prior to delivery, maternal fever and sepsis (even after delivery), preterm delivery (before 37 weeks gestation), sepsis in an older sibling after birth, and maternal GBS carriage (although the mother may not have been tested).

Physical examination – must check!

After the initial emergency assessment of the child, a more careful physical examination must be carried out. Important clues as to the cause of the collapse may be obtained from the physical examination; the Red Flag box lists the important features to assess.

⚑ Signs that may help in the diagnosis of a severe illness

Rashes, particularly petechial or purpuric (see p. 351)
Depth of coma
State of hydration (p. 417)
Vital signs (blood pressure, pulse, respiratory rate, temperature) – persistent tachycardia is a cause for concern
Signs of respiratory distress
Stridor
Signs of injury, especially bruising in a non-mobile child, which could be a sign of intracranial haemorrhage
Surface area of burns

Paediatric Early Warning Scores

Many hospitals now use a system of documenting vital signs on a chart, which is used to calculate a score to indicate severity of illness. Observations in children, however, can be affected by crying, fever, or fear, and therefore are not highly sensitive or specific. They are useful to observe a trend in observations, but you should not be reassured if a child looks unwell but does not 'score' highly. Children in hospital who have grossly abnormal observations need rapid clinical assessment to determine, and treat, the cause of this.

Investigations

Investigations are directed towards:
- *Diagnosis.* The appropriate investigations are discussed below in the relevant sections on causes of collapse.
- *A guide to appropriate management.* If the child requires respiratory support, a chest X-ray and regular blood gases are essential to guide management.

Management

Emergency treatment should occur where the child presents. In practice, this is in an Emergency Department. A guide to the immediate assessment, resuscitation and management is shown in Box 23.1. As soon as the child is stable, he or she should be moved to an intensive care or high dependency unit for further monitoring and management.

Management of the pulseless or moribund child must be prioritized into these four areas in sequence.

A	Airway	*plus*	**D** Don't
B	Breathing		**E** Ever
C	Circulation		**F** Forget
D	Disability		**G** Glucose
E	Exposure		

Management of shock is discussed on p. 408. Management of paediatric trauma is beyond this book's scope.

Support for relatives

During resuscitation, relatives must be kept closely informed. A member of the resuscitation team – usually a nurse – should stay with the relatives and keep them informed of progress and give emotional support. It is best if only one person is involved in talking to the relatives during the process of resuscitation. Once the child is stabilized, the most senior member of the team should inform the parents of the situation and answer their questions as honestly as possible.

Box 23.1 Assessment and management in an emergency

Assessment
This must be conducted rapidly
   Is the airway clear?
   Is the child breathing?
   Is there adequate circulation?
Are there obvious injuries?
- fractures
- lacerations
- burns
What is the level of consciousness?

Resuscitation
   Clear the airway
   Give inflation breaths if not breathing
   Cardiopulmonary resuscitation if cardiac output is poor
   Establish intravenous access
   Pressure to stop bleeding
   Immobilize fractured limbs, and neck if trauma
      suspected

Problem-directed management
   Blood gases
   Treat shock with fluids (p. 408)
   Investigate cause of illness
   Investigate function of other organs
   Ensure adequate hydration
   Specific drugs once a diagnosis is made

Key points: The child presenting as an emergency

- Rapidly assess the state of the child
- Stabilize the condition
- Only then take a full history and carry out a physical examination
- Assess the child for evidence of disease in other systems which may have precipitated the emergency

Cardiorespiratory arrest

Cardiorespiratory arrest is defined by apnoea (no breathing) and no effective cardiac output (pulse). In children, this is likely to be the result of hypoxia and therefore paediatric arrest algorithms emphasise the importance of oxygenation over defibrillation.

Commoner causes of cardiorespiratory arrest

Severe respiratory disease

Upper airway obstruction

Cardiac disease
Arrhythmia
Cardiac failure
Myocarditis

Neurological disorder
Birth asphyxia
Cerebral oedema
Coning
Head injury

Drug or toxin

Severe hypoxic–ischaemic insult
Suffocation
Drowning

Anaphylaxis

Electrocution

There must be a well-rehearsed protocol for cardiac arrest that occurs in hospital. All medical staff involved in resuscitation should be appropriately trained. It is beyond the scope of this book to describe the detailed approach to the management of cardiac arrest, but the important principles are shown in Box 23.2.

Management

The process of resuscitation is a team effort and requires an experienced healthcare practitioner and anaesthetist together with nursing support. The most experienced doctor on the team should take charge of the resuscitation, and if necessary be the person who decides how long resuscitation should continue if there is no response.

The principles of managing the child with cardiac arrest are the same for any critically ill child. Proceed in the sequence detailed in Box 23.1 (see Figure 23.2).

Once the initial resuscitation has been established, consideration should turn to the cause of the collapse and the child should be monitored very closely in an intensive care environment.

Box 23.2 Managing cardiorespiratory arrest

Safety – Is it safe to approach?

Stimulate the patient

Shout for help

Airway
Open airway with manoeuvres
Look, listen and feel for breathing or signs of life

Breathing
Five rescue breaths with high-concentration oxygen via a
  facemask and self-expanding resuscitation bag
Mouth-to-mouth if nothing else available

Circulation
Check for signs of life
Chest compressions at a rate of 100/min
Alternate 15 cardiac compressions with two lung inflations
Display ECG trace and defibrillate if appropriate

Drugs
Establish vascular access for drug (adrenaline) and fluid
  administration
Alternatively, some drugs can be given down the
  endotracheal tube or by direct intracardiac injection
Check blood sugar, give glucose if low
Consider, and manage, reversible causes of collapse

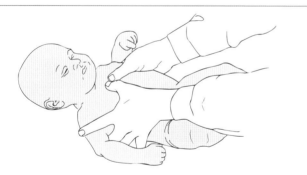

Figure 23.2 External cardiac massage in an infant. The thumbs are placed over the lower half of the sternum in the encircling technique.

See Resuscitation council UK guideline:
https://www.resus.org.uk/resuscitation-guidelines/paediatric-advanced-life-support/

Respiratory failure

Causes of respiratory failure

Upper airway obstruction
Inhaled foreign body
Croup (laryngotracheobronchitis)
Epiglottitis

Lower airway disease
Asthma
Bronchiolitis
Pneumonia
Cystic fibrosis
Neonatal lung disease
Pneumothorax
Atelectasis

Neurological
Head injury
Meningitis
Raised intracranial pressure
Muscle disorder

Cardiac
Severe cardiac failure

Toxic
Drug ingestion

Allergic
Anaphylaxis

Respiratory failure is the end result of a large number of causes, but its definition is usually based on abnormal arterial blood gases with both severe hypoxia and hypercapnia (see p. 112). A careful history and physical examination should elicit the underlying cause of the child's respiratory failure. The clinical diagnosis of respiratory failure is obvious if the child is apnoeic or severely cyanosed, but impending respiratory failure may be more difficult to recognise.

History – must ask!

Asthma and viral wheeze are the commonest causes of respiratory failure in children over 1 year of age, and a careful history of previous episodes should be taken. Wheeze and nocturnal cough are important features of these conditions. Record a list of prescribed medication and find out how much of each drug has been given in this episode.

In infants, infection, particularly bronchiolitis (p. 179), is the commonest cause, and the history should focus on exposure to infectious agents, recent fever and a history of apnoea associated with the present illness.

Physical examination – must check!

Inability to speak because of breathlessness is a worrying sign that should be carefully assessed. Signs of respiratory distress include dyspnoea, recession, cyanosis and grunting in babies, but these may all be present in children who do not go on to develop respiratory failure.

Investigations

The relevant investigations and their significance are shown in Table 23.4. Children with impending respiratory failure due to stridor may need to have their airway secured (e.g. by intubation by an experienced anaesthetist) before investigations are performed.

Management

Management is directed at the underlying cause of the respiratory failure, and supporting the respiratory physiology. If the child is hypoxic (cyanosed), but the $P\text{CO}_2$ is normal, oxygen therapy and careful observation are indicated. A rising $P\text{CO}_2$ indicates the need for respiratory support with mechanical ventilation. This should take place on an intensive care or high dependency unit. Oxygen saturation monitoring may be helpful in following the progress of the illness.

Antibiotics are required for bacterial infection (p. 177), steroids and bronchodilators for asthma (p. 169) and bronchoscopy for removal of a foreign body.

Table 23.3 Investigations and their relevance in a child with respiratory failure

Investigation	Relevance
Blood gases	Falling pH and increasing $P\text{CO}_2$ indicates respiratory failure with need for respiratory support Low $P\text{O}_2$ indicates need for additional oxygen
Oxygen saturation	Monitor progress of respiratory disease Oxygen should be given to maintain saturations >92%
Chest X-ray	Lobar or segmental collapse Aspiration

 Key points: Respiratory failure

- Assess arterial blood gases and regularly reassess
- Attach an oxygen saturation monitor and if desaturated give oxygen
- Mechanically ventilate, or offer respiratory support, if $P\text{CO}_2$ is increasing (but the need for ventilation is based on the whole clinical picture, not just blood gases)
- Investigate cause of respiratory failure
- Treat underlying cause:
- antibiotics for bacterial infection (p. 177)
- steroids and bronchodilators for asthma (p. 169)
- remove foreign body via bronchoscope

 Respiratory failure at a glance

Aetiology (see Causes box, p. 405)
Upper airway obstruction
Lower airway disease
Neurological
Toxic

Clinical features
- Dyspnoea
- Tachypnoea
- Cyanosis
- Alar flaring
- Grunting in babies
- Intercostal, subcostal and suprasternal retractions
- Symptoms and signs of underlying disease
- In severe asthma, wheezing may not be heard because of poor air entry
- Restlessness, dizziness
- Impaired consciousness and confusion

Investigations
Blood gases
Chest X-ray

Management
Oxygen saturation monitor
Consider ventilation
Investigate and treat underlying cause

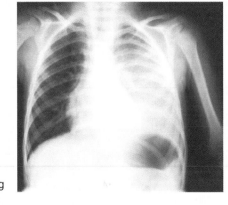

Upper airway obstruction

Acute upper airway obstruction is an acute medical emergency as death may occur rapidly if it is unrelieved. Obstruction may be within the airway, e.g. inhaled foreign body; from the wall of the airway e.g. croup or malacia; or external, e.g. compression of airway from a tumour or aberrant vessel. The major symptom of upper airway obstruction is inspiratory stridor, which is discussed fully on p. 165.

Acute upper airway obstruction is most likely to occur as the result of aspiration of a foreign body. This is particularly likely in toddlers, who tend to put small objects, such as toys or peanuts, into their mouths. Larger objects are most likely to obstruct above the level of the carina, and the symptoms are immediate and dramatic. The presentation is acute with sudden onset of choking, coughing and cyanosis.

History – must ask!

Specific questions to be asked include whether there is the possibility of aspiration of foreign body (has the child had access to plastic bags (including nappy bags), beads, peanuts, etc.?) or whether there has been a history of progressive stridor and malaise suggestive of acute epiglottitis or croup (p. 181). The sudden onset of choking and cough in an otherwise healthy child is by far the most important historical feature of inhaled foreign body.

Physical examination – must check!

If obstruction is severe, the child will be cyanosed and collapsed. Stridor may be present if the child is able to move enough air around the obstruction. Marked recession will be present. If upper airway obstruction other from an acute inhaled foreign body is suspected, the doctor must not examine the child's throat for fear of aggravating the condition.

Investigations

All investigations must be delayed until a safe airway has been established. Undertaking any painful or distressing examination or procedure such as blood tests or moving the child from the carer's arms to examine or take to an X-ray may precipitate complete airway obstruction.

Management

If an object is blocking the larynx or trachea, it must be removed as rapidly as possible as death may occur within minutes. Every effort must be made to avoid pushing the object further down as this may cause complete airway obstruction.

Tracheotomy outside hospital or in hospital tracheostomy may be necessary as a life-saving procedure.

The choking child

See Figure 23.3. If an infant or child is not able to effectively clear an airway obstruction through coughing, back blows and abdominal or chest thrusts are required.

A choking infant or small child should be managed on the carer's lap and positioned at a 45° angle, lying prone. One hand should gently open the mouth to allow any foreign body to fall out. Five back blows should be given with the heel of the hand between the shoulder blades.

In a child under a year of age this should then be followed, if needed, by chest thrusts. The operator places two fingers over the lower third of the sternum and presses firmly five times at a rate of one thrust per second.

In an older child five abdominal thrusts (Heimlich manoeuvre) may be given instead of chest thrusts. These are carried out with the operator behind the child with a fist between the xiphisternum and umbilicus. Both hands are then pulled sharply upwards and inwards increasing intra-abdominal pressure and forcing air out of the lungs.

Back blows and chest/abdominal thrusts (as appropriate) should be given alternately until the obstruction is relieved. If the child collapses, usual cardiopulmonary resuscitation (see p. 404) should be carried out.

> ### 🔑 Key points: Upper airway obstruction
>
> - If a foreign body is suspected in the trachea, use a combination of back blows and chest/abdominal thrusts as above
> - If cardiorespiratory arrest occurs, perform usual cardiopulmonary resuscitation. A tracheostomy may be rarely required to establish a patent airway
> - Avoid distressing the child until an anaesthetist arrives

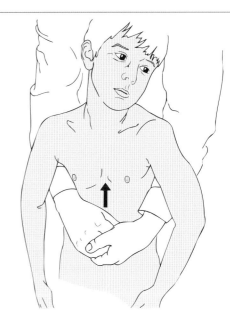

Figure 23.3 The Heimlich manoeuvre in an older child. Stand behind with hands grasping each other under the costal margin. Pull sharply inwards and upwards.

👁 Upper airway obstruction at a glance

Aetiology
Intrinsic: epiglottis, croup
Extrinsic: foreign body

Clinical features
• Choking, coughing
• Inspiratory stridor
• Decreased air movement
• Marked recession
• Cyanosis
• Collapse if complete obstruc-
  tion occurs

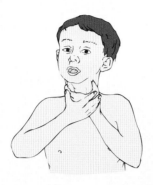

Investigations
Delay until airway is established

Older children   Younger children

Management of a choking
child depending on age

Management
Chest thrusts or abdominal
thrusts to be alternated with
back blows if foreign body
Consider intubation
CPR if necessary

Shock

Causes of shock		
Hypovolaemic	**Cardiogenic**	**Other**
Haemorrhage	Myocardial impairment	Anaphylactic
Infection/sepsis (e.g. meningococcal)	Heart failure	Neurogenic (spinal trauma)
Loss of intravascular fluid (p. 316) (e.g. vomiting, diarrhoea)		
Diabetic ketoacidosis		
Trauma		
Burns		

'Shock' is the term used to describe a state where the cardiac output is insufficient to perfuse the tissues adequately. The easiest clinical measure of shock is tachycardia combined with the capillary refill time (CRT, the time taken for the skin to turn pink again once the pressure from the observer's finger has been removed). CRT should be checked on the sternum (centrally) as well as peripherally. A central capillary refill time longer than 2 seconds is prolonged and may suggest shock. Blood pressure is maintained in the normal range by children until the very late stages of shock: once the blood pressure starts to fall, cardiac arrest is imminent unless urgent action is taken. Hypotension will cause perfusion to fall in vital organs, resulting in failure of multiple organs, of which the brain and

kidneys are the most vulnerable. The body has a variety of physiological mechanisms to protect vital organs during periods of hypotension; these include redistribution of blood flow from the skin, muscles and bowel to the vital organs, brain, myocardium and kidneys. This is why children in shock are pale with poor skin perfusion.

History – must ask!

Take a careful history to elucidate the cause of the shock. Enquire into obvious sources of fluid loss (e.g. diarrhoea, vomiting, history suggestive of diabetes). Ask whether the child has had a cardiac problem and enquire about allergies (e.g. bee stings, peanuts, etc.). Enquire whether there was a close relationship between ingesting an unusual food and the onset of shock.

Physical examination – must check!

Two distinct assessments must be made on physical examination: the severity of the shock and its underlying cause.

- *Signs of shock.* It is important to recognise the signs of shock in its relatively early stages before the child collapses. Early symptoms include restlessness, tachycardia with a thready pulse and pallor with cold clammy extremities. At this stage the blood pressure may be normal. Poor skin perfusion can be assessed by blanching the skin by pressing on it with a finger and seeing how long it takes for the capillaries to refill. Oliguria is a common feature of the shocked child. Once hypotension occurs, the child is extremely ill.
- *Signs of the underlying cause of the shock.* Signs include petechial or purpuric skin lesions in meningococcaemia, evidence of trauma, and hepatomegaly in cardiac failure.

The focus of a septicaemic illness may be otitis media (examine tympanic membranes), meningitis (assess for neck stiffness), osteomyelitis and septic arthritis (examine joints and limbs for sites of swelling and tenderness).

Investigations

The relevant investigations and their significance are shown in Table 23.4.

- *Blood gases.* Metabolic acidosis occurs as the result of anaerobic tissue metabolism.
- *Electrolytes* and *urea* to assess dehydration.
- *Blood glucose* to exclude hypoglycaemia or diabetic ketoacidosis.
- *Cardiac troponins* may be non-specifically elevated, regardless of cause of shock, but indicate increased risk of severe morbidity and mortality.
- *ECG* to evaluate cardiac function.
- A *central venous pressure* (CVP) line is helpful to assess the degree of fluid loss and to monitor replacement.
- *Blood cultures*
- *Echocardiography* to assess cardiac function
- *Chest X-ray*

Management

See Box 23.3. Time is critical in shock and there is a 'golden hour' during which the shock may still be reversible. The key to management is to give intravenous fluid irrespective of the cause. Isotonic saline should be given rapidly in repeated large volumes (20 mL/kg) to restore the blood pressure. Blood is essential if there has been acute blood loss. Drugs to improve cardiac output may also be useful. These include dobutamine, dopamine, adrenaline, and noradrenaline, which have the effect of improving cardiac output by increasing heart rate, improving myocardial contractility and causing peripheral vasoconstriction.

Specific treatment must be directed towards the cause of the shock, such as antibiotics for infection and corticosteroids for anaphylaxis.

Prognosis

Approximately 20% of children who present with hypotensive shock will die. A small proportion of the survivors will sustain irreversible brain injury as a result of failure of brain perfusion. The two most important prognostic factors are the duration of shock prior to adequate treatment and the underlying cause of the shock.

Table 23.4 Investigations in shock and their relevance

Investigation	Relevance
Full blood count (FBC)	Neutrophilia suggests infection
Blood cultures	Septicaemia
Blood pH	Metabolic acidosis suggests tissue hypoxaemia
Serum electrolytes and urea	High urea/creatinine indicates dehydration or renal impairment
Blood glucose	Hypoglycaemia Hyperglycaemia as a result of diabetic ketoacidosis
ECG and echocardiography	Cardiac function
Central venous pressure	Low in dehydration High in cardiac failure

Box 23.3 Management of shock

- Give intravenous 3rd generation cephalosporin e.g. ceftriaxone if sepsis or meningococcaemia suspected (pp. 154, 351)
- Give rapid intravenous fluid boluses of 20 mL/kg for medical causes of shock
- Give blood to replace haemorrhagic loss in 10ml/kg aliquots
- Monitor fluid replacement by central venous pressure line
- Give inotropes if cardiac performance is impaired
- Investigate and treat underlying cause(s)
- Continue monitoring in an intensive care environment
- Treat complications: coma, renal failure, etc.

Key points: Shock

- Recognise the signs of shock before the child collapses
- Elucidate the cause clinically and carry out investigations
- Give intravenous fluids

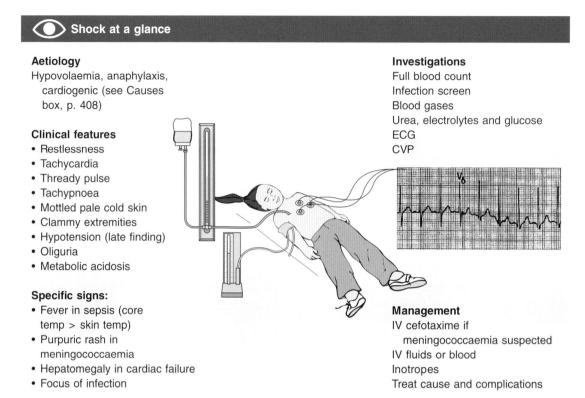

Shock at a glance

Aetiology

Hypovolaemia, anaphylaxis, cardiogenic (see Causes box, p. 408)

Clinical features
- Restlessness
- Tachycardia
- Thready pulse
- Tachypnoea
- Mottled pale cold skin
- Clammy extremities
- Hypotension (late finding)
- Oliguria
- Metabolic acidosis

Specific signs:
- Fever in sepsis (core temp > skin temp)
- Purpuric rash in meningococcaemia
- Hepatomegaly in cardiac failure
- Focus of infection

Investigations

Full blood count
Infection screen
Blood gases
Urea, electrolytes and glucose
ECG
CVP

Management

IV cefotaxime if meningococcaemia suspected
IV fluids or blood
Inotropes
Treat cause and complications

Coma

Causes of coma

Head injury (accidental or non-accidental)
Meningitis/encephalitis
Seizures, particularly status epilepticus
Cerebrovascular accident
Acute asphyxial event
   birth asphyxia
   post-cardiac arrest
Drug or alcohol-induced
Raised intracranial pressure
Metabolic disorders
   hypoglycaemia
   diabetic ketoacidosis
   inborn errors of metabolism
Drowning
Electrocution

Coma is a poorly understood condition and refers to a markedly reduced state of consciousness caused by a reduction in cerebral metabolic rate. Sometimes the terms 'encephalopathy' or 'stupor', which refers to altered state of consciousness, are used to describe a precomatose state. Prolonged epileptic seizures are an important cause of coma and are a medical emergency.

The first task is to stabilize the child (see below) prior to further evaluation.

History – must ask!

Once the child is stable, take a careful history. Focus particularly on whether there has been a prodromal illness, headache or vomiting prior to coma, alternating conscious levels, history of recent contacts with infectious diseases, possibility of drug or alcohol ingestion (either deliberate or accidental in young children) or a recent head injury. Be aware of the possibility of non-accidental injury. If there has been a seizure, ascertain its duration and whether there has been a history of previous seizures. Document the neurodevelopmental state of the child prior to the status. Clarify if there is any significant past medical history.

Physical examination – must check!

Carry out a careful neurological examination to establish the degree of coma. The Glasgow Coma Scale (GCS) is a vital standardized tool for rapid evaluation and guide to management (see Figure 23.4).

- *Vital signs.* Bradycardia with hypertension and irregular breathing (Cushing triad) suggests raised intracranial pressure, and fever with tachycardia suggests infection. Cardiac arrhythmia occurs in some types of drug overdose. Tachypnoea occurs in respiratory distress and deep sighing (Kussmaul) respirations are a feature of diabetic ketoacidosis.

Eyes open	Best verbal response	Best motor response
Spontaneously	Orientated	Obeys commands
To speech	Confused	Localizes pain
To pain	Inappropriate words	Purposeful movement to pain Withdraws from pain
None	Meaningless utterances	Extension to pain
	None	None

Figure 23.4 Glasgow Coma scale and Children's Glasgow Coma scale. The lower the score the deeper the coma (minimum 3/15).

- *Focus of infection.* Examine the child for a focus of infection that might have precipitated coma. This includes signs of consolidation in the chest, meningeal irritation and otitis media.
- *Depth of coma.* This can be determined clinically by assessing the child's best response to commands (Figure 23.4). The lighter the coma, the more appropriate the response, and the deeper the coma, the less the response. In deep coma there is no response at all. The AVPU score is the simplest classification, where the child is classified as either **A**: Alert; **V**: responds to Voice; **P**: responds to Pain; or **U**: Unresponsive.
- *Papilloedema.* Examine the fundi for papilloedema: a sign of raised intracranial pressure that may be accompanied by a slow pulse and raised blood pressure.
- *Pupillary light reflex.* A unilateral dilated pupil with impaired light reflex indicates a third nerve palsy caused by temporal lobe herniation. Unresponsive mydriasis (pupillary dilatation) or miosis (pupillary constriction) suggests drug or toxin exposure.

Investigations

Investigations required and their relevance are shown in Table 23.5. The commonest and most treatable metabolic cause of coma is hypoglycaemia, and all children with an altered level of consciousness should have an urgent fingerprick stick test for blood glucose.

All unconscious children must have a brain scan before lumbar puncture (LP) to assess for any risk of coning (p. 235). Computed tomography (CT) or magnetic resonance imaging (MRI) scans will show focal pathology (tumour, haemorrhage, infarction) and will indicate whether severe oedema is present, but cannot exclude raised intracranial pressure. If meningoencephalitis is the working diagnosis and there are no contraindications, lumbar puncture should be performed. See RCPCH guideline 'The management of children and young people with an acute decrease in conscious level'.

Table 23.5 The relevance of various investigations in elucidating the cause of coma

Investigation	Relevance
Blood glucose	Hypoglycaemia: rapid coma
	Hyperglycaemia: ketoacidosis and slower onset of coma
Full blood count	Elevated WCC and shift to left in infection
	Decreased PCV and decreased Hb in acute haemorrhage
Liver enzymes	Elevated in metabolic conditions or viral infections
Ammonia	Elevated in metabolic conditions
Blood and urine culture	Organisms identified if infection
Urea and electrolytes	Elevated urea if dehydrated
Blood gases	Indicates metabolic or respiratory acidosis (see p. 112 for interpretation)
Chest X-ray	Infection or cardiac failure
CT or MRI scan	Focal pathology (tumour, haemorrhage, abscess)
	Cerebral oedema
Lumbar puncture	Only if no cerebral oedema or features of raised ICP on imaging
	Positive in encephalo-meningitis (see Table 7.8, p. 114, for interpretation)
Urine for toxicology	Indicates the presence of common drug metabolites in the case of poisoning

WCC, white cell count; PCV, packed cell volume; Hb, haemoglobin; CT, computed tomography; MRI, magnetic resonance imaging; ICP, intracranial pressure.

Management

Specific therapy for cerebral oedema includes the use of osmotic agents (e.g. hypertonic saline, mannitol). Steroids are only used for focal oedema around a tumour. High-dose barbiturates are commonly used to reduce cerebral metabolic rate once a child is ventilated.

If the child is convulsing on admission, rapid treatment should be given to terminate the episode (see p. 415). If the child is postictal, the level of consciousness should be ascertained (see Figure 23.4). Examination for signs of head injury, pupillary reflex and formal neurological assessment should be carried out.

Drug ingestion may require specific therapy (see p. 420).

Prognosis

This depends largely on the underlying cause of the coma. The concept of brainstem death is now accepted in most countries, and life support can be withdrawn in such patients despite continued cardiac activity. Brain death should be diagnosed by two consultant doctors who are not responsible for the child's care.

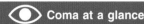

Key points: Coma

- Establish a secure airway by intubation if the child is unconscious
- Nurse child in the recovery position and aspirate any vomitus
- Check blood sugar and give 2 mL/kg 10% glucose bolus if low
- Establish the underlying cause
- Request hourly neurological observations by an experienced nurse

Coma at a glance

Aetiology
See Causes box, p. 410

Assessment
Depth of coma: AVPU
A: Alert
V: responds to Voice
P: responds to Pain
U: Unresponsive
Pulse: tachycardia, bradycardia, dysrhythmia
Breathing: depressed respiration, Kussmaul, tachypnoea
Colour: cyanosis, pallor

Blood pressure
Neurological examination: Pupils
Papilloedema, retinal haemorrhage
Focal signs
Fever
Focus of infection
Signs of trauma

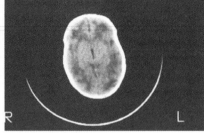
Recovery position

Investigations
Dextrostix and blood glucose
Infection screen with LP
Drug screen
Urea and electrolytes
Blood gases
Chest X-ray
CT or MRI scan (prior to LP)

Management
Intubate if unconscious
Recovery position
Treat hypoglycaemia
Hourly neurological observations

The generalised seizure

Causes of seizures in children

Febrile seizures
Meningitis
Epilepsy
Hypoglycaemia
Hypocalcaemia
Head injury
Asphyxia
Tumour
Neurodegenerative disease

Seizures are a very common symptom and occur in approximately 20% of children in the first five years of life. They are often solitary and do not indicate either that the child will have further seizures or that he or she will develop epilepsy. This section deals with the acute investigation and management of the generalised seizure. The assessment and management of epilepsy is discussed in Chapter 13. Neonatal seizures are dealt with in Chapter 24. The most common trigger factor for generalised seizures in children is fever, and these are referred to as febrile seizures (see p. 422).

Status epilepticus

Status epilepticus is defined as continuous seizure activity lasting for 30 minutes or more, or a series of shorter seizures with failure to regain consciousness between them. It may occur as the result of a febrile seizure, in a child with known epilepsy, or it may be secondary to other acute conditions. Prolonged seizure activity may lead to brain damage and therefore it needs to be terminated rapidly by administration of anticonvulsants.

History – must ask!

- *Description of the seizure.* It is very important to obtain an eyewitness account of the seizure so that a 'video' image of the episode can be visualized in the clinician's mind. Particular features to enquire about include:
  1 Duration of the seizure.
  2 Did the seizure start focally (confined to one side or one limb) and then spread to become generalised?
- *Triggers.* Was the child unwell or pyrexial before the seizure? Is drug ingestion or poisoning a possibility?
- *Past history.* Is there a previous history of seizures and any medication for these? Was the child neurologically and developmentally normal prior to the seizure?

Physical examination – must check!

- *Vital signs.* Assess the child's pulse, respiratory rate and general condition. If the child is cyanosed, immediately ascertain the patency of the airway.
- *Fever.* Record the child's temperature. Pyrexia may suggest that the child has had a febrile seizure.
- *Focus of infection.* If the child is pyrexial, look for a source of infection, including examination of the tympanic membranes, throat and chest.
- *Central nervous system examination.* Neurological examination is particularly important as a seizure may be the first sign of meningitis or other neurological disorders.

Investigations

Meningoencephalitis should be considered in all children presenting with status epilepticus who are febrile and neuroimaging and lumbar puncture are usually performed.

Investigations are not necessary in all cases of prolonged seizure, particularly if the child is having repeated febrile seizures. Advisable investigations are shown in Table 23.6.

An electroencephalogram (EEG) is not indicated, but is sometimes used to diagnose meningoencephalitis.

Computer tomography or magnetic resonance imaging brain scans are not indicated unless the child shows focal convulsive activity.

Management of the child with seizures

See Box 23.4. First place the child in the recovery position and secure the airway (Figure 23.5). The unconscious or semiconscious child should be nursed in the recovery position until he or she recovers or arrives in hospital. If the seizure is prolonged,

Table 23.6 Investigations and their relevance in the child with a first generalised seizure

Investigation	Relevance
Full blood count	Signs of bacterial infection
Throat, urine and blood culture, CXR, PCR	Occult bacterial and viral infection
Lumbar puncture and CSF PCR	Meningitis/ meningoencephalitis
Blood glucose	Hypoglycaemia (diabetic or metabolic disorder)
U&E, calcium, magnesium	Hyponatraemia, hypocalcaemia or hypomagnesaemia
CT/MRI scan	Injury, or focal neurological signs suggest intracranial bleed or tumour

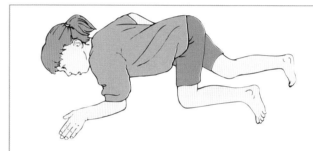

Figure 23.5 The recovery position.

it should be aborted by anticonvulsants. The next step is to ascertain the cause of the seizure.

Status epilepticus

If the child is in status epilepticus (Figure 23.6), a maximum of two doses of benzodiazepines (lorazepam, midazolam or diazepam) can be given. The intravenous route is preferable when available. A side effect of benzodiazepine administration and of a prolonged seizure itself, is respiratory depression, and if this occurs, the child will need mechanical ventilation in an intensive care setting.

Subsequent management

It is most important to spend time explaining the cause of the seizure, first-aid procedures and prognosis to the parents. Reassure them that death is extremely unlikely during a seizure and by following simple first aid measures it can be avoided. Parents whose child has had a seizure should be instructed in the first-aid management of a seizure, including the use of

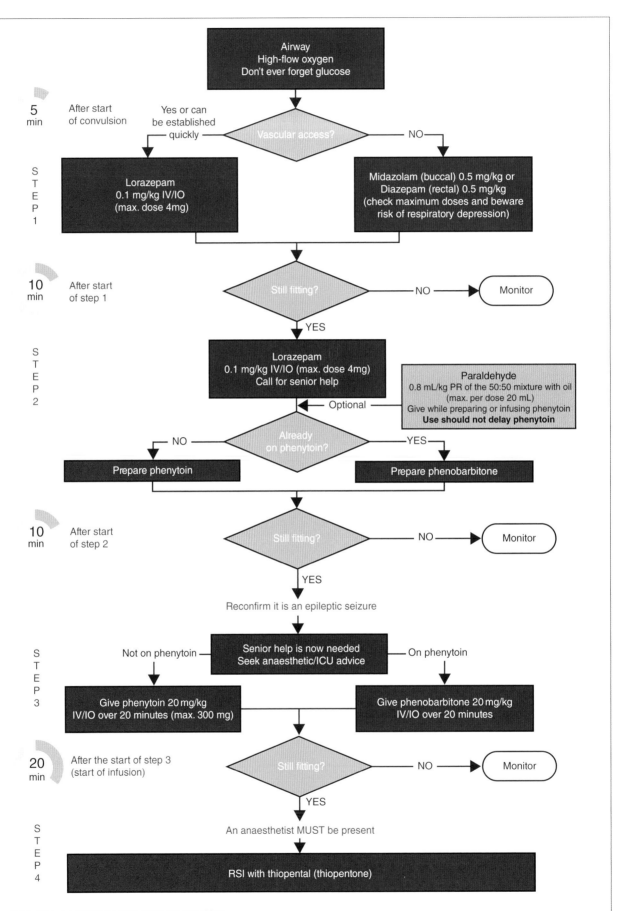

Figure 23.6 Status epilepticus management algorithm.

Box 23.4 Emergency treatment of the convulsing child

- Check airway
- Lay the child on the floor in the recovery position (Figure 23.5)
- Do not insert objects into the child's mouth
- The child needs medication to abort the seizure if it lasts longer than 5 minutes

buccal midazolam (or rarely rectal diazepam) (see Box 23.6). The management of epilepsy is covered in Chapter 13.

Prognosis

The chance of further seizures is determined by the cause of the seizure. Febrile seizures (see p. 422) occur in children aged 6 months to 6 years. Further details on epileptic seizures are discussed in Chapter 13.

Key points: Seizures

- Place the child in the recovery position and give benzodiazepines if the seizure lasts >5 minutes
- Obtain an eyewitness account of the seizure
- Exclude hypoglycaemia and hypocalcaemia
- Consider investigating for infection (including an LP)
- Don't diagnose epilepsy unless clinically appropriate
- Teach parents how to administer buccal midazolam or rectal diazepam if seizures are recurrent and/or prolonged
- Only request an EEG to support a clinical diagnosis of epilepsy or to when sedated to aid diagnosis of meningoencephalitis

Generalised convulsions at a glance

Aetiology
See Causes box, p. 412

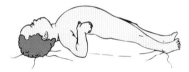

Clinical features
Obtain eyewitness account
History of:
- previous seizures
- diabetes
- trauma
- fever
- drug ingestion
- developmental disabilities
- perinatal problems

Signs of:
- focus of infection
- neurological abnormality

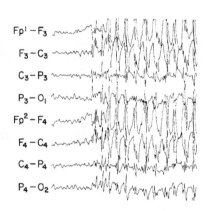

Investigations
Dextrostix and blood glucose
Electrolytes, calcium, magnesium
Drug levels (if on anticonvulsants or suspected ingestion)
Blood gases
Others as indicated: infection screen, FBC, MRI, liver function tests, toxic screen, skull X-ray, CT scan, EEG

Management
Nurse in recovery position
Suction secretions, oxygen by mask
Assess and treat hypoglycaemia
Anticonvulsants: Buccal midazolam for prolonged convulsive seizures or rectal diazepam at home
In hospital IV lorazepam is the drug of first choice
Mechanical ventilation if respiratory depression occurs

Dehydration

Commoner causes of dehydration		
	Site of loss	**Cause**
Excess losses	Stool	Gastroenteritis
	Urine	Diabetes mellitus
	Vomiting	Pyloric stenosis
		Gastroenteritis
	Sweat	High fever
		Hot climate
		Extended dancing (probably in the presence of drugs)
	Other body fluids	Acute surgical losses
		Fluid loss from burns
Decreased intake	Inability to drink	Stomatitis
		Tonsillitis

Water is the major constituent of the human body, and a reduction in body water by more than 5% represents significant dehydration. As much as 80% of an infant's body weight is made up of water, and this proportion falls to about 65% by 3 years. Loss of body fluids is therefore poorly sustained, and dehydration occurs much more readily in infants than in older children and adults. In addition, the physiological mechanisms to prevent excessive fluid losses are less efficient in infants, so further predisposing them to dehydration.

Body water is distributed between the cells (intracellular) and the extracellular compartments. The extracellular compartments can be further divided into the intravascular and the extravascular (interstitial) spaces, separated by the capillary endothelium. Dehydration may occur as the result of depletion of fluid from any of these compartments. Acute loss of fluid from the intravascular compartment may be associated with shock (see p. 408).

The clinical signs of dehydration also depend on the concentration of electrolytes in the intracellular and extracellular compartments. Sodium and bicarbonate are the major ions within the extracellular compartment, and potassium is the major intracellular cation.

Normal body fluid is maintained by a balance between intake and output and depends on the following:
- fluid intake;
- urine volume;
- stool volume;
- sweating;
- insensible loss (water vapour in breath).

Dehydration occurs where the losses exceed the input.

Gastroenteritis is the commonest cause of excessive fluid loss. Sodium may be lost in the same proportion as water; this is called isonatraemic (isotonic) dehydration. Sometimes sodium is lost but is replaced by water, so resulting in hyponatraemic dehydration. More rarely, less sodium than water is lost, or a relative excess of sodium is replaced, causing hypernatraemic dehydration.

When you evaluate a child who presents with dehydration, you need to assess how severe the dehydration is so that you can calculate how much fluid replacement is required. You also need to identify the cause of the dehydration.

The extent of the fluid loss is principally determined by clinical history and physical examination, and by the end of your assessment you should have decided if the child is:
- mildly dehydrated, in which case you can estimate that the child has experienced <4% losses
- moderately dehydrated, in which case you can estimate that the child has experienced 4–6% losses
- severely dehydrated, in which case you can estimate that the child has experienced >7% losses.

History – must ask!

- *Causes of dehydration.* Enquire about diarrhoea, vomiting or excessive drinking (polydipsia is a common symptom in acute-onset diabetes, see pp. 298, 304). Projectile vomiting in a young infant suggests pyloric stenosis.
- *Severity of dehydration.* Enquire into how many loose stools and how long the diarrhoea has persisted. Ask if the child is passing less urine, and how many wet nappies there have been in last 24 hours. If the child has been vomiting, enquire how often and for how long.

Physical examination – must check!

You need to assess both the severity of the dehydration and its most likely cause.
- *Weight.* Weighing the child is extremely important. Acute water loss can be estimated from the difference between actual weight and a recent weight made before dehydration occurred (1g of body weight is roughly equivalent to 1mL of water). Even if a recent weight is not available, regular weighing (twice daily in the acute situation) will allow accurate management of fluid replacement.
- *Causes of dehydration.* A thorough examination should identify foci of infection or other causes of dehydration. You need to examine the ears, throat, chest and abdomen. In the young infant, pay particular attention to detecting a pyloric 'olive', suggestive of pyloric stenosis, if vomiting has been a feature, although this is rare in early disease.
- *Severity of dehydration* (Figure 23.7 and Table 23.7). Examine the child for the following specific features to determine how severely dehydrated he or she is:
  - skin turgor;
  - fontanelle;
  - respiratory rate;
  - skin perfusion;
  - pulse rate and character.

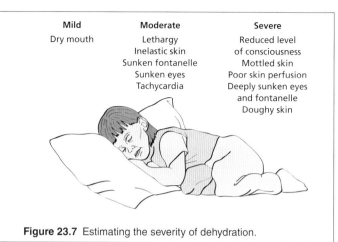

Mild	Moderate	Severe
Dry mouth	Lethargy Inelastic skin Sunken fontanelle Sunken eyes Tachycardia	Reduced level of consciousness Mottled skin Poor skin perfusion Deeply sunken eyes and fontanelle Doughy skin

Figure 23.7 Estimating the severity of dehydration.

Table 23.7 Clinical features in estimating the severity of dehydration		
Clinical feature	**Moderate**	**Severe**
Reported urine output	Reduced in last 24 h	No urine in last 12 h
Pulse	Tachycardic	Tachycardic
Blood pressure	Normal	Low
Capillary refill time	2 seconds	≥3 seconds
Fontanelle	Sunken	Very sunken
Skin turgor	Reduced	Very reduced
Percentage dehydrated	4–6%	≥7%

In *mild dehydration* the only physical sign may be reduced urine output and a concentrated urine. A dry mouth, is an unreliable indicator of dehydration as it can be influenced by mouth breathing or recent oral fluid. In *moderate dehydration* the child is lethargic, with inelastic skin, a sunken fontanelle and sunken eyes. The pulse may be fast, but is usually of normal volume, and the capillary refill time may be around 2 seconds. Skin turgor (the elasticity of the skin in response to gently lifting the skin) is reduced in dehydration, although this is a relatively late sign in hypernatraemic dehydration.

In *severe dehydration* the child may be very confused and only semiconscious. There are signs of shock in that the skin is mottled, there is delayed capillary refill time and the pulse is thread and fast. The fontanelle and eyes are deeply sunken, and the skin turgor is significantly reduced.

Investigations

In the child who is ill, investigations are required to determine the type of dehydration and the presence of acidosis, and may also be required to determine the cause.

Plasma electrolytes and blood gas   Measure the serum sodium, potassium, chloride, bicarbonate, urea and creatinine. A differential loss of sodium may occur, leading to hyper- or hyponatraemia, and the management will then differ. Bicarbonate may be lost as a result of diarrhoea, causing a metabolic acidosis. If excessive vomiting occurs, excessive hydrogen ions are lost, which may cause an initial metabolic alkalosis (see pyloric stenosis, p. 203). Disturbances in acid–base balance are discussed on p. 111.

Urine assessment   Assess the urine for specific gravity or osmolality, and consider measuring urinary electrolytes. An assessment of urinary volume over a known period of time is important and the fluid balance should be carefully monitored.

Determining the type of dehydration

Isotonic dehydration, where there are equal losses of sodium and water, is the commonest type of dehydration. Hyponatraemic and hypernatraemic dehydration may also occur.

- *Isotonic dehydration.* The serum sodium is normal, and children show physical signs commensurate with the degree of fluid loss.
- *Hyponatraemic dehydration.* This is defined as dehydration with serum sodium <130 mmol/L. It generally occurs when fluid losses have been replaced with hypotonic solutions such as water or fizzy drinks. The child is lethargic, and the skin is dry and inelastic.
- *Hypernatraemic dehydration.* This is defined as dehydration with serum sodium >150 mmol/L. It can occur through severe and acute water loss, but more commonly is seen in breast-fed babies in the first two weeks of life if there is difficulty establishing feeds, or caused by a parent giving concentrated formula feeds having incorrectly measured out scoops of powdered milk. The infant initially appears to be very hungry, but has fewer clinical signs of dehydration. The skin feels doughy. Metabolic acidosis is a common feature of this condition.

Managing the dehydrated child

Oral rehydration therapy

A child who is only mildly dehydrated may be treated using oral hydration therapy. Children with more significant dehydration need assessment in hospital. If vomiting is not a major feature, oral rehydration is usually successful and should be tried before intravenous therapy is considered. Commercially available oral rehydration solutions, such as Dioralyte or Rehidrat, should be used as they have the correct electrolyte balance. These are dispensed as oral solutions, effervescent tablets or powders, and are reconstituted with freshly boiled and cooled water. Ondansetron, or other anti-emetics, may be considered but are not routinely used.

Breast-feeding should be maintained while using these solutions. If the baby is bottle-fed, normal milk feed can be given once the diarrhoea has settled. Recurrence of diarrhoea on refeeding is most likely to be caused by transient lactose intolerance, and a lactose-free milk should be used for up to 6 weeks.

Intravenous therapy

In a child with more significant dehydration, or who has been unable to tolerate an oral fluid challenge may require intravenous fluids. It is important to assess the fluid balance frequently, including maintaining an accurate input–output chart, weighing the child twice daily and at least daily measurements of serum electrolytes.

The principles of rehydration are simple and require three calculations:

1 an estimate of the acute fluid loss;
2 an estimate of maintenance fluid requirements;
3 an assessment of ongoing losses.

These three estimates are added together to determine the volume of fluid that you need to replace over the next 24–48 hours. An example is shown in Box 23.5.

Estimate of acute fluid loss   The difference between actual weight and a recent normal weight is a good approximate method of estimating acute water loss. If the normal weight is unknown, rely on your clinical assessment of the dehydration. To calculate the volume requiring replacement:

$$(\text{actual weight in kilograms} \times \text{percent dehydration}) \times 10 = \text{deficit (mL)}$$

Example: 10kg child who is 7% dehydrated
10kg x 7% dehydrated x 10 = 700mL deficit

Estimate of maintenance requirements   Maintenance water and sodium intake depends on the weight of the child. The requirements are shown in Table 23.9.

Estimate of ongoing losses   If possible, ongoing losses must be carefully measured on an hourly basis and added to the fluid regimen every 4 hours.

Table 23.8 Calculating daily maintenance requirements of fluid based on body weight

For the first 10kg of weight	100mL/kg
For the next 10kg of weight	As above plus 50mL/kg
For subsequent kg of weight	As above plus 20mL/kg

Rehydration protocol

Therefore a 32kg child would require for maintenance $(10 \times 100) + (10 \times 50) + (12 \times 20) = 1740\text{mL}$ in 24 hours, or 72.5mL/hour

Box 23.5 Example of the calculation used for replacement fluids

A 3-year-old boy with severe gastroenteritis for 3 days is admitted. He is estimated on clinical grounds to be 6% dehydrated. On admission his weight is 15 kg.

Step 1 Assess the fluid deficit
15kg x 6% dehydrated x 10 = 900mL

Step 2 Assess the maintenance fluids required in next 24 hours
The maintenance requirements are (10kg x 100mL) + (5kg x 50mL) = 1250mL/day

Step 3 Give maintenance plus deficit
Total fluid = 900mL deficit + 1250mL maintenance = 2150mL over 24 hours (90mL/hour)
In hypernatraemic dehydration it is vital to rehydrate more slowly (e.g. to give maintenance plus half the deficit over the first 24 hours), because *if the serum sodium falls too rapidly, cerebral oedema can occur.*

If any fluid boluses have already been administered these need to be taken off the maintenance requirement.

The most appropriate fluid is usually 0.9% sodium chloride with 5% glucose. See NICE guideline (NG29) 'Intravenous fluid therapy in children and young people in hospital' for further advice.

Key points: Dehydration

- Determine the percentage dehydration on the basis of clinical signs, urine output and vital signs
- Identify the underlying reason for the dehydration
- Replace fluid according to:
  - the severity of fluid loss
  - whether dehydration is iso-, hypo-, or hypernatraemic
  - the ongoing losses and maintenance needs
- Treat the underlying cause if one is identified
- Blood glucose and urea and electrolytes need to be checked at least every 24 hours when children are on IV fluids

See NICE guideline: Intravenous fluid therapy in children and young people in hospital
https://www.nice.org.uk/guidance/ng29

Dehydration at a glance

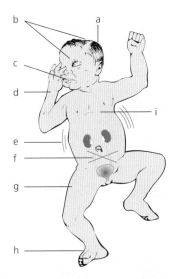

Epidemiology
Infants are the most vulnerable

Aetiology
Gastroenteritis is the commonest
  cause

Physical examination
- Excessive losses – vomiting,
  diarrhoea
- Inadequate replacement of
  fluids
- Lethargic
- ↓ level of consciousness (**a**)
- Sunken fontanelle and eyes (**b**)
- Dry mucous membranes (**c**)
- ↓ blood pressure (**d**)
- Tachypnoea (**e**)
- Oliguria (**f**)
- Reduced skin turgor (**g**)
- Cold (shut-down) peripheries (**h**)
- Tachycardia (**i**)

Confirmatory investigations
Examination findings and body
  weight
Estimate severity of dehydration
Serum and urinary electrolytes
Determine whether iso-, hypo- or
  hypernatraemic

Management
Replace deficit and ongoing
  losses and give maintenance
  fluids

Prognosis
Good
Convulsions most likely in
  hypernatraemic dehydration

Poisoning

Common poisons ingested by children

Drugs	Household agents
Aspirin	Disinfectants
Paracetamol	Bleach
Iron	Weedkiller
Antidepressants	Paraffin or white spirit
	Dishwasher tablets

Accidental drug poisoning in children has become progressively less common in recent years. This is a result of better education of parents about the risks of accidental ingestion in children and the introduction of child-proof containers for the storage of medicines. Accidental ingestion of poisonous household agents remains a problem usually caused by careless storage or putting dangerous compounds such as weedkillers into soft-drink bottles which are very attractive to small children. Poisoning is more likely to occur when a child is at the grandparents' home, where security of dangerous items may not be as strict as at home.

Accidental ingestion of poisons usually occurs in toddlers. It is common to find toddlers playing with tablets without the adult knowing whether they have ingested any or how many. Similarly, household agents such as turpentine may be smelt on the child without knowing whether he or she has swallowed any.

In older children and adolescents, deliberate overdose of medication is common.

History – must ask!

In older children who have taken a deliberate overdose, accurate information of the poisonous agent may not be forthcoming, but a friend may be able to give more reliable information. The following points must be ascertained either from the child or from a responsible adult.

- *Identify the agent.* Any tablet or medicine that may have been taken by the child must be identified. Reference manuals showing the appearance of all pharmacological agents are available, or a Poisons Reference Unit will be able to give advice by telephone or online. Chemicals and household agents should be brought for identification and analysis (pH).
- *Quantity of ingestion.* Establish from the adult what is the maximum number of tablets that the child may have taken.
- *Time from ingestion.*

Physical examination – must check!

The following points must be assessed carefully on the physical examination.

- The child's conscious level must be initially assessed and reassessed regularly (Figure 23.4, p. 411).
- Look for signs of caustic burns or skin irritation around the lips and mouth, which suggest ingestion of an irritant substance.

- Does the child smell of petrol, turpentine or glue, which would give a clue to the ingested substance?
- Cardiac dysrhythmias may occur as a result of tricyclic antidepressant ingestion. Blood pressure and heart rhythm should be regularly measured.

Investigations

If the nature of the poisonous agent is in doubt, urine should be taken for toxicology screen to eliminate or confirm possibilities. If aspirin or paracetamol overdose is suspected, measurement of serum levels of these drugs should be performed (see p. 424).

Management

- Refer to up-to-date guidance from the National Poisons Unit (e.g. www.toxbase.org for the UK).

  In the majority of cases, management consists of careful monitoring and observation. The risks of inducing vomiting usually outweigh any potential benefits and emetics are not usually recommended.

- Activated charcoal, an absorbent, is occasionally recommended to reduce the absorption of some drugs such as carbamazepine and theophylline, but is often poorly tolerated by children.
- Specific antidotes or therapy for the poison should be instituted if appropriate (e.g. naloxone for opiate poisoning).
- Supportive management. Respiratory and/or cardiovascular failure are important and common complications of many forms of poisoning. If the child is comatose, hypotensive or unwell, intravenous fluids should be given and the child nursed in an environment where he or she can be very closely observed and respiratory support can be instituted if necessary.
- Advice to parents concerning the prevention of further accidents or ingestions in the home.
- In a child who has attempted suicide or parasuicide, an appropriate psychiatric assessment (such as by the Child and Adolescent Mental Health (CAMHS) team) should be obtained after an appropriate cooling off period. Children and young people would usually stay in hospital until they have been assessed.

For the specific management of salicylate and paracetomol poisoning, see p. 424.

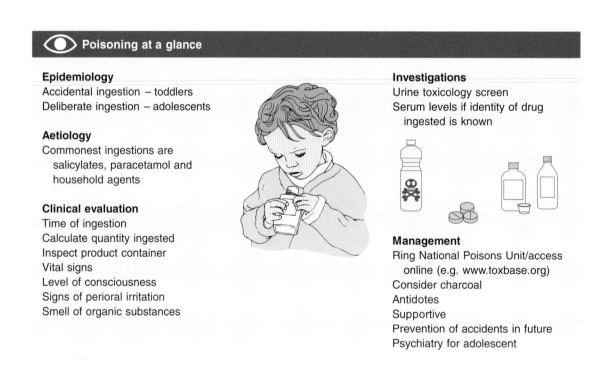

Poisoning at a glance

Epidemiology
Accidental ingestion – toddlers
Deliberate ingestion – adolescents

Aetiology
Commonest ingestions are
  salicylates, paracetamol and
  household agents

Clinical evaluation
Time of ingestion
Calculate quantity ingested
Inspect product container
Vital signs
Level of consciousness
Signs of perioral irritation
Smell of organic substances

Investigations
Urine toxicology screen
Serum levels if identity of drug
  ingested is known

Management
Ring National Poisons Unit/access
  online (e.g. www.toxbase.org)
Consider charcoal
Antidotes
Supportive
Prevention of accidents in future
Psychiatry for adolescent

Emergency paediatric conditions

Sepsis

Clinical features Sepsis is a condition where the body's response to an infection becomes over-whelming and can lead to organ failure and death. It is a spectrum and will, by definition, start with an infection, which is usually bacterial (such as urine, chest or skin infection). When the signs and symptoms of sepsis are present action must be prompt in order to treat the infection and to manage the symptoms, such as poor systemic perfusion.

Certain bacteria such as *Neisseria meningitidis* in the older child (p. 154) or Group B Streptococcus in the infant are likely to cause sepsis. Some bacteria (e.g. certain staphylococci) produce a toxin which causes massive vasodilatation and shock.

Management Infants under 3 months of age who have, or have had, a fever over 38 °C, or who have signs of sepsis, may require a lumbar puncture for suspected meningitis. Full blood count (FBC), C-reactive protein (CRP), cultures of urine, blood and/or stool, nasal secretions (as appropriate) should also be taken to assess for the source of the infection. Infants under 3 months with fever over 38 °C and suspected sepsis require prompt administration of intravenous antibiotics (such as a third-generation cephalosporin e.g. cefotaxime, as well as an antibiotic that covers for listeriosis, e.g. amoxicillin). This should be given immediately if the infant is under 1 month of age, appears unwell, or has an abnormal white cell count on FBC. The 'Rochester guidelines' or the NICE clinical guideline (CG160) 'Fever in under 5s: assessment and initial management' give further advice on management.

Older children may also present with sepsis and shock (see below) and require prompt assessment and management. Unexplained tachycardia (once the fever has settled, and where there is no other cause such as dehydration or pain) should raise concerns about sepsis and a thorough assessment carried out. Broad-spectrum antibiotics (such as ceftriaxone) should be administered within 60 minutes for children with suspected sepsis.

Anaphylactic reaction

Anaphylaxis is a very severe, life-threatening allergic reaction. It is rare and may develop rapidly to potentially fatal laryngeal oedema. It occurs as a type I allergic reaction to a large number of allergens. The most common are drugs (e.g. penicillin), blood transfusions, food (eggs, peanuts, etc.) and insect stings. In some cases, no allergen can be identified.

Clinical features The allergic reaction usually starts with pruritus, urticaria, and wheeze. In many cases the reaction is not severe and does not progress. In some cases, bronchospasm becomes very severe and laryngeal oedema causes acute stridor. Rarely, circulatory collapse occurs.

Management A severe allergic reaction should be treated rapidly. If the airway is compromised, the child should be intubated. Drug treatment includes:

- *Adrenaline* given as an emergency intramuscular injection.
- *Corticosteroids* (hydrocortisone intravenously or intramuscularly). These may take several hours to have an effect.
- *Antihistamines.*
- *Nebulized bronchodilators* if bronchospasm develops

In children who have had one episode of anaphylaxis, an adrenaline auto-injector pen should be prescribed for administration subcutaneously and oral antihistamine to keep with them to treat the child following a subsequent inadvertent exposure to the allergen. In addition, they must be taught basic life support techniques.

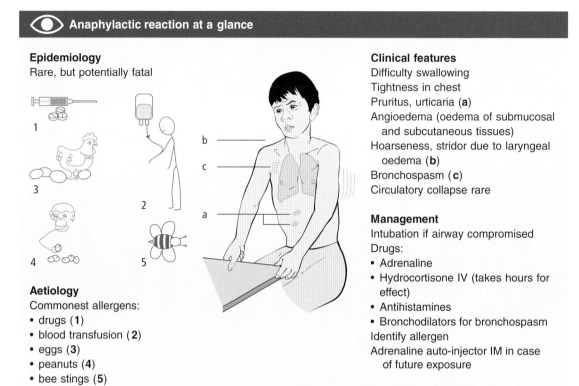

◉ Anaphylactic reaction at a glance

Epidemiology
Rare, but potentially fatal

Clinical features
Difficulty swallowing
Tightness in chest
Pruritus, urticaria (**a**)
Angioedema (oedema of submucosal
    and subcutaneous tissues)
Hoarseness, stridor due to laryngeal
    oedema (**b**)
Bronchospasm (**c**)
Circulatory collapse rare

Management
Intubation if airway compromised
Drugs:
• Adrenaline
• Hydrocortisone IV (takes hours for
  effect)
• Antihistamines
• Bronchodilators for bronchospasm
Identify allergen
Adrenaline auto-injector IM in case
  of future exposure

Aetiology
Commonest allergens:
• drugs (**1**)
• blood transfusion (**2**)
• eggs (**3**)
• peanuts (**4**)
• bee stings (**5**)

Febrile seizures

Febrile seizures are seizures which occur in children between the age of 6 months and 6 years and are caused by fever. The immature brain is more susceptible to environmental factors, and fever may precipitate a seizure. They occur in 5% of all children in this age group, and the risk is higher if there is a family history.

Clinical features   Fever precedes the seizure, but there may be a sudden rise in body temperature immediately before the seizure which may be unrecognised. The seizure is usually short-lived, lasting under five minutes. Status epilepticus occurs in only about 1% of febrile seizures. Febrile seizures are classed as 'atypical' if they last longer than 10–20 minutes; occur twice in the same illness or within 24 hours; or have focal features. In all children with febrile seizures a careful examination should be performed in order to identify the site of infection.

Management   Any seizure lasting for more than 5 minutes should be terminated with an anticonvulsant, such as buccal midazolam or rectal diazepam (Box 23.6). The child must be examined for any source of infection. In babies and very young children a lumbar puncture should be considered to rule out meningitis. Parents should be reassured, but instructed about first aid management of further seizures (see Box 23.6). They should be told that the prognosis for brief febrile seizures is

very good. Anticonvulsant medication for children with febrile seizures is not indicated. Families of children who have prolonged seizures should be discharged with buccal midazolam and trained in its use – this training will also need to be given to wider care givers, including nursery/schoolteachers.

Prognosis   There is a slight increased risk of epilepsy only if the child has atypical febrile seizures (see above); has abnormal neurodevelopment; or has a close family history of epilepsy. If none of these risk factors are present the risk of epilepsy is the same as the population risk of 1%. If one risk factor is present the risk increases to 2% and if two or more risk factors are present the risk of subsequent development of epilepsy is 10%.

Box 23.6 Advice to parents whose child has febrile seizures

• Undress the child
• Give paracetamol or ibuprofen for its antipyretic effect is the child is miserable with a fever, although this will not prevent a febrile seizure
• The child should wear minimal clothing and the environment gently cooled
• Give benzodiazepines if the seizure lasts more than 5 minutes
• Seek medical assessment following a seizure to identify focus of infection

Febrile convulsions at a glance

Epidemiology
Occurs between 6 months and
6 years in 5% of children

Aetiology
High fever of any cause,
particularly at sudden rise

History
Short-lived generalised
convulsion
Symptoms of condition
causing the fever

Physical examination
High fever
Normal neurological exam
following seizure
Signs of infection responsible
for fever*

L3
L4
L5
Vertebral
bodies
Spinous
processes
of vertebrae
Spinal
canal

Lumbar puncture

NB *Signs and symptoms are variable

Confirmatory investigations
Lumbar puncture required at
first febrile seizure in some
infants to exclude meningitis
Investigation for cause of fever
if indicated by assessment

Differential diagnosis
Meningitis
Other causes of generalised
convulsion

Management
Cannot be prevented with
antipyretics
Parental advice regarding
management of fever
Treatment of underlying
infection if identified,
Benzodiazepines for prolonged
febrile seizures

Prognosis/complications
Good
Risk of developing epilepsy
only 2% in neurologically
normal children

Head injury

Children often present to hospital acutely with head injury, however few will have any long-term complications from this. It is important to differentiate the children who have intra-cranial bleeds or skull fractures promptly using a CT head scan (see Box 23.7). Guidelines have been drawn up for the management of mild-moderate head injury regarding indications for observation, admission and CT.

 See NICE guideline: NICE clinical guideline (CG176) "Head injury: assessment and early management"). https://www.nice.org.uk/guidance/cg176

Children should have frequent assessment of consciousness following head injury using the Glasgow Coma Scale (GCS) (see Figure 23.4), and if they do not require a CT head should remain under observation for at least 4 hours in hospital. At discharge, these parents and carers should be advised to monitor the child closely and should be given written instructions on how to seek help if concerned.

Box 23.7 Indications to perform a CT head

Glasgow Coma Score (GCS) less than 15 at 2 hours after the injury
Suspicion of non-accidental injury
Post-traumatic seizure in absence of epilepsy
Suspected open or depressed skull fracture or tense fontanelle in a baby
Signs of basal skull fracture (haemotympanum, 'panda' eyes, CSF leak from ear or nose, Battle's sign (bruising behind ear))
For children under one year old a bruise, swelling or laceration on the head of more than 5cm
Focal neurological deficit
On arrival to the emergency department a GCS of less than 14, or for children under 1 year of less than 15
Witnessed loss of consciousness lasting more than 5 minutes
Abnormal drowsiness
Three or more discrete episodes of vomiting
Dangerous mechanism of injury (road traffic collision, fall from over 3 metres or high-speed injury)
Amnesia lasting more than 5 minutes

Stroke

Stroke occurs in people of all ages, but the incidence in utero and in the first year of life is especially high. Stroke is one of the top 10 causes of death in children. The presenting features may be a 'thunderclap' severe headache, weakness of the face, arm or leg, or slurred speech. An urgent CT or MRI head scan should be arranged urgently to look for a stroke, including angiography, and a full neurological assessment carried out. Sometimes focal weakness can resolve spontaneously, but these children should also have imaging of the head and cerebral vessels as they may have had a transient ischaemic event and are at risk of more severe episodes. If stroke is confirmed, the cause also needs to be identified and this may include sickle cell disease, renal disease causing high blood pressure, prothrombotic conditions or trauma.

Paracetamol poisoning

Owing to its easy availability in many homes, as well as the pleasant taste of childrens' liquid paracetamol preparations, paracetamol (acetaminophen) is the most common drug to be ingested accidentally by children. Paracetamol ingestion is rarely severe enough to cause serious problems, but liver failure is the major risk if >150 mg/kg is ingested.

Clinical features   Early symptoms are usually minimal but may include anorexia, nausea and vomiting. Signs of liver failure occur on the second day with abdominal pain, liver tenderness and hepatic failure with jaundice after 2–3 days.

Initially liver function tests are normal. The prothrombin time and liver enzymes become abnormal 12–24 hours after ingestion. The decision to treat depends on a paracetamol serum level 4 hours after ingestion.

Management   Successful treatment depends on early recognition and institution of adequate treatment. In patients with elevated paracetamol levels intravenous *N*-acetyl-cysteine reduces the severity of liver necrosis.

Salicylate poisoning

Salicylate poisoning causes initially a respiratory alkalosis caused by stimulation of the respiratory centre, and later a metabolic acidosis as a result of the acid load of the drug. Gastric bleeding may occur as the result of its effects on the mucosa.

Clinical features   The earliest sign is overbreathing, often associated with vomiting and diarrhoea. Sweating may be a feature. If the overdose has been large, metabolic acidosis occurs about 6–8 hours after ingestion, with ketosis, hyperglycaemia and glycosuria. Eventually collapse may occur with loss of consciousness. The physical and laboratory findings show a considerable similarity with those found in diabetic ketoacidosis, and blood sugar levels should be measured to exclude this possibility.

A serum salicylate level helps to establish the likely severity of the overdose.

Management   Salicylates can be retained in the stomach for a long time, and activated charcoal is often recommended. If the patient is acidotic, sodium bicarbonate is given intravenously, which promotes renal excretion of salicylate. Haemodialysis is occasionally required.

Burns and scalds

Burns are the second commonest cause of accidental childhood death after road traffic accidents. One-half of deaths are caused by smoke inhalation leading to respiratory failure (p. 405) and one-half caused by thermal damage to the skin.

Thermal injuries cause death either as a result of massive fluid loss through the denuded skin or by infection. A second major problem in children who survive is scarring, which may have major psychological consequences.

First aid   Scalds are first treated by removing the clothes over the affected area and cooling the skin with cold water. Children who are scalded or burnt should be wrapped in a clean towel or cling film and brought immediately to hospital.

Clinical assessment   The burn should be graded into superficial grade 1 (erythema only), moderate grade 2 (blistering) or severe grade 3 (full thickness). The extent of the thermal injury must also be assessed. This is done by estimating the surface area of grade 2–3 involved, as illustrated in Figure 23.7. The percentage of body area affected is calculated.

If the child has suffered smoke inhalation, respiratory failure with wheeze, cyanosis and dyspnoea may occur rapidly.

Management   See Box 23.8. Assess the airway and respiratory function. Arterial blood gases may be necessary to decide whether mechanical ventilation is required (p. 111) and can indicate carboxyhaemoglobin levels. Thermal injury to the airway may necessitate rapid endotracheal intubation or even tracheostomy before severe oedema causes obstruction.

If there are significant burns, two intravenous cannulae should be inserted to gain vascular access and give intravenous fluids to prevent or treat shock caused by fluid loss. Analgesia will be needed, and opiates may be required to control pain, with sedation administered when dressings are changed. Careful attention should be paid to nutrition and prevention of infection.

Most burns victims with greater than 20% body surface area with grade 2 or 3 burns are now treated in special burns units. Skin grafting is required for full-thickness burns. This can be assessed after a few days by testing for pain sensation: if a pinprick is not felt, the burn is full thickness. Psychological support will be needed for the child and his or her family if there is extensive scarring.

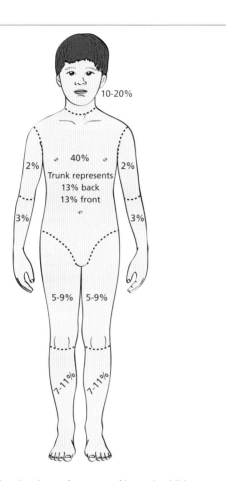

Figure 23.8 Estimating the surface area of burns in children.

Box 23.8 Management of burns

- Give intravenous fluids to compensate for severe fluid loss through burnt skin
- Analgesia to control pain
- If thermal injury to mouth or airway, assess the need for tracheostomy
- Skin grafting for full-thickness burn
- Psychological support for child and family

Drowning

Most drowning incidents in the developed world occur in fresh water (bath, river, swimming pool) and the risk of drowning is increased in males and in toddlers under 4 years old. The outcome following near-drowning in cold water (<10 °C) is traditionally thought to be better than in warm water. This is probably a result of induced hypothermia from immersion.

First aid   The child must be resuscitated at the site of the drowning incident with mouth-to-mouth resuscitation and rapidly transferred to hospital.

Management

- Clear airway and institute mechanical ventilation. Assess circulation and treat if shock is present.
- If hypothermic, slowly warm over a number of hours.

Prognosis   It is well known that children can recover fully despite a very prolonged period of cardiac arrest following a drowning incident, particularly if the child was rescued from cold water. Prolonged resuscitation efforts are therefore necessary until the child is rewarmed.

Hypoxic brain damage rarely occurs after near-drowning, and full recovery is the rule if the child can be resuscitated.

Sudden unexplained death in infancy and childhood (SUDIC) and brief resolved unexplained episodes (BRUE)

SUDIC – The definition of sudden unexplained death in infancy (SUDIC) is 'the sudden death of any infant or young child, which is unexpected by history, and in which a thorough postmortem examination fails to demonstrate an adequate cause for the death'. SUDIC affects infants below the age of 1 year, with the peak rate at 2–4 months. Other causes of sudden death in infancy include metabolic causes, non-accidental injury, and infection, and these should be considered at presentation. Risk factors for SUDIC are shown in Box 23.9.

BRUE – Some children have episodes lasting up to a minute where they appear collapsed but rapidly respond to resuscitation. These are referred to as brief resolved unexplained events (BRUE). There does not appear to be a link between BRUE and SUDIC. In the majority of cases BRUE is due to choking on food or refluxed gastric contents; it seems frightening but almost always resolves without complication. In rare cases BRUE may be due to a seizure or dysrhythmia.

Infants should be placed on the back (supine) to sleep, with the feet at the foot of the bed. They should use light bedding

Box 23.9 Risk factors for sudden unexplained death in infancy and childhood

Birth weight under 2.5kg
Socio-economic deprivation
Premature birth (under 37 weeks gestation)
Parental smoking, especially if the mother smoked during pregnancy
Co-sleeping
High environmental temperature
Sleeping in prone position
Bottle feeding
Non-use of pacifier

which will not become displaced during sleep and the head should be uncovered. Babies under 6 months old should sleep in a separate cot or Moses basket in the parents' room for the first 6 months. The room temperature should be between 16–20 °C. Breast-feeding and the use of a pacifier (dummy) reduce the risk of SUDIC.

⬤ Sudden unexplained death in infancy and childhood (SUDIC) at a glance

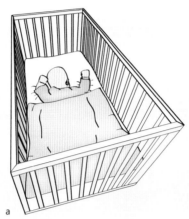

Epidemiology
Commonest cause of infant
   death (past first week)
Affects babies under 12 months,
   peak age 2–4 months

Aetiology
Related to sleep position (**a**),
   temperature (**b**), smoking (**c**)
   and environment
In 20%, a major unsuspected
   condition is found at autopsy

Prevention
Back to Sleep campaign has
   halved deaths due to sudden
   infant death syndrome

History
Normally healthy baby
   (preceding minor illness)
Full and careful history of last
   sleep required

Physical examination
Found dead
Examination usually
   unremarkable

Investigations
As guided by history and
   examination

Differential diagnosis
Sepsis
Gastro-oesophageal reflux
Neurological abnormality
Hypoglycaemia (rare)
Cardiac arrhythmia (rare)
Inborn error of metabolism
   (rare)
Suffocation (rare)

Management
Lead paediatrician for
   unexpected deaths in
   childhood informed

To test your knowledge on this part of the book, please see Chapter 26

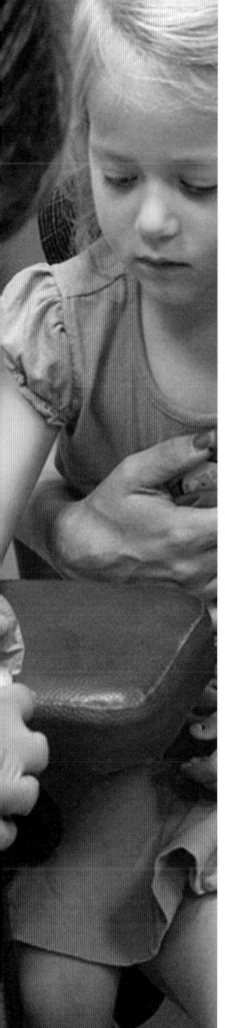

CHAPTER 24
The newborn

My mother groan'd, my father wept;
Into the dangerous world I leapt,
Helpless, naked, piping loud,
Like a fiend hid in a cloud.
Struggling in my father's hands,
Striving against my swaddling
bands,
Bound and weary, I thought best
To sulk upon my mother's breast.
William Blake, 1793

KEY COMPETENCES
You must...

Know and understand

- The difference between prematurity and growth restriction
- The basics of neonatal resuscitation
- The key congenital and perinatal conditions that present in the newborn
- When a jaundiced baby requires investigation
- The principles of establishing breast and bottle feeding

Be able to

- Examine a newborn baby and be able to assess the hips, genitalia and the red reflex
- Recognise a baby in need of resuscitation
- Recognise when a 'septic workup' is needed

Appreciate that

- The newborn is susceptible to infection but may not show classic signs
- A small baby may be either preterm or growth retarded or a combination of the two
- Congenital malformations are common and that a clear management plan should be established before discharge from hospital

Essential Paediatrics and Child Health, Fourth Edition. Mary Rudolf, Anthony Luder and Kerry Jeavons.
© 2020 John Wiley & Sons Ltd. Published 2020 by John Wiley & Sons Ltd.
Companion website: www.wiley.com/go/rudolf/paediatrics

The newborn

Finding your way around ...

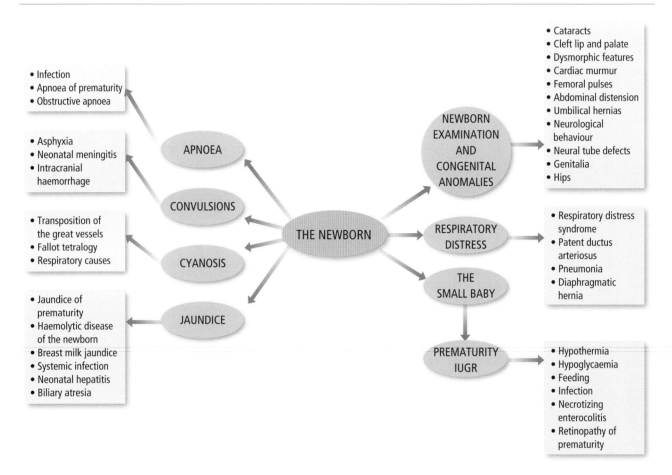

Care of the newborn infant is a very important part of paediatrics. Routine examination for occult, but treatable, abnormalities is performed for all newborn infants to prevent long-term disability. Intensive care of the sick preterm and ill full-term infant has significantly improved mortality and morbidity.

Improvement in care of the newborn over recent years is reflected in progress in perinatal and neonatal mortality rates (see below for definitions). The improvement in perinatal mortality rates (which includes stillbirths) is largely a result of improvements in obstetric care. Reduction in neonatal mortality rate (now below four per 1000 liveborn infants) has been mainly a result of improvements in the care of preterm infants with lung and other disease together with more effective management of congenital abnormalities by safer surgical techniques.

This chapter is arranged in the sequence most appropriate to the way newborn babies present to paediatricians. Only a minority of babies require resuscitation, but for those who do, this must be undertaken immediately and in an efficient and safe manner. All babies should be seen and examined by both a neonatal nurse or midwife and a doctor in the first 12–24 hours of life in order to detect occult congenital abnormalities or evidence of birth trauma in addition to assessment of the infants' acclimatization to extra-uterine life. As a medical student, you should become familiar with the newborn examination and undertake a number of such examinations on your own. You should know the common congenital abnormalities described in this section.

Only 7–9% of babies are born preterm, but these account for the much of the time that paediatricians spend caring for newborns. The small baby and his or her problems are the final and major section of this chapter.

Definitions and terminology

It is important to know the definitions of a number of widely used terms in perinatal statistics, as shown in Table 24.1.

Table 24.1 Definitions used in perinatal statistics

Term	Definition
Full-term	An infant born between 37 and 42 weeks of gestation
Preterm	An infant born before 37 weeks of gestation
Post-term (postmature)	An infant born after 42 weeks of gestation
Low birthweight	A baby born with a birthweight of 2500 g or less
Very low birthweight	A baby born with a birthweight of 1500 g or less
Extremely low birthweight	A baby born with a birthweight of 1000 g or less
Small for gestational age	A baby of birthweight below the 10th centile for the duration of gestation
Stillborn infant	A baby who shows no signs of life (including no heart beat) after delivery. 'Stillbirth' is a term used only if the infant is of 24 weeks' gestation or above
Perinatal mortality rate	The number of stillbirths and neonatal deaths in the first week of life per 1000 liveborn and stillborn infants
Neonatal mortality rate	The number of deaths of liveborn infants in the first 28 days of life per 1000 liveborn infants
Infant mortality rate	The number of deaths of all liveborn infants in the first year of life per 1000 liveborn infants

Neonatal resuscitation and asphyxia

Rapid and effective resuscitation must be available for every newborn baby, wherever birth takes place. The need for resuscitation or support of transition may often be anticipated in high risk situations and the Red Flag box shows situations a care-giver trained in neonatal resuscitation needs to be present at delivery. However, despite careful fetal surveillance in labour, babies may still be born in poor condition and unexpectedly require resuscitation.

 The most recent newborn guideline (2015) from the UK Resuscitation Council may be found at www.resus.org.uk/resuscitation-guidelines/resuscitation-and-support-of-transition-of-babies-at-birth.

 High-risk situations requiring a care-giver trained in neonatal resuscitation

Preterm birth
Fetal distress
Thick meconium staining of the amniotic fluid
Emergency caesarean section
Vacuum or forceps delivery
Major fetal abnormality
Multiple birth

The infant's condition after birth may be described by the Apgar score (Table 24.2). This records five features, each of which are scored with either 0, 1, or 2 points. The baby can obtain a maximum of 10 points or a minimum of 0 (no signs of life).

A normal score at 1 minute is 7–10, a score of 4–6 at 1 minute represents a moderately depressed baby and an Apgar score of 0–3 at 1 minute indicates severe depression. Exposure to hypoxia before or during the birth process leads to a well-recognised response.

- *Primary apnoea*. Exposure to sufficient hypoxia may lead to failure to establish spontaneous respiration, but their cardiovascular system is intact with good circulation. This corresponds to an Apgar score at 1 minute of 4–6.
- *Secondary apnoea*. Continuing hypoxia leads to anaerobic metabolism and lactic acidosis leading to failure of both circulation and respiration. Without vigorous resuscitation, these babies are at high risk. This group corresponds to a 1-minute Apgar score of 0–3.

In the newborn, the main indication for resuscitation is failure of respiration, unlike in older children and adults in whom circulatory or cardiac indications predominate. The baby is born with lungs full of fluid, much of which is expelled or absorbed around birth allowing for the rapid establishment of respiration either spontaneously or with minimal stimulation. If the infant's condition allows, cord clamping should be delayed for at least 1 minute in order to facilitate placental transfusion. After clamping, if vigorous, the infant may be placed on the mother and covered in order to be kept warm. Drying with a warm towel and skin-to-skin contact help to reduce heat loss. The care-giver assesses colour, tone, breathing and heart rate.

If the infant is not breathing, the main aim is to replace the lung fluid with air by giving inflation breaths. Open the baby's airway by laying the baby on his back and:

- put the head in a neutral position with the face up;
- hold the baby's jaw forward;
- ensure that the neck is not over-flexed or extended.

The inflation breaths are given by a self-inflating bag or a T-piece device such as a Neopuff® and a close-fitting mask applied around the baby's mouth and nose (Figure 24.1).

Table 24.2 The Apgar score			
Sign	**0**	**1**	**2**
Heart rate	Absent	<100/min	>100/min
Respiratory rate	Absent	Weak cry	Strong cry
Muscle tone	Limp	Some flexion	Good flexion
Reflex irritability (suctioning pharynx)	No response	Some motion	Cry
Colour	White	Blue periphery	Pink all over

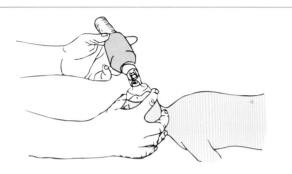

Figure 24.1 Bag and mask resuscitation.

Five inflation breaths are given and the chest movement is observed during the inflations. Consider using pulse oximetry and possibly ECG monitoring to guide care. Acceptable pre-ductal saturation is 60% at 2 minutes, 85% at 5 minutes and 90% at 10 minutes. If the chest is not moving, re-check head position and the fit of the mask on the face. Readjust and apply another five inflation breaths. If the chest wall moves, lung inflation is successful. Recheck the heart rate – if it is above 100 bpm, observe the baby for spontaneous respiratory efforts. If there are none, give short inspiratory breaths (30/minute) and await spontaneous respirations. If the heart remains low, begin cardiac compressions coordinated with ventilation in a ratio of 3:1. Intubation may be necessary for more prolonged resuscitation. If the pulse and colour do not improve, consider venous access, usually via the umbilical vein and administration of adrenaline.

Asphyxia

Physiologically asphyxia is caused by tissue hypoxia with the production of lactic acid and carbon dioxide. This results in tissue acidosis. The healthy fetus can withstand asphyxia for some time, but eventually physiological compensatory mechanisms become exhausted and the fetus decompensates, with potential irreversible injury to a number of organ systems, most importantly the brain.

Diagnosis   Asphyxia is associated with a failure of respiration before, during or after birth. Cord blood metabolic acidosis is indicative of the severity of the insult. All asphyxiated infants will show some degree of hypoxic-ischaemic

encephalopathy with abnormal neurological signs including convulsions during the first days of life. Multi-system injury is found in many asphyxiated infants.

Management   Rapid and effective resuscitation must be available wherever babies are born. Moderate induced hypothermia to 33–34 °C for 3 days significantly reduces the risk for neurodevelopmental sequelae. General supportive measures include ventilation, treatment and prevention of convulsions and blood pressure support.

Prognosis   Death and severe handicap occur in approximately 25% of all severely asphyxiated full-term infants.

 Key points: Resuscitation and asphyxia

- Resuscitation is needed rapidly and effectively
- Provide ventilatory support if the baby fails to establish adequate spontaneous respiration
- Induced moderate hypothermia reduces injury in hypoxic-ischaemic encephalopathy
- Give anticonvulsants for convulsions

The newborn examination

The first examination after birth aims to:
- Detect occult congenital abnormalities
- Define evidence of birth trauma
- Assess the infants' acclimatization to extra-uterine life

The reason for the neonatal examination must be explained to the parents, and they should be present during the examination if at all possible. The baby should be fully undressed in a warm room prior to examination.

History – must ask!

Ask the mother whether the baby is feeding well and if she has any worries about the baby, such as relating to pregnancy and family history.

Physical examination – must check!

The physical examination must be systematic. First observe the baby, then systematically start at the head and work down to the toes. Figure 24.2 summarizes the main features of the

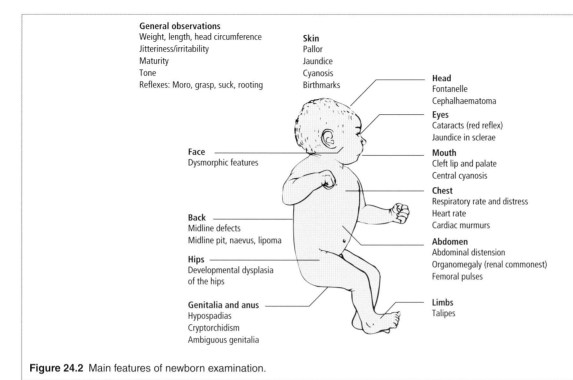

General observations
Weight, length, head circumference
Jitteriness/irritability
Maturity
Tone
Reflexes: Moro, grasp, suck, rooting

Skin
Pallor
Jaundice
Cyanosis
Birthmarks

Head
Fontanelle
Cephalhaematoma

Eyes
Cataracts (red reflex)
Jaundice in sclerae

Mouth
Cleft lip and palate
Central cyanosis

Chest
Respiratory rate and distress
Heart rate
Cardiac murmurs

Abdomen
Abdominal distension
Organomegaly (renal commonest)
Femoral pulses

Limbs
Talipes

Face
Dysmorphic features

Back
Midline defects
Midline pit, naevus, lipoma

Hips
Developmental dysplasia
of the hips

Genitalia and anus
Hypospadias
Cryptorchidism
Ambiguous genitalia

Figure 24.2 Main features of newborn examination.

newborn examination, and particular attention must be paid to potentially treatable abnormalities which, if missed, may cause irreversible damage to the baby.

Vital signs and general observation

- *Respiratory rate*. Count the respirations. A rate above 60 breaths per minute (tachypnoea) may be abnormal, but is normal transiently after a feed or if the baby has been crying.
- *Colour*. Central cyanosis (involving the tongue) is always abnormal, and if it is present the baby must be rapidly investigated (see p. 438). Jaundice in the first 24 hours is always abnormal and suggests haemolytic disease (see p. 448).
- *Spontaneous movements*. Normally full-term babies have frequent smooth movements. They may be reciprocal so that when a leg extends the other flexes.
- *Jitteriness*. This refers to spontaneous movements which are stimulus-independent; jitteriness is not necessarily abnormal, but, if persistent, hypocalcaemia and hypoglycaemia should be excluded as a cause.
- *Irritability* Irritability is a stimulus-sensitive phenomenon and is always abnormal, suggesting a neurological problem, although neonatal sepsis must also be considered.

Measurement

Carefully measure the head circumference, length and birth-weight, record the measurements in the notes and plot them onto centile charts to ensure that the baby has grown

symmetrically. Accurate measurements of occipitofrontal head circumference and length in the newborn are not easy to make and require some training. These techniques are discussed in Chapter 5.

Dysmorphic features

A *dysmorphic feature* is a variation from normal and is often subtle. Many normal people have at least one or two dysmorphic features, but the more such features coexist, the more likely it is that a recognizable dysmorphic syndrome is present. A *syndrome* is a consistent pattern of dysmorphic features which is usually recognised to be of genetic origin. The commonest syndrome recognizable in the neonatal period is Down syndrome (p. 270).

Head

Palpate the head and feel for the anterior and posterior fontanelles. A cephalhaematoma may be present due to subperiosteal bleeding. These resolve without treatment.

Eyes

Newborn infants keep their eyes closed much of the time. They can see, respond to changes in light and can fix their gaze on objects. The red reflex examination for detection of cataracts is described in detail on p. 32. If abnormal, ophthalmologic referral is critical as early treatment is essential for normal visual development.

Mouth

Look for central cyanosis and examine the palate for a cleft. The most reliable way is to insert your *clean* little finger into the baby's mouth and palpate with the soft part of your finger. A cleft is easily felt, and this method may also detect the rare submucous cleft with a bony defect but intact mucosa. Assessment under direct vision is also required.

Chest

Cardiac murmurs are commonly heard in the neonatal period and are usually innocent. In contrast, some very severe cardiac anomalies may not be associated with a murmur at the 24-hour examination. The following features suggest that a murmur is more likely to indicate cardiac pathology:

- the presence of cyanosis or breathlessness
- an active praecordium
- absent femoral pulses (see below)
- diastolic or gallop murmur.

Femoral pulses

Palpate the femoral pulses in the groin. Absence of a femoral pulse suggests severe *coarctation of the aorta* (see Figure 12.5) and requires immediate cardiologic assessment. Less severe coarctation, which leads to hypertension in later life, is not associated with absent pulses at the neonatal examination.

The abdomen

A distended abdomen suggests bowel obstruction, while a scaphoid abdomen is characteristic of congenital diaphragmatic hernia. Bile-stained vomiting must always be rapidly investigated as it may be the first sign of obstruction. The causes of bowel obstruction are discussed on p. 444.

Organomegaly is detected by careful abdominal examination. Enlargement of a single kidney as a result of pyeloureteric junction obstruction is the most common cause of a mass in the abdomen. Hepatosplenomegaly is not a common finding in the newborn infant.

The back and limbs

Examine the spine carefully. Look for midline defects, naevi and lipomas. When severe, *neural tube defects* (see p. 451) are obvious.

However, spina bifida occulta is harder to detect and, if missed, may lead to severe complications. Examine the limbs for deformities and extra digits.

Genitalia and anus

The testes are present in the scrotum in 95% of full-term male infants. Most *undescended testes* (see p. 342) enter the scrotum during the first year of life with no treatment. Persistent undescended testes should be assessed for intervention in order to prevent impaired fertility. *Hypospadias* is a condition where the urethra is abnormally sited, with the meatal opening lying anywhere from the ventral aspect of the glans penis to the perineum (see p. 342 and Figure 18.3). With severe hypospadias, the penis is curved ventrally (chordee). Rarely, babies are born with *ambiguous genitalia* and indeterminate sex. This should be considered to be a medical emergency because of the risk of severe electrolyte imbalance secondary to congenital adrenal hyperplasia and also for social and psychological reasons (see p. 343).

Abnormal neurological behaviour

Abnormal findings on neurological examination are rarely specific for particular forms of central nervous system pathology. The main features suggestive of serious neurological abnormality are the following:

- hypotonia (floppiness) or hypertonia (spasticity)
- irritability
- loss or asymmetry of the Moro reflex
- feeding problems.

The skin

Look for birth marks.

The hips

Leave the examination of the hips to the end as it usually causes the baby to cry. It is important to detect if a hip is dislocated or dislocatable. Both these abnormalities require early treatment to prevent permanent maldevelopment of the hip joints. The Ortolani and Barlow tests are described in Figures 24.10 and 24.11 and should be performed one hip at a time.

Signs and problems presenting in the newborn period

The small baby

The low birthweight infant may have three causes for being abnormally small:

- prematurity;
- intrauterine growth retardation (IUGR);
- a combination of both of these.

As the causes, management and prognosis of these conditions are different, it is important to determine into which of these three categories any small baby falls.

Prematurity

A preterm baby is one whose gestation falls short of 37 weeks. Approximately 7–9% of all babies are preterm, and 1% of births are severely preterm with birthweight below 1500 g (very low birthweight).

Assessment of gestation

Gestational age is determined by the following techniques:

- Calculation of gestational age from the maternal last menstrual period.
- Assessment of fetal maturity from early antenatal ultrasound scans.
- Assessment of neonatal maturity by clinical assessment of gestation after birth. This is based on standardized observation of both external physical criteria and neurological criteria. External criteria include skin development, nipple and genitalia appearance and ear form. Neurological criteria include posture, neck and limb tone and joint mobility. Neonatal examination is relatively inaccurate when compared with early obstetric measurements.

Disorders of prematurity

Table 24.3 lists the conditions most likely to occur in premature infants. It is generally the case that the more severe the prematurity, the more likely it will be that these complications will occur and the more severe they are likely to be.

Table 24.3 A comparison of the risk of problems for premature babies and those who have intrauterine growth retardation (IUGR)

	Prematurity	Intrauterine growth retardation
Hypothermia	++	+++
Hypoglycaemia	++	+++
Jaundice	++	–
Infection	++	+
Respiratory distress syndrome	+++	Reduced risk
Necrotizing enterocolitis	++	++
Retinopathy of prematurity	+++	–
Intracranial haemorrhage	+++	–
Feeding difficulties	+++	–

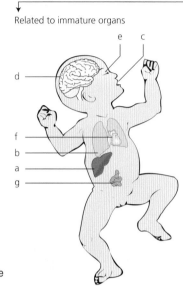

Prematurity at a glance

Definition
Birth at less than 37 weeks' gestation

Epidemiology
7% of births are premature
1% are severely premature

Clinical features
Thin, transparent skin
Immature nipples, genitalia and ear shape
Hypotonic posture with limbs in extension
Increased joint mobility

Management
Maintain environmental temperature
Non-oral feeding if too immature or sick
Management of complications as indicated

Related to immature organs

Complications
• Hypothermia
Metabolic: hypoglycaemia, hypocalcaemia, jaundice (**a**)
Respiratory: respiratory distress (**b**) syndrome, apnoea and bradycardia
• Feeding problems (**c**)
• Intracranial haemorrhage (**d**)
• Infection
• Retinopathy of prematurity (**e**)
• Patent ductus arteriosus (**f**)
• Necrotizing enterocolitis **g**)

Prognosis
Excellent if born beyond 32 weeks' gestation
Premature babies are now viable from 23 weeks' gestation

Intrauterine growth retardation

Impaired fetal growth will cause the baby to be born smaller than expected for the duration of gestation. These babies are referred to as 'small for gestational age' (SGA). In order to make the diagnosis of an SGA baby, it is necessary to make a careful assessment of gestational age and to plot the baby's weight on a centile chart to determine whether the baby's weight is below the 10th centile for the gestational age. SGA infants can be described as symmetrically or asymmetrically small.

Symmetrical growth retardation

A symmetrically small infant is one whose weight, head circumference and length all fall below the 10th centile in the same proportion (Figure 24.3). It is possible that a symmetrically small baby is simply a normal baby whose measurements happen to fall below the 10th centile: by definition, 10% of normal babies will have weight and other measurements below the 10th centile. The further the measurements are below the 10th centile, the more likely it is that the baby has a pathological reason for being small. The baby who is symmetrically growth retarded suggests that an insult causing impaired growth of both body and head occurred *early* in gestation. The commonest identifiable cause for this is infection, such as Cytomegalovirus, in early pregnancy. Other causes for symmetrical intrauterine growth retardation (IUGR) are shown in Table 24.4.

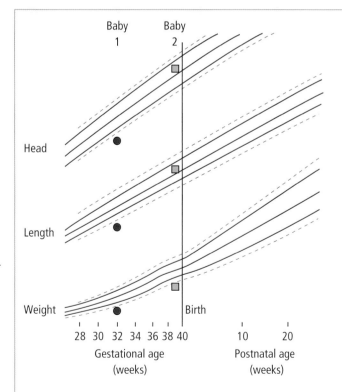

Figure 24.3 Growth chart showing baby 1 born at 32 weeks of gestation with symmetrical growth retardation and baby 2 born at 39 weeks of gestation with asymmetrical growth retardation.

Table 24.4 Causes of symmetrical and asymmetrical growth retardation

Symmetrical intrauterine growth retardation	Asymmetrical intrauterine growth retardation
Chromosomal abnormalities	Toxaemia of pregnancy
Prenatal infection	Multiple pregnancy
Maternal disease	Placental insufficiency
Maternal alcoholism	Maternal smoking

Prenatal infection

Prenatal infection occurs as the result of a number of organisms. These are usually described by the acronym TORCH infection:

Toxoplasma
Other (syphilis)
Rubella
Cytomegalovirus
Herpes.

Toxoplasma, syphilis and rubella are now very rare in Britain as causes of significant illness in the newborn. Cytomegalovirus is much more common, but rarely causes severe disabling sequelae. Most babies are asymptomatic but occasionally babies may present in the neonatal period with hepatosplenomegaly, purpura (caused by thrombocytopenia) and conjugated hyperbilirubinaemia.

Congenital CMV is the commonest cause of acquired sensorineural deafness. Less common sequelae include developmental delay, microcephaly, cerebral palsy, mental retardation and blindness. Diagnosis of congenital CMV infection is important, as therapy with ganciclovir or valgancyclovir reduces sensorineural deafness and developmental delay.

Asymmetrical growth retardation

In asymmetrical growth retardation the baby's weight is affected most, followed by length, with head growth being least impaired (Figure 24.3, baby 2). In this case the cause of the growth retardation has occurred relatively *late* in fetal development, most usually as a result of placental insufficiency. Weight gain is affected first, and fat is not laid down. Brain growth is affected least, as in the presence of relative starvation the brain is spared and continues to obtain the major share of available nutrition.

The asymmetrically growth-retarded infant looks long and thin. There is little subcutaneous fat and the baby is scrawny. His or her skin is dry and often cracks and peels in the days after birth.

Management of the SGA infant

After delivery, the main problem to anticipate in the SGA infant is the development of hypoglycaemia. Early and effective feeding is also important to allow for reasonable catch-up growth aiming to return the infant to the normal percentile range.

The SGA baby has a reduced risk of developing respiratory distress syndrome. The reason for this is that prenatal stress resulting from the underlying cause of the growth retardation causes endogenous corticosteroid release that enhances fetal lung maturation and surfactant production (see p. 445).

Outcome of SGA babies

Very severely growth-retarded babies may never catch up in terms of growth despite attempts at optimal postnatal feeding. Severe IUGR is a cause of short stature in children (p. 279) and some may benefit from growth hormone therapy.

There is evidence that severe growth retardation, particularly where there has been restriction in brain growth, is associated with long-term intellectual impairment.

Problems of the small baby

The small baby is particularly prone to a number of problems, depending on the degree of prematurity and the severity of the growth retardation (see Table 24.3).

Hypothermia

A small baby has a larger surface area from which heat can be lost. Heat loss must be minimized by drying the baby at birth and nursing in an incubator. Very immature babies have little or no waterproofing keratin layer and water is easily lost through the skin. Nursing in high ambient humidity minimizes this effect.

Hypoglycaemia

The definition of hypoglycaemia is a blood sugar <2.6 mmol/L. It is a particular problem for small babies because of their lack of glycogen and fat stores. They have fewer reserves of mobilisable glucose on which to draw. Hypoglycaemia is particularly a problem in babies who have suffered IUGR as they have fewer fat stores than babies who are premature alone. Hypoglycaemia must be anticipated in small infants and regular assessment of blood sugar made. This is most conveniently carried out on capillary blood by glucose-sensitive stick tests. Low levels of blood sugar must be treated rapidly with additional milk feeds or intravenous glucose (dextrose) solution.

The prognosis of hypoglycaemia depends on whether the baby was symptomatic. Infants with asymptomatic hypoglycaemia have an excellent prognosis, but those with severe neurological symptoms and convulsions have a poor prognosis that may include cerebral palsy (p. 262) and/or disorders of intellectual development (p. 267).

Feeding

Immaturity of the gastrointestinal tract is a common problem that prevents early gastric feeding in small babies. The suck reflex does not develop until 34–35 weeks of gestation. Therefore, premature babies cannot breast- or bottle-feed and the milk must be given through a nasogastric tube. Initial nutritional support routinely starts with parenteral nutrition combined with gradually increasing enteral feeds.

Infection

Both preterm and growth-retarded newborns have impairment of their immune function and are more prone to infection than full-term and appropriately grown infants. Great attention must be paid to avoidance of cross infection, and broad-spectrum antibiotics must be used if infection is suspected (see p. 447).

Apnoea of prematurity

Premature babies may experience apnoea, which results from immaturity of the respiratory system. They usually show a periodic pattern of respiration, with periods of hyperventilation alternating with periods of hypoventilation eventually leading to brief apnoeic episodes. Apnoea of prematurity is diagnosed by excluding other causes of apnoea in otherwise well premature infants. The management is with a xanthine-based drug, such as caffeine and non-invasive respiratory support. Apnoea of prematurity is not a risk factor for Sudden Infant Death. The prognosis is excellent.

👁 Small for gestational age (intrauterine growth retardation) at a glance

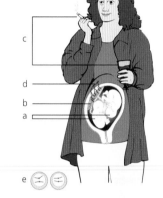

Definition
Weight less than 10% for gestational age (but problems are more common if less than 3rd centile). Growth retardation may be symmetrical or asymmetrical

Aetiology
Multiple pregnancy (**a**)
Placental insufficiency (**b**)
Maternal smoking/alcohol intake (**c**)
Congenital infection (TORCH infections) (**d**)
Genetic syndromes (**e**)
Normal small babies

Clinical features
Low birthweight
Mature ears, genitalia, breast tissue
Good muscle tone
Symmetrical IUGR: length and head circumference proportional to weight
Asymmetrical : long and thin, little subcutaneous fat, dry peeling skin, sparing of head growth

Investigations
TORCH screen

Complications
Hypoglycaemia
Birth asphyxia
Hypothermia

Management
Monitor blood glucose
Early and increased feeds

Prognosis
At risk for poor growth in childhood
At risk for intellectual impairment if poor head growth has occurred

---

Respiratory distress

Causes of acute respiratory distress in neonates

Respiratory distress syndrome
Pneumonia (congenital or acquired)
Pneumothorax
Surgical conditions (diaphragmatic hernia)
Cardiac causes

Respiratory distress is a very common symptom in preterm infants and requires careful assessment in all cases in order to determine the diagnosis and whether specific treatment is required. Respiratory distress occurs in approximately 5% of full-term infants and in over 50% of very low birthweight infants.

In preterm infants, respiratory distress syndrome is the most common diagnosis, although infection must also be considered. The commonest surgical cause is diaphragmatic hernia (p. 450).

Clinical evaluation – must check!

The clinical features of respiratory distress include the following:

- tachypnoea
- recession (subcostal, intercostal, sternal)
- nasal flaring
- cyanosis
- expiratory grunting.

Chest X-ray is the best method to distinguish between the various causes and to make a definitive diagnosis. Respiratory distress syndrome has a characteristic radiological appearance (see Figure 24.6), and an X-ray will distinguish it from other common causes.

Management

Management depends on the diagnosis, but there are general principles of management of the baby with respiratory distress. These include:

- *Monitoring vital signs.* Babies with respiratory distress are potentially if not actually very ill. Early deterioration may be detected by monitoring respiratory rate, heart rate, and blood pressure. Maintenance of normal blood pressure is particularly important in avoiding cerebral complications.
- *Monitoring blood gases.* This is essential in all infants with respiratory distress. Pulse oximetry guides oxygen requirement. Transcutaneous CO_2 measurement allows for intermittent use of capillary or arterial blood gasses that define the need for mechanical ventilation and its settings.
- *Respiratory support.* Babies with deteriorating lung disease, particularly those who are very small and weak, require respiratory support. This takes the form of either nasal continuous positive airway pressure (CPAP) or nasal intermittent positive pressure ventilation (IPPV). If insufficient, intubation and endotracheal ventilation are required.
- *Treat infection.* The possibility of infection must always be considered. Blood cultures are taken, and antibiotics are given until the cultures are known to be negative. If a pathogen is identified, antibiotic therapy may be tailored accordingly.

Cyanosis in the neonatal period

Causes of neonatal cyanosis

Cardiac
Transposition of the great arteries
Other right to left shunt defects

Respiratory
Respiratory distress syndrome
Pneumonia
Pneumothorax
Diaphragmatic hernia
Pulmonary hypertension

 Neonatal respiratory distress at a glance

Epidemiology
50% premature infants
5% full-term infants

Aetiology
- Respiratory distress syndrome (surfactant deficiency) in premature infants (**a**)
- Pneumonia (**b**)
- Pneumothorax (**c**)
- Diaphragmatic hernia (**d**)
- Cardiac causes (**e**)
- Meconium aspiration

Clinical features
- Tachypnoea
- Recession (intercostal, subcostal, sternal)
- Cyanosis
- Expiratory grunting

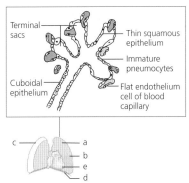

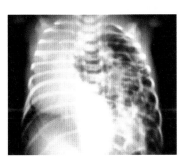

Diaphragmatic hernia

Confirmatory investigations
Chest X-ray
Infection screen
Blood gases

Management
Monitor vital signs
Titrate inspired oxygen concentration against baby's oxygen saturation
Surfactant in respiratory distress syndrome
CPAP and/or IPPV for respiratory failure
Antibiotics for infection
Monitor function of other organ systems

Prognosis
Depends on underlying causes and infant's maturity

Peripheral cyanosis involving hands and feet is very common in the neonatal period, and is referred to as acrocyanosis. This is of no clinical significance providing the baby has no central cyanosis (tongue involvement). Central cyanosis is always significant and indicates respiratory or cardiac disease. It must be rapidly investigated. If there is doubt about clinical cyanosis, a short period of oxygen saturation monitoring is required.

The most common cardiac causes of cyanosis presenting in the neonatal period are transposition of the great vessels and Tetralogy of Fallot (p. 226). These are surgically remediable conditions with a good prognosis. Cardiac failure rarely presents in the neonatal period other than in premature infants with patent ductus arteriosus (p. 449).

Clinical evaluation – must check!

Cyanosis caused by respiratory disease can be differentiated in most cases from that caused by cardiac disease by the presence of respiratory distress, which suggests the presence of lung disease. Occasionally, babies (particularly those born preterm) may have both respiratory and cardiac disease.

Investigations of a child with suspected cyanotic heart disease include chest X-ray, electrocardiogram (ECG), and echocardiography, which should define the structural anatomy. In the absence of a cardiological assessment, a hyperoxia or nitrogen wash-out test may help to distinguish between cyanotic heart disease and lung disease (Figure 24.4). The baby is administered oxygen as close to 100% as possible and the response is assessed either by pulse oximetry or arterial PO_2. Marked rise in oxygenation serves to rule out a cyanotic congenital heart condition.

Management

The management of cyanotic lesions depends on the underlying diagnosis. Oxygen, CPAP and mechanical ventilation

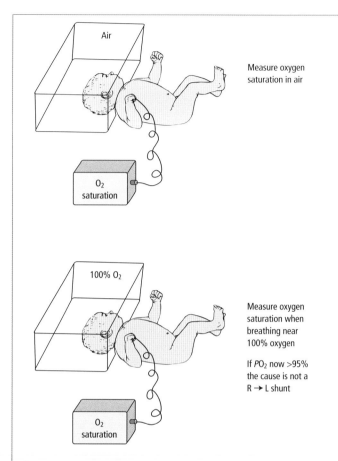

Measure oxygen saturation in air

Measure oxygen saturation when breathing near 100% oxygen

If PO_2 now >95% the cause is not a R → L shunt

Figure 24.4 The hyperoxia or nitrogen wash-out test.

(p. 437) may be of considerable benefit for respiratory disease, but are usually of little benefit in cardiac disease. Prostaglandin infusion to keep the ductus arteriosus open may be life-saving in infants with a duct-dependent cyanotic cardiac lesion.

Clues to the differential diagnosis of cyanosis

Causes of cyanosis	Features on clinical evaluation
Cardiac	
Transposition of the great vessels	Murmur Characteristic chest X-ray Echocardiogram
Other congenital cardiac lesions with right to left shunt	Murmur Echocardiography Chest X-ray may be diagnostic
Respiratory	
Respiratory distress syndrome	Signs of respiratory distress Characteristic chest X-ray
Other causes of respiratory distress	Chest X-ray Blood cultures

Convulsions

Convulsions are not uncommon in neonates, particularly preterm. They may be clonic and fragmentary, often involving different limbs for a short time. Less commonly, neonatal convulsions may be tonic or myoclonic. There may also be subtle events such as rhythmic lip-smacking, blinking, staring, or sucking. It is sometimes very difficult to interpret whether unusual movements in premature infants are convulsive in nature. Jitteriness is not a sign of cerebral dysfunction and is described on p. 431. Idiopathic epilepsy does not occur in the neonatal period.

Causes of neonatal convulsions

Asphyxia
Hypoglycaemia
Hypocalcaemia
Meningitis
Congenital brain anomalies
Intracranial haemorrhage
Maternal drug withdrawal (neonatal abstinence
   syndrome)
Inborn errors of metabolism (rare)
Unknown (idiopathic)

 Cyanosis in the newborn period at a glance

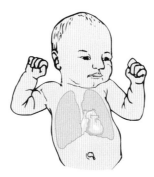

Epidemiology
Cyanosis due to respiratory
   disease is common; due to
   cardiac disease is rare. See
   Causes box, p. 437

Clinical features
Cyanosis of the lips and tongue
   (distinguish from
   acrocyanosis)
Respiratory distress if cyanosis
   is respiratory
Heart murmur if cyanosis is
   cardiac*

NB *Signs and symptoms are variable.

Confirmatory investigations
Blood gases – low arterial O_2
Nitrogen wash-out to distinguish
   cardiac from respiratory
   disease
Chest X-rays
ECG and echocardiography if
   cardiac cyanosis is suspected

Management
Oxygen, CPAP and ventilation
   for respiratory cyanosis
Investigate cardiac disease
Cardiac surgery usually
   required for cyanotic heart
   disease

Prognosis
Good for most respiratory
   causes and operable cardiac
   lesion

History – must ask!

A careful maternal and perinatal history is required in all cases. Pay particular attention to maternal illness (diabetes predisposes the baby to hypoglycaemia), evidence of fetal distress, symptoms of neurological abnormality prior to the convulsion (feeding problems, irritability, stiffness) and whether there is a family history of neonatal convulsions. Ask the mother if she took any illicit drugs in pregnancy.

Physical examination – must check!

- *Abnormal neurological findings.* Non-responsiveness, hypotonicity.
- *Extensive bruising.* This may be suggestive of birth trauma.

- *Dysmorphic features.* These are suggestive of an underlying brain anomaly.
- *Intrauterine growth retardation.* If the baby is SGA this increases the risk of hypoglycaemia and hypocalcaemia.
- *Hepatosplenomegaly and purpura.* These suggest prenatal infection (TORCH).

Investigations

The investigations listed in Table 24.5 should be undertaken in all neonates with convulsions. These include:
- Amplitude-integrated (bedside) EEG or Full EEG
- Metabolic tests
- Tests for infection
- Brain imaging – ultrasound and/or MRI

Table 24.5 Investigations and their significance in neonates with convulsions

Investigations	Significance
Full blood count	Abnormal white cell count suggestive of infection
Blood cultures	Infection
Lumbar puncture	Meningitis
Blood glucose	Hypoglycaemia
Serum calcium	Hypocalcaemia
Amplitude-integrated EEG	Confirm and monitor convulsions and response to therapy
Ultrasound brain imaging	Intracranial haemorrhage Periventricular leucomalacia Congenital anomaly
Metabolic screen	Inborn error of metabolism

Management

Management should be directed towards treating the underlying cause of the convulsions (meningitis, hypoglycaemia, etc.) as well as therapy to prevent further convulsions if a specific cause cannot be found.

Phenobarbitone is the first-line anticonvulsant used in the neonatal period.

Prognosis

The prognosis depends on the underlying cause for the convulsions. A very poor prognosis is likely if a major congenital brain anomaly is detected, and there is a significant chance of poor outcome if the convulsions are caused by meningitis, asphyxia or major intracranial haemorrhage.

Neonatal convulsions at a glance

Epidemiology
0.5–1% of all neonates

Aetiology
Causes are intracranial (asphyxia, meningitis, malformation or haemorrhage), metabolic (hypoglycaemia, hypocalcaemia) or idiopathic

Clinical features
Usually clonic and fragmentary movements
Less commonly tonic or myoclonic
May be difficult to differentiate from jitteriness*
Apnoea and bradycardia*
History of intrapartum asphyxia*
Bilateral intraventricular haemorrhage

NB * Signs and symptoms are variable.

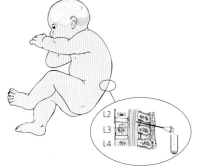

Confirmatory investigations
• Blood glucose, electrolytes, calcium
• Infection screen, including lumbar puncture to exclude meningitis
• Ultrasound for haemorrhage or cerebral malformations
• Metabolic screen

Management
Treat underlying cause
Prevent further convulsions with phenobarbitone

Prognosis
Depends on underlying cause
If none identified, the prognosis is usually good

Apnoea

Causes of apnoea in the neonate

Central apnoea
Apnoea of prematurity
Hypoglycaemia
Infection
Intracranial haemorrhage
Necrotizing enterocolitis
Convulsions

Obstructive apnoea
Pharyngeal closure in preterm infants
Small jaw
Thick oropharyngeal secretions
Congenital blockage of the posterior nares (very rare)

Apnoea is a very common symptom in the neonatal period and is particularly seen in preterm infants. The definition of apnoea is a pause in respiration lasting for 20 seconds or more. It is a non-specific symptom and the baby requires careful assessment to discover the underlying cause.

Apnoea may be central or obstructive in origin. Central causes may involve the brainstem or higher cortical structures. Obstructive causes occur as a result of airway obstruction and can sometimes be recognised by observing the episode. Both forms may co-exist in preterm infants. Apnoea of prematurity is a diagnosis of exclusion.

Clinical evaluation – must check!

In *obstructive apnoea,* the baby continues to make respiratory efforts despite increasing cyanosis or bradycardia, suggesting that the airway is becoming blocked and the baby is fighting to overcome this effect. Obstructive apnoea can be excluded by passing a tube through the nares and evaluating whether the baby has a small jaw. The obstructive component in preterm infants is difficult to assess in clinical practice.

In *central apnoea,* the baby usually shows periodic respiration with slowing in the respiratory rate until apnoea occurs. It is always important to consider infection as the cause of apnoeic episodes and to investigate this rapidly and institute treatment as early as possible. Other investigations should be performed to exclude or confirm the causes of the apnoea.

Management

The acute apnoeic episode should be treated rapidly. Infants presenting with a significant apnoea should normally be admitted for careful observation. The management depends on the severity and frequency of the attacks. Initially, tactile stimulation is effective, and nasopharyngeal suction may be necessary in obstructive causes. Severe apnoeic episodes may require bag and mask ventilation.

Treatment should also be directed towards the cause of the condition if this is known. Where the cause is thought to be apnoea of prematurity, non-specific therapy involves administration of a xanthine-based drug, such as caffeine, to stimulate the respiratory system. Non-invasive ventilatory support with nasal continuous positive airway pressure or nasal intermittent positive pressure ventilation may be useful in more refractory cases, and the most severe cases occasionally require mechanical ventilation.

 Apnoea at a glance

Epidemiology
Common symptom, particularly in premature infants

Aetiology
Apnoea may be due to partial obstruction of the airway or central causes (see Causes box, above)

Clinical features
Pause in breathing lasting longer than 20 seconds
Often associated with periodic breathing
Bradycardia
Cyanosis*

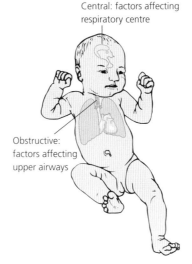

Central: factors affecting respiratory centre

Obstructive: factors affecting upper airways

Confirmatory investigations
Infection screen in all cases
Assess for anatomic problems of upper airway
Assess for brain pathology

Management
Treat all apnoeic episodes with stimulation
Treat underlying cause, where possible
Xanthine derivatives, e.g. caffeine if apnoea is persistent
CPAP or IPPV if apnoea is very severe
Home apnoea monitors are rarely indicated except for severe life-threatening apnoeic episodes

Prognosis
Good except where there is major central pathology

NB *Signs and symptoms are variable.

Neonatal jaundice

Causes of neonatal jaundice

Unconjugated hyperbilirubinaemia
Rhesus and ABO incompatibility
G6PD deficiency
Bacterial infection
Excessive bruising
Internal haemorrhage
Prematurity
Hypothyroidism
Breast-milk jaundice
Physiological

Conjugated hyperbilirubinaemia
Neonatal hepatitis
Cystic fibrosis
Biliary atresia

Jaundice in the neonatal period is a very common feature; it is usually caused by the physiological immaturity of the liver, and is self-limiting over the first week of life as liver function matures. Neonatal jaundice (hyperbilirubinaemia) can be classified depending on whether it is conjugated or unconjugated.

Jaundice occurs as a result of the build-up of bilirubin – which may be caused by prehepatic, hepatic or posthepatic causes.

- *Prehepatic.* This is a result of excessive breakdown of red blood cells, as occurs in haemolysis. The bilirubin is all unconjugated.
- *Hepatic.* An abnormality in liver function, such as occurs in neonatal hepatitis, will cause a build-up of conjugated bilirubin.
- *Posthepatic.* This is a result of absent or atretic bile ductules extending to main branches of the bile ducts, and causes conjugated hyperbilirubinaemia. This condition is referred to as biliary atresia (see below).

Jaundice may be clinically significant for two reasons:

1. High levels of unconjugated bilirubin may cause irreversible brain damage, referred to as kernicterus or Bilirubin-Induced Neurologic Damage (BIND) that includes kernicterus in the neonate and sensorineural deafness, choreoathetoid cerebral palsy and mental retardation.
2. Prolonged jaundice may indicate severe underlying disease.

History – must ask!

Neonatal jaundice occurs in almost all newborn infants to some degree. At high levels, jaundice may cause the baby to become lethargic and feed less well. Conversely, those babies who become somewhat dehydrated appear more jaundiced as a result of haemoconcentration and so may feed less well, thus causing more severe dehydration.

In conjugated hyperbilirubinaemia, specific enquiries include family history of cystic fibrosis, metabolic disorders and liver disease.

Physical examination – must check!

On examination, the distribution of the jaundice may help in estimating the total bilirubin level:

- Limited to head and neck: mild.
- Over lower trunk and thighs: moderate.
- Extending to hands and feet: may require treatment.

Examination should also identify petechial or purpuric lesions, pallor, and hepatosplenomegaly.

Investigations

Transcutaneous bilirubinometry is a useful screening tool for monitoring jaundice and timing serum bilirubin measurements. Total and unconjugated levels of bilirubin should be measured. The Coombs' test determines whether there is antibody on the red blood cell membrane. It is positive in incompatibility conditions.

There are four circumstances which indicate that a baby should be investigated rapidly for serious causes of the jaundice:

- Early evidence of jaundice appearing in the first 24 hours of life. This suggests that there is underlying haemolysis.
- Marked hyperbilirubinemia requiring phototherapy.
- Prolonged conjugated jaundice lasting more than one to two weeks, which suggests a serious underlying cause.
- Increasing levels of conjugated bilirubin. This suggests a severe hepatic cause of the jaundice.

Further investigations are indicated for prolonged jaundice and increasing conjugated bilirubinaemia to diagnose the causes listed in Table 24.6.

Management

The aim of treatment for unconjugated hyperbilirubinaemia is to avoid kernicterus or BIND. The level of unconjugated bilirubin which causes brain damage is not known for certain and depends on the gestational age of the baby and how sick the baby is. Charts are available which indicate the level of unconjugated bilirubin at which babies of different gestational age should be treated.

Treatment is initially by phototherapy, which degrades the unconjugated bilirubin to non-toxic soluble compounds and these are excreted in the urine. If levels continue to rise to a potentially toxic level, exchange transfusion may be required. However, the advent of modern powerful phototherapy units and maternal treatment with Anti-D to prevent rhesus diseases have made exchange transfusion a rare necessity. The management of conjugated hyperbilirubinaemia depends on the underlying cause.

Table 24.6 Investigations to be considered in severe or prolonged jaundice

Investigations	Relevance
Full blood count (routine)	Neutrophilia or neutropenia suggests infection Thrombocytopenia suggests TORCH infection
Maternal and neonatal blood groups and Coombs' test (routine)	ABO and rhesus incompatibility
Urine cultures (if sepsis suspected)	Infection
Lumbar puncture (if sepsis suspected)	Meningitis
Ultrasound scans (if severe or prolonged or evidence of cholestasis)	Internal haemorrhage Biliary atresia
Thyroid function tests (if prolonged)	Hypothyroidism
Hepatitis B antigen (if evidence of hepatitis)	Hepatitis B infection
Metabolic screen (rare)	Inborn errors of metabolism
Sweat test (rare)	Cystic fibrosis

Neonatal jaundice at a glance

Epidemiology
All premature infants, also common in full-term infants
1–2% of babies require treatment

Aetiology
Jaundice may be caused by conjugated or unconjugated hyperbilirubinaemia
See Causes box, p. 442

Clinical features
Yellow pigmentation of skin
Yellow sclerae
Lethargy*
Bruising*
Poor feeding*
Hepatomegaly*

Confirmatory investigations
Conjugated and unconjugated bilirubin
FBC and smear
Blood group
Coombs' test

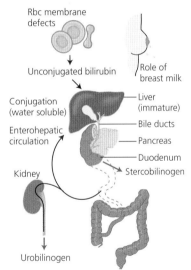

Features of concern
Presentation less than 24 hours
Severe jaundice
Prolonged (greater than 2 weeks) jaundice
Increased conjugated bilirubin

Management
Identify cause
Unconjugated hyperbilirubinaemia:
Phototherapy
Exchange transfusion to avert kernicterus if very high bilirubin
Hearing assessment if levels indicate risk of kernicterus
Conjugated hyperbilirubinaemia:
Treatment depends on cause

Prognosis/complications
Danger of kernicterus (athetoid cerebral palsy) and neurosensory deafness if unconjugated bilirubinaemia rises to high levels
Prognosis for severe conjugated bilirubinaemia is poor

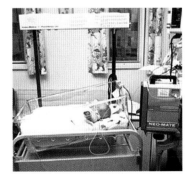

NB *Signs and symptoms are variable.

Bowel obstruction

Causes of bowel obstruction in the neonate

Anatomical abnormalities
Oesophageal atresia
Duodenal atresia
Jejunal atresia
Anal atresia / imperforate anus

Functional abnormalities
Hirschsprung's disease
Meconium ileus
Volvulus secondary to malrotation

Congenital intestinal obstruction occurs in one in 1000 babies. Causes can be divided into anatomical obstruction (e.g. duodenal atresia) and functional obstruction, where the bowel is patent, but the peristaltic function is abnormal (e.g. Hirschsprung disease, see below).

Clinical features – must check!

There are four major features of intestinal obstruction:
- bile-stained vomiting;
- failure to pass meconium;

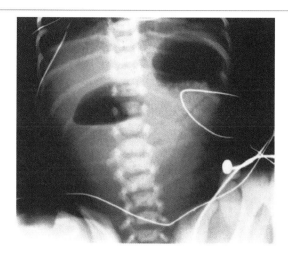

Figure 24.5 Abdominal X-ray showing the 'double bubble' in duodenal atresia.

- abdominal distension;
- visible peristalsis (rare in neonate).

If the obstruction is high in the gastrointestinal tract, abdominal distension may not be obvious, and the infant may pass meconium from below the obstruction. The stool, however, does not show a change from meconium to products of milk digestion (the changing stool).

Bile-stained vomiting is always abnormal and strongly suggests obstruction. An emergency surgical opinion is required.

Investigations and management

Assessment for dehydration with serum electrolytes and assessment for infection are important in the vomiting neonate. A plain abdominal X-ray shows fluid levels and dilated bowel in complete obstruction. In duodenal atresia the classical 'double bubble' is seen (Figure 24.5), with air in the stomach and first part of duodenum.

Surgery is required to relieve the site of obstruction.

🔍 Clues to the differential diagnosis of neonatal bowel obstruction

Anatomical abnormalities	
Oesophageal atresia	Drooling saliva, choking Associated with tracheo-oesophageal fistula in 95% of cases
Duodenal atresia	Bile-stained vomiting, 'double bubble' seen on abdominal X-ray
Jejunal atresia	Abdominal distension and bile-stained vomiting
Anal atresia	Detected on routine examination
Functional abnormalities	
Hirschsprung disease	Delayed passage of meconium and abdominal distension
Meconium ileus	Delayed passage of meconium. Very thick tenacious meconium
Volvulus secondary to malrotation	Intermittent episodes of partial obstruction Bile-stained vomiting

Neonatal conditions

Respiratory distress syndrome

Respiratory distress syndrome (RDS) has in the past been referred to as hyaline membrane disease (HMD), a condition recognised on histological examination. The condition is primarily caused by surfactant deficiency in the immature lung. Although babies now rarely die in the acute phase of RDS, complications such as brain damage and chronic lung disease are still common.

The incidence of RDS is inversely related to gestational age. Approximately 70% of infants born at 26 weeks' gestation will develop RDS, 25% at 32 weeks and 0.5% at term.

Aetiology

Respiratory distress syndrome is caused by surfactant deficiency. Surfactant is a phospholipid which reduces surface tension in the alveolus. It is produced by type II alveolar cells, which, although they are present from an early stage in fetal development, do not produce adequate amounts of surfactant until late in gestation. Consequently, preterm birth is associated with deficiency of surfactant and the development of RDS. The stress of preterm birth and developing RDS causes release of corticosteroids from the infant's own adrenal glands which together with catecholamine release and lung stretches will in turn lead to increased surfactant production. RDS is therefore a self-limiting condition as endogenous surfactant will eventually resolve the clinical condition, but it may take 5–7 days or more for sufficient endogenous surfactant to be produced to resolve the lung disorder. The challenge of neonatology is to support the baby in optimal condition and prevent any complications in the meantime.

The fetal lung is a stiff structure as a result of lack of surfactant. At birth the baby takes a deep breath which expands the lungs with air, but if surfactant is not present the stiff alveoli collapse down to their fetal size and the next breath is another massive inspiratory effort. This increased work of breathing continues until the baby becomes exhausted. Surfactant molecules produce a molecular monolayer within the alveolus and prevent the alveolus from collapsing down to its unexpanded state.

The antenatal administration of a corticosteroid for 48 hours to the mother who is at risk of delivering a premature infant is the most effective treatment in preventing RDS in her baby by stimulating surfactant release. Endogenous corticosteroid release, as occurs in the growth-retarded fetus, also reduces the risk of the SGA baby developing RDS. Infants of diabetic mothers are at increased risk of RDS because intrauterine exposure to the combination of hyperglycemia and hyperinsulinaemia inhibits surfactant development.

Clinical features

The baby presents with signs of respiratory distress as described above. There is no specific clinical feature of RDS, but a major feature is recession, which may be very severe in small infants with a soft rib cage. Sternal recession is marked, with the appearance of the sternum meeting the spine.

Investigations

Diagnosis of RDS is confirmed by chest X-ray which is usually diagnostic (Figure 24.6). It shows two characteristic features:

1. An air bronchogram (radiolucent air in the bronchi seen against the airless lung)
2. Ground glass appearance of the lung fields as a result of alveolar collapse.

Management

Specific treatment for this condition includes the following:

- *Titration of the inspired oxygen level against oxygen saturations measured by pulse oximetry.* If the baby is breathing spontaneously, the oxygen can be administered directly in the incubator or via a headbox.
- *Continuous positive airway pressure.* Respiratory support can be given in a spontaneously breathing baby by applying CPAP via either a facemask or nasal prongs. This technique

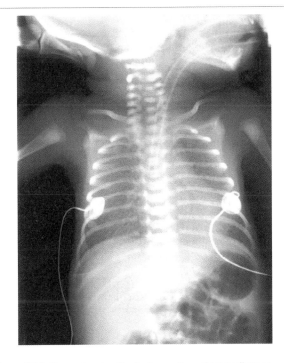

Figure 24.6 X-ray showing the features of respiratory distress syndrome (RDS).

Table 24.7 Complications of respiratory distress syndrome
Pneumothorax / pulmonary interstitial emphysema
Pneumonia
Intracranial haemorrhage
Hydrocephalus
Patent ductus arteriosus
Necrotizing enterocolitis
Retinopathy of prematurity
Chronic lung disease
Cerebral palsy

maintains constant positive distending pressure on expiration, which prevents alveolar collapse. Nasal Intermittent Positive Pressure ventilation may help to prevent the need for endotracheal ventilation.

- *Mechanical ventilation.* Very small babies will require immediate mechanical ventilation because they are too weak to breathe spontaneously. Larger babies who do not improve on CPAP or those having severe apnoeic episodes will also require mechanical ventilation (IPPV). Mechanical ventilation is applied by intubating the baby and connecting the endotracheal tube to a ventilator.

- *Administration of exogenous surfactant.* Exogenous surfactant is given directly into the baby's lungs by instillation either via an endotracheal tube or through a thin catheter during Nasal ventilation (Minimally-Invasive Surfactant Administration). This therapy has markedly reduced the mortality of RDS.

Complications

The major complications of RDS and its treatment are listed in Table 24.7.

Prognosis

Although most babies recover fully from RDS, some develop chronic lung disease or bronchopulmonary dysplasia. This chronic condition is characterised by respiratory difficulties requiring oxygen and sometimes ventilatory support and is most commonly defined as the requirement for oxygen at 36 weeks gestational age. The major contributing factors are preterm birth, oxygen toxicity and barotrauma due to ventilation. Treatment is mostly symptomatic with caffeine, diuretics and steroids, either systemic or inhaled. A small proportion may be sent home on additional oxygen. Most will recover although growth failure and neurodevelopmental delay are common. Babies with chronic lung disease are much more likely to wheeze in the first 2 years of life and a few may develop long-term respiratory problems.

👁 Respiratory distress syndrome at a glance

Epidemiology
Increasing risk with degree of prematurity
70% of 28-week infants,
0.5% of full-terms

Aetiology
Due to surfactant deficiency

Prevention
Corticosteroids for mother 48 hours prior to delivery if at risk for premature birth

Clinical features
Tachypnoea
Intercostal, subcostal, sternal recession
Cyanosis
Expiratory grunting

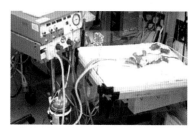

Confirmatory investigations
Chest X-ray shows air bronchogram, ground glass appearance of lung fields

Differential diagnosis
Infection
Pneumothorax
Diaphragmatic hernia
Cardiac causes

Management
Titration of inspired O_2 against baby's O_2 saturation
CPAP or IPPV for respiratory failure
Surfactant for intubated infants
Monitor vital signs and blood pressure

Complications
See Table 24.7

Prognosis
Babies who are ventilated are at risk for bronchopulmonary dysplasia (chronic lung disease)
Very premature babies receiving high PO_2 are at risk of retinopathy
80% of babies survive severe respiratory distress syndrome, but 5% develop severe cerebral palsy

Infection

The newborn, and particularly the premature infant, is particularly susceptible to infection because of immaturity of the immune system. An important factor in the integrity of the immune response is maternal IgG, which crosses the placenta to the fetus in the last three months of pregnancy. Babies who are born severely preterm miss the maternal IgG contribution.

Infection in the newborn is usually bacterial and may be acquired either at birth from the maternal genital tract during delivery (perinatally) or by cross-infection (nosocomial) from medical and nursing staff. Perinatally acquired early infection is most commonly caused by group B beta-haemolytic Streptococcus and *E. coli*. Nosocomial infection is most commonly caused by *Staphylococcus epidermidis* and *Gram-negative Bacilli*.

Clinical features

There are no specific signs of infection in the newborn, and infection must always be considered to be a possible cause of any compromise in all newborn infants. Signs of infection are shown in the Red Flag box.

Clinical signs suggestive of neonatal infection

Unstable temperature
Lethargy
Apnoeic or bradycardic episodes
Hypotonia
Irritability
Convulsions
Poor feeding
Respiratory distress
Jaundice
Vomiting
Abdominal distension

Investigations

Infection must be considered to be a cause of almost any acute symptom or sign in the neonate and requires rapid investigation. Infection screen includes the following:

- full blood count;
- C-reactive protein
- blood cultures
- swabs from skin, throat, trachea and rectum;
- lumbar puncture (after day 1)
- Urine culture (after day 1–2)
- Chest X-ray (as clinically indicated)

Management

Antibiotic treatment is most effective if started early. Bacteriological confirmation of infection will take 24–48 hours from taking the specimens and consequently, if infection is suspected, broad-spectrum antibiotics should be started immediately. They can be stopped if microbiological surveillance is negative. If it is positive, a full course should be given for 7–10 days.

Meningitis

Meningitis occurring in the neonatal period is sufficiently different from meningitis in older children to be considered separately. The incidence of neonatal meningitis is one in 4000 babies. The neonate is relatively immunocompromised by immaturity, which predisposes to meningitis. Any organism may cause neonatal meningitis, but the most common are group B beta-haemolytic streptococci and *Escherichia coli*.

The neonate does not develop specific symptoms of meningitis such as a stiff neck, and the signs of infection are often very non-specific. This is why meningitis must be considered in any baby with unexpected deterioration. Lumbar puncture is essential in any neonate with unexplained deterioration to confirm or exclude the diagnosis.

Treatment is directed towards the causal organisms. Broad-spectrum antibiotics should be given prior to isolation of the infecting bacterium. The prognosis depends on how quickly the diagnosis is made and appropriate antibiotic treatment started. In general, it is not good. Approximately 25% of babies die and a further 25% become handicapped. Hydrocephalus is a common complication after neonatal meningitis.

Pneumonia

Pneumonia develops shortly after birth if infection is acquired from the mother during passage down the genital tract (perinatal infection). Group B beta-haemolytic Streptococcus or Gram-negative bacilli are the common causative organism. Pneumonia may also occur in mechanically ventilated babies who acquire nosocomial infection from their carers.

Clinical features   The baby presents early with respiratory distress and shock. The chest X-ray may show an identical appearance to that of RDS, so pneumonia must always be considered as a differential diagnosis in RDS. Pneumonia must always be considered in any infant who deteriorates on mechanical ventilation.

Management and prognosis   An appropriate antibiotic is curative if given early enough. Supportive care is necessary to manage respiration and the circulation until the baby recovers. Prognosis is good with early diagnosis. Death occurs in rapidly progressive cases.

Intracranial haemorrhage

Intracranial haemorrhage is common in premature newborn infants. In particular, intraventricular haemorrhage (IVH) occurs in many very low birthweight infants. Intraventricular haemorrhage develops in the floor of the lateral ventricle and then may rupture into the lateral ventricle. In the most severe form, corresponding intra-parenchymal haemorrhage occurs. This is thought to be primarily a periventricular hemorrhagic infarction, although extension from the ventricle has also been proposed. This form of parenchymal haemorrhage is the most severe, and if the child survives there is a high risk of cerebral palsy (p. 262).

Periventricular leucomalacia (PVL) is caused by cerebral ischaemia and frequently occurs in babies with IVH although it may appear alone in the absence of IVH. Exposure to chorioamnionitis is a contributing factor. It is less common than IVH, but PVL is the commonest cause of severe cerebral palsy in surviving preterm infants. Poor outcome is particularly likely if the baby develops cystic PVL.

Clinical features   Many babies who develop IVH show no symptoms, but convulsions are not uncommon in babies with parenchymal haemorrhage. The diagnosis is made by ultrasound examination.

Management and prognosis   There is no specific treatment, but post-haemorrhagic hydrocephalus occurs in 10% of babies following IVH and may require temporary or permanent ventricular shunting in order to reduce pressure on the periventricular white matter. Cerebral palsy (see p. 262) occurs in 80% of babies with cystic PVL, and is usually severe. Cerebral palsy may also occur in infants with parenchymal haemorrhage, but this is usually less severe than that seen with PVL.

Necrotizing enterocolitis

This is a rare complication of preterm infants. It is related to impaired intestinal blood flow which predisposes the mucosa to invasion by enteric organisms. The babies present with acute deterioration, abdominal distension, and bloody in the stools and respiratory distress. In 20% of cases bowel perforation occurs, followed by signs of peritonitis.

The diagnosis is confirmed on abdominal X-ray, when gas produced by the invading organisms can be seen in the wall of the bowel. Management is initially expectant. Enteral feeds are stopped, and broad-spectrum antibiotics started. If bowel perforation has occurred, laparotomy is indicated although peritoneal drainage may be an acceptable alterna-tive in extremely small infants. Most babies make a full recovery, but 10% later develop bowel stricture in the affected area of bowel.

Jaundice of prematurity

All premature infants become visibly jaundiced in the few days after birth. This is caused by immaturity of the liver and failure of the hepatocytes to conjugate the bilirubin adequately. Other causes of jaundice may co-exist.

Haemolytic disease of the newborn

Haemolysis occurs in the fetus as a result of maternal antibod-ies reacting with antigen on the fetal red blood cell. The two commonest reasons for this are ABO blood group incompati-bility and rhesus incompatibility.

In ABO blood group incompatibility, the mother is most commonly blood group O and the baby is blood group A. The mother's natural anti-A antibodies react with the fetal cells causing, haemolysis and jaundice. This condition cannot be detected antenatally.

In rhesus disease the mother is rhesus negative and the fetus rhesus positive. The mother has been sensitized to rhesus-positive cells in earlier pregnancies, when fetal cells cross into the maternal circulation. This causes the mother to develop anti-rhesus antibodies, which cross the placenta and cause hae-molysis of fetal red blood cells. This tends to be worse in suc-cessive pregnancies.

Clinical features   Haemolysis due to ABO incompatibility usually presents with jaundice in the first 24 hours after birth.

Rhesus incompatibility may cause fetal haemolysis, anaemia, and if untreated, severe oedema (hydrops) occurs. At birth the severely affected baby is very oedematous and anaemic with rapid development of jaundice.

Management   The treatment of infants with ABO incom-patibility requires intensive early phototherapy. In severe cases, intravenous immunoglobulin reduces the need for exchange transfusion which is rare nowadays. Late anaemia (6–8 weeks after birth) may occur in haemolytic conditions, and the baby may require a top-up blood transfusion.

In Rhesus incompatibility, the aim of management is to deliver the baby before severe haemolysis has occurred and then perform exchange transfusion to wash out the antibodies as well as the toxic bilirubin. Rhesus-negative women are now immunised with anti-D antibody and consequently rhesus haemolytic disease is now very rare.

Prognosis If kernicterus is avoided, the prognosis is excellent. Sensorineural hearing impairment may be the only sign of bilirubin toxicity.

Breast-milk jaundice

This is a benign condition and requires no treatment. It is generally diagnosed by excluding other more serious conditions. In this condition the baby is being breast-fed, develops mild to moderate hyperbilirubinaemia in the second week of life and remains well. Breast-feeding should continue with appropriate reassurance for the parents.

Neonatal hepatitis

This is a rare condition. It is usually caused by either a virus (hepatitis B, cytomegalovirus), cystic fibrosis or a metabolic cause. There is no specific treatment.

An avoidable cause of morbidity from hepatitis B is when the baby contracts the infection from the mother. The baby is most at risk if the mother contracts hepatitis B in the last trimester of pregnancy. The baby should be immunised immediately after birth with hepatitis B vaccine together with hepatitis B immunoglobulin.

Biliary atresia

Biliary atresia is an important but rare condition that is caused by atresia of intrahepatic or extrahepatic bile ducts. The babies present with increasing conjugated hyperbilirubinaemia from 2–4 weeks of life. If undiagnosed, there is rapid progression to liver failure and death, but if the diagnosis is made within three months of birth, surgery may restore liver function to near normal. This condition should be considered in any baby presenting with conjugated jaundice beyond 2 weeks of age.

Patent ductus arteriosus

Patent ductus arteriosus (Figure 24.7) is a common complication of infants who require mechanical ventilation. During fetal life, the ductus arteriosus shunts blood from right to left away from the unexpanded lungs. In preterm infants with lung disease, particularly RDS, the increased pulmonary resistance and hypoxia makes it more likely that the ductus will reopen. In neonatal life, the direction of the blood shunt is reversed and is more likely to be left to right, leading to pulmonary oedema and increased work of breathing. This may make it difficult to wean the baby from the ventilator.

In preterm infants, PDA may be asymptomatic although there may be a systolic murmur and collapsing pulses (p. 220).

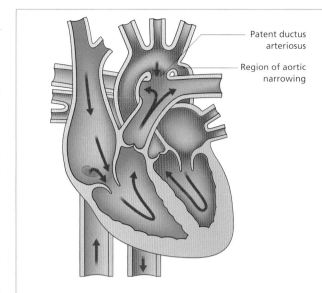

Figure 24.7 Patent ductus arteriosus.

If the left to right shunt is large, the chest X-ray shows plethoric lung fields. Diagnosis is confirmed by echocardiography.

Indomethacin or ibuprofen are prostaglandin synthetase inhibitors that promote ductal closure. Rarely, surgical ligation may be required. With appropriate treatment the prognosis is excellent.

Obstructive apnoea

This condition occurs in babies with either anatomical or functional problems.

Anatomical obstruction of upper airway structures occurs, for example, in posterior nasal obstruction (choanal atresia). Babies born with a small jaw (micrognathia) are subject to obstructive apnoea when the tongue falls back and causes the upper airway to be occluded.

Functional obstruction occurs in preterm infants who may have hypotonia of the oropharyngeal musculature, which predisposes to collapse of the upper airway structures during breathing.

Obstructive apnoea may be recognised by the effort of breathing that the baby makes to overcome upper airway obstruction. Anatomical obstruction caused by choanal atresia is diagnosed by an inability to pass a cannula through both nostrils. You can see if the baby has micrognathia by looking at the face in profile.

Anatomical obstruction requires surgical correction, and the prognosis is generally good. Obstruction in premature infants is best treated by nasal CPAP. This improves the patency of the upper airway until the baby grows and the tone improves spontaneously. Premature babies usually grow out of the problem.

Diaphragmatic hernia

This is a congenital defect usually in the left hemidiaphragm that allows bowel to herniate into the left chest, with compression of the lungs and deviation of the heart to the right. If herniation occurs early in pregnancy, severe lung hypoplasia and pulmonary hypertension develops as a result of the compression and the baby dies rapidly in the neonatal period. Management is directed towards respiratory support, and surgical repair of the hernia is performed once the lung is stabilized and pulmonary vascular resistance falls in the days after birth.

Hirschsprung disease

Hirschsprung disease is caused by the absence of ganglion cells in the bowel wall nerve plexus. The colon is most commonly affected, and although presentation in the neonatal period is most common, mild cases may present later in infancy with severe constipation (p. 198).

The baby presents with delay in passage of meconium and abdominal distension. Rectal examination reveals an empty rectum. The diagnosis is suspected by abdominal X-ray, which shows dilated loops of bowel with an airless rectum, but can only be confirmed at biopsy when the abnormal nerve plexus is identified.

Management is surgical and in one or two stages depending on the severity and extent of the condition.

⊙ Hirschsprung disease at a glance

Epidemiology
One in 4500 births

Aetiology
Absence of ganglion cells in a segment of the bowel wall leads to aperistalsis and functional obstruction

History
Delay in passage of meconium
Constipation
Eventual bile-stained vomiting

Physical examination
Abdominal distension
Empty rectum on rectal examination

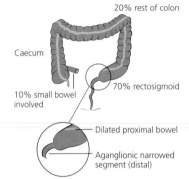

Caecum
20% rest of colon
70% rectosigmoid
10% small bowel involved
Dilated proximal bowel
Aganglionic narrowed segment (distal)

Confirmatory investigations
Abdominal X-ray shows dilated loops of bowel and airless rectum
Anorectal manometry
Rectal biopsy shows an absence of ganglion cells in the nerve plexus

Differential diagnosis
In neonates: other causes of intestinal obstruction (see Clues box, p. 444)
In older child: functional constipation

Management
Defunctioning colostomy followed at a later stage by resection of the abnormal bowel and closure of colostomy

Prognosis
Good following surgery
Milder cases may present with constipation and failure to thrive later

---

Hydronephrosis

'Hydronephrosis' refers to a grossly enlarged kidney caused by urinary tract obstruction. It is the commonest cause of abdominal organomegaly. Commonest sites of obstruction are:
- pelviureteric junction (usually unilateral);
- junction of ureter and bladder (ureterocoele);
- posterior urethra.

Unilateral hydronephrosis is common, as a result of obstruction at the pelviureteric junction (PUJ obstruction). Bilateral hydronephrosis and distended bladder in a boy is caused by bladder neck obstruction that results from obstruction at the posterior urethra (posterior urethral valves). Severe reflux may cause hydronephrosis.

Nephromegaly is usually the only sign of hydronephrosis. Ultrasound examination is particularly good at defining the diagnosis and site of obstruction. Surgical excision of the obstruction is curative in most cases. Severe renal impairment may occur if the obstruction has been long-standing.

Cleft palate and lip

Cleft lip (Figure 24.8), a distressing congenital abnormality in view of the cosmetic implications, occurs in one in 1000 children and tends to recur in families, although there is no single gene inheritance. Cleft palate is seen in association with a cleft lip in 70% of cases although may also appear in the absence of cleft lip.

The parents of children with cleft palate must be seen as soon after birth as possible and the nature of the condition discussed with them. Cleft palate is associated with the problems listed in Table 24.8.

The cosmetic appearance is excellent following plastic surgery and photographs of treated cases are particularly helpful in allaying parents' anxieties (see Figure 24.8). Surgical correction is usually undertaken at about 3–6 months of age for cleft lip and 12–18 months for cleft palate. The parents may need specialised advice to ensure effective feeding. It is important to involve speech therapists, an orthodontic and plastic surgeon and to arrange regular audiology assessment to prevent sequelae of the disorder.

Neural tube defects (spina bifida)

Spina bifida is a very important cause of severe disability and is a result of the failure of the neural tube to close normally in early pregnancy. The introduction of periconceptual folic acid supplementation has reduced the incidence of spina bifida lesions by 75%. Routine screening of almost all women in early pregnancy by either ultrasound or alpha-fetoprotein with selective termination of pregnancy has made open spina bifida a rare condition.

Various degrees of severity of neural tube disorder exist and are illustrated in Figure 24.9.

- *Anencephaly.* This is the most severe form of neural tube disorder, where there is complete failure of the development of the cranial part of the neural tube and the brain does not develop.
- *Myelomeningocoele.* This refers to an open lesion with the malformed and exposed spinal cord (myelocoele) being covered by a thin membrane of meninges (meningocoele). This is associated with severe neurological abnormality of the lower limbs, bladder, and anal innervation together with hydrocephalus in 90%. Surviving children have major disabilities requiring lifelong supervision.

Table 24.8 Problems to be anticipated in babies with cleft palate
Difficulties in establishing milk feeding
Milk aspiration
Speech difficulties caused by nasal escape
Conductive hearing loss as a result of eustachian tube dysfunction
Dental problems as a result of gingival margin maldevelopment

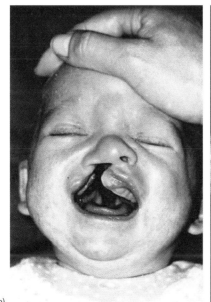
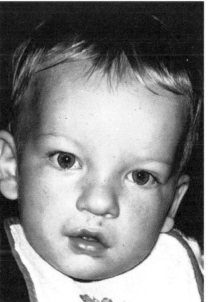

(a)

(b)

Figure 24.8 (a) Baby with cleft lip and (b) the same baby after plastic surgical repair.

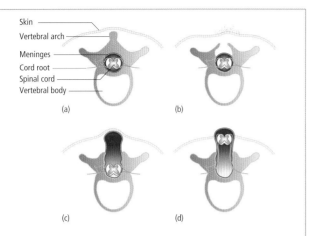

Figure 24.9 Varieties of neural tube disorders: (a) normal, (b) spina bifida occulta, (c) meningocoele with intact cord, (d) meningomyelocoele.

- *Meningocoele.* In this condition the spinal cord is intact and functions normally, but the defect involves an exposed bag of meningeal membranes which ruptures easily. Meningitis and hydrocephalus are a major risk in these cases. Rapid surgical closure is necessary to avoid infection.

- *Spina bifida occulta.* This refers to a 'hidden' abnormality of the developing neural tube which, if unrecognised and untreated, may later cause serious neurological disability.

The first three conditions are very obvious at birth and the mother will draw them immediately to medical attention. Spina bifida occulta may be missed on cursory examination and has very severe implications.

Spina bifida occulta

Spina bifida occulta (SBO) may be the only visible feature of tethering of the spinal cord within the spinal canal, with eventual stretching of the cord. This is associated with the development of bladder dysfunction and pyramidal tract signs in the lower limbs as the child grows. Spina bifida occulta is suggested by a subtle abnormality of the midline over the spine. In particular these include:

- a deep pit over the lower back;
- a tuft of hair;
- a naevus;
- a fatty tumour (lipoma) at or near the midline.

Ultrasound is the best investigative technique to exclude tethering of the spinal cord, and all babies with the possibility of SBO should be referred for scanning.

Neural tube defects (spina bifida) at a glance

Epidemiology
Now rare as a result of antenatal screening and folic acid supplementation preconceptually

Aetiology/pathophysiology
Failure of neural tube closure early in pregnancy. The defects range from anencephaly to spina bifida occulta (Figure 24.9), with complications related to the severity of the lesion

Clinical features
Open midline lesion with malformed and exposed spinal cord and meninges
Variable paralysis and sensory loss of legs
In spina bifida occulta a pit, hair tuft, naevus or lipoma may be found in the midline of the back (**a**)

Confirmatory investigations
Ultrasound can detect significant spina bifida occulta

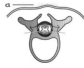
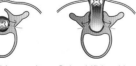
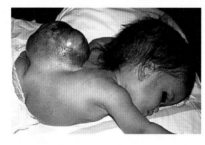

Spina bifida occulta   Spina bifida with meningomyelocele

Complications
(Vary according to severity of lesion)
Neurogenic bladder
Neurogenic bowel
Hydrocephalus (in 90% with meningomyelocoele)
Scoliosis

Management
Immediate surgical closure
Mobility:
Physiotherapy to prevent joint contractures
Walking aids
Bladder and bowel:
Intermittent urinary catheterisation to allow regular, complete emptying of the bladder
Prophylactic antibiotics for UTI
Regular toileting, laxatives, suppositories
Hydrocephalus:
Ventriculoperitoneal shunt
Skin care:
Avoidance of ulceration due to sensory loss

Prognosis
If the defect is severe there is likely to be significant physical and some intellectual impairment

Developmental dislocation of the hips

Developmental Dislocation of the Hip (DDH) may be diagnosed at birth and occurs in 0.2% of neonates. Factors associated with increased risk of DDH are shown in Table 24.9. Routine examination of the hips at birth will detect babies in whom the hips are either dislocated or dislocatable, and both these abnormalities require early treatment to prevent permanent maldevelopment of the hip joints with severe impairment in walking. The hips are also routinely checked at 6 weeks and 6–9 months (p. 29). Increasingly, assessment of hip

stability is performed by ultrasound screening. If any abnormality is detected on clinical examination, the baby should be referred for ultrasound assessment.

There are three components of the clinical examination:
- *Observation.* Is there any asymmetry of gluteal folds around the buttocks? Is there any difference in leg length or posture?
- *The Ortolani test* (Figure 24.10). This is a test to see whether the hip is already dislocated. Examine the baby on his or her back with the knees flexed. Grasp the infant's thigh with your middle finger on the greater trochanter and the thumb on the lesser trochanter and gently abduct the hip. If the hip is dislocated, you will be unable to do this. The Ortolani test attempts to relocate the already dislocated hip by lifting the thigh upwards and gently abducting it to bring the hip from its dislocated position back into the acetabulum. This is associated with a 'clunk' as the head of the femur is relocated in the acetabulum. Examine each hip separately while anchoring the other leg.
- *The Barlow test* (Figure 24.11). This test detects the hip that is in joint but is dislocatable because of underdevelopment

Table 24.9 Factors associated with increased risk of DDH

Family history
Multiple pregnancy
Breech delivery
Neurological defects associated with impaired lower limb movement, e.g. spina bifida

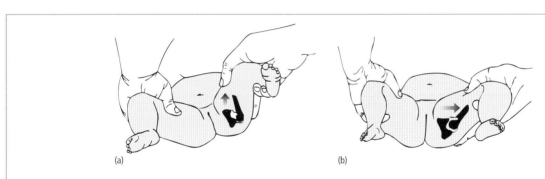

(a)   (b)

Figure 24.10 The Ortolani test.

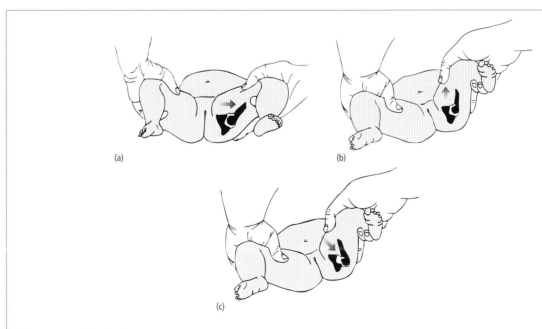

(a)   (b)

(c)

Figure 24.11 The Barlow test.

of the acetabulum. Place the baby in the same position as for the Ortolani test and grasp the thigh in the same way. Place the hip an abducted position. The aim of the test is to use downward and lateral force via your thumb to attempt to dislocate the hip posteriorly. You will feel the femoral head slip over the posterior lip of the acetabulum.

If an abnormality is detected, or if the hip feels stable but there is a ligamentous 'click' on abduction, an ultrasound scan of the hip is performed to look for an abnormally shallow acetabulum. In addition, ultrasound examination at age 4–6 weeks is indicated in the high risk groups in Table 24.9. There is no value in X-raying the neonatal hip as the hip joint is not ossified until 3–4 months of age.

Treatment involves immobilizing the hip joint in abduction by a special splint for 3–6 months, in order to allow normal development of the acetabular rim.

👁 Developmental dislocation of the hips at a glance

Epidemiology
One and a half per 1000 births
Commoner in girls and breech births

Aetiology/pathophysiology
Dysplasia of the acetabulum leading to laxity, subluxation or dislocation

Clinical features
Positive Ortolani/Barlow screening test
Restricted hip abduction if the hip is dislocated
Asymmetric leg skin folds*
Shortening of the affected leg*

Confirmatory investigations
Ultrasound of the hip

Management
Immobilization of the hip in abduction by splinting for several months
Monitor progress by ultrasound or X-ray
Surgery if conservative measures fail

Prognosis
Good with treatment
If undetected, leads to permanent limp or waddling gait

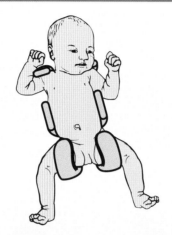

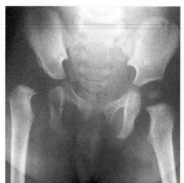

NB *Signs and symptoms are variable.

Retinopathy of prematurity

Retinopathy of prematurity is a common condition of very preterm infants. It occurs in 50% of babies with birthweight <1500 g, but resolves spontaneously in the vast majority of cases, only occasionally leading to blindness.

The cause of ROP is incompletely understood, but iatrogenic oxygen toxicity is a factor. The retina becomes ischaemic, and vascular endothelial growth factor is released leading to abnormal neo-vascularization in the nearby retina. This may lead to retinal detachment.

The condition can only be recognised by regular ophthalmoscopy. If the condition appears to be rapidly progressive, retinal detachment can be avoided by laser therapy or intraocular injection of VEGF antagonists. However, most babies require no treatment and the prognosis is good.

To test your knowledge on this part of the book, see Chapter 26

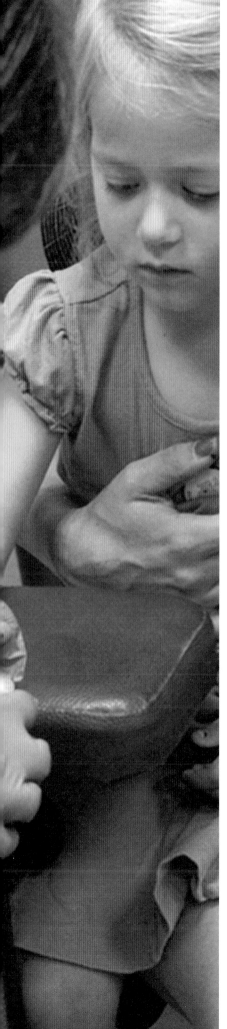

CHAPTER 25

Adolescence and puberty

Adolescence is the interruption of peaceful growth.

Anna Freud

KEY COMPETENCES

You must ...

Know and understand

- The common and important pubertal, gynaecological, emotional and psychological conditions affecting adolescents
- The increasing importance of abuse of social media, alcohol, tobacco and other substances
- How sexually transmitted diseases present and are managed
- The importance of HPV vaccination
- The tasks that characterise adolescence
- The physical changes that occur and how they are 'staged'
- The role and approach taken by adolescent health clinics

Be able to

- Relate to adolescent patients
- Take a history including HEADSS
- Discuss birth control and responsible sexual behaviour
- Undertake health promotion discussions

Appreciate that

- Adolescents can agree to treatment without parental consent if the doctor deems that they are mature enough to understand the implications
- Adolescence is a time when individuals often feel reticent about doctors
- Adolescence can be a stormy time characterised by high-risk behaviours and sexuality exploration

Essential Paediatrics and Child Health, Fourth Edition. Mary Rudolf, Anthony Luder and Kerry Jeavons.
© 2020 John Wiley & Sons Ltd. Published 2020 by John Wiley & Sons Ltd.
Companion website: www.wiley.com/go/rudolf/paediatrics

Finding your way around …

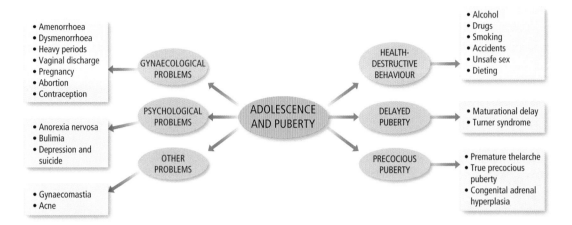

Until recently, the health care of adolescents has been somewhat neglected in many countries including Britain, with the responsibility for this age group falling somewhere between the paediatrician and the physician. Even in general practice, adolescents gain little attention between the needs and demands of young children and the elderly. The problem is compounded by the fact that, as a group, adolescents tend not to seek out health care, although they often have considerable needs which are not being met.

In paediatrics, there is increasing awareness that these needs should be met, and it is important that you develop an awareness of the health issues facing adolescents, and acquire the special skills needed in relating to them.

As adolescents infrequently present with a 'problem' which requires a differential diagnostic approach, the issues covered in this chapter for the most part are not problem orientated.

Changes occurring in adolescence

Adolescence can be defined as the period between childhood and adulthood during which the process of maturity occurs. During this period the individual undergoes physical, psychological and social changes.

Physical changes

The adolescent's body undergoes rapid change, and over the course of a few years secondary sexual characteristics are acquired, fertility is achieved and there is an accompanying growth spurt.

Psychological changes

Psychological changes occur of both an emotional and intellectual nature. Cognitively, adolescents develop a widening scope of intellectual activity and a capacity for insight. As compared with younger children, they begin to use abstract reasoning and logic, and develop an increased sophistication

in moral reasoning. These skills are used in questioning the fundamental values of parents and other adults, and developing a critical awareness of social challenges and the world around.

Emotional changes also occur, often with conflict and turmoil. There is a search for independence and relationships change with both parents and peers. Experimentation and exploration occur and may result in risk-taking behaviour and a need to test limits. Psychological and psychiatric problems are not infrequent including self-image problems, eating disturbances, anxiety and depression and unfortunately suicidal ideation.

Adolesence is the period during which individuals become intensely aware of their sexuality. Medical issues are common and important, including sexually-transmitted diseases and HIV. Contraception and safe sex guidance are critical as are coping with the large variety of non-heterosexual identifications, attractions and roles (see Table 25.1). Many doctors have not been trained in these issues and feel incompetent to deal with them.

Table 25.1 Medical issues and sexuality variance

Variant	Medical issues
Heterosexuals	Safe sex Contraception STD
Homosexuals	Family adjustment disorders Anxiety HIV and anorectal trauma
Transexuals	Gender identification Surgical and endocrine treatment
Transgender	Exposure to violence and abuse
Asexuals	Loneliness and adjustment disorder

Table 25.2 Tasks of adolescence

Establishing a sense of identity

Achieving a degree of independence

Achieving sexual maturity

Taking on adult responsibility

Development of an adult thinking pattern

Table 25.3 Vulnerable adolescents

Chronic illness

Physical and mental handicap

Victims of physical, emotional and sexual abuse

Homeless, poor and unemployed

Pregnant

Disrupted homes

Minority groups

Social changes

Significant changes occur for the individual socially, although most adolescents today remain financially and physically dependent on their parents. At school adolescents are given greater freedom and flexibility, and more emphasis is placed on self-motivation and self-discipline. Peer relationships gain increasing importance. By the end of adolescence, the individual has to face leaving school and moving towards further education, earning and financial independence, or unemployment. In recent years the ability of the adolescent to play a responsible and proportionate role in the virtual world of social media has become increasingly central to healthy adjustment.

The tasks of adolescence

By the end of adolescence, it is expected that the individual will have succeeded in completing the tasks required to become a competent adult. In order to do so, all of the physical, cognitive, emotional, and social changes must have been integrated into some sort of meaningful whole. The individual should have achieved sexual maturity, established a stable sense of identity, achieved a degree of independence, developed an adult pattern of thinking, and taken on adult responsibilities (Table 25.2).

Health care for the adolescent

Adolescence is in general a healthy period of life, and the incidence of illness in this age group is lower than at any other time. As a result, there is a very low rate of contact with doctors.

Health issues during adolescence

The health issues of this age group can be divided into medical problems, health concerns (which may well not be related to those perceived by health professionals), and health promotion. The medical problems broadly relate to health-destructive behaviour, psychological problems, skin and cosmetic issues, concerns around pubertal changes, and gynaecological issues especially abdominal pain and menstrual problems. The extent of adolescents' worries is often underestimated and seem to focus particularly on weight gain, nutrition, exercise, and sexual matters. Health promotion is an important issue, in part because destructive and high-risk behaviour is particularly prevalent at this age, and also because adolescents are more amenable to changes in lifestyle than they are likely to be later in life.

Box 25.1 Goals of adolescent health clinics

- Comprehensive health mapping and solution provision for all health issues – 'one-stop'
- Counselling for emotional and personal problems
- Advice about sexually transmitted diseases and safer sex
- Contraceptive advice and availability
- Pregnancy testing and counselling

There are certain adolescents who are especially vulnerable, either for medical or psychosocial reasons (Table 25.3). These are the very individuals who are likely to have difficulty in accessing health care and it is important that efforts are made to reach them.

Health care facilities

Adolescents' health care may be delivered via their GP's surgery and clinics, at school, in hospital outpatients, family planning clinics or in special adolescent centres. Whatever the facility, the service needs to be relevant and specific to adolescents' particular needs (see Box 25.1).

The ideal service needs to be comprehensive friendly, discreet, multidisciplinary, attractive and easily accessible. Adolescents may not come twice so as much as possible should be done on the first visit. Outpatients clinics in hospital often fail, in that they are faced with an alienating clinical, institutional atmosphere, toys and toddlers in the waiting room, and inadequate attention is paid to their need for privacy. The GP may also fail in that adolescents may not believe that the doctor they have known since infancy is going to supply them with confidential care. Schools too may fail through lack of facilities and personnel. In recognition of the particular needs for this age group, a new concept of the 'drop-in' clinic is developing, whereby adolescents can attend a conveniently located, easy-to-find centre, at times that fit in with school and where anonymity is more likely to be attained. These centres aim to provide immediate help and advice on all health matters, counselling for emotional and personal problems, and contraceptive advice and supplies.

Approach to the adolescent

More important than the physical facility is the approach to be taken by health personnel in seeing an adolescent in any health context (see Box 25.2). Principles include a respect for the adolescent's emerging maturity and his or her need for privacy. Time must be allowed for concerns to be expressed and the effort made to listen well. A sympathetic, non-judgemental but firm approach is usually appreciated. Confidentiality should be provided and made explicit, although the adolescent should know that this would have to be broken if his or her own wellbeing or that of another is jeopardized.

Adolescents often do not initially state the problems that are most troubling them, even though they may be very depressed, and troubled by delay in puberty or bad acne. They may be grateful if the doctor broadens the context of any visit to address these concerns.

HEADSS is an approach which is widely used as a way to structure a consultation with adolescents that facilitates communication and aims to create a sympathetic, confidential, respectful environment. The acronym relates to six key areas: **H**ome, **E**ducation/employment, peer group **A**ctivities, **D**rugs, **S**exuality, and **S**uicide/depression, and specific open-ended developmentally appropriate questions are recommended for each area of enquiry.

If the adolescent is accompanied by a parent, as commonly occurs in the hospital setting, it is important that the patient is always given the opportunity to see the doctor alone, both to address private concerns and to encourage them to take responsibility for their own health needs. The doctor may need to strike a balance between adolescents' needs for autonomy, privacy, and confidentiality and their parent's concerns and wishes to be informed.

Consent to treatment

In most circumstances consent is not a problematic issue, although the doctor should be aware that legally a young person under the age of 16, in the absence of mental incapacity, or a younger child who in the doctor's view is of sufficient understanding to make an informed decision, is entitled to refuse to submit to any examination, assessment or treatment

('Fraser (previously Gillick) competence'). If a young person under 18 years refuses treatment, which may lead to their death or a severe permanent injury, their decision can be overruled by the Court of Protection. This is the legal body that oversees the operation of the Mental Capacity Act (2005). The parents of a young person who has refused treatment may consent for them, but it is usually thought best to go through the courts in this situation.

The problem for doctors tends to centre on the prescription of contraceptives, treatment for sexually transmitted diseases and abortion in cases where adolescents do not wish their parents to be involved. Although the doctor may be uncomfortable, the law indicates that an individual under the age of 16 years is capable of giving his or her own consent, provided the doctor deems the individual to be mature enough to make an informed decision regarding risks and benefits. Nevertheless, strenuous efforts should be made to convince the patient that parents should be informed and if possible, consent.

Physical changes in adolescence

Puberty can be defined as the process of gonadal maturation which results in the acquisition of secondary sexual characteristics, a growth spurt and fertility. These occur under the influence of the sex hormones (Figure 25.1). Gonodotrophin-releasing hormone (GnRH) is released from the hypothalamus and stimulates the synthesis of follicle-stimulating hormone (FSH) and luteinizing hormone (LH), which in turn stimulate the gonads to produce testosterone or oestrogen. These hormones are responsible for development of breasts and the uterus in girls and the testicles, penis, body hair, and all the other secondary sexual characteristics in boys. Androgens secreted by the adrenal glands are responsible for sexual hair in girls and contribute to sexual hair development in boys. The key ages at which pubertal events are usually seen are shown in Table 25.4.

Box 25.2 Guidelines for relating to adolescents

- Take time to listen
- Show respect for the adolescent's emerging maturity
- Allow the adolescent to express his or her concerns
- Avoid judgemental statements
- Assure confidentiality (provided the wellbeing of the patient or another is not jeopardized)
- Respect the need for privacy
- HEADSS is a good framework for taking a psychosocial history and facilitating communication

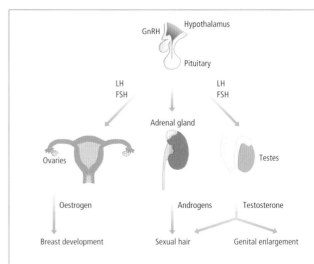

Figure 25.1 Hormonal events leading to the development of secondary sexual characteristics.

Table 25.4 Key ages in puberty		
	Boys	**Girls**
Normal pubertal range from start to completion	11–16 years	10–14 years
First signs of puberty	Testicular enlargement	Breast budding
Precocious puberty	Onset <9.5 years*	Onset <8.5 years
Delayed puberty	Onset >14 years	Onset >13 years
Delayed menarche	–	Onset >16 years

* High likelihood of pathological rather than physiological cause for precocious puberty in boys.

For the purpose of clinical description, puberty has been divided into five stages, known as Tanner stages. These range from Tanner stage 1 (prepuberty) to Tanner stage 5 (full maturity). They are useful for monitoring the progress of puberty in children where there are concerns about growth or puberty. The five stages for breast, gonadal and pubic hair development are illustrated in Figure 25.2.

Pubertal development in boys

Puberty in boys usually starts between the ages of 11 and 14 years. The first sign is testicular enlargement, which is followed by pigmentation and thinning of the scrotum and growth of the penis. As puberty progresses, pubic, axillary and facial hair develop, the voice deepens and the ability to ejaculate develops. The growth spurt, which is accompanied by an increase in body size and muscle bulk, occurs when puberty is well under way and is maximal from 14 to 16 years, reaching its peak 2 years after that of girls.

Pubertal development in girls

Puberty tends to start earlier in girls than boys. The first sign is usually breast budding, which develops at around 10–11 years, and is followed by pubic and axillary hair development. The growth spurt occurs early, and is virtually completed by menarche (the onset of periods) which usually occurs at 11–13 years. The interval between onset of puberty and menarche is, on average, 2.0–2.5 years.

Health-destructive behaviour

Many of the medical problems incurred by this age group relate to health-destructive behaviour, which includes alcohol, smoking, substance abuse, injuries and unsafe sex. This behaviour results from the desire to explore and experiment, which is characteristic of adolescents in their challenge to achieve independence and assert their individuality.

Alcohol

Surveys show that children become familiar with alcohol at an early age, and by their teens drinking is a regular part of their lives. Alcohol has a greater effect on judgement and control in young, inexperienced drinkers. Binge drinking leading to drunkenness and behavioural disinhibition is a serious risk, especially when the adolescent reaches driving age. Interestingly, the principal place where alcohol is obtained is the home.

Drugs

Studies of drug and solvent misuse among secondary school children in the UK suggest misuse levels of 11% in 11-year-olds

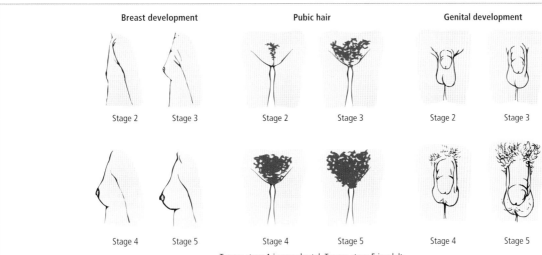

Tanner stage 1 is prepubertal. Tanner stage 5 is adult.
Breast or genital development should be staged independently of pubic hair development

Figure 25.2 Tanner staging of secondary sexual characteristics.

increasing to 37% in 15-year-olds. Peer group influence is important in terms of experimentation. Misusers are more likely to come from single-parent families and be involved in truancy, vandalism, smoking, and drinking. Most involvement is temporary, but a minority progress to multiple drug use, chronic use and addiction. Table 25.4 summarizes the signs of drug taking, and Table 25.5 describes the commoner drugs of abuse, their effects and clinical features.

Educational initiatives are provided in schools and focus on providing information on the abuse and misuse of drugs, promoting self-esteem, decision-making skills and coping with adverse situations.

Smoking

The earlier a person begins to smoke, the greater the risk of chronic bronchitis, emphysema, cardiovascular disease and lung cancer. As compared with adults, where the prevalence of smoking is decreasing, it is increasing in this age group. Girls are more likely to be smokers than boys, and those who smoke are more likely to try other drugs, sniff solvents, drink alcohol and go out partying. Smokers are often underachievers and truants.

Table 25.4 Signs of drug taking

Sudden changes of mood

Loss of appetite

Loss of interest in appearance, school work, leisure interests

Drowsiness or sleeplessness

Furtive behaviour

Unusual stains/smells on clothing

Accidents

Car and motorcycle accidents are the leading causes of adolescent morbidity and mortality. The majority of these incidents involve vehicles driven by adolescents. Alcohol and failure to wear seat belts and motorcycle helmets are factors underlying most fatalities. Sports injuries and drowning are additional prominent causes of serious injury.

Unsafe sex

Sexual activity is occurring at younger ages. Thirty per cent of girls and 50% of boys have had sexual intercourse before the age of 16. The majority do not seek contraceptive advice for some time, and casual sexual relationships are particularly likely to be unprotected. Unsafe sex can lead to pregnancy and sexually transmitted diseases including HIV, and have a deleterious effect on future fertility. These problems can all lead to serious psychological problems as well.

The highest rate of sexually transmitted disease is found amongst adolescents. This is in part a result of the sexual behaviour characteristic of this age group, which includes multiple partners, failure to use barrier contraception, reluctance to consider that a partner may have venereal disease, and lack of communication skills to discuss the issue. There are also physiological differences that render the adolescent vaginal epithelium more susceptible to infection.

Gonorrhoea, chlamydia and human papilloma virus are the commonest sexually transmitted diseases in adolescence, although syphilis is still a threat. HIV infection is on the increase, although because of the long latency period it may not manifest itself in the adolescent years. Risk factors for contraction of HIV include unprotected intercourse and intravenous drug use.

Table 25.5 Common forms of substance abuse

Substance	Epidemiology	Effects	Physical signs
Solvent (sniffing) – toluene based glues, aerosols, fuel gases and solvents	Mainly boys 100 deaths per year from heart failure, suffocation and injuries	Intoxication, excitement, hallucination	Disorientation, slurred speech, blurred vision Skin irritation around the nose and mouth Solvent smells on breath or clothing
Cannabis (generally smoked as a hand-rolled cigarette)	Most widely used illicit drug	Pleasurable feelings of relaxation, altered sensory perception	Red eyes and tachycardia
Cocaine (sniffed through a tube or injected). 'Crack' refers to a less refined form of cocaine		Exhilaration, indifference to pain and hunger, residual depression and fatigue	Tachycardia, hypertension, hyperthermia Teratogenic effect on the fetus
Opiates (swallowing, injecting, sniffing and smoking)	Leading cause of drug-related death Consequences of injecting include thrombophlebitis, HIV and hepatitis B	Euphoria and contentment	Sedation, depression of respiration, heart rate and bowel activity Skin scars

Dieting

A preoccupation with appearance and body shape is characteristic of adolescence. Dieting is an almost universal activity among adolescent girls, and often takes the form of extreme starvation diets. Eating disorders are an increasing problem. A further concern is that girls as young as 8 or 9 years commonly have a distorted sense of body image, and are increasingly involved in dieting behaviour. Recent evidence has shown that media images especially idealized notions of professional models' appearance are a significant promoter of these problems.

Problems of puberty

Delayed puberty

Puberty is defined as being delayed if there are no signs of puberty by the age of 14 in a boy, 13 in a girl or if menarche has not occurred by the age of 16 (Table 25.3). Adolescents may present either because of concerns about the absence of sexual development or because of short stature (see p. 279). The causes of delayed puberty are shown in Table 25.6. The commonest cause of pubertal delay is constitutional delay, which is commonly familial. Other causes to be considered are Turner syndrome in girls, and anorexia nervosa or intense athletic training, both of which can suppress the hypothalamus. Any chronic and severe disease can delay puberty, and rare causes include pituitary or gonadal failure.

Constitutional delay

Constitutional delay of puberty (see p. 291) is commonly familial. Although a normal variant, it can cause considerable distress, particularly in boys. The diagnosis is based on the pattern of growth (short but steady, see p. 282), a family history of delayed menarche in the women or delayed growth in the men of the family, a delayed bone age and the absence of any evidence of central nervous system pathology. Reassurance is usually all that is required, but if the adolescent

(nearly always a boy) is suffering socially, puberty can be triggered by a low dose of testosterone given for a few months.

Turner syndrome (see p. 297)

In Turner syndrome, which is caused by an abnormality or absence of one of the X-chromosomes, puberty does not occur, as the gonads, which are streaks of fibrous tissue, fail to secrete oestrogen. Girls with Turner syndrome should have been identified earlier in childhood because of short stature, but still occasionally present with delayed puberty. It is important to remember that many girls with Turner syndrome are normal phenotypically and do not have the classic features of the syndrome, so a karyotype is indicated in any girl with either delayed puberty or short stature. Rare cases of pregnancy have been reported in Turner therefore this syndrome is not a guarantee of infertility.

Precocious puberty

Puberty is defined as being precocious if secondary sexual characteristics occur before the age of 8.5 years in a girl or 9.5 years in a boy (Table 25.3). The causes of precocious puberty are shown in Table 25.7. Precocious puberty in girls is usually idiopathic; boys are far more likely to have an underlying pathological lesion, and so require especially thorough evaluation.

Children with precocious puberty suffer on two accounts. First, they have to contend with physical, emotional and social changes at an inappropriately young age and, secondly, adult height is jeopardized as a result of premature fusion of the bones.

Pubertal signs may occur precociously as a result of premature activation of the hypothalamic–pituitary axis ('true' precocious puberty) or inappropriate secretion of oestrogen or androgens. These can be distinguished clinically. In the former, the full picture of puberty occurs. In the latter, oestrogen secretion causes breast development (thelarche) but no pubic hair; androgen secretion causes pubic hair but no testicular or breast enlargement.

Table 25.6 Causes of delayed puberty

Boys and girls

Constitutional delay (commonly familial)

Pituitary lesions

Gonadal failure

Chronic and severe disease

Girls

Turner syndrome

Intense athletic training

Anorexia nervosa

Table 25.7 Causes of precocious puberty

Hypothalamic–pituitary

Constitutional advance (true precocious puberty)

Central nervous system lesions

Ovarian

Premature thelarche

Adrenal

Congenital adrenal hyperplasia

Adrenal tumours

Accompanying features of precocious puberty (with the exception of premature thelarche) include acceleration of growth, advance of skeletal maturation and emotional changes.

Investigations should be directed by the findings on physical examination and should include hormone levels, a karyotype in girls, X-ray for bone age, pelvic ultrasound, and computed tomography (CT) or magnetic resonance imaging (MRI) of the head.

Premature thelarche

Premature thelarche (isolated premature breast development) is not uncommon and occurs in the first 2 years of life. It is a benign condition thought to be caused by a maturational aberration of the hypothalamic–pituitary axis. It does not cause acceleration of growth, and investigations are normal, although ovarian ultrasound may show a few small cysts. The breasts regress spontaneously over some months. Accidental ingestion of maternal contraceptive pills can also cause thelarche. Neonates commonly have transient breast engorgement due to maternal hormones.

True precocious puberty

True precocious puberty refers to puberty that is triggered early by premature activation of the hypothalamic–pituitary axis. In girls, the underlying cause is usually idiopathic, but in boys there is commonly an underlying central nervous system lesion such as a tumour or trauma. Treatment includes therapy for the underlying lesion if there is one, and administration of a hormonal analogue which suppresses the secretion of the gonadotrophins.

Congenital adrenal hyperplasia

Congenital adrenal hyperplasia is an autosomal recessive disorder which results in a block in the adrenal production of corticosteroids. As a consequence, a build-up of androgenic precursors occurs, which can result in either ambiguous genitalia (detected at birth, see p. 343) or precocious development of pubic hair. Diagnosis is confirmed by the finding of elevated corticosteroid precursors, and treatment consists of life-long steroid replacement therapy. This condition is a medical emergency in neonates because of the concomitant Addison syndrome that may develop.

Gynaecomastia

Gynaecomastia (breast development in boys) is very common, occurring in 65% of adolescent boys, and is thought to be caused by an oestrogen–androgen imbalance which occurs at puberty. It may be unilateral or bilateral, and spontaneous regression occurs over time. Reassurance is usually all that is required, but if there is significant social embarrassment, rarely hormonal or surgical treatment can be given.

Acne

Acne is virtually universal in adolescence. Its development is linked to the onset of sebaceous gland activity and the production of free fatty acids. Inflammation occurs as a result of colonization by micro-organisms.

Clinical features   The skin lesions consist of a mixture of comedones (white heads and black heads), pustules and nodulocystic lesions, which may be interspersed with scarring. Lesions may be confined to the face or involve the chest and upper back. As adolescents become preoccupied with their appearance, acne assumes great importance. It can cause much distress, may dominate life and may even give rise to self-imposed isolation.

Management   Offering treatment for even mild acne can enhance self-image and is therefore important. Diet plays no significant part in the development of acne, although a healthy diet should be encouraged for reasons of general health. Greasy cosmetic and hair preparations should be discontinued. Mild cleansing agents can help by drying the skin and suppressing skin flora. In more severe cases topical antibiotics and topical or oral retinoic acid, which acts by eliminating the keratinous plug, may be required. The adolescent should be warned that all topical treatment requires several weeks to have an effect. In severe pustular or nodulocystic acne, oral retinoic acid and/or antibiotics (usually tetracycline or a macrolide antibiotic) are indicated.

Psychological problems of adolescence

Eating disorders

Eating disorders commonly begin as innocent dieting behaviour, which progresses to become a serious condition which may be life-threatening. Girls are far more commonly affected than boys, and the age of onset is decreasing so that as many as one-fifth are under the age of 13 years. The eating disorders are characterised by intense fear of becoming obese, and a distorted body image, so that even emaciated affected individuals perceive themselves as being fat. In an attempt to achieve the desired weight, there is a denial of hunger, preoccupation with food and bizarre eating behaviours.

👁 Eating disorders at a glance

Epidemiology
Girls principally affected
Prepubertal onset now more
common

Aetiology/pathophysiology
Bizarre eating behaviour
associated with a distorted
body image and fear of
becoming obese

Clinical features

Anorexia nervosa
History

- extreme dieting (**a**)
- excessive physical activity (**b**)
- weight loss
- amenorrhoea
- constipation

Physical examination

- emaciation
- dry skin
- lanugo hair
- hair loss
- if severe – bradycardia, hypotension and hypothermia

NB *Signs and symptoms are variable.

Anorexia   Bulimia

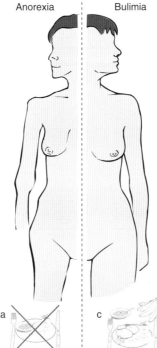
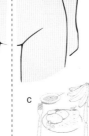
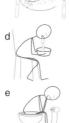
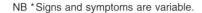

a

b

c

d

e

Clinical features

Bulimia
History

- eating in binges (**c**)
- followed by induced vomiting
(**d**) or laxatives (**e**)
- symptoms of oesophagitis
Physical examination
- usually normal weight
- staining of inner surface of
teeth*
- parotid swelling*

Confirmatory investigations
Not required
Severe weight loss may be
complicated by biochemical
derangement
(e.g. hypophosphataemia)
which makes re-feeding hazardous

Differential diagnosis
Other causes of weight loss
Other causes of amenorrhoea

Management
Psychotherapy
Behaviour modification
techniques
Nutritional rehabilitation

Prognosis
Can be life-threatening
(mortality rates up to 10%)

Anorexia nervosa

Young people with anorexia nervosa restrict their intake of carbohydrate- and fat-containing foods by extreme dieting in order to control their weight. This is usually accompanied by excessive physical activity.

An arbitrary definition of anorexia nervosa has been taken to be a loss of more than 20% body weight in relation to height. The clinical features found are those of malnutrition, with emaciation, amenorrhoea, constipation, dry skin, lanugo hair and hair loss. As body weight decreases, bradycardia, hypotension and hypothermia are found.

Bulimia

Young people with bulimia have bouts of eating in binges and then purge themselves by inducing vomiting or using laxatives.

These young people, in contrast to those with anorexia, are often of normal weight or slightly obese. Oesophagitis, parotid swelling and staining of the internal surface of the teeth can occur as a result of frequent vomiting.

Eating disorders, particularly anorexia, can be life-threatening and mortality rates are as high as 10%, so the condition must be taken seriously. The approach involves a combination of psychotherapy, behaviour modification techniques, selective pharmacotherapy and nutritional rehabilitation. Initially re-feeding is required, which may demand hospitalization and nasogastric feeding. The cornerstone of management is family therapy.

Depression and suicide

Adolescence is naturally a time of moods which swing from the depths of depression to the heights of elation. It is often difficult therefore to decide which adolescent is at risk for true depression. Factors associated with an increased risk include a disturbed or disrupted home life, poor functioning at school, low self-esteem, antisocial and aggressive behaviour, substance misuse, stressful life events and a family history of affective disorder.

Suicide is increasing in incidence and is a leading cause of death in this age group. The method most commonly used in adolescence is ingestion of medication, either their own or a parent's. The seriousness of an attempt cannot be related to the lethality of the dose, but is related to the degree of premeditation and the likelihood of rescue.

Depression and suicide at a glance

Epidemiology
Suicide: a leading cause of
  death in teenagers
Commonest method is drug
  ingestion
Risk factors
• disturbed home life
• poor functioning at school
• low self-esteem
• antisocial behaviour
• substance misuse
• family history of affective disorder

Clinical features
Insomnia and difficulty falling
  asleep*
Altered appetite*
School failure and absenteeism*
Alcohol and drug use*

NB *Signs and symptoms are variable.

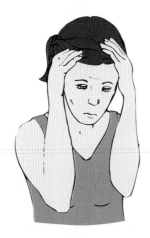

Management
Identify sources of stress
Counselling/psychotherapy for
  adolescent and family
Antidepressants with caution
Attempted suicide: hospitalize
  for medical treatment and
  psychosocial assessment

Prognosis
Seriousness of attempted
  suicide is related to the degree
  of premeditation and likelihood
  of rescue, rather than
  drug dose
Most successful suicides follow
  an earlier attempt

Clinical features.   Depression has been defined as a persistently lowered mood and misery that is severe enough to interfere with everyday life. It is accompanied by feelings of worthlessness, a sense of hopelessness, anxiety, pessimistic thoughts and often suicidal ideas or acts. Depressed adolescents may experience insomnia and difficulty falling asleep, sometimes to the extent of being awake all night and sleeping through the day, and appetite may be altered. Falling school grades, increase in school absenteeism, and the use of alcohol and drugs are common. Most successful suicides occur among those who have made earlier attempts. Many failed suicide attempts are ominous signs of genuine intent and should not be dismissed as childish impetuousness or attention-seeking behaviour.

Management   Sources of stress should be identified and dealt with as far as possible. Counselling, psychotherapy and where appropriate, family therapy may be helpful. The parents, too, need help, especially in dealing with uncooperative behaviour, and providing additional care and affection. At this age, treatment with antidepressants should only be prescribed by specialists.

Short-term hospitalization is usually indicated to attend to pharmacological sequelae, to assess the psychosocial situation and to impress on the family the need to attend to underlying problems.

Gynaecological problems

Menstrual complaints

Amenorrhoea

Amenorrhoea, or the absence of periods, may be primary or secondary. The term 'primary amenorrhoea' indicates that menarche has never occurred, and is discussed on p. 461 ('Delayed puberty'). Secondary amenorrhoea refers to the cessation of periods for more than 3 months after regular cycles have been established. Its causes are listed in Table 25.8.

Most amenorrhoea in adolescence is physiological. After menarche it is usual for periods to be scanty or irregular for several months, and several months may elapse between periods. Stress, such as starting a new school, can disrupt periods, and girls undergoing intense athletic training can experience amenorrhoea as a result of hypothalamic–pituitary axis suppression. Pregnancy should always be considered as a cause of amenorrhoea in adolescent girls.

The commonest pathological cause of amenorrhoea is anorexia nervosa or dieting. Interestingly, amenorrhoea can precede the weight loss. Any chronic illness can cause amenorrhoea, but particularly those associated with malnutrition or tissue hypoxia, such as diabetes mellitus, inflammatory bowel disease, cystic fibrosis or cyanotic congenital heart disease. Turner syndrome, endocrine disorders and uro-genital malformations are all important although less common causes of amenorrhoea.

When evaluating a girl with amenorrhoea, you should take a complete history, focusing on diet, potentially stressful events, exercise, sexual activity, medical history and neurological symptoms. You need to look for signs of anorexia nervosa, pregnancy and neurological abnormality on physical examination. Baseline investigations include a full blood count, plasma viscosity and pregnancy test, and if these are negative, consider gonadotrophin levels, thyroid function tests, pelvic ultrasound and imaging of the head.

Table 25.8 Causes of secondary amenorrhoea

Physiological

Hormonal cycle immaturity

Stress

Intense athletic training

Pregnancy

Pathological

Anorexia nervosa

Chronic illness

Brain tumour

Hyperthyroidism

Dysmenorrhoea

Adolescent girls commonly experience painful menstrual cramps, and dysmenorrhoea is the commonest cause of short-term school absenteeism. The mechanism is thought to be caused by high levels of endometrial prostaglandins. Effective treatment can be given prophylactically using non-steroidal anti-inflammatory drugs such as ibuprofen. An alternative is the oral contraceptive pill, if contraception is desired.

Heavy periods

Excessive menstrual bleeding is most often secondary to the anovulatory cycles that normally occur in the first year postmenarche. Without ovulation, oestrogen unopposed by progesterone causes endometrial proliferation with eventual massive shedding. Hormonal treatment is required if there is anaemia or hypovolaemia. Other causes of heavy periods include bleeding disorders and aspirin ingestion.

Vaginal discharge

A normal physiological increase in vaginal discharge (Table 25.9) occurs in the year prior to menarche. In childhood, discharge secondary to poor perineal hygiene is common and may be accompanied by dysuria, frequency, and pruritus. The treatment is as described for dysuria (p. 320). If the discharge is persistent and foul smelling, a foreign body (usually toilet paper or a retained tampon) should be suspected. In prepubertal girls, candida is not common, although it may follow antibiotic or steroid therapy. Sexually transmitted diseases must be suspected in sexually active girls, and a high index of suspicion maintained even in prepubertal children as, if found, it is indicative of sexual abuse.

Sexually transmitted diseases

Coverage of sexually transmitted diseases is beyond the scope of this book. However, they are a significant and prevalent cause of morbidity in the adolescent years, and should not be overlooked when working with adolescents.

Table 25.9 Causes of vaginal discharge

Physiological

Poor perineal hygiene

Foreign body

Candida

Sexually transmitted diseases*

* Indicative of sexual abuse if found in a prepubertal child.

Pregnancy

Adolescent pregnancy carries risks for both mother and baby. Contributing factors obstetrically include late booking for antenatal care, poor attendance at clinic and antenatal classes, and poor nutrition. The babies tend to suffer from higher infant and perinatal mortality rates, an increased incidence of sudden unexplained death in infancy or childhood (SUDIC), low birthweight (both pre- and post-term), gastrointestinal problems, accidental and non-accidental injury, behaviour problems and delayed psychomotor development.

Girls most at risk are those who lack self-esteem, become sexually active early, come from unhappy or unstable backgrounds and those in care. Adolescent mothers are more likely to suffer from postnatal depression, and are less likely to marry ultimately, finish secondary school education or gain employment.

It is always wise to consider pregnancy in any female patient with abdominal or urinary symptoms, and before prescribing medications with a potential for teratogenicity.

Abortion

Abortion remains a major form of contraception in this age group, and in the UK about 60% of adolescent pregnancies end in legal abortion. Apart from the medical risks of abortion, there are considerable emotional effects. Follow-up, careful counselling and support are particularly important as many become pregnant again within a year.

Contraception

More adolescents are engaging in sexual intercourse at younger ages, often without any form of contraception. Studies show that fewer than 50% of adolescents use any form of contraception at the time of first intercourse, and the lag between becoming sexually active and seeking effective contraception usually exceeds 1 year. Unfortunately, the first visit to a family planning clinic is frequently because of a pregnancy scare.

Reasons why adolescents commonly fail to seek contraceptive advice include their conviction that sexual intercourse is an unpremeditated and infrequent act, fear that their parents will find out and doubt that any advice they seek will be confidential.

Information, access to contraception and motivation are all necessary for successful pregnancy prevention. Interestingly, in contrast to common expectations, sex education, far from increasing sexual activity, has been shown to delay the onset of first intercourse, increase contraceptive use and reduce numbers of pregnancies. Advice to adolescents should be based on frequency and circumstances of sexual activity, past experience, and compliance with both contraceptive and non-contraceptive chronic medications. Emphasis needs to be placed on the need

Table 25.10 The advantages and disadvantages of various contraceptive methods during adolescence

Contraceptive method	Advantages	Disadvantages
Condom	Effective in preventing transmission of STD including HIV Low price Available without prescription Little need for advanced planning No side effects	Inadequate protection in preventing pregnancy if used alone Acceptance low in younger adolescents
Oral contraceptive pill	Reliable method if taken effectively Method unrelated to episode of intercourse Relief of dysmenorrhoea Decreased risks of benign breast disease, anaemia and ovarian cysts	Not good for chaotic adolescents Less suitable if intercourse is infrequent Post-pill amenorrhoea more common in adolescence Raises levels of high-density lipoproteins (major side effects are exceedingly rare in adolescents)
Depot (parenteral) contraceptive	Reliable with the advantage that compliance is not an issue. Some preparations give protection for as much as 3 years	Maybe unsuitable if intercourse is infrequent Some concern regarding osteoporosis in the long term
Intrauterine contraceptive systems (IUS)	Effective in preventing pregnancy Requires no motivation	Dysmenorrhoea Increased risk of pelvic infection and future infertility
Post-coital contraception 'morning after pill' and IUD	Taken after unprotected sex has taken place	Adolescent needs to know how to access service

STD, sexually transmitted disease.

for protection against sexually transmitted disease as well as pregnancy. The risk of any contraceptive method should be weighed against the risk of pregnancy, which for young adolescents is a significant one. If contraception is to be successful, every effort must be made to individualize the method to the needs of the patient. The advantages and disadvantages of the various types of contraception for adolescents are shown in Table 25.10.

Parental consent is not required for the prescription of contraception, provided the doctor has grounds to believe that the adolescent is mature enough to appreciate the risks (and benefits) of contraception.

To test your knowledge on this part of the book, see Chapter 26

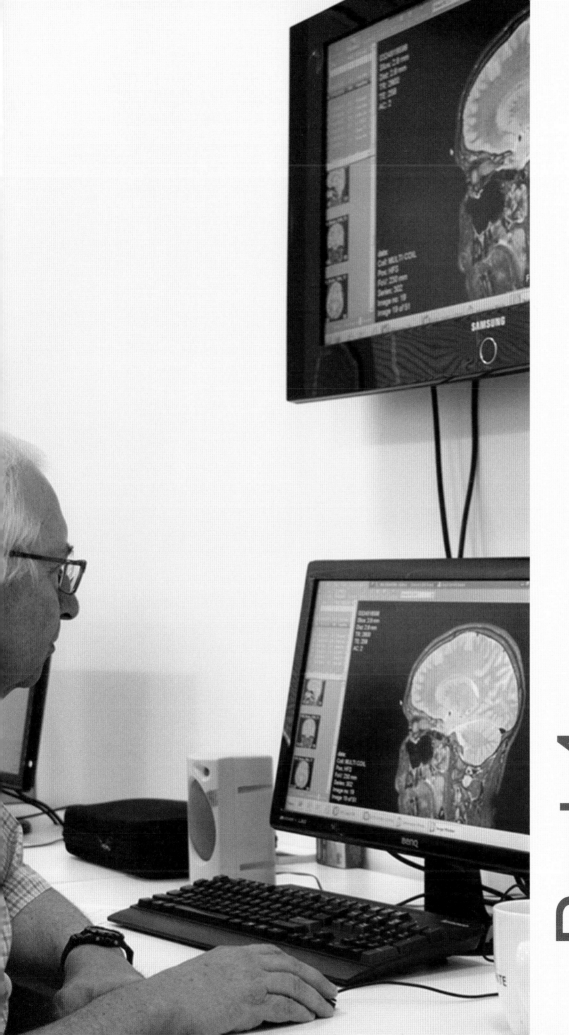

Part 4
Testing your knowledge

CHAPTER 26

Practice MCQ and examination questions

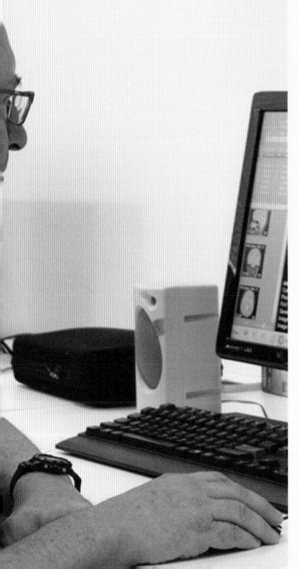

This chapter provides you with the opportunity to test your knowledge by working through multiple choice questions. The aim is to help you identify what you have yet to learn as well as serving as an aid to help you pass examinations. The first set of questions covers each section of the book. Two practice papers follow, covering the full range of topics that you are likely to receive in a paediatric examination.

Please note that there is only one correct answer for each statement ('*Single Best Answer*' format). Answers are provided at the end of the chapter, along with a reference that will lead you back to the topic for more information.

Multiple choice questions

PART 1 ABOUT CHILDREN (CHAPTER 1 TO CHAPTER 3)

Answers on page 484

MULTIPLE CHOICE QUESTION

1 **The terms growth and development are often confused. What is the correct definition?**
   a. growth refers to an increase in number and size of cells, whereas development refers to an increase in complexity and maturation of the nervous system
   b. growth refers to increase in height whereas development refers to pubertal changes
   c. growth is a physical attribute whereas development is psychological
   d. growth is a biological term whereas development is a social construct
   e. growth refers to early childhood whereas development refers to adolescence

2 **Which of the following statements is true?**
   a. Young children should be encouraged to eat a low-fat, high-fibre diet
   b. Iron deficiency is a common problem as young children often fail to eat iron-rich foods
   c. Children should have at least 900 mL milk per day
   d. Adolescents should be encouraged to eat snacks during the day to meet their increased nutritional requirements
   e. Children should be encouraged to eat at least three portions of fruit or vegetables each day.

3 **Which of the following statements concerning weaning is/are correct:?**
   a. Weaning should be delayed until the infant is 12 months old
   b. Breast milk is the only food a baby requires for the first 6 months
   c. Avoid introducing too many new tastes to the baby in its first year
   d. Multivitamins should be started at birth
   e. The baby should not eat with the family until he or she can feed him- or herself with a spoon

4 **Which of the following is an important influence on a child's eventual height?**
   a. Weight of the mother during pregnancy
   b. Whether the child is breast-fed or formula fed
   c. Height of the father
   d. A family history of thyroid disease
   e. The child's consumption of fruit and vegetables

5 **Principles of good nutrition in childhood include:**
   a. Toddlers should not be given snacks between meals
   b. Added salt should be avoided
   c. The child should be encouraged to finish all meals
   d. Add a level teaspoon of sugar to a bottle of cow's milk each day
   e. Avoid giving fatty foods such as cheese before the child is 18 months old

6 **Which of the following is true regarding the development of babies and children's sleep patterns?**
   a. Newborns spend only 7–8 hours per day awake
   b. Most babies are sleeping through the night by the time they are 6 months old
   c. Primary school-age children need on average 8 hours sleep per night
   d. Adolescents need substantially less sleep than primary school-age children
   e. Toddlers should be discouraged from day time naps to make them sleep better at night

7 **Which of the following physical activity is recommendations is correct?**
   a. 'Tummytime' should be started once a baby is ready to crawl
   b. Television should be restricted to <3 hours per day
   c. School children should engage in at least 1 hour physical activity each day
   d. Preschool children should be physically active for 2 hours spread throughout the day
   e. Parents should engage in at least 90 minutes physical activity per week

MULTIPLE CHOICE QUESTION

8 **Which one of the following statements about a child's development is true?**
   a. Bonding difficulties only occur if a newborn is separated from the mother for more than 3 days
   b. A baby begins to sustain eye contact by 6 months
   c. Sleep–wake cycles emerge within the first week of life
   d. Babies begin to smile by 6 weeks
   e. Children only begin to learn rules of games once they are school age

9 **Which of the following is a definite contraindication to breast-feeding?**
   a. Maternal administration of penicillin
   b. Maternal depression
   c. Severe maternal hypertension
   d. Anti-retroviral medication given to the mother
   e. Mastitis

10 **Which of the following practices are against the law?**
   a. Giving morphine with the intention of ending life
   b. Not treating a fatal condition
   c. Prescribing contraception to a 12-year-old
   d. Giving diamorphine to a premature neonate for pain relief
   e. Treating adolescents without parental permission

11 **At the 6- to 8-week child health assessment the following should be checked:**
   a. Hips for developmental dysplasia
   b. Oto-acoustic emissions
   c. Tooth decay
   d. PKU
   e. Visual acuity

12 **Which of the following is a principal component of the UK Healthy Child Programme?**
   a. Annual height and weight on all children
   b. Progressive universalism
   c. Supervision of childminders
   d. Employment of health visitors
   e. Call-in service for sick children

13 **Contraindications to immunisation include which of these?**
   a. The child has a cold
   b. The child has missed the previous immunisation
   c. The child is unwell with fever
   d. An older sibling developed diarrhoea following the immunisation
   e. Treated epilepsy

14 **The following have been considered to be new morbidities affecting children today, except:**
   a. Emotional and behavioural problems
   b. Childhood obesity
   c. Child abuse and neglect
   d. Febrile illnesses
   e. Social and health inequalities

15 **Which of the following statements is true regarding the Personal Child Health Record (PCHR)?**
   a. The PCHR is primarily for children with potential developmental problems
   b. Parents are generally poor at ensuring the record is up-to-date
   c. It consists of a record of health checks, a growth chart, and medical visits
   d. It is issued by the family doctor at the baby's first visit
   e. Parents prefer that the record is held by health professionals

PART 2 A PAEDIATRIC TOOLKIT (CHAPTER 4 TO CHAPTER 8)

Answers on page 484

MULTIPLE CHOICE QUESTION

1 **Which of the following is an important principle when children require invasive procedures?**
   a. Avoiding talking through the procedure with the child
   b. Blood tests should be taken in the hospital bed as it provides a sense of security
   c. Sedation prior to a procedure is not necessary for patients aged <12 months
   d. Ensuring the child agrees where possible before starting a procedure
   e. Excluding parents from the room as they may upset the child

2 **The first step in supporting families over time should be:**
   a. Questioning and helping patients talk
   b. Identifying goals and helping families achieve them
   c. Exploring concerns
   d. Approaches to support
   e. Reviewing progress

3 **In making decisions about treatment options, who is likely to know best what works for the family:**
   a. Parents
   b. Social worker
   c. Nurse

    d. Doctor

    e. Psychologist

4 **SOAP is an acronym for writing information according to a standard format. It stands for:**

    a. Sensitively; Organized; Actively, Predictively

    b. Simply; Objectively; Accurately; Precisely

    c. Symptoms; Orders; Appraisal; Proposed action

    d. Solutions; Obstructions; Aids; Problems

    e. Symptoms; Observations; Assessment; Plan

5 **Which of the following is an important principle of history taking in paediatrics?**

    a. Don't ask leading questions about specific fears so as not to put ideas in the heads of the parents

    b. Children should not be part of the history taking process since they are too young to understand

    c. Parents should not be present when taking an adolescent history to avoid embarrassment

    d. It is better to disregard a referral letter in order to gain an objective and unbiased view

    e. Observation of the child during history taking may give valuable information

6 **In drawing up a family tree and social history, which item is best avoided?**

    a. Were there any dead children in the family

    b. Is the father in gainful employment

    c. Is this a one-parent or one gender parent family

    d. Has the mother been the victim of sexual abuse

    e. To what ethnic group does the family belong

7 **When examining a child it is best to:**

    a. Begin by breaking the ice with some general questions and comments

    b. Allow the child to remain mainly dressed in order to avoid resistance and embarrassment

    c. Follow a strict routine in order to prevent omissions

    d. Examine from the side of the bed most comfortable for the child

    e. Hide the stethoscope from view to prevent anxiety

8 **Which statement is correct regarding growth charts?**

    a. Children grow along the same centile from 1 year onwards

    b. Height weight and head circumference centiles are expected to be the same in normal children

    c. Growth charts for breast-fed infants are different from those of bottle-fed babies

    d. Growth charts based on US populations are the most reliable because of large sample size

    e. Premature babies should be age corrected on a chart until 6 months postnatal age

9 **Which of the following is a cause of clubbing in children?**

    a. Coeliac disease

    b. Asthma

    c. Methaemoglobinaemia

    d. Familial

    e. Aortic stenosis

10 **In the cardiac examination what is always a pathological finding?**

    a. A systolic murmur

    b. Second sound split widens on expiration

    c. A grade II cardiac murmur

    d. Pulse rate accelerates during inspiration

    e. Ectopic beats

11 **A bimanual examination technique is required to examine which abdominal organ?**

    a. Kidney

    b. Liver

    c. Pancreas

    d. Spleen

    e. Urinary bladder

12 **Which of the following suggests that a swelling in the inguinal area is due to an undescended testis?**

    a. Positive transillumination

    b. Pulsatility

    c. Increases on straining

    d. Poorly developed ipsilateral scrotum

    e. Erythema and tenderness over an immobile oval mass

13 **Which primitive reflex typically disappears at the age of 1 month?**

    a. Plantar reflex

    b. Stepping reflex

    c. Moro reflex

    d. Sucking reflex

    e. Parachute reflex

14 **Which among the following signs is clear evidence of acute purulent otitis media?**

    a. A red ear drum

    b. Bubbles behind the ear drum

    c. A bulging oedematous ear drum

    d. An obvious malleus

    e. A lost light reflex

15 **An abnormal eye cover test and abnormal corneal reflex suggest what?**

    a. Nystagmus

    b. Conjunctivitis

    c. Corneal ulcer

    d. Ptosis

    e. Squint

16 **Occipital lymphadenopathy would be expected in which circumstance?**

    a. Tonsillitis

    b. Roseola

    c. Otitis media

    d. Rubella

    e. EBV

17 A normal child of 9 months should have achieved the following milestones:
   a. Cruises
   b. Walks with one hand held
   c. Finger feeds
   d. Builds a tower of two blocks
   e. Has three words with meaning

18 Which of the following is a normal developmental milestone?
   a. Smile for the first time at 8 weeks
   b. Sitting unsupported at 5 months
   c. Pincer grip by 9 months
   d. First words by 12 months
   e. Two- to three-word sentences at 18 months

19 Which of the following is a warning sign that development is not progressing normally?
   a. Stranger anxiety at 7 months
   b. First smiling at 6 weeks
   c. Unintelligible speech at 2 years
   d. Not crawling at 8 months
   e. Persistent primitive reflexes

20 The following is the most useful tool for examining fine motor skills in a 3-year-old
   a. a rattle
   b. a skipping rope
   c. a formboard with circle, square and triangle
   d. a doll
   e. 1 inch bricks

21 In carrying out a developmental assessment, what should guide the examiner?
   a. Do this after physical examination so that the child is used to you
   b. Best done when the child is tired to prevent attention seeking
   c. Parents' reports are especially unreliable when there is delay
   d. Parents' anxieties are misleading since they always tend to be anxious
   e. Identifying any regressing skills is particularly important

22 A 4-year-old girl in hospital requires blood tests. Which is the best approach to perform the procedure?
   a. Take the bloods at her bedside so that she is in a familiar environment
   b. Make sure that the carers are not present as they may become distressed
   c. Engage the help of a play therapist
   d. Try to avoid topical analgesia as this may upset her in advance
   e. Use oral sucrose drops for analgesia

23 The following blood count is obtained from a 2-year-old boy. Haemoglobin 10 g/dL (11–14 g/dL), mean cell volume 68 fL (76–88 fL), mean cell haemoglobin 22 pg (24-30 pg), ferritin <2 (10-250 microgram/l). There is no history of pica, nor any family history of haemoglobinopathy.
   What is the best management plan?
   a. Check lead levels
   b. Start iron supplementation then repeat blood tests in 4-6 weeks
   c. Request haemoglobinopathy screening
   d. Give dietary advice on increasing folate
   e. Check coeliac status

24 Which of the following is the blood gas picture most likely to be seen in a child with diabetic ketoacidosis?
   a. pH 7.30, $P\text{co}_2$ 6.8 (51 mm Hg), bicarbonate 20 mmol/L
   b. pH 7.41, $P\text{co}_2$ 4.8 (36 mm Hg), bicarbonate 12 mmol/L
   c. pH 7.16, $P\text{co}_2$ 9.8 (74 mm Hg), bicarbonate 17 mmol/L
   d. pH 7.35, $P\text{co}_2$ 4.5 (34 mm Hg), bicarbonate 20 mmol/L
   e. pH 7.2, $P\text{co}_2$ 2.2 (17 mm Hg), bicarbonate 9 mmol/L

25 Which statement regarding peak flow measurements is correct?
   a. It indicates the maximal flow generated by one forceful expiration
   b. The average of three attempts should be recorded
   c. It is not possible in children under 6 years old
   d. An increased peak flow suggests that asthma management is suboptimal
   e. Scores are independent of height or age

26 Which imaging technique is most likely to be used when screening a premature baby for the risk of hydrocephalus?
   a. MRI brain
   b. CT head
   c. Lateral skull x-ray
   d. CSF manometry
   e. Cranial ultrasound

27 What could explain a serum sodium of 153 mmol/L in a 4-month-old infant?
   a. Cystic fibrosis on a hot day
   b. Compulsive water drinking
   c. Syndrome of inappropriate ADH secretion
   d. Inappropriate milk-feed preparation
   e. Administration of DDAVP (desmopressin)

28 Which of the following is a cause of microcytic anaemia in children?
   a. Lead poisoning
   b. Sickle cell disease
   c. Folate deficiency
   d. Renal failure
   e. Viral infection

29 The following are supportive findings for a urinary tract infection
   a. Cola-coloured urine
   b. The absence of nitrates
   c. Urinary white blood cells >50/mm³
   d. Positive ketones
   e. 104 cfu/mL *E. coli* in a bag urine

30 Which of the following best describes prescribing for children?
   a. Doses and indications can be extrapolated easily from adult usage
   b. Generally the mechanisms of action of drugs are similar in children and adults
   c. Little has changed in the way new drugs are developed for children
   d. Paediatric doses are small therefore errors are less serious
   e. Basic pharmacological science differs between children and adults

31 Which of the following is a drug complication specific to children?
   a. Ibuprofen induced interstitial nephritis
   b. Penicillin allergy
   c. Chloramphenicol induced aplastic anaemia
   d. Tetracycline induced tooth discolouration
   e. Steroid induced hypertension

32 Which of the following may displace protein-bound drugs and increase risk for toxicity?
   a. Bilirubin
   b. Urea
   c. Glucose
   d. Sodium
   e. Calcium

33 Regarding drug clearance and metabolism in children, which statement is true?
   a. The main liver metabolic effect is drug decarboxylation
   b. The lower the P450 level in a child, the higher the consequent plasma drug level
   c. Immature metabolism can sometimes reduce the potential for toxicity

   d. Renal clearance is entirely dependent on glomerular function
   e. Pro-drugs are less affected by age than other drugs

34 A Greek child has developed anaemia and jaundice following treatment with co-trimoxazole. What is the most likely explanation?
   a. Auto-immune hepatitis with cholestasis
   b. Severe type I drug allergy
   c. Beta-thalassaemia intermedia and splenomegaly
   d. Bone marrow depression with iron deficiency
   e. Glucose-6-phosphate dehydrogenase deficiency

35 A 1-year-old boy presents to a clinic with moderate dehydration due to 2 days of watery diarrhoea and two vomits. What would be the recommended management?
   a. Administration of normal saline intravenously in the clinic
   b. Immediate referral to hospital for investigation and treatment
   c. Prescribing oral rehydration fluids and follow-up
   d. Prescription of anti-emetic drugs
   e. Recommend fasting and sips of cold water

36 A child with asthma is prescribed and given nebulized salbutamol at home but does not respond. However, in the clinic there is a rapid response to the same drug and dose. What is the best explanation?
   a. Mechanical fault with the nebulizer and/or technique, at home
   b. The child is more nervous at home thus exacerbating the asthma
   c. The drug at home may have passed its due date
   d. Despite the mother's assurances there was non-compliance
   e. Salbutamol effect is unpredictable and fickle

37 What is the best advice for a breast-feeding mother who has been prescribed a pain-killer drug?
   a. Stop breast-feeding to avoid toxic effects in the baby
   b. Don't take the drug but carry on breast-feeding
   c. There are no concerns as drugs do not enter the milk in large amounts
   d. Carefully monitor the baby for any effects but do as prescribed
   e. Take the drug immediately before breast-feeding

PART 3a AN APPROACH TO PROBLEM BASED PAEDIATRICS (CHAPTER 9 TO CHAPTER 16)

Answers on page 484

1 A baby of 2 weeks develops a temperature of 38.1 degrees per rectum at home. The child is feeding but a little irritable. Which is the correct advice to give the parents?
  a. Paracetamol should be given, and the baby brought to the clinic for a check
  b. This is a normal temperature for a baby and no action is needed
  c. The temperature should be re-checked in 4 hours and if elevated the baby brought to the clinic
  d. The baby should come to the hospital immediately for a full evaluation
  e. The baby should be wrapped in wet towels and the temperature re-checked

2 Which sign indicates acute purulent acute otitis media?
  a. A bulging ear drum
  b. Erythema of ear drum
  c. Tenderness of the ear pinna
  d. Prominent malleus process
  e. Oedematous ear canal

3 What would be the correct diagnostic investigation for a 5-year-old boy with headache, fever, vomiting, drowsiness and a positive Kernig sign?
  a. A CT scan of the brain
  b. An ultrasound of the abdomen
  c. A lumbar puncture
  d. An ECG
  e. An EEG

4 A 2-week-old baby is generally well but a firm rubbery mass has been found in the mid-lateral zone of the neck. It is immobile in the rostral-caudal dimension but not red, warm or fluctuant. Transillumination is negative. Which is the most likely diagnosis?
  a. Acute lymphadenitis
  b. Parotiditis
  c. Branchial cyst
  d. Cystic lymphangioma
  e. Sternocleidomastoid tumour

5 Which feature would be suggestive of a habitual cough in a school-aged child?
  a. Wheezy quality
  b. Poor growth
  c. Only during the day
  d. Nasal flaring
  e. Worse on exercise

6 Which noise is characteristic of bronchitis?
  a. Rhonchi
  b. Snoring
  c. Whooping
  d. Barking
  e. Stridor

7 A 2-year-old boy suffers from wheeze. Which is a true statement?
  a. There is narrowing of extra-thoracic airways
  b. He is suffering from bronchial asthma
  c. About 60% of children at this age suffer from wheezing
  d. Previous RSV infection is a known antecedent
  e. A chest X-ray will be necessary before treatment

8 A 1-year-old child has acute stridor. What is the most important risk factor or feature that may be related to acute epiglottitis?
  a. Very restless
  b. Mild fever
  c. Non-immunised
  d. Barking cough
  e. Hoarseness

9 What is true about screening for cystic fibrosis (CF)?
  a. 98% of cases are diagnosed via screening
  b. Screening is best carried out using a postnatal sweat test
  c. Screening has not had an impact on the incidence of CF
  d. Screening can be pre-natal and postnatal
  e. A negative screen excludes CF

10 In children with asthma which statement is true?
  a. Dry powder inhalers are preferred to metered dose inhalers
  b. Spacers should only be used in older children and not infants
  c. Ipratropium bromide is usually required as a reliever therapy
  d. Children with a severe asthma attack may benefit from IV magnesium
  e. Leukotriene receptor agonists can be helpful in asthma management

11 The following are causes of blood in the stool except for:
  a. *Salmonella* infection
  b. Giardia lamblia infection
  c. Crohn disease
  d. Henoch–Schönlein purpura
  e. Anal fissure

12 Management of children experiencing idiopathic recurrent abdominal pain should involve which one of the following?
  a. Prescription of vitamin C as a placebo
  b. Explaining to the parent that the child is malingering
  c. A letter to school suggesting that the child is allowed home when the pain starts
  d. Checking a blood count periodically
  e. Scheduling a return appointment

13 Only one of the following measures is appropriate in the management of a 9-month-old infant suspected of having mild gastroenteritis:
   a. Stop breastfeeding or formula feeds until the diarrhoea stops
   b. Prescribe anti-emetics to control vomiting
   c. Prescribe an anti-peristaltic agent to reduce gut motility
   d. Prescribe amoxicillin if a stool culture shows a growth of enteropathic *E. coli*
   e. Prescribe oral rehydration therapy (ORT) to ensure adequate hydration

14 A 4-month-old baby has vomiting precipitated by episodes of severe prolonged coughing with gasping. There is no dehydration and the abdomen is soft. What is the most likely diagnosis?
   a. Reflux
   b. Pertussis
   c. Bowel obstruction
   d. Asthma
   e. Aspirated foreign body

15 An 18-month-old presents with chronic watery gassy diarrhoea for 6 weeks. It started with 2 days of diarrhea and vomiting and fever. The vomiting and fever have resolved but the diarrhea has persisted. On examination the child looks well, and the abdomen is non-tender. The skin is excoriated around the anus. What is the most likely diagnosis?
   a. Lactose intolerance
   b. Coeliac disease
   c. Toddler diarrhoea
   d. Inflammatory bowel disease
   e. Cystic fibrosis

16 An 8-year-old girl attends the clinic with recurrent abdominal pain. Which of the following is most consistent with a functional origin to her symptoms?
   a. Nocturnal pain
   b. Weight loss
   c. Periumbilical pain
   d. Recurrent fever
   e. Ill appearance

17 Which is correct relating to ventricular septal defect?
   a. Cardiac failure does not occur at birth
   b. Commonly causes central cyanosis
   c. Typically has a marked diastolic murmur
   d. Surgery is required in most cases
   e. Ventricular fibrillation is common

18 A 15-year-old girl has fainted a number of times. What would suggest a cardiac cause?
   a. Occurred during a sports lesson at school
   b. A soft systolic murmur on lying down
   c. Dizziness on rising from bed in the morning
   d. Feeling of nausea when seeing blood
   e. Blood pressure 110/70

19 What would be a typical indication of congestive heart failure in an infant?
   a. Bradycardia
   b. Splenomegaly
   c. Pulmonary crepitations
   d. Peripheral oedema
   e. Polydipsia

20 What of the following is **not** a typical feature of raised intracranial pressure?
   a. Headache waking at night
   b. Headache worse on standing
   c. Bradycardia with hypertension and sighing respirations
   d. Seizure
   e. Papilloedema

21 Which one of the following developmental stages is of concern?
   a. Not walking by 15 months
   b. Not sitting by 8 months
   c. Unintelligible speech at 3 years
   d. Not smiling by 10 weeks
   e. Poor focusing on objects at birth

22 In a child of 18 months, the following may be a sign of neurodevelopmental disability:
   a. Not walking independently
   b. Only six words with meaning
   c. Not talking in sentences
   d. Inability to eat with a fork
   e. Unable to hop

23 A 3-year-old presents with language delay. He has poor eye contact and his parents report that he never was a cuddly baby. The history is suggestive of which of the following diagnoses?
   a. Autism
   b. Attention deficit disorder
   c. Visual impairment
   d. Mild cerebral palsy
   e. Phenylketonuria

24 One of the following statements is inconsistent with a diagnosis of cerebral palsy:
   a. Cerebral palsy is a disorder of movement
   b. Spasticity is the commonest form
   c. Cerebral palsy is due to an insult in the developing brain
   d. The physical signs vary as childhood progresses
   e. It is a form of neurodegenerative disorder

25 What feature would strengthen your suspicion that delayed walking is due to muscular dystrophy?
   a. No family members affected
   b. Large calf muscles

c. Other developmental issues

d. Positive Romberg sign

e. Weakness of hand small muscles

26 The following are recognised associated disabilities in children with cerebral palsy EXCEPT:

a. Epilepsy

b. Hearing impairment

c. Cortical visual impairment

d. Asthma

e. Speech and language problems

27 Which of the following statements is true of severe sensorineural hearing impairment:

a. The prognosis for hearing is best if the diagnosis is made before the child is 3 months old

b. Deaf children should be discouraged from learning sign language

c. Severely deaf children do best if educated with normal hearing peers

d. The incidence is 1%

e. Glue ear is a common cause

28 Which is true regarding stammering or stuttering?

a. Is a form of articulation difficulty

b. Is due to delayed language development

c. Usually becomes persistent and aggravates

d. Most common at the ages of 6-8 years

e. Speech therapy is not useful

29 Which of the following is a common cause of global developmental delay?

a. Neonatal jaundice

b. Turner syndrome

c. Congenital HIV infection

d. Alcohol during pregnancy

e. Muscular dystrophy

30 The following are common causes of cerebral palsy:

a. Muscular dystrophy

b. Epilepsy

c. Birth asphyxia (hypoxic–ischaemic insult)

d. *E. coli* infection

e. Neonatal respiratory distress syndrome

31 Which of the following is the commonest complication of obesity in childhood?

a. Non-alcoholic fatty liver disease

b. Poor self-esteem

c. Type 2 diabetes

d. Dyslipidaemia

e. Hypertension

32 Which one of the following is a symptom of diabetic hypoglycemia?

a. Shakiness

b. Polydipsia

c. Polyuria

d. Vomiting

e. Abdominal pain

33 A 13-year-old girl presents with swelling in the neck. Which feature is unusual in hypothyroidism at this age?

a. Poor growth

b. Dry hair

c. Constipation

d. Underachievement at school

e. Umbilical hernia

34 In-toeing is common in early childhood and most causes resolve spontaneously by age 4 or 5 years. Which of the following causes requires surgical correction?

a. Femoral anteversion

b. Tibial torsion

c. Bowing of the legs

d. Metatarsus adductus

e. Diplegic cerebral palsy

35 Which of the following features makes growing pains an unlikely diagnosis?

a. Age 3 to 6 years

b. Fever

c. Accompanying headaches and abdominal pains

d. Bilateral pain

e. Normal gait

36 A 3-year-old child presents with a limp. There is no fever, but he has had a URTI (upper respiratory tract infection) for the last few days. What is the most likely diagnosis?

a. Juvenile idiopathic arthritis

b. Septic arthritis

c. Transient synovitis

d. Slipped capital femoral epiphysis

e. Legg-Calve-Perthes disease

37 Which of these joint diseases can present without any joint symptoms?

a. Systemic JIA (Still disease)

b. Poly articular JIA

c. Pauciarticular JIA

d. Psoriatic arthritis

e. Septic arthritis

38 Obese children may experience musculoskeletal problems. Which of the following is classically associated with obesity?

a. Transient synovitis

b. Neoplastic disease affecting the bones

c. Legg-Calve Perthes disease

d. Rupture of the anterior cruciate ligament

e. Slipped capital femoral epiphysis

39 When would you first expect to see X-ray changes in osteomyelitis?

a. From the onset of the fever

b. 10 days following onset of symptoms

c. 3 weeks following onset of symptoms

MULTIPLE CHOICE QUESTION

d. 2 days after onset of symptoms

e. X-rays are not helpful in the diagnosis of osteomyelitis

40 **Which one of these findings are suggestive of septic arthritis of the hip?**

a. Limited movement of the leg

b. Narrowing of the joint space on ultrasound

c. Absence of organisms on gram stain of the aspirate

d. Leg held in extension and adduction

e. Nocturnal pain in the knee

PART 3b AN APPROACH TO PROBLEM BASED PAEDIATRICS (CHAPTER 17 TO CHAPTER 25)

Answers on page 485

MULTIPLE CHOICE QUESTION

1 **Which is a true statement regarding dysuria?**
   a. Commonest in infants under 1 year of age
   b. More common in boys than girls
   c. Suggests a neurogenic bladder
   d. Candida is the most likely cause
   e. Should prompt a search for threadworms

2 **Which feature of haematuria suggests a non-renal origin?**
   a. A pink or bright-red colour
   b. Proteinuria
   c. Leg oedema
   d. Red-cell casts
   e. Hypertension

3 **Nocturnal enuresis is best initially treated by:**
   a. Psychotherapy
   b. Star charts
   c. Water deprivation
   d. Enuresis alarms
   e. Tricyclic antidepressants

4 **A 5-year-old-boy develops haematuria 2 weeks after acute tonsillitis. What is the test most likely to establish the correct aetiological diagnosis?**
   a. Complement studies
   b. Serum IgA levels
   c. Urine culture
   d. Renal ultrasound
   e. Creatinine clearance

5 **A 6-year-old girl presents with hypoproteinaemia, oedema and proteinuria, but not haematuria or hypertension. What is the correct next step?**
   a. Renal dialysis
   b. Steroid therapy
   c. Diuretics
   d. Renal biopsy
   e. Cyclophosphamide treatment

6 **A newborn baby is found to have a hypospadias with the urethral opening at the penoscrotal junction. Both testes are present, and he has a normal urine stream.**

What would you advise parents?
   a. There is a risk of disorders of sex development (DSD)
   b. Renal function tests are required before discharge.
   c. Surgery may be required after the age of 5 years if symptoms persist
   d. Circumcision should not be performed
   e. Sexual function is likely to be limited in adulthood

7 **Which of the following is associated with polycystic ovaries?**
   a. Alopecia
   b. Pelvic pain
   c. Glucose intolerance
   d. Dysrhythmias
   e. Anorexia

8 **A baby is born with genitalia that are indeterminate between male and female. Which is the correct statement?**
   a. The baby will grow up with indeterminate sexual identity
   b. The genetic sex is the determining factor in sex rearing
   c. The baby may become seriously ill in a short time
   d. A name should be given as soon as possible
   e. Usually no aetiology for this clinical problem can be found

9 **A girl is examined because of labial adhesions of the labia majora. Which of the following is correct?**
   a. If treatment is required, surgery is the best choice
   b. The prognosis is poor in most cases
   c. High oestrogen levels are associated
   d. Nappy rash may be aetiological
   e. One should suspect sexual abuse

10 **Which statement is true of strawberry naevi?**
   a. They are red, hard and stony lumps under the skin
   b. They occur in patients allergic to strawberries
   c. Their borders are diffuse and ill-defined
   d. They tend to enlarge after 1 year of age
   e. They can be treated with drugs

MULTIPLE CHOICE QUESTION

11 **A Mongolian blue spot is:**
 a. Usually located in the sacral area
 b. More common in Down syndrome ('mongolism')
 c. A large bruise
 d. Tends to darken with age
 e. Is best treated with emollient creams

12 **What is characteristic of seborrheic dermatitis?**
 a. Red weeping lesions
 b. Papular lesions in the axillae
 c. Cradle cap
 d. Nail pitting
 e. Oral thrush

13 **A well 3-year-old girl complains of severe peri-anal itching at night and early in the morning. She is generally healthy and physical examination is normal. What is the likely cause?**
 a. Chickenpox
 b. Atopic dermatitis
 c. Cholestasis
 d. Threadworms
 e. *Tinea capitis*

14 **A 16-year-old boy presents with intensely itchy wheals of different sizes. His physical examination is otherwise normal, and he feels well. What is true about this condition?**
 a. Lesions usually resolve in 2-4 hours
 b. Anxiety is a well-recognised cause
 c. It is a likely to be a post-infectious exanthema
 d. The best treatment is a non-steroidal anti-inflammatory drug
 e. Systemic signs do not occur with this rash

15 **A 14-year-old girl has had scaly silvery lesions on her elbows for 6 months. They are non-itchy, and she is otherwise healthy. Her father has had a similar problem since adolescence. What physical sign is expected?**
 a. Enlarged tonsils
 b. Splenomegaly
 c. Absent knee reflexes
 d. Nail pitting
 e. Clubbing

16 **A 2-year-old boy with normocytic normochromic anaemia has failed to respond to a course of iron. Which among the following tests would be appropriate as a next step?**
 a. Blood lead levels
 b. Urea and electrolytes
 c. Vitamin B12 levels
 d. Haemoglobin electrophoresis
 e. Red cell folate

17 **Which is the initial laboratory finding in iron-deficiency?**
 a. Poikilocytosis
 b. Anaemia
 c. Hypochromia
 d. Reduced red cell count
 e. Reduced ferritin

18 **Desferrioxamine is of value in paediatric haematology since it:**
 a. Decreases iron levels
 b. Increases beta chain synthesis
 c. Increases fetal haemoglobin
 d. Decreases hypochromia
 e. Prevents aplasia of the bone marrow

19 **A 3-year-old girl presents with severe chronic anaemia, attacks of afebrile back pain, pain in her hands and feet and marked splenomegaly. Apart from anaemia, her blood count is unremarkable. What is the most likely diagnosis?**
 a. Leukaemia
 b. Thalassaemia
 c. Iron deficiency
 d. Sickle cell disease
 e. Chronic infection

20 **Regarding childhood behaviour, which of the following statements is true?**
 a. Masturbation is a sign of sexual abuse
 b. Temper tantrums become a feature at 12 months
 c. Most babies sleep through the night by 4 months
 d. Rewarding positive behavior is more effective than punishing bad
 e. Attention deficit disorder is always accompanied by hyperactivity

21 **Which of the following statements are true regarding school bullying?**
 a. One in four children are bullied at school once a week
 b. Bullies should be suspended until the problem has been resolved
 c. The school often colludes with bullying
 d. The bullying child usually has inappropriately high self-esteem
 e. Bullying is a common cause of school avoidance

22 **A 4-year-old boy has frequent temper tantrums. Which of the following is an appropriate strategy for encouraging more positive behavior?**
 a. 10 minutes 'time-out' in a quiet place
 b. Punish him by not allowing television for the following week
 c. Avoid high sugar foods
 d. Praise him for positive behaviour
 e. Refer him for a psychological evaluation

23 **A 2-year-old has developed food refusal and fussy eating. She is well and is growing satisfactorily. What advice is appropriate?**
 a. Give snacks between meals to avoid her becoming excessively hungry
 b. Feed her on her own to give her extra attention

c. Give her extra milk to ensure she has adequate nutrients

d. Devise games to encourage her to eat

e. Encourage family meals with minimal attention to her food refusal

24 **Which of the following statements is true regarding dyslexia?**

a. The reading level is appropriate for the level of intelligence

b. It is a condition that resolves naturally over time

c. The history indicates advanced language milestones as a young child

d. Myopia commonly underlies the problem and must be corrected

e. An educational psychology referral is required to make the diagnosis

25 **A 2-year-old child presents to your clinic with six round erythematous lesions on her arm some of which have scabs. The mother thought they were insect bites and the father that she had fallen on a toy. On examination you find bruising on her face. You suspect the lesions are cigarette burns. What is the most appropriate first course of action?**

a. Admit to hospital for investigations

b. Make comprehensive notes and take photographs

c. Write a referral to the hospital social worker

d. Arrange for her to go to the local social services nursery

e. Request a return appointment in one week

26 **Which of the following is the most important factor in uncovering the possibility that a child has been physical abused?**

a. The clinical history and examination

b. Clotting screen for blood dyscrasias

c. Skeletal survey

d. Urine test for haematuria

e. CT scan of the head

27 **A child presents with apathy, poor weight gain and signs of physical neglect. There are no signs of physical abuse. You involve the health visitor and the social worker. A case conference is held. What is the most likely action at this stage?**

a. Admit to hospital for urgent shelter

b. Place in foster care for 6 months

c. Provide a day nursery placement

d. Weekly visits to the Health Visiting clinic

e. Provide the mother with nutritional guidance

28 **A 2-year-old boy is seen for a burn. Which feature would indicate that the burn may have been non-accidental?**

a. Irregular shape

b. Superficial in depth

c. Symmetric across the midline

d. Additional 'splash' burns present

e. Presents early after the event

29 **A 14-year-old girl attends after a deliberate overdose of paracetamol at 60mg/kg 1 hour ago. What is the appropriate management?**

a. Admit for mental health assessment

b. Give ipecac to induce vomiting

c. Check liver function tests, clotting and paracetamol levels 6 hours after ingestion

d. Give N-acetylcysteine

e. Give activated charcoal

30 **Which of the following is a risk factor for severe and acute illness in childhood?**

a. Previous antibiotic treatment

b. Being overweight

c. Hospitalization

d. Post-maturity

e. Splenomegaly

31 **In the ABCDDEFG acronym for managing a moribund child, what does the B stand for?**

a. Blood clot

b. Breathing

c. Bone fracture

d. Brachycardia

e. Bladder size

32 **A 5-year-old with asthma is in severe distress and not responding well to drug therapy. Which is a clear indication for assisted ventilation?**

a. Moderate hypoxia

b. Tachypnoea

c. Severe thirst

d. Progressive hypercapnia

e. Segmental collapse

33 **A 10-year-old is urgently admitted with high fever and signs of hypotensive shock. What is the most ominous prognostic factor?**

a. Tachycardia of 160/min

b. Tachypnoea of 50/min

c. Capillary filling time 3 seconds

d. Onset of shock 3 hours prior to admission

e. Urine output <0.5 cc/kg/hour

34 **A 3-year-old girl is known to have severe allergy to peanuts. Which is the most important step in management?**

a. Supply the family with an adrenaline auto-injector syringe

b. Advise on the need to keep antihistamines at near reach

c. Instruct the family how to give inhaled steroids

d. Forbid the child to participate in activities like parties

e. Give graded injections of peanut extract

35 Complications of respiratory distress syndrome include all of the following except?
   a. Patent ductus arteriosus
   b. Bronchopulmonary dysplasia
   c. Obstructive apnoea
   d. Intraventricular haemorrhage
   e. Pulmonary interstitial emphysema

36 Risk factors for Developmental Dysplasia of the Hip include all of the following except?
   a. Breech delivery
   b. Twins
   c. Family history of DDH
   d. Prematurity
   e. Spina bifida

37 An acceptable oxygen saturation by oximetry at age 5 minutes after birth is?
   a. 100%
   b. 97%
   c. 95%
   d. 90%
   e. 85%

38 Surfactant is mainly produced in:
   a. Bronchial epithelium
   b. Lung macrophages
   c. Alveolar Type I cells
   d. Alveolar Type II cells
   e. Pulmonary fibroblasts

39 Which sign is compatible with an innocent murmur?
   a. Diastolic murmur
   b. Absent femoral pulses
   c. Hyperactive praecordium
   d. Fixed split second sound
   e. Ejection systolic murmur at left sternal border

40 All of the following are true regarding necrotizing enterocolitis except?
   a. Intramural gas is often seen on X-ray
   b. Bloody stools are common
   c. Bilious vomiting often seen
   d. Peritoneal drainage may be used in extremely small infants
   e. Bowel stricture occurs in the majority of infants

41 Spina bifida occulta may be suspected in the presence of which finding?
   a. Anal stenosis
   b. Neurological bladder
   c. A naevus over lower lumbar spine
   d. Ambiguous genitalia
   e. A Mongolian blue spot over lower lumbar spine

42 Which common problem is associated with cleft palate?
   a. Intolerance of formula milk
   b. Obesity
   c. Tongue tie
   d. Sensorineural hearing loss
   e. Dental problems due to gingival margin maldevelopment

43 Which of the following statements is true of puberty:
   a. The first sign in girls is menstruation
   b. The growth spurt occurs prior to the onset of puberty
   c. The interval between the onset and menarche is on average 5 years
   d. The first sign in boys is testicular enlargement
   e. It is significantly delayed if not started by 12 years in boys

44 Which of the following is a cause of precocious puberty?
   a. Anorexia nervosa
   b. Intense athletic training
   c. Down syndrome
   d. Chronic disease
   e. Central nervous system lesions

45 Which of the following is a cause of secondary amenorrhoea?
   a. Turner syndrome
   b. Anorexia nervosa
   c. Epilepsy
   d. Urinary tract infection
   e. HIV infection

46 Which of the following is true regarding care of adolescent patients?
   a. Confidentiality is paramount in all circumstances
   b. They should always have a chaperone
   c. Adolescents under the age of 14 cannot refuse to submit to physical examination
   d. Adolescents under the age of 16 always require parental consent for treatment
   e. Adolescents should be given the opportunity to be seen alone in a hospital consultation

Answers to multiple choice questions

References to boxes, tables and/or relevant pages are provided to lead you back to the topic for more information and an explanation for the answers

Part 1 ABOUT CHILDREN (CHAPTER 1 TO CHAPTER 3)

1. a p14
2. b p20
3. b p19   Box 1.3 and 1.4
4. c p14
5. b p20
6. a p23
7. c pp22-3
8. d p13
9. d p17
10. a p41
11. a p29   Table 2.1
12. b p28
13. c p36
14. d p382
15. c p30, pp63-4

Part 2 A PAEDIATRIC TOOLKIT (CHAPTER 4 TO CHAPTER 8)

1. d p63
2. c p65
3. a p474
4. e p65
5. e p68
6. d p69
7. a p70
8. c p73
9. d p76   Table 5.1
10. b pp77-8
11. a p83
12. d p85
13. b p93   Fig 5.33
14. c p95   Fig 5.37
15. e p97
16. d p84-5
17. c pp102-3, Fig 6.4a
18. d p100   Table 6.1
19. e p105   Table 6.2
20. e p100
21. e p100, Table 6.2
22. c p108
23. b p109
24. e p113

25. a p119
26. e p120   Fig 7.11
27. d p111   Table 7.4
28. a pp108-9
29. c p115   Table 7.9
30. b p124
31. d p124
32. a p125
33. c p125
34. e p125
35. c p125
36. a p127
37. d p130

Part 3a AN APPROACH TO PROBLEM BASED PAEDIATRICS (CHAPTER 9 TO CHAPTER 16)

1. d p135
2. a p136, 145
3. c p137 Clues box
4. e p139
5. c p161   Table 10.1
6. a p163
7. d p163
8. c p165
9. d p175
10. d pp168-74
11. b p199
12. e p195   Box 11.1
13. e p417
14. b p38
15. a p192   Clues box
16. c p193   Table 11.4
17. a p222-3
18. a pp224-5
19. c p220
20. b p234 Clues box
21. d p252
22. a p252
23. e pp255-6
24. e p262
25. a p258 Clues box
26. d p263
27. a pp272-4
28. a pp255-6
29. d p258

30. c   p262   Table 14.3
31. b   p286
32. a   p302
33. e   p294-6
34. d   p312
35. b   p310   Clues box
36. c   p308, pp314-15
37. a   p316
38. e   pp315-16
39. b   p313
40. a   p315

Part 3b AN APPROACH TO PROBLEM BASED PAEDIATRICS (CHAPTER 17 TO CHAPTER 25)

1. e   p320
2. a   p324
3. d   p330
4. a   p324, p325   Table 17.1
5. b   pp332-3
6. d   p342, p343
7. c   p343
8. c   p343
9. d   p343
10. e   p368, p369
11. a   p368, p369
12. c   p360, p361
13. d   p368
14. b   p361
15. d   p361
16. b   Fig 20.1 and p372

17. e   p374
18. a   p374
19. d   p376
20. d   pp382-3
21. e   p388
22. d   p387
23. e   p385, p386, Box 21.3
24. e   p389
25. b   p395
26. a   p392
27. c   p397
28. c   p393, Fig 22.1
29. a   pp419-20
30. c   p401, Table 23.1
31. b   p403
32. d   p405-6
33. d   p409
34. a   p421
35. c   pp445-6   Table 24.7
36. d   p453   Table 24.9
37. e   p430
38. d   p445
39. e   p220, Table 12.1
40. e   p448
41. c   p452
42. e   p451
43. d   p459   Table 25.4
44. e   p461   Table 25.7
45. b   p465   Table 25.8
46. e   p458

Practice examination papers

In this section, you have the opportunity to take an exam under exam conditions. Allow yourself 45 minutes to complete each paper. *Note that there is only one correct answer for each statement.*

Mark the paper by giving yourself one mark for each correct answer, and do not subtract marks for incorrect answers. There are 36 questions in each paper. Answers are provided at the end of the chapter, along with a reference that will lead you back to the topic for more information.

MCQ EXAM 1

Answers on page 492

EXAM QUESTION

1 **Which of the following advice is helpful to a mother who wishes to breast-feed?**
   a. Place the baby on the breast immediately after delivery
   b. Feed the baby every 4 hours to establish a schedule
   c. Have the father give a bottle overnight so the mother can rest and build up her strength
   d. If mastitis seems to be developing, give the breast a rest from sucking
   e. If the baby seems hungry after a feed give a bottle of formula to make sure the breast fills up for the next feed

2 **Immunisations should not be given in the following circumstance:**
   a. Live attenuated vaccines to severely immunocompromised children
   b. If the child is older than the age indicated on the schedule
   c. A parent is not present
   d. If there has been a fever following a previous dose of the same vaccine
   e. A history of developmental delay

3 **Which of the following is correct regarding medical management of children with cancer?**
   a. The most appropriate place for treatment is the child's local hospital as it allows for greater support from family, friends and school
   b. Surgery is the first-line treatment for solid tumours
   c. The use of several chemotherapeutic agents simultaneously increases the likelihood of chemo-resistance developing
   d. Allopurinol is prescribed to reduce the impact that breakdown of malignant tissue has on renal tubular function
   e. Patients who are immunosuppressed should receive all the childhood immunisations to protect them from disease

4 **The traditional 'problem-focused' approach used by the medical profession to examine issues and difficulties is now considered limited because**
   a. It identifies families' strengths and expertise, rather than the problem
   b. It may inappropriately build parents' belief in their ability to cope and make change.
   c. It maintains an overly negative focus which affects patients' ability to cope.
   d. It tends to result in doctor and patient becoming more expert about a problem but is less helpful in guiding patients to take effective action.
   e. It comes across as dismissive which patients find is unacceptable

5 **Which of the following is a sign of respiratory disease?**
   a. Bronchial breathing heard over the trachea
   b. Upper airway noises heard over the chest
   c. Dullness to percussion beneath the right nipple
   d. Pectus carinatum
   e. Respiratory rate of 35 in a 6-year-old

6 **A normal child of 15 months should have achieved the following milestones:**
   a. Copies a circle
   b. Builds a tower of two blocks
   c. Can recognise three different colours
   d. Runs
   e. Plays interactively with other children of the same age

7 **Which imaging technique is most likely to be used when screening a premature baby for the risk of hydrocephalus?**
   a. MRI brain
   b. CT head
   c. Lateral skull X-ray
   d. CSF manometry
   e. Cranial ultrasound

8 **Which of the following is the blood gas pictures is most likely to be seen in a child with diabetic ketoacidosis?**
   a. pH 7.30, $P\text{co}_2$ 6.8 (51 mm Hg), bicarbonate 20 mmol/L
   b. pH 7.41, $P\text{co}_2$ 4.8 (36 mm Hg), bicarbonate 12 mmol/L
   c. pH 7.16, $P\text{co}_2$ 9.8 (74 mm Hg), bicarbonate 17 mmol/L
   d. pH 7.35, $P\text{co}_2$ 4.5 (34 mm Hg), bicarbonate 20 mmol/L
   e. pH 7.2, $P\text{co}_2$ 2.2 (17 mm Hg), bicarbonate 9 mmol/L

9 **Which is correct when prescribing a drug for a child?**
a. Syrups are invariably preferred to solid formulations by children
b. If a child vomits a dose, it is best to repeat the dose
c. In the face of drug refusal, the best policy is wait and watch
d. Prescribe liquids in millilitres as this is easier for parents
e. If the mother doesn't succeed giving a drug, no one else is likely to

10 **Which of the following is a marker for a serious bacterial infection?**
a. Poor fever response to antipyretics
b. A fever above 39.5 degrees pr.
c. A red flushed appearance
d. Fever for more than 48 hours
e. A raised C-reactive protein in infants

11 **A 2-year-old child presents with high fever and cough, a runny nose and conjunctivitis. Which sign would suggest pneumonia?**
a. Stridor
b. Tachypnoea
c. Anorexia
d. Sleepiness
e. Exanthema

12 **A 3-year-old girl has recurrent cough and fever. Two weeks ago she was seen by her doctor after she had a choking episode at the kindergarten, but the doctor found nothing concerning. A week ago she had cough and fever and received antibiotics. Now she has atelectasis of her right middle lobe. What is the correct management?**
a. Order a chest CT
b. Arrange for bronchoscopy
c. Give different antibiotics and follow-up
d. Treat with a cough syrup and antipyretic
e. Give bronchodilators and steroids

13 **Which feature in a child with chronic wheezing would suggest a cardiac aetiology?**
a. Lymphocytosis
b. Unilateral wheezing
c. Responds to bronchodilators
d. Family history of atopy
e. Hepatomegaly

14 **Which one of the following is true about constipation?**
a. It is likely to be the diagnosis if a breast-fed baby does not pass a stool for 5 days
b. It may cause an anal fissure
c. Prescribing laxatives may cause long-term dependency
d. Recurrent urine infections commonly accompany the constipation
e. The development of Hirschsprung disease should be considered if the problem begins when the patient is a toddler

15 **Which one of the following is true regarding coeliac disease?**
a. Usually starts in infancy before solid foods are introduced
b. Diarrhoea can be provoked by rice and potatoes
c. Crypt atrophy is seen in jejunal biopsy
d. Requires adherence to a gluten free diet for 6 months
e. When untreated is often accompanied by anaemia

16 **A 6-year-old boy at a routine examination has a soft systolic murmur and a fixed split second sound. What is the most likely diagnosis?**
a. Mitral valve prolapse
b. Tetralogy of Fallot
c. Atrial septal defect
d. Pericarditis
e. Functional flow murmur

17 **A 3-month-old infant presents with attacks of cyanosis and irritability. On examination he has a right parasternal heave and a pan-systolic murmur. What is the most likely diagnosis?**
a. Transposition of the great vessels
b. Anomalous drainage of pulmonary veins
c. Patent ductus arteriosus
d. Fallot tetralogy
e. Pulmonary stenosis

18 **A 10-year-old boy is seen in clinic with headaches over the right side of the face, associated with watering of the right eye. The headaches start suddenly, and his parents note that he is incapacitated by them – writhing and rolling around on the floor. He has experienced some bullying at school recently and is not good at wearing his spectacles. What is the most likely diagnosis?**
a. Tension headaches
b. Migraines
c. School avoidance
d. Cluster headaches
e. Eye strain

19 **A 12-year-old boy presents with episodes of staring spells, noted over the last few months. The staring spells are noted a few times a day, at home and school and are uninterruptable. He is doing well at school, but the family noted that the absences were more frequent when it is a sunny day. He recently had a generalised tonic seizure when the family was setting off for an early morning flight. What is the most likely epilepsy syndrome diagnosis?**
a. Childhood Absence Epilepsy
b. Childhood Epilepsy with Centro-Temporal Spikes (CECTS)
c. West syndrome
d. Focal epilepsy
e. Juvenile Absence Epilepsy

20 Spastic cerebral palsy is characterised by:
a. Increased limb tone
b. Athetoid movements
c. Persistence of a grasp reflex in an 2-month-old infant
d. Parkinsonism
e. Delayed deep tendon reflexes

21 Which of the following is an unlikely cause of severe sensorineural hearing impairment:
a. Very high levels of unconjugated bilirubin
b. Secretory otitis media
c. Meningitis
d. Head injury
e. Exposure to excessive noise levels

22 At routine follow up a 12-year-old girl with diabetes shows poor growth. Her diabetic control is reasonable, and she feels generally well. Which investigation is most likely to be helpful?
a. CT of the brain
b. Serum lactate level
c. Coeliac antibodies
d. Ultrasound of the ovaries
e. Insulin C peptide

23 A 2-year-old girl has poor weight gain and poor appetite. Which of the following causes is commonest in the toddler age group?
a. Cystic fibrosis
b. Coeliac disease
c. Environmental (psychosocial)
d. Constipation
e. Renal failure

24 A 6-year-old presents with a swollen knee which developed 3 days previously. There was no history of trauma. What is the most appropriate action to take?
a. Adopt a policy of 'watch and wait'
b. Suspect non-accidental injury
c. Aspirate the joint
d. X-ray both knees
e. Investigate by blood tests

25 A continuous day-time dribble of urine in a 3-year-old suggests:
a. Urinary tract infection
b. A congenital anomaly
c. Psychological stress
d. Vaginal foreign body
e. Constipation

26 A 1-year-old girl has a first urinary tract infection. What is the recommended management?
a. Immediate ultrasound of the urinary tract
b. Prophylactic antibiotics after recovery
c. Routine micturating cystourethrography
d. A DMSA renal scan to detect scarring
e. Initial antibiotic therapy guided by local guidelines

27 A 2-month-old boy is brought in by his parents with an intermittent swelling to the right groin, which they have noticed occurs when he cries. The examination in clinic is normal. Which is the most likely diagnosis?
a. Testicular torsion
b. Hydrocoele
c. Inguinal hernia
d. Normal child
e. Undescended testis

28 Which disease is associated with a vesicular eruption?
a. Measles
b. Rubella
c. Kawasaki
d. Varicella zoster
e. Group A Streptococcus

29 A breast-fed baby presents with a stubborn nappy rash. She has white plaques in her mouth. The mother's nipples are red and itchy. What is the diagnosis?
a. Candida
b. Ammoniacal dermatitis
c. Psoriasis
d. Seborrheic dermatitis
e. Impetigo

30 What is an important factor in the development of iron deficiency in young children?
a. Immunisations
b. Growth slowdown in the third year
c. Consumption of iron-poor foods
d. Abuse of antibiotics
e. Chronic constipation

31 A 2-year-old child wakes several times at night and will not go back to sleep. Which of the following strategies is appropriate for worried parents?
a. Prescription of chloral hydrate
b. Keep him up until he falls asleep again
c. Take him to sleep in the parents' bed
d. Check him but give no positive attention
e. Give him a milky drink when he wakes

32 Which one of the following features would usually be a normal finding and not suggest the possibility of abuse or non-accidental injury?
a. Extensive bruising on a 5-year-old child's shins
b. Unexplained failure to thrive
c. Spiral fracture of the femur in an 18-month-old
d. Torn frenulum of the tongue in a 6-month-old
e. Two different explanations from the parents as to how the injury happened

33 You are at your aunt's house when your 3-year-old nephew starts choking on some sausage. He starts coughing but this doesn't seem to help, and your aunt is calling the emergency services.
Which is the most appropriate course of action?
 a. Alternate 5 chest thrusts, then 5 back blows
 b. Alternate 5 back blows, then 5 chest thrusts
 c. Alternate 5 back blows, then 5 abdominal blows
 d. Alternate 5 abdominal thrusts, then 5 back blows
 e. Give 2 rescue breaths then 15 chest thrusts

34 A 12-year old girl is brought into hospital unconscious. She has a fever of 40 °C and a purpuric rash to the trunk. She withdraws from pain, groans and her eyes remain shut. Her glucose is 3.5 mmol/L (63 mg/dL). Her heart rate is 180, respiratory rate 30, capillary refill time 4 seconds peripherally and her blood pressure 100/55.
Which is the first steps in management?
 a. Give a cephalosporin antibiotic
 b. Secure airway and consider intubation

 c. Give 20mL/kg 0.9% sodium chloride fluid bolus
 d. Give 2mL/kg 10% glucose bolus
 e. Obtain further history

35 The most common causes of early neonatal sepsis are?
 a. Group B Streptococcus and *E. coli*
 b. *Staphylococcus aureus* and *epidermidis*
 c. *Klebsiella* and *Pseudomonas*
 d. *Haemophilus* and *Candida*
 e. *Pneumococcus* and *Staphylococcus aureus*

36 Which of the following statements about puberty in girls is true?
 a. Menstruation usually occurs within 1 year of onset of puberty
 b. The growth spurt occurs late in puberty
 c. Menarche is delayed if it has not occurred by age 14
 d. First sign in girls is usually breast budding
 e. It is precocious if it starts at 9 years of age

MCQ EXAM 2

Answers begin on page 492

1 Poverty is known to be associated with an increased risk for which of the following conditions?
 a. High birthweight
 b. Hydrocephalus
 c. Tay-sachs disease
 d. Recurrent abdominal pain
 e. Respiratory infections

2 Which of the following is true regarding screening tests?
 a. They accurately identify unrecognised disease or defects
 b. They identify children with high-risk for a health problem
 c. A good screening test should be the gold standard test for the condition.
 d. The condition must be already evident in order for it to be picked up by screening
 e. Cost effectiveness of the test is not significant as screening always leads to savings.

3 Palliative care services in childhood:
 a. Are confined to children with terminal cancer
 b. Are primarily aimed at children of school age who need support in coming to terms with their shortened life expectancy
 c. Protecting the child from too much information is one of palliative care's principles

 d. Palliative care is available at any time during a serious illness, whereas hospice care focuses on a person's final months of life,
 e. Palliative care should be delayed until curative options have been exhausted

4 Open questions, as compared to closed questions, help patients to think and reflect. Which of the following is an example of an open question?
 a. What time did the seizure occur…?
 b. What do you think might be going on …?'
 c. What did he eat before the seizure happened?
 d. What medications are there in the household?
 e. Did the seizure take place at home?

5 Spastic cerebral palsy is suggested by:
 a. Positive Babinski reflex
 b. Gower sign
 c. Romberg positive
 d. Lead-pipe rigidity
 e. Muscle hypertrophy

6 Which of the following indicates that development may not be progressing normally?
 a. Regression of skills that have been acquired
 b. First smiling at 6 weeks
 c. Unintelligible speech at 3 years
 d. Not walking by 15 months
 e. Immature pincer grip at 12 months

7 **Which statement is true regarding ECGs in young children?**
   a. An absent P wave prior to the QRS complex is consistent with sinus arrhythmia
   b. A QTc of 0.5ms is normal in newborns.
   c. Inverted T waves are normal in leads V1-3.
   d. Right axis deviation in the neonatal period suggests congenital cardiac disease.
   e. Lead V4R is obtained by placing electrodes on the infant's back

8 **A child is suspected clinically of having Prader-Willi syndrome, a disorder which can be caused by the absence of paternally derived segments of chromosome 15. Which genetic test is initially recommended to be used to assess this possibility?**
   a. Fluorescence in situ hybridization (FISH)
   b. Comparative genomic hybridization (CGH array)
   c. Whole exome sequencing
   d. Karyotype
   e. Developmental disorders gene panel

9 **What is true regarding off-label prescription of drugs for children?**
   a. It is not legal and therefore must never be done
   b. Refers to prescribing a drug package with a hand-written sticky label
   c. Is mostly due to the lack of efficacy expected in children
   d. Will probably increase significantly in future years
   e. May be unavoidable in many clinical situations

10 **A 5-month-old baby presents with extreme irritability and a fever of 40 degrees. Physical examination is unrevealing. The next day he has a short seizure. Three days later the fever suddenly drops, and a red, punctate, centrifugal macular rash appears on the trunk and back. What is the most likely causative organism?**
   a. Meningococcus
   b. Measles
   c. Varicella
   d. Human herpes virus 6
   e. Parvovirus

11 **What statement is true regarding temperature reduction in a febrile infant?**
   a. This is obligatory if the child has had febrile seizures in the past
   b. The best method is to use cold wet towels and sponges
   c. Aspirin is effective but may cause renal complications
   d. Reducing the temperature improves prognosis in viral disease
   e. Treatment of fever is for subjective wellbeing

12 **Concerning acute bronchiolitis, which statement is correct?**
   a. Most infants require hospitalization
   b. There is no effective preventative therapy
   c. Babies can be sent home only when pO2 > 97% in air
   d. Immunity against the causative virus is life-long
   e. High flow humidified oxygen can reduce ICU admission rates

13 **A young child with asthma is recommended inhaler treatment with a spacer device. What explanation is correct for the parents?**
   a. The device ensures drug delivery to the lungs
   b. The child should breathe via the device for 5 minutes
   c. Spacers are used to give extra oxygen
   d. Spacers enable leukotriene antagonists to be given
   e. Only children over 3 years can use a spacer

14 **Which one of the following is a feature of pyloric stenosis?**
   a. Anaemia due to blood in the vomitus
   b. Bile in the vomitus
   c. Presents on the first day of life
   d. Projectile vomiting
   e. Typically causes hyperchloraemic acidosis

15 **In a 2-year-old child with chronic faecal soiling, which one of the following is a possible cause:**
   a. Threadworms
   b. Constipation
   c. Gastrointestinal reflux
   d. Irritable bowel syndrome
   e. Appendicitis

16 **Which of the following would be expected in severe aortic stenosis?**
   a. Right axis deviation on ECG
   b. Dizziness on exertion
   c. Harsh pan-systolic mumur
   d. Systolic hypertension
   e. Atrial fibrillation

17 **Sub-acute infective endocarditis is characterised by:**
   a. Sudden onset of high fever
   b. Maculo-papular skin rash
   c. Mostly caused by gram negative rods
   d. Often complicates atrial septal defect
   e. Hepatosplenomegaly

18 **A 7-year-old girl is seen having presented with a 3-month history of staring spells, noted at home and at school, which are uninterruptable. In clinic you demonstrate absences triggered by hyperventilation, and her EEG is reported to show 3Hz spike and wave absences in keeping with Childhood Absence Epilepsy.**

Which antiepileptic medication is most appropriate?
a. Carbamazepine
b. Lamotrigine
c. Ethosuximide
d. Topiramate
e. Phenytoin

19 **A 15-year-old girl presents with sudden onset, left-sided facial weakness and a headache. She has slurred speech and is afebrile.**
Which is the most important test?
a. MRI head scan with angiography
b. Pregnancy test
c. 24-hour urinary catecholamines
d. Full (complete) blood count, ESR and CRP
e. Urea and electrolytes, and renin

20 **Which one of the following complications is common in children with severe cerebral palsy?**
a. Obesity
b. Dislocation of the hip joints
c. Colour blindness
d. Migraine
e. Attention deficit disorder

21 **In regard to severe learning disability, which of the following statements is correct?**
a. The child never develops speech or language
b. The aetiology of the condition is usually obvious
c. Down syndrome is a cause
d. Diagnosis is usually made in the first month of life
e. Few of these children will lead independent adult lives

22 **Which one the following conditions is not associated with a fall-off in growth?**
a. Hypothyroidism
b. Cushing syndrome
c. Growth hormone deficiency
d. Chronic illness
e. Corticosteroid deficiency

23 **A 15-year-old girl presents with short stature. What feature would make you consider a diagnosis of Turner syndrome?**
a. Amenorrhoea
b. Short parents
c. Decline in growth from the age of 5 years
d. Abdominal pain
e. Chronic cough

24 **Which of the following is a normal variant for a 3-year-old?**
a. Genu varum (bow legs)
b. Genu valgum (knock-knees)
c. Toe-walking
d. Asymmetry in leg length
e. Discordant shoe size

25 **Which statement regarding vesicoureteric reflux is true?**
a. It is best diagnosed by pre-natal ultrasound
b. Tends to aggravate with age

c. Long-term antibiotic prophylaxis is indicated
d. Severe reflux is associated with renal scars in 5% of cases
e. Surgical treatment is no longer recommended

26 **Which is true regarding nocturnal enuresis?**
a. The aetiology of secondary enuresis is usually different from primary
b. Genetic factors are important causes
c. Physical examination is usually abnormal
d. Neurogenic bladder is a common pathophysiology
e. Commoner in girls due to their short urethra

27 **A 15-year-old afebrile adolescent presents with acute scrotal pain and swelling. Examination is limited due to pain but the cremasteric reflex is absent on the right. Which is the most important step in management?**
a. Ultrasound scan to aid in diagnosis
b. Surgical exploration to treat the cause definitively
c. Urinalysis
d. Analgesia and reassess in a few hours
e. Urethral swabs in case of sexually transmitted infections

28 **What is the correct advice for a child with atopic eczema?**
a. A strict exclusion diet until the itching resolves
b. Damp warm rooms are helpful
c. Bleach baths can ameliorate the lesions
d. Steroid creams should be avoided due to side effects
e. Skin patch testing is the best diagnostic test

29 **Small purple skin lesions that are non-fading with pressure are best described as:**
a. Macules
b. Café-au-lait patches
c. Petechiae
d. Wheals
e. Target lesions

30 **Which statement is true of idiopathic thrombocytopenic purpura?**
a. Bone marrow examination is routinely required
b. Marked splenomegaly is typical
c. The prognosis is usually poor
d. Drug therapy may not be required
e. Onset is usually insidious

31 **Which of the following statements is true of attention deficit disorder?**
a. It is more common in girls than boys
b. There is often a history of sensitivity to food additives
c. It is usually associated with impaired intelligence
d. Symptoms deteriorate during adolescence
e. Methylphenidate is of proven benefit in selected cases

32 **Which radiological finding is particularly suggestive of non-accidental injury in a child?**
a. A skull fracture in a 12-year-old child
b. Spiral fracture of the femur
c. Slipped capital femoral epiphysis

d. Colles fracture of the wrist in a 3-year-old

e. Greenstick fracture in a 7-year-old

33 **A 15-month-old girl is brought into hospital with profuse diarrhoea and vomiting. She has a capillary refill time of 2 seconds, her skin turgor is reduced, and she has had one wet nappy in the last 12 hours. What is the best management plan?**

a. IV 0.9% sodium chloride maintenance fluid for the next 4 hours

b. Oral rehydration fluid for 24 hours

c. IV 0.9% sodium chloride fluid bolus over 30 minutes

d. Oral rehydration fluid, and IV fluid if unable to tolerate oral fluid challenge

e. IV 0.9% sodium chloride fluid bolus, followed by 0.9% sodium chloride maintenance fluid

34 **What is the maintenance fluid volume rate required for a 23 kg child?**

a. 25 mL/hour

b. 58 mL/hour

c. 33 mL/hour

d. 49 mL/hour

e. 65 mL/hour

35 **The most common cause of significant jaundice on the first day of life is?**

a. Rhesus incompatibility

b. G6PD deficiency

c. ABO incompatibility

d. Breast milk jaundice

e. Biliary atresia

36 **Which of the following is characteristic of anorexia nervosa?**

a. Staining of the inside of the teeth

b. Reduced physical activity

c. Diarrhoea

d. Distorted body image

e. Tachycardia

Answers to practice examination papers

References to boxes, tables and/or relevant pages are provided to lead you back to the topic for more information and an explanation for the answers

MCQ EXAM 1

1. a   p17   Box 1.2
2. a   p36
3. d   p54
4. d   p65
5. e   pp79-80
6. b   p102, Figs 6.3-6.6
7. e   pp119-20
8. e   pp111-13
9. b   pp126-7
10. e   pp135-6
11. b   pp177-8
12. b   pp161-2   Table 10.2
13. e   pp163-4
14. b   pp198-9
15. e   pp207-8
16. c   p220, Clues box
17. d   p76, pp226-7
18. d   pp232-4
19. e   pp238
20. a   pp262-3
21. b   p272   Table 14.6
22. c   p303
23. c   p291
24. e   pp310-11   Table 16.2

25. b   p321
26. e   p326
27. c   p341
28. d   p347   Table 19.1 and p353 Clues box
29. a   p363
30. c   p374
31. d   p385
32. a   p393
33. c   p407
34. b   p412
35. a   p447
36. d   p459   Table 25.4

MCQ EXAM 2

1. e   p25   Box 1.6
2. b   p32
3. d   pp55-7
4. b   p65
5. a   pp86-8
6. a   p105   Table 6.2
7. c   p118
8. a   p121
9. e   p129
10. d   p151
11. e   p136

12. e   p179
13. a   pp169-70
14. d   p203
15. b   p198
16. b   pp224-5
17. e   p227
18. c   p239   Table 13.3
19. a   p250
20. b   p263
21. c   p258
22. e   p282
23. a   p297
24. b   p312

25. c   p328
26. b   pp321-3
27. b   p339 Clues box   p342
28. c   p358   Box 19.1
29. c   pp347-9   Table 19.1
30. d   p378
31. e   p261
32. b   p394   Fig 22.3
33. d   pp417-18
34. e   p418
35. c   p442
36. d   p462, p463

Index

In this index, tables, figures, and boxes are indicated in **bold** type

Essential Paediatrics and Child Health, Fourth Edition. Mary Rudolf, Anthony Luder and Kerry Jeavons.
© 2020 John Wiley & Sons Ltd. Published 2020 by John Wiley & Sons Ltd.
Companion website: www.wiley.com/go/rudolf/paediatrics

muscular dystrophy 257, **258**
musculoskeletal disorders 307, 313–318
   see also specific disorders (as listed page 307)
musculoskeletal pain, chest 167
musculoskeletal system
   examination 93–94, **94**, 311
   problems in obesity 286
   symptoms/signs 308–312
Mycobacterium tuberculosis 17, 39
Mycoplasma pneumoniae 177, 178
myelocoele 451
myelomeningocele 451, **452**
myoclonic seizures **232**, 237, **239**, **243**
myoclonus 237
myopia 34, **248**, 249

N
naevi
   pigmented 368, 369
   spider 82, **347**
   strawberry 368, **369**
naevus flammeus 368, **369**
nail bed angle 75, **75**
nail-biting 386
nappy rash **354**, **355**, **356**
   ammoniacal 355, **355**, **356**, 362, **362**
   Candida **355**, **356**, 363, **363**
   at a glance **362**
   psoriatic **355**, **356**, 361, **362**
   seborrhoeic dermatitis 355, **355**,
      356, 360
nasal obstruction 144
National Child Measurement Programme
   (NCMP) **35**
National Institute for Health and Care
   Excellence (NICE) *see* NICE
nature and nurture 9–25
   see also development, child
nebulizers 169–170, **170**
neck
   anterior/posterior triangles 84–85
   asymmetrical tonic reflex **92**, **93**
   examination 219
   examination of lymph nodes 84–85
   stiffness, meningitis 235
   swelling in, fever with **139**,
      139–140, **140**
   webbing 297, **297**
necrotizing enterocolitis 448
neglect 40, 259, 392, 397
   abnormal brain development after
      11, **11**
   child, long-term outcomes **25**
   examination 393
   failure to thrive 284, **286**, 291, 397
   global developmental delay 259,
      260, 268
   investigations 394–395
   medical 397–398
   weight/growth faltering **286**
   see also child abuse

neglectful parenting style 12, **12**
Neisseria meningitidis 39, 154, 236, 421
neonatal onset multi-system inflammatory
   disease (NOMID) **143**
neonates 427–454
   asphyxia 430
   breast engorgement 462
   breathing 429–430, 445
   conditions 428, 445–454
      acute kidney injury 335
      biliary atresia 449
      breast-milk jaundice 449
      cleft palate and lip 432, 451, **451**
      DDH *see* developmental dislocation of
         the hips (DDH)
      diaphragmatic hernia 450
      haemolytic disease of newborn
         448–449
      hepatitis 449
      Hirschsprung disease 450, **450**
      hydronephrosis 450–451
      infections 400, 436, 447, **447**
      intracranial haemorrhage 448
      jaundice of prematurity 448
      meningitis 235, 236, 447
      necrotizing enterocolitis 448
      neural tube defects 451–452, **452**
      obstructive apnoea 449–450
      patent ductus arteriosus 449, **449**
      pneumonia 447
      respiratory distress *see* respiratory
         distress syndrome (RDS)
      retinopathy of prematurity 454
      septic arthritis 315
   cranial ultrasound **120**
   examination 428, 430–432, **431**
      for developmental dislocation of hips
         33, 432, 453, **453**
   The Health Child Programme **29**
   heart rate 430, **430**
   hypoxia 429
   maturity, assessment 433
   measurement 431
   mortality rates 428, **429**
   resuscitation 428, **429**, 429–430,
      430
   screening tests 32, 32–34, **33**, **34**, 175
   signs and problems 433–444
      apnoea 441, **441**
      bowel obstruction 444, **444**
      convulsions **439**, 439–440, **440**
      cyanosis **437**, 437–438, **438**, **439**
      jaundice *see* jaundice
      respiratory distress **433**, **435**, **436**,
         436–437, **437**
      small infants **433**, 433–436, **434**,
         435, **436**
      see also intrauterine growth retardation
         (IUGR); prematurity
neoplastic disease *see* cancer, child with
nephromegaly 450, 451

nephropathy, diabetic 298
nephrotic syndrome 116, 325, 332,
   332, **333**
   minimal change 332
neural tube 451, **452**
neural tube defects 432, 451–452, **452**
neuroblastoma **53**
neurocutaneous syndromes 259, **260**, 271
neurodegenerative conditions 258, **260**,
   268, 290
neurological behaviour, abnormal in
   neonates 432
neurological disorders 229, 235–250
   see also specific disorders (as listed page 229)
neurological examination 253
   in babies 90–93, **91**, **92**, **93**
   of children **86**, 86–90, **87**
      cerebellar signs 89
      cranial nerves 89, **90**
      gait 87, **87**
      motor 87–88, **88**
      sensation 89
   in global developmental delay 259
   large head 289
neurological symptoms/signs 230–234
   fits, faints and funny turns **230**,
      230–231, **231**, **232**
   headaches *see* headache(s)
   squint (strabismus) 234, **234**
neuromuscular disease 266, **267**
neuronal circuits, development 10, **10**
neutropenia 110
   febrile 54, 110
'new morbidities of childhood' 382
newborn infants *see* neonates
NICE
   traffic light system, serious illness
      400–401, **402**
   TV/screen time recommendation 22
NICE guidelines
   asthma 168, 173
   atopic dermatitis 359
   attention deficit disorder 262
   autism spectrum disorder 261
   bedwetting 331
   child maltreatment 395
   constipation 199, 214
   diabetes mellitus 305
   diarrhoea and vomiting 189
   epilepsies 242
   feverish illness in children under 5 years
      400–401, **402**, 421
   head injury 423
   meningitis 237
   UTI diagnosis/management 115, 328
night terrors **231**, 247, 385
nightmares 385
nipples, development, and trauma 16
Nissen fundoplication 202
nitrites **115**
nitrogen wash-out test 438, **438**